INTRAEPITHELIAL NEOPLASIA

Edited by **Supriya Srivastava**

Intraepithelial Neoplasia
Edited by Supriya Srivastava

Published by InTech

Janeza Trdine 9, 51000 Rijeka, Croatia

Publishing Process Manager Sasa Leporic

Technical Editor Teodora Smiljanic

Cover Designer InTech Design Team

Additional hard copies can be obtained from orders@intechopen.com

Intraepithelial Neoplasia, Edited by Supriya Srivastava
p. cm.
ISBN 978-953-307-987-5

Meet the editor

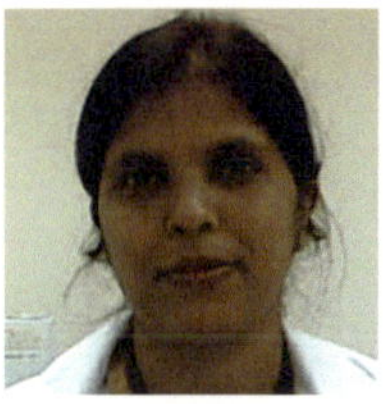

Dr Supriya Srivastava is a pathologist at the Cancer Science Institute, National University of Singapore. She attended medical school in India (Meerut, UP) and graduated in 2001. She then specialized in Pathology at King Georges' Medical University, Lucknow (UP), receiving her postgraduate medical degree (MD) in 2007. As a medical student she received various recognitions in academic circles. For more than three years, she has been actively engaged in research at the National University of Singapore. Her areas of research include identifying biomarkers in patients at high risk of gastric cancer, prognostic biomarkers in hepatocellular carcinoma and cervical carcinoma and identifying the origin of Barrett's Oesophagus. She is also involved in research projects involving confocal laser endomicroscopy of the gastrointestinal tract and Laser Capture Microdissection, and has been an author and co-author in various papers on topics within her research interest.

Contents

Preface

Intraepithelial neoplasias (IEN) are preinvasive lesions which are confined to the basement membrane. In developing countries worldwide, where the costs of modern sophisticated healthcare are a problem and issues of cost constraints are becoming widespread, the importance of early and timely diagnosis has become an imperative. Needless to say, accurate and thorough, macroscopic and histologic examination remains the gold standard, and every other method has to be assessed accordingly. To aid the clinicians and the pathologists, the esteemed and eminent panel of authors are pleased to bring to you a book which is relevant not only to the clinicians to understand and identify preinvasive lesions but also to the researchers and medical students. There is a vast sea of knowledge available in molecular genetic data, concerning a wide variety of IEN, and much of these data, at least where applicable, have been incorporated in this book. The extent to which this information directly influences patients is variable and is dependent on both the type of intraepithelial lesion and the resources available.

Through each chapter, this book discusses in detail the aetiology, pathogenesis, molecular and genetic profile, diagnosis and possible treatments of IEN of an organ. The organs discussed in this book include the oral cavity, the eye and the ocular adnexa, breast, prostate, uterus, cervix and vulva. Each chapter is illustrated with colored images of the preinvasive lesions of that particular organ. Differential diagnosis has been provided wherever required. All of the chapters contain a considerable amount of new information, with latest references and technical advances. This book has been extensively reviewed to take account of the latest developments and the standard WHO system of classification has also been included.

I am deeply obliged to the contributors for their hard work and enthusiasm in supplying such excellent material for the purpose of this book. I would also like to express my gratitude to the publishers for offering me to be a part of this book. I am grateful to Ms Sasa Leporic and the technical staff for their invaluable effort and support provided in the preparation of this book. Lastly, I would like to thank my spouse, Dr Sudeep Saxena and my family, for being a supporting pillar throughout this period.

Supriya Srivastava
Cancer Science Institute, National University Of Singapore
Singapore

Part 1

Intraepithelial Neoplasia of Oral Cavity

1

Novel Markers for Diagnosis and Prognosis of Oral Intraepithelial Neoplasia

Angela Celetti[1], Francesco Merolla[1,2], Chiara Luise[1], Maria Siano[2] and Stefania Staibano[2]
[1]*Istituto di Endocrinologia e Oncologia Sperimentale, CNR, c/o Dipartimento di Biologia e Patologia Cellulare e Molecolare, Università Federico II, Napoli,*
[2]*Dipartimento di Scienze Biomorfologiche e Funzionali, Università Federico II, Napoli*
Italy

1. Introduction

Squamous carcinoma of the oral cavity is a slow multi-steps process, based on progressive accumulation of genetic events leading to the selection of clonal populations of transformed epithelial cells (Ha&Califano, 2002) The spectrum of histological changes occurring in this process ranges from atypical squamous hyperplasia to carcinoma in situ (CIS), and is grouped under the designation of oral intraepithelial lesions (OILs) (Gale et al, 2005; Gale et al 2006). In their evolution, most cases of OILs are self-limiting and reversible, whereas some persist and may progress to SCC in spite of careful follow-up and treatment (Kambicˇ&Gale, 1986; Crissman et al, 1993).

As for the largest group of head and neck intraepithelial lesions, in the last years, various aspects of oral carcinogenesis have been investigated, including the aetiology, histological classification, treatment, frequency of malignant transformation and predictive factors. Particular attention has been directed to the analysis of the interrelationship between histological parameters and their biological behaviour (Gale et al 2005, Gale et al 2006; Kambicˇ&Gale, 1986; Putney&O'Keefe 1953; Kambicˇ 1978; Crissman 1979; Henry 1979; Hellquist et al, 1982; Gillis et al, 1983; Grundmann 1983; Goodman 1984; Crissman&Fu 1986; Velasco et al 1987; Olde-Kalter et al 1987; Crissman&Zarbo 1989; Sllamniku et al 1989; Bouquot et al, 1991a; Kambic&Gale 1995; Hellquist et al 1999; Gale et al, 2000; Gallo et al 2001; Ricci et al 2003). These analyses have been recently further supplemented by molecular genetic investigations trying to include the molecular events involved in the pathogenesis of oral squamous cell carcinoma (OSCC) to improve the prognostic evaluation of OIN (Ha&Califano 2002; Somers et al 1992; Saglam et al 2007).

A precise and uniform terminology of squamous intraepithelia lesions is essential for successful collaboration among pathologists, as well as for proper communication with clinicians. The terminology used in clinical and pathological reports has changed significantly over the last six decades. Common agreement has recently been achieved for terms that are used only for the clinical appearance and do not have any histopathological and prognostic implications. The most frequently applied clinical diagnoses are oral leukoplakia and erythroplakia (Kambicˇ&Gale 1995; Gale et al 2000; Gallo et al 2001). In contrast, keratosis remains a controversial term, since it is often wrongly applied interchangeably to macroscopic and microscopic features, whereas it really represents a histological term denoting the appearance of a keratin layer on the surface of the squamous epithelium.

Unfortunately, inconsistent terminology still exists for the histological classification of OIN. The spectrum of epithelial changes has been variously described as keratosis, dysplasia, squamous intraepithelial neoplasia (SIN), oral intraepithelial neoplasia (OIN), etc, to list only the most commonly used terms. Because of our inability to harmonize different views and establish a single classification of squamous intraepithelial lesions, there are three classification schemes in the most recent edition of the World Health Organization (WHO) classification of tumours, pathology of the head and neck tumours, as follows: (i) dysplasia system, (ii) SIN system, and (iii) Ljubljana classification (Gale et al 2005). These classifications differ conceptually and terminologically, and analogy between them can only be approximate.

Chronic inflammation, leukoplakia or, occasionally, erythroplakia, appear mainly in the buccal mucosa, labial commissure, gingiva/alveolar ridge, tongue, floor of the mouth. Lesions can be either sharply circumscribed and grow exophytically, or be predominantly flat and diffuse, related in part to the amount of keratin layer. Their surface is rough, may be muddy brown to red (erythroplakia), perhaps with increasingly visible vascularity, or coated with diffuse or dispersed circumscribed whitish plaques. A circumscribed whitish thickening of the mucosa may be observed, covered by irregularly exophytic warty plaques. A speckled appearance of lesions can also be present, caused by an unequal thickness of the keratin layer (Gale et al 2005; Kambic&Gale 1995). Some leukoplakic lesions are ulcerated (6.5%) or combined with erythroplakia (15%) (Bouquot et al 1991a). In general, leukoplakic lesions are thought to have a low risk of malignant transformation, mixed white and red lesions, or speckled leukoplakia, an intermediate risk, and pure erythroplakia (red lesions) the highest risk of cancer development. However, none of these features can be used as an indicator of the overlying changes of the epithelium, and histological analysis of these lesions is mandatory to determine their biological potential.

Symptoms depend on the location and severity of the disease and usually last a few months before clinical notice.

2. Clinical classification of leukoplakia and epithelial dysplasia

Leukoplakia, erythroplakia and palatal keratosis, associated with reverse smoking, are categorized as precancerous lesions (Axell et al 1996; Pindborg JJ et al 1997). Oral leukoplakia is the most common disease among precancerous lesions, whereas erythroplakia is relatively uncommon, and palatal keratosis associated with reverse smoking is rarely reported in Japan (Warnakulasuriya et al 2007). Pindborg et al (1963) confirmed that speckled leukoplakia, which is characterized by the presence of white nodular patches or white lesions interspersed with erythematous areas, was often associated with epithelial dysplasia or carcinoma. These findings were supported by subsequent reports showing the association of nonhomogeneous leukoplakia with epithelial dysplasia (Silverman et al 1976; Gupta et al 1980). The two-tiered clinical classification system, used to divide oral leukoplakia into homogeneous and nonhomogeneous leukoplakia, was created by an international symposium (Axell et al 1996; Pindborg et al 1997). Under this system, homogeneous leukoplakia is further divided into four subtypes: flat, corrugated, wrinkled, or pumice; and similarly nonhomogeneous leukoplakia is subdivided into four types: verrucous, nodular (speckled), ulcerated, or erythroleukoplakia. The adjective "nonhomogeneous" refers to the color (i.e., a mixture of white and red changes for erythroleukoplakia) and texture (i.e., exophytic, papillary, or verrucous) of the lesion (van der Waal et al 1997). However, with regard to nonhomologous lesions, there are no reproducible criteria under this system for the clinical differentiation of proliferative verrucous leukoplakia from verrucous hyperplasia or verrucous carcinoma (van der Waal et al 1997; Shear&Pindborg 1980).

Sugar& Banoczy (1969) reported that leukoplakia erosiva and leukoplakia verrucosa were more often associated with epithelial dysplasia than leukoplakia simplex. Furthermore, because the clinical features of oral leukoplakia in Japan did not correlate with the two aforementioned systems, Amagasa et al (1977) developed a clinical classification system of oral leukoplakia in Japan, which was subsequently further developed in 2006 (Amagasa et al 2006). Under this system, oral leukoplakia is classified into four clinical types: type I, a flat white patch or plaque without red components; type II, a flat white patch or plaque with red components; type III, a slightly raised or elevated white plaque; and type IV, a markedly raised or elevated white plaque. Using this classification system, it was found that type II leukoplakia was significantly associated with epithelial dysplasia.

3. Histopathological features of Squamous Intraepithelial Lesions (SILs)

Traditional light microscopic examination, in spite of a certain subjectivity in interpretation, remains the most reliable method for determining an accurate diagnosis of SILs. Jackson first defined chronic laryngitis and keratosis as precancerous lesions (Jackson C, 1923); later, numerous studies and classifications have attempted to correlate phenotypic and genetic changes with the biological behaviour of the lesions (Michaels&Hellquist 2001). Regrettably, neither generally accepted criteria nor unified terminology have to date been provided for a histological grading system of oral SILs. Evidence of the inability of pathologists to set up a single, unified classification of SILs was manifest in the WHO Classification of head and neck tumours, published in 2005, where the dysplasia system is presented as the 2005 WHO classification simultaneously with the classification of SIN and the Ljubljana classification (Gale et al 2005). The majority of current classifications, such as the traditional dysplasia system (Hellquist et al 1982; Blackwell et al 1995), keratosis without (KWA) and with atypia/ in situ carcinoma (CIS) (Crissman 1979; Crissman 1982), Squamous Intraepithelial Neoplasia (SIN) (Crissman et al 1993; Crissman&Zarbo 1989) and Laryngeal Intraepithelial Neoplasia (LIN), (Friedmann&Ferlito 1993; Resta et al 1992) follow criteria similar to those commonly used for epithelial lesions of the uterine cervix. However, the different aetiology of oral lesions and their particular clinical and histological features require a grading system more appropriate to this region (Hellquist et al 1999). One can object that grading SILs, in spite of the clear histological criteria, is an attempt to impose arbitrary distinct categories of a continually progressing process without naturally and sharply defined borders (Bosman 2001; Kujan et al 2011). However, this continuous process, which is of long duration, may eventually stop, regress or progress, depending above all on the influence of various detrimental factors causing genetic and, consequently, phenotypic epithelial changes. When a biopsy is performed with a representative tissue sample, the established histological changes still serve at present as the main guidance for clinicians on how to treat the patient, as well as being the most reliable prognostic factor of the biological behaviour of the disease.

4. A lesson from premalignant lesions of the uterine cervix

One of the most significant advances in oncology has been the realization that cervical carcinoma arises from precursor lesions. There is probably more known about cervical neoplasia and its natural history than about any other human epithelial neoplasm. Most medical authorities now agree that cervical cancer is the end stage of a continuum of progressively more atypical changes in which one stage merges imperceptibility with the next. The first and apparently earliest change is the appearance of atypical cells in the basal layers of the squamous epithelium, but this occurs alongside normal differentiation toward the prickle and keratinizing cell layers. As the lesion evolves, there is progressive involvement of more and more layers of the epithelium, until it is totally replaced by atypical cells, exhibiting no surface differentiation (Robbins&Cortran 1979).

The most widely used term for the various stages in the evolution of these precursor lesions is "dysplasia" (Reagan&Hamonic 1956), which literally means bad molding or, in more scientific terms, disordered development. In WHO's 1975 "Histological Typing of Female Genital Tract Tumours" (Poulsen et al 1975), dysplasia is subdivided into mild, moderate and severe, depending on the thickness of the squamous epithelium involved by atypical cells. When there is full-thickness involvement, we use the term "carcinoma in situ", which was coined by Broders in 1932 in relation to head and neck lesions (Bouquot et al 2006; Broders 1932).

A newer terminology, "cervical intraepithelial neoplasia" (CIN), was subsequently proposed in an attempt to emphasize that these dysplastic changes represent a spectrum of the same basic changes (Richart 1966; 1973). CIN involves one or more clones of transformed cells slowly replacing normal keratinocytes, starting from the basal and parabasal layers to progressively invading the entire epithelial height. Richart subdivided CIN into three grades, CIN I, CIN II and CIN III, corresponding to mild, moderate and severe dysplasia, respectively, which then progresses to CIS.

The classifications and concepts of premalignant lesions of the uterine cervix have been extended to all other mucosal sites covered by squamous epithelial as oral mucosa.

5. WHO classification

In 1973, WHO defined an oral premalignant lesion as "a morphologically altered tissue in which oral cancer was more likely to occur than in its apparently normal counterpart"; more recently, researchers have recommended use of the term "potentially malignant disorder" (Warnakulasuriya et al 2007). Under the WHO classification, atypical epithelium is divided into two pathological entities, one with progression to SCC and the other without progression. Although the former is a true premalignant lesion and the latter is a reactive atypical epithelium, the concept of epithelial dysplasia (mild, moderate or severe) includes both lesions and is a borderline category which can be placed in neither of the WHO's classifications.

As mentioned earlier, the dysplasia–carcinoma sequence theory as applied to the oral mucosa was adopted from the case of the uterine cervix, and the fundamental view of the WHO classification for oral cancer remained unchanged for more than three decades, from the first edition in 1971 (Wahi et al 1971, Napier&Speight 2008) to the latest version in 2005 (Gale et al 2005). WHO's "Histo-pathological Typing of Cancer and Precancer of the Oral Mucosa" (Pindborg et al 1997), is now used as a worldwide standard guide to diagnosis. The dysplastic features of oral mucosa are characterized by cellular atypia and loss of normal maturation and stratification, and the more severe the dysplasia, the greater the likelihood of malignant transformation. On the basis of the various criteria thought to be typical for the transformation of a dysplastic lesion to carcinoma, lesions are most frequently graded into one of four different groups: mild, moderate or severe dysplasia, or CIS, with the latter considered to be pre-invasive malignancy at the extreme end of epithelial dysplasia. Several histopathological changes may occur in epithelial dysplasia (Pindborg 1980). The criteria used for diagnosing dysplasia are provided in the form of a table in the WHO classification of tumours for the head and neck. Within the frame-work of the grading system of dysplasia, the more prominent or more numerous these factors are, the more severe the grade. These factors are limited to the lower third of the epithelium in mild dysplasia and extend to lower two-thirds of the epithelium in moderate dysplasia upward to the outer layer (Gale et al 2005). The use of the terms full thickness or almost full thickness architectural abnormalities is also recommended for the diagnosis of CIS.

This grading system of one-third, two-thirds and full thickness was described for the first time in the latest version of WHO's classification of head and neck tumours although it had been clearly referred to in the classification of uterine cervix since 1975 (Poulsen et al 1975). The large number of factors in this grading system would appear to be the basis of the many problems associated with the subjectivity of diagnosis (Pindborg 1980; Karabulut et al 1995; Holmstrup et al 2006). Accordingly, examination of the universality (inter-observer variability) and reproducibility (intra-observer variability) of this grading system for diagnosis has been carried out in recent years (Warnakulasuriya et al 2007; Kujan et al 2006; Kujan et al 2007; Ficher et al 2004; Tabor et al 2003; Abbey et al 1995; Brothwell et al 2003; Speight et al 1996) to sharply discriminate "indolent" low grade lesions, potentially reversible, from throughly preneoplastic high grade lesions. To this end, a novel binary grading system (low risk and high risk) designed to simplify the WHO classification and to raise the reproducibility of diagnosis has been advocated (Jares et al 1994; Califano et al 1996).

The histopathological criteria of dysplasia in the WHO classification are widely accepted among pathologists, and the concept of epithelial dysplasia outlined in the classification is considered to be correct in many cases (Crissman et al 1993; Putney&O'Keefe 1953; Ricci et al 2003; Franchi et al 2001). The notion that atypical cells progress from the basal layer to the surface is widely accepted in terms of the universality and reproducibility of diagnosis. However, it has become clear that there is a fatal flaw in this grading system as it does not, in practice, accurately reflect the clinical behaviour (Crissman&Zarbo 1989; Voravud et al 1993; Nadal&Cardesa 2003; Sanz-Ortega et al 2003; Chatrath et al 2003). The grades do not offer clear therapeutic guidelines to clinicians for appropriate management. For CIS at least, the WHO grading system diagnoses CIS showing maturation and differentiation as lower risk lesions, and these lesions account for a large proportion of cases in the oral mucosa (Hellquist et al 1982; Gillis et al 1983; Yoo et al 2004; Kleist&Poetsh 2004; Jeannon et al 2004; Chi et al 2004).

6. SIN/dysplasia classification

In response to the concept of CIN in the uterine cervix, a similar view developed for the oral mucosa. In 2002, Kuffer&Lombardi stated that malignant transformation is a multistep process that should be approached from the histological—not merely clinical—standpoint. Intraepithelial neoplasia, a concept created in relation to the uterine cervix and already extended to other mucosae, should also be adapted for the case of the oral mucosa and used as diagnostic term: the use of the term oral intraepithelial neoplasia represents not only a change in terminology, but also progress in unifying the concept of the precursors of squamous cell carcinoma, while at the same time suppressing the futile debate about severe dysplasia and CIS. Furthermore, grading lesions as low- and high-grade OIN increases diagnostic consistency.

SIN/dysplasia in the oral cavity has been found to take two distinct morphological forms, at opposite ends of the SIN/ dysplasia spectrum: hyperplastic keratinizing SIN/dysplasia and atrophic SIN/dysplasia, which are clinically compatible with leukoplakia and erythroplakia, respectively. The former is keratinizing dysplasia and the latter is the classic (WHO type) form of dysplasia. As a complication, the features of these extremes overlap. Caution must be exercised as the admixture type of these two ends of the spectrum is commonly underdiagnosed and may not be recognized as high-grade SIN/dysplasia.

The SIN/dysplasia classification, a modification of the WHO grading system, proposes a category of keratinizing dysplasia to designate lesions showing superficial keratinization in association with high-grade cytological atypia in the lower epithelium (Crissman et al 1988; Blackwell et al 1995; Kambicˇ et al 1992; Kambicˇ 1997; Hellquist et al 1999; Crissman 1982). The authors suggesting this modification reported that these lesions have a high incidence of local relapse and a high progression rate to invasive SCC and, as such, they are included in the high-grade group as high-grade keratinizing SIN (Crissman&Sakr 2001; Sakr et al 2009). The authors further stressed that abnormal differentiation is present in these lesions in the form of aberrant keratinization (dyskeratosis), manifesting as single-cell keratinization and keratin pearls, occurring in the midst of the epithelium. The histopathological features used for grading OIN according to WHO are listed below:

1. Loss of polarity of the basal cells
2. Proliferation of the basal cells
3. Increased nucleus-to-cytoplasm ratio
4. Epithelial hyperplasia with drop-shaped submucosal rete extension
5. Irregular epithelial stratification and cellular pleomorphism
6. Premature keratinization of single cells (dyskeratosis) or keratin pearls in the rete pegs
7. Increased mitotic figures and abnormally superficial mitoses
8. Presence of abnormal mitotic figures
9. Variation in nucleus size, shape, and hyperchromatism; increased nucleus size

10. Increased number and size of nucleoli
11. Abnormal variation in cell shape and size.

The transition from normal epithelium to atypical epithelium and SCC is related to the progressive accumulation of genetic changes leading to a clonal population of transformed epithelial cells. Despite extensive research into these genetic changes in oral carcinogenesis, reliable genetic markers with diagnostic and prognostic value are still lacking (Gale et al 2009).

7. Ljubljana classification and SIL classification

The Ljubljana classification was devised by laryngeal pathologists Kambic and Lenart in 1971 (Hellquist et al 1999; Gale et al 2009; Kambic&Lenart 1971, Gale et al 2000). Based on clinical and histological observations, these authors adapted the classification to the specific demands of the oral cavity. The Ljubljana system nominally recognizes four grades: simple hyperplasia and basal/parabasal cell hyperplasia include mainly benign categories with a minimum risk of malignant alteration; atypical hyperplasia is potentially a malignant lesion; CIS is actually a malignant lesion (Kambic 1997; Gale et al 2000; Michaels 1997; Eversole 2009; Fleskens&Slootweg 2009; Koren et al, 2002). The main features that differentiate the Ljubljana grading system from other classifications are the distinction between mainly benign (squamous hyperplasia and basal-parabasal hyperplasia) and potentially malignant (atypical hyperplasia) lesions, and the positive separation of CIS from atypical hyperplasia. These two entities differ in morphology and progression to invasive carcinoma. In this classification, all histopathological change is included until it results in SCC (Crissman et al 1988; Sllamniku et al 1988; Crissman 1982). Although many studies have focused on the usefulness of this classification in relation to the larynx (Blackwell et al, 1995; Michaels 1997; Gale et al 2000; Kambic 1997; Frangez I et al, 1997), there is currently almost no verification of this in the oral mucosa (Mahajan&Hazarey 2004; Zerdoner 2003) so its usefulness cannot be discussed as yet.

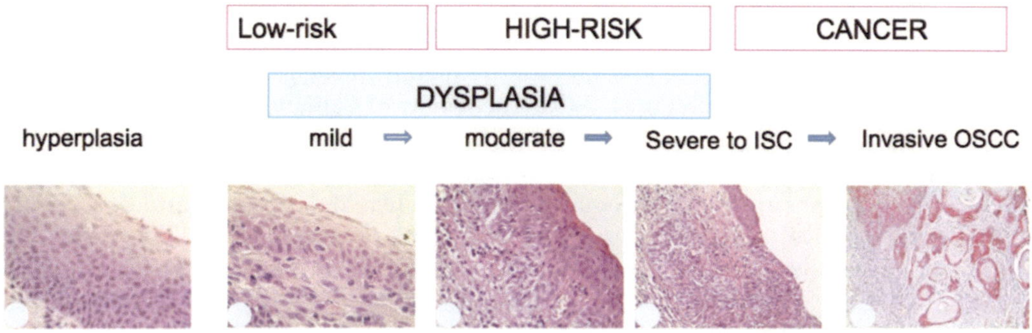

a) Oral mucosa with epithelial hyperplasia without dysplasia. This is not to be considered a preneoplastic lesion.
b) Oral mucosa with mild dysplastic changes. Rare mitoses are appreciable at the basal third of the epithelium.
c) Mild dysplasia of the epithelium of oral mucosa.
d) Severe dysplasia of oral mucosal epithelium (top-right), flanking an area of in situ- and microinfiltrating carcinoma.
e) Deeply infiltrating OSCC
(a-d: hematoxylin and eosin stain; e: immunohistochemical staining for CD44v6)

Fig. 1. Progression of Oral Cancer

The binary system which unites the SIN classification and the Ljubljana classification is advocated mainly by laryngeal pathologists. This system encompasses the Ljubljana classification into the SIN classification, with the concept of SILs being fundamentally the same (Gale et al 2009). The whole spectrum of histological changes, both reversible and irreversible, has recently been cumulatively designated as SIL, ranging from squamous hyperplasia to CIS. In terms of their evolution, some cases of SIL are self-limiting and reversible, some persist, and some progress to SCC despite careful follow-up and treatment. Although it would appear that both classifications can be unified, verification in the case of the oral mucosa remains to be determined.

8. Mechanisms of developing OIN

The genetic changes and the sequence of genetic events underlying the progression of normal mucosa to oral neoplastic tissue are still not entirely recognized. Between six and ten independent genetic events within a single cell have been estimated to be necessary for SCC development in the head and neck region. They are believed to be morphologically expressed as different grades of epithelial abnormality. The latency period between carcinogen exposure and appearance of malignancy may last up to 25 years.

The process of tumorigenesis of solid tumours, including oral neoplasia, involves both activation of proto-oncogene products that stimulate growth, and inactivation of tumour-suppressor genes (TSGs), the products of which normally inhibit cell proliferation (Califano et al 1996; Field 1996; Gallo et al 1997; Califano et al 2000). The identification and characterization of the comprehensive spectrum of genetic aberrations in SCC development may not only elucidate the process of carcinogenesis, but also provide promising diagnostic tools for early detection, prevention and assessment of cancer risk from precursor lesions.

9. Genetic progression model

Califano and co-workers have made two studies of cytogenetic alterations in head and neck carcinogenesis, which showed an increasing number of chromosomal alterations with the progression of Oral Intraepithelial Neoplasia (OILs), ranging from hyperplasia to CIS and invasive SCC. The areas of allelic loss, and less frequently allelic gain, are decisive elements in the progression model involving HNSCC. The results of Califano's studies have revealed that the spectrum of chromosomal loss progressively increases at each histopathological step of squamous intraepithelial lesions from benign hyperplasia to CIS and invasive SCC. The earliest alterations appear on chromosomes 9p21, where the p16 gene resides, at 3p with at least three putative tumour-supressor loci, and at 17p13 where the p53 gene is located. Loss of chromosome region 9p21-22 appeared to be the most common of all genetic changes in HNSCC, with a frequency of 70% (van der Riet P et al 1994). Additional studies of microsatellite DNA allelic imbalance in oral carcinogenesis have confirmed that dysplasia correlates with loss of heterozygosity (LOH) at 3p21, 5q21, 9p21 and 17q13 (Sanz-Ortega J, 2003). Yoo et al. have suggested that 9p21 is the earliest event, already appearing in squamous metaplasia, as well as in invasive and metastatic SCC. LOH at 17p13, 3p35 and 3p14 was observed as an intermediate event, occurring from dysplasia to metastatic SCC (Yoo et al 2004). Micro-satellite instability (MSI), a novel marker of genetic instability, was also applied in a study to assess the risk of malignant progression in laryngeal preinvasive lesions. The authors concluded that MSI is more common in preneoplastic oral lesions that have progressed to invasive SCC. They suggest that MSI assessment may be useful in determining the risk of malignant alteration in patients for whom chemopreventive and multiple endoscopic protocols can be attempted (Sardi et al 2006).

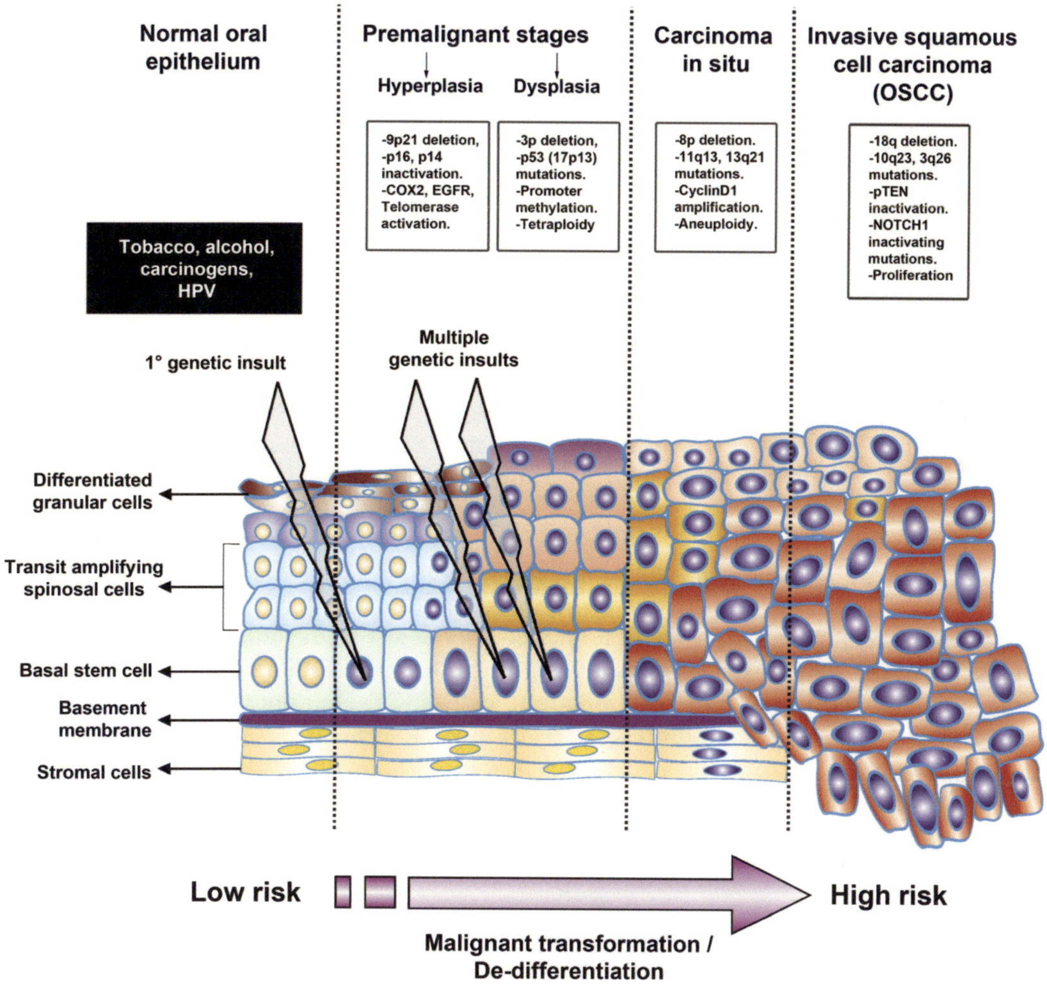

Fig. 2. Genetic Progression Model

10. Key tumour-suppressor genes in oral carcinogenesis

Gene p16 can be inactivated by a variety of mechanisms, such as mutation, homozygous deletion and promoter hypermethylation (Kamb et al 1994; Merlo et al 1995). The p16 gene functions as an inhibitor of cyclin-dependent kinase 4 and 6, with subsequent abrogation of retinoblastoma (Rb) phosphorylation and G1 cell cycle arrest (Serrano et al 1993; Kim et al 2004). Loss of chromosome region 9p21-22 occurs prior to the development of histological atypia, already at the level of hyperplastic mucosa, and is regarded as an early event in the development of HNSCC (Hasina&Lingen 2004).

Another important region identified by allelic loss is chromosome 17p, the site of the p53 gene. It is involved in several key cell functions such as gene transcription, DNA synthesis and repair, cell-cycle coordination and apoptosis. Mutation/inactivation of the p53 gene has been detected in approximately 50%, but may be present in as high as 80% of HNSCCs (Balz et al 2003). It remains unclear whether p53 gene inactivation is an early or late event of oral carcinogenesis. According to Boyle and co-workers, it occurs in the transition from the preinvasive to invasive form (Boyle et al 1993). Some others argue the opposite, presenting alterations of p53 among early steps of neoplastic transformation. Furthermore, gene p53 mutation has been hypothesized to be the earliest event in the development of a genetically altered field in oral mucosa, identifying an area of clonally related cells with malignant potential (Braakhuis et al 2003).

Although LOH frequently appears in head and neck carcinogenesis at chromosome 3p, the genes at this region have not been well defined (Ha&Califano 2002). The fragile histidine triad (FHIT) gene has been identified on chromosome 3p14 as one candidate for TSG, altered by deletions in human tumours. The expression of FHIT protein has recently been studied in HNSCC and premalignant lesions (Yuge et al 2005). Loss of FHIT protein was observed in 42% of SCCs and 23% of premalignant lesions. There was no significant difference among the three grades of dysplasia and FHIT expression. The results of this study indicate that FHIT alterations may play an important role in early events of carcinogenesis.

11. Key oncogenes in malignant alteration of SILs

Chromosome region 11q13 has been identified as the site of several putative oncogenes, such as Bcl-1, int-2, hst-1, EMS-1 and cyclin D1/PRAD1 (Kim&Califano 2004). Amplification of 11q13 is detected in approximately one-third of HNSCCs, but only cyclin D1 has shown consistent overexpression/amplification (Jares et al 1994, Callender et al 1994). The function of proto-oncogene cyclin D1 is to activate Rb via phosphorylation, thus facilitating progression from the G1 phase to the S phase (Kim&Califano 2004).

12. HPV-linked OSCC and OIN

Besides the evident epidemiological meaning, HPV infection linked to OSCC development shows clinical implications as these patients have about half the risk of death with respect to HPV-negative OSCC ones (Fakhry et al 2006). Moreover, the incidence of the subsets of OSCC more frequently found associated with HPV infection, i.e. tongue and tonsillar cancers, has been rising in youngs with men and women 18 to 44 years old (67% of increase) for the past three decades, and the trend is actually most evident for young white women (Patel et al, 2011), whereas the OSCC incidence is declining for nonwhite men, for all age groups. These findings have been justified with the decrease of alcohol and smoke abuse, and the relative prevalence of infection with high-risk HPV strains, particularly in youngs.

This identifies then distinct risk factor profiles for HPV-positive and HPV-negative OIN patients, and justifies the designation of clinical trials to assess the optimal treatment for these groups. From a histopathological point-of-view, the HPV-linked OIN are mostly undifferentiated (Carpenter et al 2011).

This is particularly intriguing, considerating that traditionally undifferentiated cancers have a very worse clinical outcome, being radio- and chemo-resistant, whereas HPV-linked undifferentiated OIN seems to have a better overall prognosis and a good response to post-surgical therapy.

For this reason, it seems fundamental to easily detect this subgroup of cancers and precancerous lesions, to preserve patients from overtreatment of their lesions.

Since high-risk HPVs lead to the intracellular accumulation of p16INK4a protein, due to the E7 block of pRb, it has been proposed to utilize the immunohistochemical evaluation of p16 for the screening of lesional tissue obtained from diagnostic biopsies. This has been shown to reliably predict the high-risk HPV infection in oral biopsies (Hoffmann et al 2010).

The screening with IHC for p16 INK4a protein, then, may be regarded as a precious tool for the proper evaluation of the outcome and responsiveness to therapy of oral cancer and precancerous lesions.

13. Key protein-based alterations in oral carcinogenesis

Protein overexpression can appear as a consequence of gene amplification, increased DNA transcription and translation. Several gene products can influence cancer progression in this manner (Ha&Califano 2002).

Epidermal growth factor receptor (EGFR), located on chromosome 7p12, codes for transmembrane growth-regulating receptor glycoprotein, which influences cell division, migration, adhesion, differentiation and apoptosis through a tyrosine kinase pathway (Pomerantz&Grandis 2004). The EGFR gene was found to be amplified in 25%, and its mRNA was overexpressed in 43% of oral SCCs. Half of the expressed cases occurred in the absence of detectable gene amplification. Both alterations appeared in advanced HNSCC (Irish&Bernstein 1993). Furthermore, overexpression of EGFR protein is an early event in carcinogenesis, rising with increasing degree of epithelial abnormalities, mainly in the progression of oral intraepithelial lesions to SCC (Shin et al 1994; Gale et al 1997).

Eucaryotic initiation factor 4E (eIF4E) is a 24-kDa protein, which binds to mRNA as the initial rate-limiting step in protein synthesis. Amplification and overexpression of the eIF4E gene, located at chromosome 4q21, has been associated with malignant transformation in breast cancer and HNSCC. The proto-oncogene eIF4E was found to be elevated in 100% of HNSCCs and is of prognostic value in predicting recurrence (Sorrells et al 1999).

14. Field cancerization

In early 1953, Slaughter et al. proposed the clinical concept of field cancerization to explain the development of multiple cancers and precursor lesions in the head and neck area, particularly in the oral cavity. Their concept is based on long-term carcinogenic exposure, which causes the independent transformation of multiple epithelial cells at separate sites. Polyclonal tumours may independently arise from these spots. The so called histologically-based field cancerization model has been gradually succeeded by a new one established on the basis of molecular changes of the affected mucosa. This hypothesis advocates a micrometastatic spread or a monoclonal theory, suggesting that a precancerous field of mucosa may derive from an early genetic event that has undergone clonal expansion and lateral migration or expansion (Ha&Califano 2002, Califano et al 1996; 2000; Bedi et al 1996). Subsequent genetic alterations produce genetic divergence and various phenotypic alterations, resulting in a variety of histopathologically diverse regions in the local anatomical area and in the selection of various subclones. The theory, therefore, proposes a clonal origin of premalignant cells with successive lateral migration, and possible multiple primary tumours would not be monoclonal, but clonally related (Almadori et al 2004).

15. Telomerase reactivation in malignant alteration of OIN

The telomerase enzyme is a specialized multisubunit complex, with telomerase catalytic subunit (hTERT) functioning as a reverse transcriptase that can synthesize the telomeric ends at each cell division. Telomerase has been found to be re-activated in 90% of malignant neoplasms, including oral SCC (Meyerson et al 1996; Shay &Wright 1996, Luzar et al 2001). Recent studies have confirmed a close relationship between hTERT mRNA expression and telomerase activity, suggesting that quantification of hTERT gene expression can be used as an alternative to measurement of telomerase activity (De Kok et al 2000). These results suggest that telomerase re-activation is an early event in oral carcinogenesis, already detectable at the stage of precancerous oral epithelial changes.

16. Additional markers of malignant alterations of oral intraepithelial neoplasia

Several studies of OIN generally agree that the severity of epithelial abnormality reflects the degree of risk of SCC development (Jeannon et al 2004). No marker or group of markers has so far been identified as a reliable predictor of malignant progression of SILs. It is therefore under-standable that numerous studies have been devoted to the progression of OIN to invasive SCC. The role of cell-cycle proteins such as p16, p21, p27, p53, cyclin D1 and E have been extensively studied over the last two decades (Shin et al 1994; Fraczek et al 2007; Gorgoulis et al 1994; Gale et al 1997; Dolcetti et al 1992; Barbatis et al 1995; Nadal et al 1995; Poljak et al 1996; Uhlman et al 1996; Hirai et al 2003; Ioachim et al 2004; Wayne&Robinson 2006). However, none of these markers has been found to have reliable predictive value. In addition, detection of proliferative activity, mainly as immunohistochemical labelling for pCNA and Ki67 antigens, can be used only as adjuncts to light microscopy for more objective and reliable histological grading of OIN (Leopardi et al 2001; Peschos et al 2005). Recent study of the transforming growth factor-beta (TGF-bRII) has indicated that its down-regulation is an early event in oral carcinogenesis, which may occur in the loss of TGF- b-mediated inhibition, thereby facilitating progression of precancerous lesions to SCC (Franchi A, 2001). Promising biomarkers for improving cancer detection include minichromosome maintenance proteins (Mcm-2-7), which assemble in the prereplication complex and are essential for DNA replication in eucaryotic cells. All six proteins are abundant throughout the cell cycle, being broken down rapidly on differentiation and more slowly in quiescence. In 2003 Chatrath et al found that Mcm-2 is expressed within the most superficial surface layer in cases of oral CIS and SCC and with minimal expression in basal-parabasal (abnormal) and atypical hyperplasia. The authors suggest that Mcm-2 would be a good biomarker for distinguishing premalignant from malignant lesions. Quantification of cellular DNA by image or flow cytometry has achieved acceptance as an objective and reproducible component in diagnostic pathology. Several studies of oral intraepithelial lesions have shown that a proportion of these lesions show abnormal DNA content and that the incidence of this finding correlates with the degree of oral intraepithelial leions (Bracˇko 1997; Munck-Wikland et al 1991; Crissman&Zarbo 1991). Bracˇko has additionally noted that lack of abnormal DNA does not exclude malignant alteration, since malignant tumours exhibit minimal chromosomal abnormalities resulting in DNA changes, which are below the threshold of sensitivity of measurement with the use of image analysis or flow cytometry. In 2004, Kim and co-workers performed a study of quantitative PCR for genes specific to mitochondrial abundance in a spectrum of dysplastic head and neck lesions (Kim et al 2004b). Their study shows that mitochondrial DNA is directly proportional to histo-pathological grade.

17. Next-generation sequencing reveals NOTCH1 as an important tumor suppressor gene in head and neck cancer

Recently (Brakenhoff 2011; License Number 2756960749906), two papers came out on Science (Agrawal 2011; Stransky 2011). Their aim has been to provide new insight into the genetic changes of Head&Neck-SCC that may suggest the development of alternative treatment strategies. By using a high-throughput technique called massively parallel sequencing or next-generation sequencing to analyze the genomes of head and neck cancers in great detail. Both groups sequenced the exons of all known human genes in tumor DNA and compared the sequence to that of the corresponding normal DNA of the same patient. In total, the genomic landscapes of 32 (Agrawal 2011) and 74 (Stransky 2011) tumors were examined, including tumors that were positive or negative for the human papillomavirus. Agrawal et al. also provided genetic profiling data on chromosomal changes, verified the mutations by classical Sanger sequencing, and validated some mutations in an additional panel of tumor and normal tissues. Mutations were found in many of the genes already known to play a role in HNSCC, such as TP53, CDKN2A, PIK3CA, PTEN, and HRAS, but at least one new cancer gene previously not known to be involved in HNSCC, NOTCH1, was identified. In both studies, inactivating mutations of NOTCH1 were found in 10 to 15% of the head and neck tumors, and it was the second most frequently mutated gene after TP53 (which is mutated in 50 to 80% of the tumors). In several tumors, both alleles harbored mutations in NOTCH1.

Why was NOTCH1 not found before in this type of cancer or even in other malignancies (Klinakis et al 2011,) as an important tumor suppressor? Functional studies had identified a role for NOTCH1 in squamous cell carcinogenesis, at least in the skin (Dotto 2008), but robust mutational data in clinical samples were missing. NOTCH1 is a very large gene consisting of 34 coding exons, which hampers classical (Sanger) DNA sequencing, thus demonstrating the major improvement afforded by next- generation sequencing platforms.

The finding of numerous inactivating mutations in NOTCH1 in HNSCCs and the observation that mice with a disrupted NOTCH1 gene in the skin show a skin cancer phenotype (Nicolas et al 2003; Proweller et al 2006) provide strong evidence that NOTCH1 is an important tumor suppressor gene in HNSCC. NOTCH1 encodes a transmembrane receptor that functions in cell-to-cell communication (Ranganathan et al 2011) and is in the skin typically located in the cilia of the squamous cells, the dermal keratinocytes (Okuyama et al 2008; Ezratty et al 2011).

After ligand binding, the cytoplasmic tail of NOTCH is cleaved by a secretase enzyme, translocates to the nucleus, and functions as a transcription factor, driving the expression of numerous genes. All four NOTCH receptors encoded in the human genome are important for cell differentiation. Stransky et al. also found mutations in other cell differentiation-related genes, such as NOTCH2, NOTCH3, and TP63, suggesting that deregulation of the terminal differentiation program of mucosal keratinocytes is critical for squamous cancer development. This is not unexpected because terminal differentiation of normal keratinocytes in skin and mucosal epithelia is characterized by loss of cell organelles and even the nucleus during cornification—events that support the barrier function of squamous epithelia but which would inhibit malignant transformation.

However, some questions remain. A high-throughput sequencing approach can reveal many mutations in a large number of genes, but this does not necessarily imply that these are all "driver mutations" causally related to the malignant transformation process. Tumors are genetically unstable and acquire many mutations including so-called "passenger mutations" (Sjoblom et al 2006; Wood et al 2007) that are a result of malignant transformation and not the cause. Functional studies in animal models are required to elucidate the exact role of the NOTCH receptors and the other genes that are mutated in HNSCC. As an example, Agrawal et al. indicated that they also found mutations in FBXW7 in tumors that lack inactivating NOTCH1 mutations. The FBXW7 protein is a component of a ubiquitin ligase complex that targets NOTCH receptors for degradation by the proteasome, the protein degradation system of the cell, and this could be considered an inhibitory regulatory system of NOTCH1. Surprisingly, these FBXW7 mutations were also inactivating. One would have expected activating mutations in this inhibitory down- stream pathway, assuming that NOTCH1 is the target. Hence, this requires more detailed investigation. Relating mutations to phenotypic consequences is a challenge for all potential cancer genes identified by these high-throughput methods. Even non-synonymous mutations in established cancer genes may not always be driving, unless supported by functional testing in relevant models.

An issue even more relevant to clinical application is that identification of a cancer gene does not mean that it is druggable. As Agrawal et al. note, proteins encoded by oncogenes (genes that, when activated, cause a normal cell to become cancerous) are most suited for treatments because inhibitory drugs will result in a reduction of cellular proliferation. However, in the case of inactivated or lost tumor suppressor proteins, inhibitors are of no use, and reactivation is complex or impossible. Instead, one has to make use of the principal of synthetic lethality—finding another pathway that compensates the effect of, for example, NOTCH pathway inactivation (Iglehart&Silver 2009). Cancer-associated signaling pathways are often so critical for cellular homeostasis that there are mechanisms of redundancy to compensate inactivation, and these take over in tumor cells. Blocking this compensating pathway is then lethal for tumor cells, whereas in normal cells this has less effect as both pathways are active. This principle of synthetic lethality is a highly successful strategy, as shown by the application of poly(ADP-ribose) polymerase inhibitors in BRCA1- and BRCA2-deficient breast cancers (Fong et al 2009). However, the presence of such compensating pathways and their synthetic lethal character need to be identified. Hence, there is more work to be done, but the studies by Agrawal et al and Stransky et alindicate that there are more candidate cancer genes to be identified and we should keep searching for them.

18. Cancer stem cells in oral cancer

The cancer stem cell hypothesis suggests that neoplastic clones are maintained exclusively by a rare fraction of cells with stem cell properties. Stem cells are defined as cells which are able to both extensively self-renew and differentiate into progenitors. Furthermore, stem cells are also attractive candidates as origin of cancers, as in their long lifespan they can acquire mutations and epigenetic changes that could favour the evolution toward malignancy. We discuss the evidences reported in literature on existence of cancer stem cells in oral cancer and mechanisms of the extrinsic and intrinsic circuitry controlling stem cell fate as well as their possible connections to cancer.

Oral cancer is a culmination of continued hyperplasia or uncontrolled proliferation of basal epithelial stem cells. In a well differentiated tumor tissue, the suprabasal cells exhibits basal stem-like phenotype and differ from the terminal highly keratinized cells. Many experiments have compared the expression patterns of epidermal and oral epithelial stem cells (Kaur&Li 2000; Evander et al 1997). Up to now, no true stem cell population could be identified from both normal and tumor tissue of oral epithelium purely based on sorting for stem cell specific surface markers reported from epidermal tissue (Prince&Ailles 2008). The stratified squamous epithelia of the oesophagus and epidermis have different functions and embryological origins. The pursuit for specific oral epithelial stem cell surface markers lead to the identification of CD markers such as CD44 (Prince et al 2007; Naor et al 2008), CD147 (Kose et al 2007; Toole et al 2008), integrins (Evander et al 1997), cytokeratins (Lindberg et al 1989, Presland et al 2002), EpCAM/ESA (Trzpis et al 2007; Munz et al 2004), E-cadherin (Kudo et al 2004), along with transcription factors Oct-4, Nanog (Chiou et al 2008) and Bmi-1 (Prince et al 2007). p75NGFR, a potential oral keratinocyte stem cell marker also co-localizes with BrdU incorporated stem cells and functions to mediate intercellular signaling in cell survival and apoptosis (Hatakeyama et al 2007; Nakamura et al 2007). An ideal cancer stem cell marker should impart all the acquired hallmarks of self-sufficiency in growth signals, anchorage-independent growth, apoptotic/drug resistance, invasiveness, metastatic potential in addition to primacy of high self- renewal conferred by cell of its origin, the normal stem cell. We discuss below several such stem cell markers representing the putative CSCs in oral squamous cell carcinoma and functional attributes bestowed by the expression pattern.

Methods for the identification of CSCs in solid malignancies mirror those strategies employed to differentiate normal stem cells from their differentiated progeny. These include the efflux of vital dyes by multidrug transporters, the enzymatic activity of aldehyde dehydrogenase, colony and sphere-forming assays utilizing specific culture conditions and the most widely used method—the expression of specific cell surface antigens known to enrich for stem cells. Once the subpopulation of tumor cells has been identified and isolated, functional characterization through quantitative xenotransplantation assays, the gold-standard for identification of CSCs, are used to assess the tumorigenicity and self- renewing potential of the putative CSC population in vivo

18.1 Surface antigens

By far the most common method of identifying CSCs has relied on the expression of specific cell-surface antigens that enrich for cells with CSC properties. Many of these antigens were initially targeted because of their known expression on endogenous stem cells. While a multitude of studies have identified CSC markers across a variety of solid malignancies, relatively few of these markers have been studied in HNSCC. **CD133**. A pentaspan transmembrane glycoprotein localized on cell membrane protrusions (Costea et al 2006; Prince&Alley 2008), is a putative CSC marker for a number of epithelial malignancies including brain, prostate, colorectal, and lung (Chiou et al 2008; Kelly et al 2007). In HNSCC cell lines, CD133hi cells display increased clonogenicity, tumor sphere formation and tumorigenicity in xenograft models when compared to their CD133 low counterparts (Ramalho-Santos&Willenbring 2007; Singh et al 2004; Ricci-Vitiani et al 2007). **CD44.** A large cell surface glycoprotein involved in cell adhesion and migration. It is a known receptor for hyaluronic acid and interacts with other ligands such as matrix metalloproteases (Tan&Coussens 2007; Mimeault M, 2007). Initially identified as a solid malignancy CSC marker in breast cancer (Tabor et al 2002), Prince et al. demonstrated that CD44 expression could also be used to isolate a tumor subpopulation with increased tumorigenicity in HNSCC (Pillai&Nair 2000). Although CD44 expression enriches for cells with CSC properties, the relatively high number of cells required for tumor formation as compared with known CSC populations from other epithelial malignancies raises questions about whether CD44 expression alone is sufficient for isolation of a pure CSC population. Using primary human tumor samples as well as utilizing a more natural host microenvironment through an orthotopic xenograft model (Phesse&Clarke 2009) might reduce the number of cells needed to generate tumors.

18.2 Aldehyde dehydrogenase activity

Aldehyde dehydrogenase (ALDH) is an intracellular enzyme normally present in the liver. Its known functions include the conversion of retinol to retinoic acids and the oxidation of toxic aldehyde metabolites, like those formed during alcohol metabolism and with certain chemotherapeutics such as cyclophosphamide and cisplatin (Bosron et al 1988; Thomasson et al 1991; Visus et al 2007). ALDH activity is known to enrich hematopoetic stem/progenitor cells (Chute et al 2006) and more recently has been shown to enrich cells with increased stem-like properties in solid malignancies (Carpentino et al 2009; Croker et al 2009, Deng et al 2010; Ma et al 2008). Chen et al. showed that ALDH activity correlated with disease staging in HNSCC and that higher enzymatic activity correlated with expression of epithelial-to-mesenchymal transition (EMT) genes as well as enriching cells with CSC properties (Chen et al 2009). **Side Population.** Hoechst 33342 is a fluorescent DNA- binding dye that preferentially binds to A-T rich regions. It is actively pumped out of cells by members of the ATP-binding cassette (ABC) transporter superfamily. Once stained with Hoechst dye, cells can be sorted by fluorescent-activated cell sorting (FACS) based upon the activity level of these multidrug transporters. Originally noted to enrich bone marrow for long-term hematopoetic stem cells (Clay et al 2010), this method has also been used to identify cells within solid tumors with increased tumorigenicity (Ho et al 2007; Szotek et al 2006; Wang et al 2007). Side population (SP) cells from oral squamous cell carcinoma have been shown to have increased clonogenicity and tumorigenicity in xenotransplantation assays (Loebinger et al 2008). Furthermore, HNSCC SP cells displayed higher expression of known stem cell related genes—Oct4, CK19, BMI-1 and CD44—and lower expression of involucrin and CK13, genes associated with a differentiated status (Zhang et al 2009).

18.3 Tumor sphere formation

Under serum-free culture conditions CSCs can be maintained in an undifferentiated state, and when driven toward proliferation by the addition of growth factors, form clonally derived aggregates of cells termed tumor spheres (Singh et al 2003). The ability of CSCs—but not the remaining tumor bulk—to form tumor spheres has been used extensively in neural tumors to identify populations enriched for CSCs. In HNSCC, these spheres have been shown to be enriched for stem markers, including CD44hi (Okamoto et al 2009), Oct-4, Nanog, Nestin, and CD133hi (Zhang et al 2009), as well as exhibiting increased tumorigenicity in orthotopic xenografts (Chiou et al 2008).

19. Cancer stem cells and disease progression

While there exists significant data defining the presence of CSCs within a variety of tumor types and many aspects of the cell and molecular biology of CSC have been elucidated, the manner in which this unique cell population influences clinical disease progression remains unclear. Given that metastases can be formed from implantation of a single tumor cell (Fidler&Talmadge 1986), it seems likely that CSCs, as the progenitor of all tumor cell types, would be responsible for metastatic spread. Central to the CSC hypothesis is the presence of a unique stem cell "niche" or environment necessary to support the growth of stem cells (Li&Xie 2005). It has been shown that a premetastatic niche is established by the attraction of bone marrow derived cells to the future site of metastases by the secretion of factors from cancer cells and that blocking the creation of this premetastatic niche prevents metastases (Kaplan et al 2005). What these secreted factors are and whether they are secreted by CSCs or one of their progeny remains an open question; however, creation of this niche, possibly for the arrival of CSCs to form a metastasis, appears to be a crucial step in metastatic spread.

Another stem cell marker, CD44, has also been implicated in metastatic spread and disease progression in HNSCC (Celetti et al 2005), although the CD44 story is more complex. Recently, three different isoforms, CD44 v3, v6, and v10, have been shown to be associated with progression and metastasis of HNSCC (Wang et al 2009). Increased CD44 v3 expression in primary tumors was associated with lymph node metastasis, while CD44 v10 expression was associated with distant metastasis and CD44 v6 expression was associated with perineural spread. In cell culture, blockade of these CD44 isoforms with isoform-specific antibodies inhibited cellular proliferation, with the greatest inhibition seen with blockade of CD44 v6. Finally, increased expression of CD44 v6 and v10 was associated with shortened disease-free survival (Staibano et al 2007). These studies suggest that alteration in CSC phenotype through variation in CD44 isoform expression may alter the interaction of CSCs with the surrounding microenvironment. This may allow CSCs to more readily invade surrounding tissues or metastasize, thereby promoting disease progression.

20. Treatment and evolution to malignancy

To date, many researchers have reported that the risk of developing cancer from oral leukoplakia could not be significantly reduced by surgical intervention (Holmstrup et al 2006; Vedtofte et al 1987; Schoelch et al 1999). Moreover, some review papers have stated that it is actually unclear whether removal of the lesion decreases malignant transformation of oral leukoplakia because there is a lack of randomized controlled trials comparing the different treatment modalities (Lodi et al 2006, Lodi&Porter 2008).

Nevertheless, the research by Amagasa et al. (2006; 2011a; 2011b) showed that the malignant transformation rate of leukoplakia treated by surgery was significantly lower than that without any treatment or that without surgery, so we believe that surgical excision with an adequate safety margin, coupled with well-timed evaluation of oral leukoplakia on follow-up, is effective in preventing the malignant transformation of these lesions.

21. References

Abbey L, Kaugars GE, Gunsolley JC et al (1995) Intraexaminer and interexaminer reliability in the diagnosis of oral epithelial dysplasia. Oral Surg Oral Med Oral Pathol 80:188–191

Agrawal N, Frederick MJ, Pickering CR, Bettegowda C, Chang K, Li RJ, et al (2011) Exome Sequencing of Head and Neck Squamous Cell Carcinoma Reveals Inactivating Mutations in NOTCH1, Science 333, 1154.

Almadori G, Bussu F, Cadoni G et al (2004) Multistep laryngeal carcinogenesis helps our understanding of the field cancerisation phenomenon: a review. Eur. J. Cancer 40; 2383- 2388.

Amagasa T, Yamashiro M, Ishikawa H (2006) Oral leukoplakia related to malignant transformation. Oral Sci Int 3:45–55

Amagasa T (2011a) Oral premalignant lesions Int J Clin Oncol 16:1–4

Amagasa T, Yamashiro M, Uzawa N (2011b) "Oral premalignant lesions: from a clinical perspective" Int J Clin Oncol 16:5–14

Axell T, Pindborg JJ, Smith CJ et al (1996) Oral white lesions with special reference to precancerous and tobacco-related lesions. J Oral Pathol Med 25:49–54

Balz V, Scheckenbach K, Gotte K, Bockmuhl U, Petersen I, Bier H (2003) Is the p53 inactivation frequency in squamous cell carcinomas of the head and neck underestimated? Analysis of p53 exons 2-11 and human papillomavirus 16 / 18 E6 tran- scripts in 123 unselected tumor specimens. Cancer Res 63; 1188–1191.

Barbatis C, Loukas L, Grigoriou M et al (1995) p53 overexpression in laryngeal squamous cell carcinoma and dysplasia. Clin. Mol. Pathol 48; M194–M197.

Bedi GC, Westra WH, Gabrielson E, Koch W, Sidransky D. (1996) Multiple head and neck tumors: evidence for a common clonal origin. Cancer Res. 56; 2484–2487.

Blackwell KB, Calcaterra TC, Fu YS (1995) Laryngeal dysplasia: epidemiology and treatment outcome. Ann Otol Rhinol Laryngol 104:596–602

Blackwell KE, Fu YS, Calcaterra TC (1995) Laryngeal dysplasia. A clinicopathologic study. Cancer 75; 457–463.

Bonneretal JA, N.Engl.J.Med.354,567(2006).

Bosman FT (2001) Dysplasia classification: pathology in disgrace? J. Pathol. 194; 143–144.

Bosron WF, Lumeng L, and Li TK (1988) "Genetic polymorphism of enzymes of alcohol metabolism and susceptibility to alcoholic liver disease," Molecular Aspects of Medicine, vol. 10, no. 2, pp. 147–158

Bouquot JE, Gnepp DR (1991) Laryngeal precancer: a review of the literature, commentary, and comparison with oral leukoplakia. Head Neck 13; 488–497.

Bouquot JE, Speight PM, Farthing PM (2006) Epithelial dysplasia of the oral mucosa-diagnostic problems and prognostic features. Curr Diagn Pathol 12:11–21

Boyle JO, Hakim J, Koch W et al (1993) The incidence of p53 mutations increases with progression of head and neck cancer. Cancer Res 53; 4477–4480.

Braakhuis BJ, Tabor MP, Kummer JA, Leemans CR, Brakenhoff RH (2003) A genetic explanation of Slaughter's concept of field cancerization: evidence and clinical implications. Cancer Res 63; 1727–1730.

Brac˘ko M. Evaluation of DNA content in epithelial hyperplastic lesions of the larynx (1997) Acta Otolaryngol 527(Suppl.); 62–65.

Brakenhoff RH (2011) Another NOTCH for Cancer, Science 333, 1102-1103

Broders AC (1932) Carcinoma in situ contrasted with benign penetrating epithelium. J Am Med Assoc 99:1670–1674

Brothwell DJ, Lewis DW, Bradley G et al (2003) Observer agreement in the grading of oral epithelial dysplasia. Commun Dent Oral Epidemiol 31:300–305

Callender T, el-Naggar AK, Lee MS, Frankenthaler R, Luna MA, Batsakis JG (1994) PRAD-1 (CCND1) / cyclin D1 oncogene amplification in primary head and neck squamous cell carcinoma. Cancer 74; 152–158.

Califano J, van der Riet P, Westra W et al (1996) Genetic progression model for head and neck cancer: implications for field cancerization. Cancer Res 56; 2488–2492.

Califano J, Westra WH, Meininger G, Corio R, Koch WM, Sidransky D (2000) Genetic progression and clonal relationship of recurrent premalignant head and neck lesions. Clin. Cancer Res 6; 347–352.

Carpenter DH, El-Mofty SK, Lewis JS Jr (2011) Undifferentiated carcinoma of the oropharynx: a human papillomavirus-associated tumor with a favorable prognosis. Mod Pathol 24(10):1306-12.

Carpentino JE, Hynes MJ, Appelman HD et al (2009) Aldehyde dehydrogenase-expressing colon stem cells contribute to tumorigenesis in the transition from colitis to cancer Cancer Research, vol. 69, no. 20, pp. 8208–8215

Celetti A, Testa D, Staibano S, Merolla F, Guarino V, Castellone MD, et al (2005) Overexpression of the cytokine osteopontin identifies aggressive laryngeal squamous cell carcinomas and enhances carcinoma cell proliferation and invasiveness. Clin Cancer Res 15;11(22):8019-27.

Chatrath P, Scott IS, Morris LS et al (2003) Aberrant expression of minichromosome maintenance protein-2 and Ki67 in laryngeal squamous epithelial lesions. Br. J. Cancer 89; 1048– 1054.

Chen Y-C, Chen Y-W, Hsu H-S et al (2009) Aldehyde dehydrogenase 1 is a putative marker for cancer stem cells in head and neck squamous cancer Biochemical and Biophysical Research Communications, vol. 385, no. 3, pp. 307–313.

Chi FL, Yuan YS, Wang SY, Wang ZM (2004) Study on ceramide expression and DNA content in patients with healthy mucosa, leukoplakia, and carcinoma of the larynx. Arch. Otolaryngol. Head Neck Surg 130; 307–310.

Chiou S-H, Yu C-C, Huang C-Y, Lin S-C, Liu C-J, Tsai T-H et al (2008) Positive correlations of Oct-4 and Nanog in oral cancer stem-like cells and high-grade oral squamous cell carcinoma, Clinical Cancer Research 14 4085–4095.

Chute JP, Muramoto GG, Whitesides J et al (2006) Inhibition of aldehyde dehydrogenase and retinoid signaling induces the expansion of human hematopoietic stem cells," Proceedings of the National Academy of Sciences of the United States of America, vol. 103, no. 31, pp. 11707–11712.

Clay MR, Tabor M, Owen JH et al (2010) Single-marker identification of head and neck squamous cell carcinoma cancer stem cells with aldehyde dehydrogenase Head Neck, vol. 32, no. 9, pp. 1195–1201.

Costea D, Tsinkalovsky O, Vintermyr O, Johannessen A, Mackenzie I (2006) Cancer stem cells new and potentially important targets for the therapy of oral squamous cell carcinoma, Oral Diseases 12 443–454.

Crissman JD (1979) Laryngeal keratosis and subsequent carcinoma. Head Neck Surg 1; 386–391.

Crissman JD (1982) Laryngeal keratosis preceding laryngeal carcinoma. A report of four cases. Arch Otolaryngol 108:445–448

Crissman JD, Fu YS (1986) Intraepithelial neoplasia of the larynx. Arch. Otolaryngol. Head Neck Surg. 112; 522–528.

Crissman JD, Zarbo RJ, Drozdowicz S et al (1988) Carcinoma in situ and microinvasive squamous carcinoma of the laryngeal glottis. Arch Otolaryngol Head Neck Surg 114:299–307

Crissman JD, Zarbo RJ (1989) Dysplasia, in situ carcinoma, and progression to invasive squamous cell carcinoma of the upper aerodigestive tract. Am. J. Surg. Pathol. 13(Suppl. I); 5- 16.

Crissman JD, Zarbo RJ (1991) Quantitation of DNA ploidy in squamous intraepithelial neoplasia of the laryngeal glottis. Arch. Otolaryngol. Head Neck Surg. 117; 182–188.

Crissman JD, Visscher DW, Sakr W (1993) Premalignant lesions of the upper aerodigestive tract: pathologic classification. J. Cell. Biochem. Suppl. 17F; 49–56.

Crissman JD, Sakr WA (2001) Squamous intraepithelial neoplasia of upper aerodigestive tract. In: Gnepp DR (ed) Diagnostic surgical pathology of the head and neck. Saunders, Philadelphia, pp 1–17

Croker AK, Goodale D, Chu J et al (2009) High aldehyde dehydrogenase and expression of cancer stem cell markers selects for breast cancer cells with enhanced malignant and metastatic ability," Journal of Cellular and Molecular Medicine, vol. 13, no. 8 B, pp. 2236–2252 .

De Kok JB, Schalken JA, Aalders TW, Reurs TJM, Willems HL, Swinkels DW (2000) Quantitative measurement of telomerase reverse trascriptase (hTERT) mRNA in urothelial cell carcinomas. Int. J. Cancer 87; 217–220.

Deng S, Yang X, Lassus H et al (2010) Distinct expression levels and patterns of stem cell marker, aldehyde dehydrogenase isoform 1 (ALDH1), in human epithelial cancers," PLoS ONE, vol. 5, no. 4, Article ID e10277, pp. 1–11.

Dolcetti R, Doglioni C, Maestro R et al (1992) p53 over-expression is an early event in the development of human squamous-cell carcinoma of the larynx: genetic and prognostic implications. Int. J. Cancer 52; 178–182.

Dotto GP (2008) Notch tumor suppressor function Oncogene 27,5115.

Ezratty EJ, Stokes N, Chai S, Shah AS, Williams SE, Fuchs E (2011) A role for the primary cilium in Notch signaling and epidermal differentiation during skin development Cell 145, 1129-41.

Evander M, Frazer I, Payne E, Qi Y, Hengst K, McMillan N (1997) Identification of the alpha6 integrin as a candidate receptor for papillomaviruses Journal of Virology 71 2449–2456.

Eversole LR (2009) Dysplasia of the upper aerodigestive tract squamous epithelium. Head Neck Pathol 3:63–68

Fakhry C, D'souza G, Sugar E, Weber K, Goshu E, Minkoff H et al (2006) Relationship between prevalent oral and cervical human papillomavirus infections in human immunodeficiency virus-positive and -negative women. J Clin Microbiol 44(12):4479-85

Field JK (1996) Genomic instability in squamous cell carcinoma of the head and neck. Anticancer Res 16; 2421–2431.

Ficher DJ, Epstein JB, Morton TH et al (2004) Interobserver reliability in the histopathologic diagnosis of oral pre-malignant and malignant lesions. J Oral Pathol Med 33:65–70

Fidler IJ and Talmadge JE (1986) Evidence that intravenously derived murine pulmonary melanoma metastases can originate from the expansion of a single tumor cell Cancer Research, vol. 46, no. 10, pp. 5167–5171

Fong PC, Boss DS, Yap TA, Tutt A, Wu P, Mergui-Roelvink M et al (2009) N.Engl.J.Med. 361, 123-34.

Fleskens S, Slootweg P (2009) Grading systems in head and neck dysplasia: their prognostic value, weakness and utility. Head Neck Oncol 1:1–8

Fraczek M, Wozniak Z, Ramsey D, Krecicki T (2007) Epression patterns of cyclin E, cyclin A and CDC25 phosphatases in laryngeal carcinogenesis. Eur. Arch. Otorhinolaryngol 264; 923–928.

Franchi A, Gallo O, Sardi I, Santucci M (2001) Downregulation of transforming growth factor beta type II receptor in laryngeal carcinogenesis. J. Clin. Pathol 54; 201–204.

Frangez I, Gale N, Luzar B (1997) The interpretation of leukoplakia in laryngeal pathology. Acta Otolaryngol 527:142–144

Friedmann I, Ferlito A (1993) Precursors of squamous cell carcinoma. In Ferlito A ed. Neoplasms of the laryn. Edinburgh: Churchill Livingstone 97–111.

Gale N, Zidar N, Kambic V, Poljak M et al (1997) Epidermal growth factor receptor, c-erbB-2 and p53 overexpressions in epithelial hyperplastic lesions of the larynx. Acta Otolaryngol. 527(Suppl.); 105–110.

Gale N, Kambicˇ V, Michaels L et al (2000) The Ljubljana classification: a practical strategy for the diagnosis of laryngeal precancerous lesions. Adv. Anat. Pathol 7; 240–251.

Gale N, Kambic V, Poljak M, Cor A, Velkavrh D, Mlacak B (2000) Chromosomes 7,17 polysomies and overexpression of epidermal growth factor receptor and p53 protein in epithelial hyperplastic laryngeal lesions. Oncology 58; 117–125.

Gale N, Pilch BZ, Sidransky D, Westra WH, Califano J (2005) Epithelial precursor lesions. In Barnes L, Eveson JW, Reichart P, Sidransky D eds. World Health Organization classification of tumour. Pathology and genetics of head and neck tumours. Lyon: IARC, 140–143.

Gale N, Michaels L, Luzar B et al (2009) Current review on squamous intraepithelial lesions of the larynx. Histopathology 54:639–656

Gallo O, Santucci M, Franchi A (1997) Cumulative prognostic value of p16/CDKN2 and p53 oncoprotein expression in premalignant laryngeal lesions. J. Natl Cancer Inst. 89; 1161–1163.

Gallo A, de Vincentiis M, Della Rocca C et al (2001) Evolution of precancerous laryngeal lesions: a clinicopathologic study with long-term follow-up on 259 patients. Head Neck 23; 42– 47.

Gillis TM, Incze J, Strong MS, Vaughan CW, Simpson GT (1983) Natural history and management of keratosis, atypia, car- cinoma in situ, and microinvasive cancer of the larynx. Am. J. Surg 146; 512–516.

Goodman ML. Keratosis (leukoplakia) of the larynx Otolaryngol (1984) Clin. North Am. 17; 179–183.

Gorgoulis V, Rassidakis G, Karameris A, Giatromanolaki A, Barbatis C, Kittas C (1994) Expression of p53 protein in laryngeal squamous cell carcinoma and dysplasia: possible correlation with human papillomavirus infection and clinicopathological findings. Virchows Arch 425; 481–489.

Grundmann E (1983) Classification and clinical consequences of precancerous lesions in the digestive and respiratory tracts. Acta Pathol. Jpn. 33; 195–217.

Gupta PC, Mehta FS, Daftary DR et al (1980) Incidence rates of oral cancer and natural history of oral precancerous lesions in a 10 year follow-up study of Indian villagers. Community Dent Oral Epidemiol 8:287–333

Ha PK, Califano J (2002) The molecular biology of laryngeal cancer. Otolaryngol. Clin. North Am 3; 993–1012.

Hasina R, Lingen MW (2004) Head and neck cancer: the pursuit of molecular diagnostic markers. Semin. Oncol 31; 718–725.

Hatakeyama S, Yaegashi T, Takeda Y, Kunimatsu K (2007) Localization of bromo-deoxyuridine-incorporating, p63- and p75NGFR- expressing cells in the human gingival epithelium, Journal of Oral Science 49, 287–291.

Hellquist H, Lundgren J, Olofsson J (1982) Hyperplasia, keratosis, dysplasia and carcinoma in situ of the vocal cords–a follow-up study. Clin. Otolaryngol 7; 11–27.

Hellquist H, Cardesa A, Gale N, Kambicˇ V, Michaels L (1999) Criteria for grading in the Ljubljana classification of epithelial hyperplastic laryngeal lesions. A study by members of the Working group on Epithelial Hyperplastic Laryngeal Lesions of the European Society of Pathology. Histopathology 34; 226–233.

Henry RC (1979) The transformation of laryngeal leucoplakia to cancer. J. Laryngol. Otol 93; 447–459

Hirai T, Hayashi K, Takumida M, Ueda T, Hirakawa K, Yajin K (2003) Reduced expression of p27 is correlated with progression in precancerous lesions of the larynx. Auris Nasus Larynx 30; 163–168.

Ho M M, Ng AV, Lam S, and Hung JY (2007) Side population in human lung cancer cell lines and tumors is enriched with stem-like cancer cells Cancer Research, vol. 67, no. 10, pp. 4827–4833.

Hoffmann M, Ihloff AS, Görögh T, Weise JB, Fazel A, Krams M et al (2010) p16(INK4a) overexpression predicts translational active human papillomavirus infection in tonsillar cancer. Int J Cancer Oct 1;127(7):1595-602.

Holmstrup P, Vedtofte P, Reibel J et al (2006) Long-term treat- ment outcome of oral premalignant lesions. Oral Oncol 42:461–474

Iglehart JD, Silver DP (2009) Synthetic lethality--a new direction in cancer-drug development. N.Engl.J.Med. 361, 189.

Ioachim E, Peschos D, Goussia A et al (2004) Expression patterns of cyclins D1, E in laryngeal epithelial lesions: correlation with other cell cycle regulators (p53, pRb, Ki-67 and PCNA) and clinicopathological features. J. Exp. Clin. Cancer Res 23; 277–283.

Irish JC, Bernstein A (1993) Oncogenes in head and neck cancer Laryngoscope 103; 42–52.

Jackson C (1923) Cancer of the larynx: is it preceded by a recognizable precancerous condition? Ann. Surg 77; 1–14.

Jares P, Fernandez PL, Campo E et al (1994) PRAD-1 / cyclin D1 gene amplification correlates with messenger RNA overexpression and tumor progression in human laryngeal carcinomas. Cancer Res 54; 4813–4817.

Jeannon JP, Soames JV, Aston V, Stafford FW, Wilson JA (2004) Molecular markers in dysplasia of the larynx: expression of cyclin-dependent kinase inhibitors p21, p27 and p53 tumour suppressor gene in predicting cancer risk. Clin. Otolaryngol. Allied Sci 29; 698–704.

Kamb A, Shattuck-Eidens D, Eeles R et al (1994) Analysis of the p16 gene (CDKN2) as a candidate for the chromosome 9p melanoma susceptibility locus. Nat. Genet 8; 23–26.

Kambic V, Lenart I (1971) Notre classification des hyperplasies de l'epithelium du larynx au point de vue prognostic. JFORL 20:1145–1150

Kambicˇ V (1978) Difficulties in management of vocal cord precancer- ous lesions. J. Laryngol. Otol 92; 305

KambicˇV, Gale N, Ferluga D (1992) Laryngeal hyperplastic lesions, follow-up study and application of lectins and anticytokeratins for their evaluation. Path. Res. Pract 188; 1067–1077.

KambicˇV, Gale N (1995) Epithelial hyperplastic lesions of the larynx. Amsterdam: Elsevier 1–265.

Kambicˇ V (1997) Epithelial hyperplastic lesions – a challenging topicin laryngology. Acta Otolaryngol. (Stockh) 527(Suppl.); 7–11.

Kaplan RN, Riba RD, Zacharoulis S et al (2005) VEGFR1- positive haematopoietic bone marrow progenitors initiate the pre-metastatic niche Nature, vol. 438, no. 7069, pp. 820–827.

Karabulut A, Reibel J, Therkildsen MH et al (1995) Observer variability in the histologic assessment of oral premalignant lesions. J Oral Pathol Med 24:198–200

Kaur P, Li A (2000) Adhesive properties of human basal epidermal cells: an analysis of keratinocyte stem cells, Transit amplifying cells and postmitotic differentiating cells 114 413–420.

Kelly PN, Dakic A, Adams JM, Nutt SL, Strasser A (2007) Tumor growth need not be driven by rare cancer stem cells, Science 317, 337-.

Kim MM, Califano JA (2004) Molecular pathology of head-and-neck cancer. Int. J. Cancer 112; 545–553.

Kim MM, Clinger JD, Masayesva BG et al (2004) Mitochondrial DNA quantity increases with histopathologic grade in premalignant and malignant head and neck lesions. Clin. Cancer Res 10; 8512–8515.

Klinakis A Lobry C, Abdel-Wahab O, Oh P, Haeno H, Buonamici S, van De Walle I et al (2011) A novel tumour-suppressor function for the Notch pathway in myeloid leukaemia. Nature 473, 230-3.

Kleist B, Poetsch M (2004) Divergent patterns of allelic alterations in premalignant laryngeal lesions indicate differences in the impact of morphological grading characteristics. Oncology 67; 420–427.

Koren R, Kristt D, Shvero J et al (2002) The spectrum of laryngeal neoplasia: the pathologist's view. Pathol Res Pract 198:709–715

Kose O, Lalli A, Kutulola AO, Odell EW, Waseem A (2007) Changes in the expression of stem cell markers in oral lichen planus and hyperkeratotic lesions, Journal of Oral Science 49 133–139.

Kramer IRH, Lucas RB, Pindborg JJ et al (1978) Definition of leukoplakia and related lesions: an aid to studies on oral pre- cancer. Oral Surg Oral Med Oral Pathol 46:518–539

Kudo Y, Kitajima S, Ogawa I, Hiraoka M, Sargolzaei S. Keikhaee MR et al (2004) Invasion and metastasis of oral cancer cells require methylation of E-cadherin and/or degradation of membranous a-catenin, Clinical Cancer Research 10 5455–5463.

Kuffer R, Lombardi T (2002) Premalignant lesions of the oral mucosa. A discussion about the place of oral intraepithelial neoplasia (OIN). Oral Oncol 38:125–130

Kujan O, Oliver RJ, Khattab A et al (2007) Why oral histopa- thology suffers inter-observer variability on grading oral epi- thelial dysplasia: an attempt to understand the sources of variation. Oral Oncol 43:224–231

Kujan O, Oliver RJ, Khattab A, Roberts SA, Thakker N, Sloan P (2006) Evaluation of binary system of grading oral epithelial dysplasia for prediction of malignant transformation. Oral Oncol 42; 987–993.

Leopardi G, Serafini G, Simoncelli C, Ludovini V, Pistola L, Altissimi G (2001) Ki67 and p53 in laryngeal epithelial lesions: correlations with risk factors. Acta Otorhinolaryngol. Ital 21; 243–247.

Li L and Xie T (2005) Stem cell niche: structure and function Annual Review of Cell and Developmental Biology, vol. 21, pp. 605–631.

Lindberg K, Rheinwald J (1989) Suprabasal 40 kd keratin (K19) expression as an immunohistologic marker of premalignancy in oral epithelium, The American Journal of Pathology 134, 89–98.

Loebinger MR, Giangreco A, Groot KR et al (2008) Squamous cell cancers contain a side population of stem-like cells that are made chemosensitive by ABC transporter blockade," British Journal of Cancer, vol. 98, no. 2, pp. 380–387.

Lodi G, Sardella A, Bez C et al (2006) Interventions for treating oral leukoplakia. Cochrane Database Syst Rev; CD001829

Lodi G, Porter S (2008) Management of potentially malignant disorders: evidence and critique. J Oral Pathol Med 37(2):63–69

Luzar B, Poljak M, Marin IJ, Fischinger J, Gale N (2001) Quantitative measurement of telomerase catalytic subunit (hTERT) mRNA in laryngeal squamous cell carcinomas. Anticancer Res. 21; 4011–4015.

Ma S, Kwok W C, Lee T KW et al (2008) Aldehyde dehy- drogenase discriminates the CD133 liver cancer stem cell populations Molecular Cancer Research, vol. 6, no. 7, pp. 1146–1153.

Mahajan M, Hazarey VK (2004) An assessment of oral epithelial dysplasia using criteria of 'Smith & Pindborg grading system' & 'Ljubljana grading system' in oral precancerous lesions'. J Oral Maxillofac Pathol 8:73–81

Merlo A, Herman JG, Mao L et al (1995) CpG island methylation is associated with transcriptional silencing of the tumour sup- pressor p16 / CDKN2 / MTS1 in human cancers. Nat. Med 1; 686–692.

Meyerson M, Counter CM, Eaton EN et al (1996) Telomerase activity in human cancer. Curr. Opin. Oncol 8; 66–71.

Michaels L (1997) The Kambic–Gale method of assessment of epithelial hyperplastic lesions of the larynx in comparison with the dysplasia grade method. Acta Otolaryngol 527:17–20

Michaels L, Hellquist HB (2001) Ear, nose and throat histopathology, 2nd edn. London: Springer, 378–387.

Mimeault M, Hauke R, Mehta PP, Batra SK (2007) Recent advances in cancer stem/progenitor cell research: therapeutic implications for overcoming resistance to the most aggressive cancers, Journal of Cellular and Molecular Medicine 11, 981–1011.

Munck-Wikland E, Kuylenstierna R, Lindholm J, Auer G (1991) Image cytometry DNA analysis of dysplastic squamous epithelial lesions in the larynx. Anticancer Res 11; 597–600.

Munz M, Kieu C, Mack B, Schmitt B, Zeidler R, Gires O (2004) The carcinoma- associated antigen EpCAM upregulates c-myc and induces cell proliferation, Oncogene 23, 5748–5758.

Nadal A, Campo E, Pinto J et al (1995) p53 expression in normal, dysplastic, and neoplastic laryngeal epithelium. Absence of a correlation with prognostic factors. J. Pathol 175; 181–

Nadal A, Cardesa A. Molecular biology of laryngeal squamous cell carcinoma. Virchows Arch. 2003; 442; 1–7.

Nakamura T, Endo K.i, Kinoshita S (2007) Identification of human oral keratinocyte stem/progenitor cells by neurotrophin receptor p75 and the role of neurotrophin/p75 signaling, Stem Cells 25, 628–638.

Naor D, Wallach-Dayan SB, Zahalka MA, Sionov RV (2008) Involvement of CD44, a molecule with a thousand faces, in cancer dissemination, Seminars in Cancer Biology 18, 260–267.

Napier SS, Speight PM (2008) Natural history of potentially malignant oral lesions and conditions: an overview of the lit- erature. J Oral Pathol Med 37:1–10

Nicolas M, Wolfer A, Raj K, Kummer JA, Mill P, van Noort M, et al (2003) Nat. Genet. 33, 416-21.

Olde Kalter P, Lubsen H, Delemarre JFM, Snow GB (1987) Squamous cell hyperplasia of the larynx. A clinical follow-up study. J. Laryngol. Otol 101; 579–588.

Okamoto A, Chikamatsu K, Sakakura K, Hatsushika K, Takahashi G, and Masuyama K (2009) Expansion and characterization of cancer stem-like cells in squamous cell carcinoma of the head and neck Oral Oncology, vol. 45, no. 7, pp. 633–639.

Patel SC, Carpenter WR, Tyree S, Couch ME, Weissler M, Hackman T et al (2011) Increasing incidence of oral tongue squamous cell carcinoma in young white women, age 18 to 44 years. J Clin Oncol 29(11):1488-94.

Peschos D, Stefanou D, Vougiouklakis T, Assimakopoulos DA, Agnantis NJ (2005) Cell cycle proteins in laryngeal cancer: role in proliferation and prognosis. J. Exp. Clin. Cancer Res. 24; 431–437.

Phesse TJ, Clarke AR (2009) Normal stem cells in cancer prone epithelial tissues, British Journal of Cancer 100 221–227.

Pillai MR, Nair MK (2000) Development of a condemned mucosa syndrome and pathogenesis of human papillomavirus-associated upper aerodigestive tract and uterine cervical tumors, Experimental and Molecular Pathology 69, 233–241.

Pindborg JJ, Renstrup G, Poulsen HE et al (1963) Studies in oral leukoplakias. V. Clinical and histologic signs of malignancy. Acta Odont Scand 21:407–414.

Pindborg JJ (1980) Oral cancer and precancer. John Wright & Sons, Bristol

Pindborg JJ, Reichart PA, Smith CJ et al (1997) World Health Organization: Histological typing of cancer and precancer of the oral mucosa, 2nd edn. Springer, Berlin

Pomerantz RG, Grandis JR (2004) The epidermal growth factor receptor signaling network in head and neck carcinogenesis and implications for targeted therapy. Semin. Oncol 31; 734–443.

Poljak M, Gale N, Kambic V, Ferluga D, Fischinger J (1996) Over- expression of p53 protein in benign and malignant laryngeal epithelial lesions. Anticancer Res. 16; 1947–1951.

Poulsen HE, Taylor CW, Sobin LH (1975) Histological typing of female genital tract tumours, International histological classification of tumours, No. 13. World Health Organization, Geneva

Proweller A, Tu L, Lepore JJ, Cheng L, Lu MM, Seykora J et al (2006) CancerRes. 66, 7438-44.

Presland R, Jurevic R (2002) Making sense of the epithelial barrier: what molecular biology and genetics tell us about the functions of oral mucosal and epidermal tissues, Journal of Dental Education 66, 564–574.

Prince ME, Sivanandan R, Kaczorowski A, Wolf GT, Kaplan MJ, Dalerba P et al (2007) Identification of a subpopulation of cells with cancer stem cell properties in head and neck squamous cell carcinoma, Proceedings of the National Academy of Science 104, 973–978.

Prince ME, Ailles LE (2008) Cancer stem cells in head and neck squamous cell cancer, Journal of Clinical Oncology 26 2871–2875.

Putney FJ, O'Keefe JJ (1953) The clinical significance of keratosis of the larynx as a premalignant lesion. Ann. Otol. Rhinol. Laryngol 62; 348–357.

Ramalho-Santos M, Willenbring H (2007) On the origin of the term "stem cell", Cell Stem Cell 1 35–38.

Renan MJ (1993) How many mutations are required for tumorigen- esis? Implications from human cancer data. Mol. Carcinog 7; 139–146.

Ranganathan P, Weaver KL, Capobianco AJ (2011), Nat.Rev. Cancer 11, 338-51.

Reagan JW, Hamonic MJ (1956) Dysplasia of the uterine cervix. Ann N Y Acad Sci 63:1236–1244

Resta L, Colucci GA, Troia M, Russo S, Vacca E, Pesce Delfino V (1992) Laryngeal intraepithelial neoplasia (LIN). An analytical mor- phometric approach. Path. Res. Pract.; 188; 517–523.

Ricci G, Molini E, Faralli M, Simoncelli C. (2003) Retrospective study on precancerous laryngeal lesions: long-term follow-up. Acta Otorhinolaryngol. Ital 23; 362–367.

Ricci-Vitiani L, Lombardi DG, Pilozzi E, Biffoni M, Todaro M, Peschle C (2007) Identification and expansion of human colon-cancer-initiating cells, Nature 445 111–115.

Richart RM (1966) Influence of diagnostic and therapeutic procedures on the distribution of cervical intraepithelial neo- plasia. Cancer 19:1635–1638

Richart RM (1973) Cervical intraepithelial neoplasia. Pathol Ann 8:301–328

Robbins SL, Cortran RS (1979) Pathologic basis of disease, 2nd edn. Saunders, Philadelphia

Saglam O, Shah V, Worsham MJ (2007) Molecular differentiation of early and late stage laryngeal squamous cell carcinoma: an exploratory analysis. Diagn. Mol. Pathol 16; 218–221.

Sakr WA, Gale N, Gnepp DR et al (2009) Squamous intraepi- thelial neoplasia of the upper aerodigestive tract. In: Gnepp DR (ed) Diagnostic surgical pathology of the head and neck, 2nd edn. Saunders, Philadelphia, pp 1–44

Sanz-Ortega J, Valor C, Saez MC et al (2003) 3p21, 5q21, 9p21 and 17p13 allelic deletions accumulate in the dysplastic spectrum of laryngeal carcinogenesis and precede malignant transforma- tion. Histol. Histopathol 18; 1053–1057.

Sardi I, Franchi A, De Campora L, Passali GC, Gallo O (2006) Microsatellite instability as an indicator of malignant progres sion in laryngeal premalignancy. Head Neck 28; 730–739.

Shafer WG (1975) Oral carcinoma in situ. Oral Surg 39:227–238

Shear M, Pindborg JJ (1980) Verrucous hyperplasia of the oral mucosa. Cancer (Phila) 46:1855–1962

Schoelch ML, Sekandari N, Regezi JA et al (1999) Laser management of oral leukoplakias: a follow-up study of 70 patients. Laryngoscope 109:949–953

Serrano M, Hannon GJ, Beach D (1993) A new regulatory motif in cell-cycle control causing specific inhibition of cyclin D/CDK4. Nature 366; 704–707.

Shay JW, Wright WE (1996) Telomerase activity in human cancer. Curr. Opin. Oncol 8; 66–71.

Shin DM, Kim J, Ro JY et al (1994) Activation of p53 gene expression in premalignant lesions during head and neck tumorigenesis. Cancer Res 54; 321–326.

Silverman S Jr, Bhargava K, Mani NJ et al (1976) Malignant transformation and natural history of oral leukoplakia in 57518 industrial workers of Gujarat, India. Cancer (Phila) 38:1790–1795

Singh SK, Clarke ID, Terasaki M et al (2003) Identification of a cancer stem cell in human brain tumors," Cancer Research, vol. 63, no. 18, pp. 5821–5828.

Singh SK, Hawkins C, Clarke ID, Squire JA, Bayani J, Hide T et al (2004) Identification of human brain tumour initiating cells, Nature 432 396–401.

Sjoblom T, Jones S, Wood LD, Parsons DW, Lin J, Barber TD, et al , Science 314, 268-74 (2006).

Sllamniku B, Bauer W, Painter C, Sessions D (1989) The transformation of laryngeal keratosis into invasive carcinoma. Am. J. Otolaryngol 10; 42–54.

Somers KD, Merrick MA, Lopez ME, Incognito LS, Schechter GL, Casey G (1992) Frequent p53 mutations in head and neck cancer Cancer Res 52; 5997–6000.

Sorrells DL Jr, Ghali GE, De Benedetti A, Nathan CA, Li BD (1999) Progressive amplification and overexpression of the eukaryotic initiation factor 4E gene in different zones of head and neck cancers J. Oral Maxillofac. Surg 57; 294–299.

Speight PM, Farthing PM, Bouquot JE (1996) The pathology of oral cancer and precancer. Curr Diagn Pathol 3:165–176

Staibano S, Merolla F, Testa D, Iovine R, Mascolo M, Guarino V et al (2007) OPN/CD44v6 overexpression in laryngeal dysplasia and correlation with clinical outcome. Br J Cancer 97(11):1545-51

Stransky N, Egloff AM, Tward AD, Kostic AD, Cibulskis K, Sivachenko A, et al (2011) The Mutational Landscape of Head and Neck Squamous Cell Carcinoma, Science 333, 1157 10.1126/ science.1208130.

Szotek PP, Pieretti-Vanmarcke R, Masiakos PT et al (2006) Ovarian cancer side population defines cells with stem cell-like characteristics and Mullerian inhibiting substance respon- siveness Proceedings of the National Academy of Sciences of the United States of America, vol. 103, no. 30, pp. 11154–11159,.

Tabor MP, Brakenhoff RH, Ruijter-Schippers HJ, Van Der Wal JE, Snow GB, Leemans CR, et al (2002) Multiple head and neck tumours frequently originate from a single preneoplastic lesion. Am J Pathol 161: 1051–1060

Tabor MP, Braakhuis BJM, Van der Waal JE et al (2003) Comparative molecular and histological grading of epithelial dysplasia of the oral cavity and the oropharynx. J Pathol 199:354–360

Tan T-T, Coussens LM (2007) Humoral immunity, inflammation and cancer, Current Opinion in Immunology 19 209–216.

Thomasson HR, Edenberg HJ, Crabb DW et al (1991) Alcohol and aldehyde dehydrogenase genotypes and alcoholism in Chinese men American Journal of Human Genetics, vol. 48, no. 4, pp. 677–681.

Toole BP, Wight TN, Tammi MI (2002) Hyaluronan-cell interactions in cancer and vascular disease, The Journal of Biological Chemistry 277 4593–4596.

Trzpis M, McLaughlin PMJ, de Leij LMFH, Harmsen MC (2007) Epithelial cell adhesion molecule: more than a carcinoma marker and adhesion molecule, The American Journal of Pathology 171, 386–395.

Uhlman DL, Adams G, Knapp D, Aeppli DM, Niehans G (1996) Immunohistochemical staining for markers of future neoplastic progression in the larynx. Cancer Res 56; 2199–2205.

van der Riet P, Nawroz H, Hruban RH et al (1994) Frequent loss of chromosome 9p21-22 early in head and neck cancer progres- sion. Cancer Res 54; 1156–1158.

van der Waal I, Schepman KP, van der Meiji EH et al (1997) Oral leukoplakia: a clinicopathological review. Oral Oncol 33:291-301

Vedtofte P, Holmstrup P, Hjorting-Hansen E et al (1987) Surgical treatment of premalignant lesions of the oral mucosa. Int J Oral Maxillofac Surg 16:656–664

Velasco JRR, Nieto CS, de Bustos CP, Marcos CA (1987) Premalignant lesions of the larynx: pathological prognostic factors. J. Otolaryngol 16; 367–370.

Vinitha Richard, M. Radhakrishna Pillai (2010) The stem cell code in oral epithelial tumorigenesis: "The cancer stem cell shift hypothesis" Biochimica et Biophysica Acta 1806 146–162

Visus C, Ito D, Amoscato A et al (2007) Identification of human aldehyde dehydrogenase 1 family member a1 as a novel CD8+ T-cell-defined tumor antigen in squamous cell carcinoma of the head and neck Cancer Research, vol. 67, no. 21, pp. 10538–10545.

Voravud N, Shin DM, Ro JY, Lee JS, Hong WK, Hittelman WN (1993) Increased polysomies of chromosomes 7 and 17 during head and neck multistage tumorigenesis. Cancer Res 53; 2874–2883.

Wahi PN, Cohen B, Luthra UK et al (1971) Histological typing of oral and oropharyngeal tumours. International histological classification of tumours no. 4. World Health Organization, Geneva

Wang SJ, Wong G, De Heer AM, Xia W, and Bourguignon LYW (2009) CD44 Variant isoforms in head and neck squamous cell carcinoma progression Laryngoscope, vol. 119, no. 8, pp. 1518–1530.

Wang J, Guo LP, Chen LZ, Zeng YX, and Shih HL (2007) Identification of cancer stem cell-like side population cells in human nasopharyngeal carcinoma cell line Cancer Research, vol. 67, no. 8, pp. 3716–3724.

Warnakulasuriya S (2001) Histological grading of oral epithelial dysplasia: revisited. J Pathol 194:294–297

Warnakulasuriya S, Johnson NW, van der Wall I (2007) Nomenclature and classification of potentially malignant disorders of the oral mucosa. J Oral Pathol Med 36:575–580

Warnakulasuriya S, Reibel J, Bouquot J et al (2008) Oral epithelial dysplasia classification system: predictive value, utility, weakness and scope for improvement. J Oral Pathol Med 37:127–133

Wayne S, Robinson RA (2006) Upper aerodigestive tract squamous dysplasia: correlation with p16, p53, pRb, and Ki-67 expres- sion. Arch. Pathol. Lab. Med 130; 1309-1314.

Wood LD, Parsons DW, Jones S, Lin J, Sjöblom T, Leary RJ, et al (2007) Science 318, 1108-13.

Yoo WJ, Cho SH, Lee YS et al (2004) Loss of heterozygosity on chromosomes 3p,8p,9p and 17p in the progression of squamous cell carcinoma of the larynx. J. Korean Med. Sci 19; 345–351.

Yuge T, Nibu K, Kondo K, Shibahara J, Tayama N, Sugasawa M (2005) Loss of FHIT expression in squamous cell carcinoma and premalignant lesions of the larynx. Ann. Otol. Rhinol. Laryngol 114; 127–131.

Zerdoner D (2003) The Ljubljana classification: its application to grading oral epithelial hyperplasia. J Craniomaxillofacial Surg 31:75–79

Zhang P, Zhang Y, Mao L, Zhang Z, and Chen W (2009) Side population in oral squamous cell carcinoma possesses tumor stem cell phenotypes Cancer Letters, vol. 277, no. 2, pp. 227- 234.

Zhang Q, Shi S, Yen Y, Brown J, Ta JQ, and Le AD (2009) A subpopulation of CD133+ cancer stem-like cells characterized in human oral squamous cell carcinoma confer resistance to chemotherapy Cancer Letters, vol. 289, no. 2, pp. 151–160.

Part 2

Intraepithelial Neoplasia of Eye and Ocular Adnexa

2

Ocular Surface Squamous Neoplasia

Napaporn Tananuvat[1] and Nirush Lertprasertsuke[2]
Departments of [1]Ophthalmology and [2]Pathology,
Faculty of Medicine, Chiang Mai University,
Thailand

1. Introduction

The ocular surface is composed of the conjunctiva and the cornea. The conjunctiva is a mucous membrane which covers the globe and inner part of the eyelids. The morphology of conjunctival epithelial cells are nonkeratinized stratified epithelia which vary from cuboidal over the tarsus, to columnar in the fornices, to squamous epithelia on the globe. Goblet cells account for up to 10% of the basal cells of the conjunctival epithelia. The substantia propia of the conjunctiva consists of loose connective tissue. The cornea is a transparent, avascular tissue which acts as both the anterior eye wall and an optical media for light to enter the eye. The corneal epithelium layer is composed of stratified squamous epithelial cells and makeup about 5 % (0.05 mm) of the total corneal thickness. The corneal epithelial stem cells located at the basal layer of the limbal epithelia proliferate continuously and give rise to the superficial layer that subsequently differentiate into superficial cells. Regulation of cell growth and metabolism are critical to maintain an intact ocular surface and transparent cornea.

Primary tumors of the conjunctiva and cornea can be grouped into two major categories: congenital and acquired. The acquired lesions are composed of a variety of neoplasms which originate from squamous epithelia, melanocytes, and lymphocyte cells. Tumors of squamous epithelium occupy a large spectrum of lesions, ranging from benign lesions like squamous papilloma, to precancerous lesions which are confined to the surface epithelium (intraepithelial neoplasia or dysplasia, previously known as Bowen's disease). There are even more invasive squamous cell carcinomas that break through the basement membrane to the underlying substantria propia of the conjunctiva or corneal stroma.

The term ocular surface squamous neoplasia (OSSN) was first described in 1995 by Lee and Hirst to denote a spectrum of neoplasm originate from squamous epithelium ranging from simple dysplasia to invasive squamous cell carcinoma(SCC), involving the conjunctiva, the limbus, and the cornea.(Lee & Hirst 1995) Similar to cancer of cervix, it has a relative high recurrence after treatment and may metastasize. This tumor is considered as a low grade malignancy but invasive lesion can spread to the globe or orbit. This chapter highlights the epidemiology, etiologies and related factors, clinical manifestations, diagnostic tools, and standard care of management of these tumors. Squamous papilloma is also included as some conjunctival papilloma may have dysplastic potential.

2. Epidemiology and pathogenesis

OSSN is considered an uncommon disease with geographic incidences which vary from 0.2 to 3.5 per 100,000, with greater frequency near the equator. (Lee & Hirst 1995) It is the most common ocular surface tumor in many series.(Lee & Hirst 1995; Shields et al. 2004; Shields & Shields 2004) Prior to HIV pandemic, OSSN was noted to occur predominantly in the elderly for whom it was the third most common oculo-orbital tumor after malignant melanoma and lymphoma. (Lee & Hirst 1995) This tumor is rare in the United States, with an incidence rate of 0.03 per 100,000 persons, although the rate was approximately 5-fold higher in males and Caucasians (Sun et al. 1997).

Pathogenesis of OSSN has yet to be attributed to specific etiologic factors, the main associated factors being exposure to ultraviolet (UV) radiation, human papilloma virus infection, and human immunodeficiency virus (HIV) seropositivity.

2.1 Ultraviolet-B

Chronic exposure to UV–B radiation (290-320 nm) is an established cause of many eye diseases such as pingecular, pterygium, cataract, and age-related macular degeneration. (Taylor et al. 1992) Evidence from epidemiologic studies and worldwide cancer registries have confirmed that the incidence rate of OSSN increased with proximity to the equator, presumably from increased solar UV radiation. (Lee et al. 1994; Newton et al. 1996) One population-based cancer study found that the incidence of squamous cell carcinoma(SCC) of the eye declined by 49% for each 10 degree increase in latitude, falling from more than 12 cases per million per year in Uganda, to less than 0.2 cases per million per year in the UK. The incidence of SCC decreased by 29% per unit reduction in UV exposure. (Newton et al. 1996) There is considerable evidence linking cutaneous malignancy and UV exposure. (English et al. 1997) These lesions occur predominantly in sun-exposured areas of the skin. Lesions of OSSN are often found at the corneal limbus in the interpalpebral area, where sun-exposure is greater. The corneal limbus is a transitional area, from the conjunctival to corneal epithelial, analogous to the squamocollumnar junction of the uterine cervix which is prone to dysplastic change. The role of limbal stem cells in development of OSSN is controversial. These cells are long-lived and have great potential to clonagenic division. OSSN may arise from dysfunction limbal stem cells and from mutagenic agents such as UV radiation leading to mutations in the P53 tumor suppressor gene, also known as *TP*53 gene. One pilot case-control study found that the *TP*53 mutation was detected in 56% of cancer cases (SCC) and 14% of control. 50% of mutations were CC-TT transition which was a molecular signature of mutagenesis by solar UV rays. This prevalence was high compared to any cancer type (not exceed 6%), but matched that of skin cancer in subjects with xeroderma pigmentosum.(Ateenyi-Agaba et al. 2004) Solar elastosis was also found more frequently in pathological specimens from the conjunctival squamous cell neoplasia (53.3% of cases and 3.3% of controls). (Tulvatana et al. 2003) One immunohistochemical study showed that UV radiation may play a role as a stimulating agent in the expression of some proteolytic enzymes, such as matrix metalloproteinases (MMPs) and their tissue inhibitors (TIMPs), which are relevant to neoplasia. (Ng et al. 2008)

2.2 Human papilloma virus

Human papilloma viruses (HPV) are oncogenic viruses and their role in human cervical carcinoma is well-established, however, their role in OSSN is unclear. Nakamura demonstrated that 50% of squamous tumors of the ocular surface and lacrimal sac were associated with HPV. (Nakamura et al. 1997) Biopsy specimens together with analyses of archrival embedded tissue revealed that the low risk HPV type 6 and 11 were the most common types of viruses associated with conjunctival papilloma. (Sjo et al. 2007; Verma et al. 2008) The high risk HPV type 16 and 18 have also been demonstrated in conjunctival papilloma, however, both are commonly found in high grade dysplasia, or invasive squamous cell carcinoma of the conjunctiva. (Sjo et al. 2007; Verma et al. 2008) One study identified the DNA of HPV 16, 18, and mRNA from the *E6* region, which represented active transcribed viruses from all specimens of conjunctival intraepithelial neoplasia by using the PCR technique (n = 10). (Scott et al. 2002)

In contrast, several studies have failed to demonstrate HPV in malignant conjunctival epithelial tumors and suggested that HPV was not associated with malignant conjunctival lesions and posed other mechanism, such as UVB being more important to the etiology of these lesions. (Eng et al. 2002; Tulvatana et al. 2003; Sen et al. 2007; Manderwad et al. 2009) Thus, the association between HPV and OSSN is variable in different geographic areas, and perhaps depends on the method of detection used. (Eng et al. 2002; Sen et al. 2007; Guthoff et al. 2009; Manderwad et al. 2009)

2.3 Human immunodeficiency virus

OSSN is now recognized as an AIDS-related cancer and its incidence has increased with the HIV pandemic in Africa. (Porges & Groisman 2003) One study revealed that HIV was strongly associated with conjunctival squamous neoplasia in Africa with an odds ratio of 13 (HIV was positive in 71% of cases and 16% of controls). (Waddell et al. 1996) A case-control study of conjunctival SCC in Uganda demonstrated a 10 fold increased risk of conjunctival SCC in HIV-infected patients. (Newton et al. 2002) These tumors occurred at an earlier age in HIV-infected individuals and was often more aggressive than immunocompetent patients. OSSN may be the primary or only apparent manifestation of HIV infection in sub-Saharan Africa. (Spitzer et al. 2008) SCC can also involve other non-ocular sites such as the oropharynx, cervix, and anorectum.(Jeng et al. 2007) One study from the US found that there was an increased prevalence of HIV among patients with CIN who were younger than 50 years of age. (Karp et al. 1996) A HIV/AIDS Cancer Match Registry Study in the USA, however, demonstrated that the risk of conjunctival SCC was elevated regardless of HIV category, CD4 lymphocyte count, and time relative to AID-onset. The risk was highest with age≥ 50, Hispanic ethnicity, and residence in regions with high solar-UV radiation. (Guech-Ongey et al. 2008) Tissue analysis from OSSN specimens in HIV-1 patients identified multiple oncogenic viruses including HPV, EBV, and KSHV, suggested that these infectious agents may contribute to the development of this malignancy in HIV patients. (Simbiri et al. 2010)

2.4 Immunosuppression

Of note, OSSN shares some striking similarities to skin neoplasm. It is believed that localized immune suppression of the skin from sun damage may lead to increased susceptibility to HPV infection, causing neoplasia. Additional risks have also been reported in immunosuppressed cancer patients and organ transplant patients. (Shelil et al. 2003; Shome et al. 2006) As well, there have been reports of OSSN after corneal grafts, which may partly be related to local immunosuppression, HPV, or possibly that neoplastic cells had been in the donor corneal epithelia at the time of transplantation. (Ramasubramanian et al. 2010)

2.5 Others

Other factors associated with this condition include old age, the male sex (Lee & Hirst 1995; Sun et al. 1997), and fair skin pigmentation (Lee et al. 1994; Sun et al. 1997), as well as heavy cigarette smoking (Napora et al. 1990), exposure to petroleum products (Napora et al. 1990), and some genetic conditions like xeroderma pigmentosum. The latter is an uncommon genetic disorder, where excessive reactivity to UV light-induced damage results in a more malignant course. It is common in early childhood with severe photosensitivity and photophobia. (Kraemer et al. 1987; Chidzonga et al. 2009) Long standing use of ocular prosthesis (Jain et al. 2010)and contact lens wear (Guex-Crosier & Herbort 1993) have also been implicated in the pathogenesis of OSSN, although evidence is scant.

3. Clinical manifestations

The clinical spectrum of OSSN varies from benign lesions like squamous papilloma, precancerous lesions like conjunctiva-corneal intraepithelial dysplasia (CCIN), carcinoma in situ, and invasive squamous cell carcinoma (SCC).

3.1 Conjunctival papilloma

Squamous papillomas are among the most common benign acquired lesions of the conjunctiva. There are two forms of conjunctival papilloma: pendunculated and sessile. Both have different etiology and clinical courses. A pedunculated conjunctival papilloma is a fleshy, exophytic mass with a fibrovascular core which gives rise to a stalk. (Fig.1) It often arises in the inferior fornix, but can be present on the tarsus or bulbar conjunctiva. This lesion is associated with HPV subtype 6 or 11 (Sjo et al. 2007), and often occurs in children. It can regress spontaneously, or may recur after surgical excision.

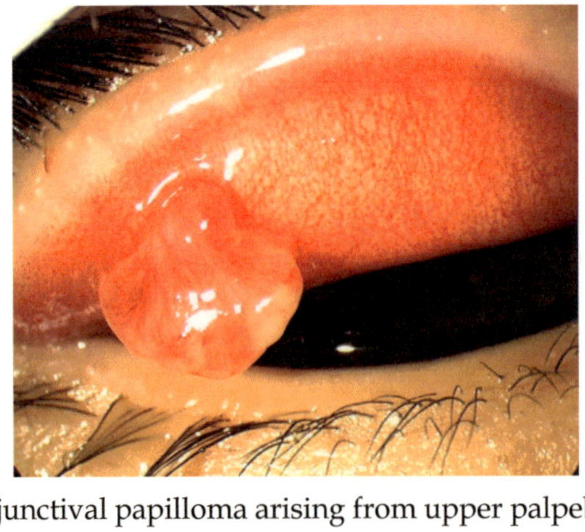

Fig. 1. Penduculate conjunctival papilloma arising from upper palpebral conjunctiva.

A sessile papilloma is more typically found at the limbus and has a broad base. The glistening surface and numerous red dots resemble a strawberry. (Fig.2) In contrast, a sessile lesion usually occurs in adults and more prone to dysplastic change. This lesion is related to HPV subtype 16 or 18. The latter oncogenic virus strains are strongly associated with human cervical carcinoma.

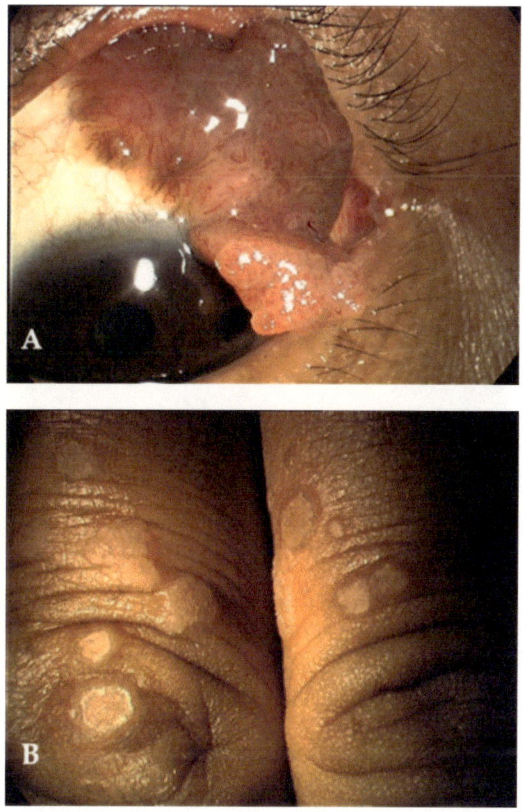

Fig. 2. A. Sessile mass arising from bulbar conjunctiva. B. Multiple papillomas involve skin of two fingers in the same patient.

3.2 Conjunctival-corneal intraepithelial neoplasia

The clinical symptoms are generally nonspecific, vary from asymptomatic to chronic irritation, redness, and varying degrees of visual involvement determine by the extension of lesions to the visual axis. Clinical patterns may be in a papilliform, as well as velvety, gelatinous, leukoplakic, nodular or even diffuse fashion. (Fig. 3-5) The lesions most commonly arise in the interpalpebral area of perilimbal conjunctiva, but are less common in the forniceal or palpebral conjunctiva. A white plaque (leukoplakia) may occur on the surface of the lesion, representing secondary hyperkeratosis, which results from squamous cell dysfunction. The conjunctival lesion is mobile with feeder vessels supplying the mass. These tumors may appear as slowly growing localized lesions that mimic benign conjunctival degenerations, and sometimes coexist with pterygia or pingecula. (Hirst et al. 2009) Sometimes, the lesions can have pigmentation and masquerade as malignant melanoma. (Shields et al. 2008) (Fig.6) OSSN can be diffused or have bilateral involvement. (Fig.7) Corneal OSSN is usually an extension of conjunctival squamous neoplasia. Rarely, isolated corneal involvement has been reported with the potentially aggressive form. (Fig.8) Bowman's layer usually is a barrier to invasive lesions. (Cha et al. 1993)

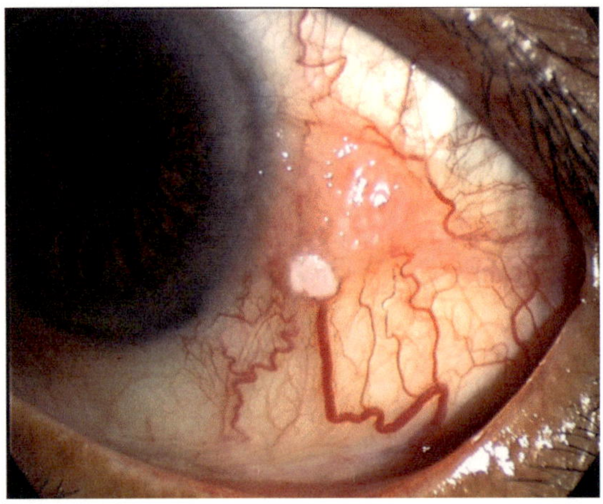

Fig. 3. Conjunctival intraepithelial neoplasia is present as a nodular mass with foci of leukoplakia on the surface of the lesion.

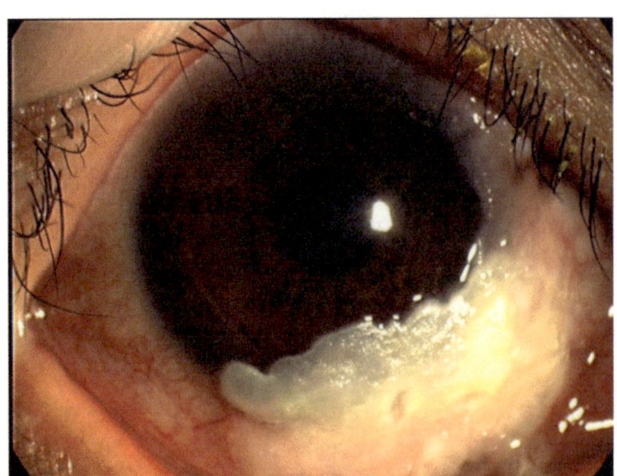

Fig. 4. Conjunctival-corneal intraepithelial neoplasia: a flat gelatinous mass with surface leukoplakia involves 2 quadrants of limbus.

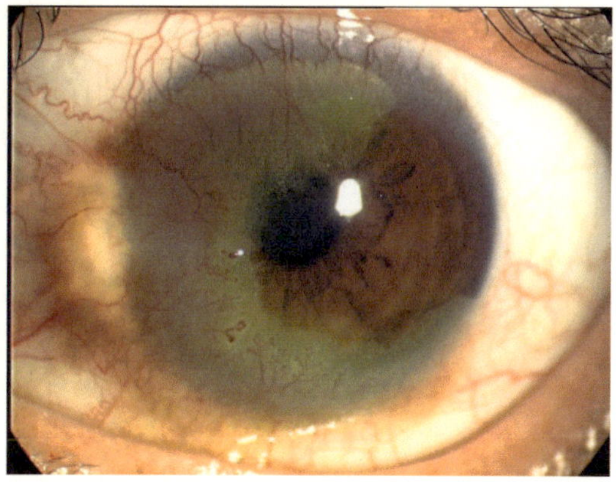

Fig. 5. Corneal intraepithelial neoplasia involving 270 degrees of the limbus (note vascular tuffs present on the mass)

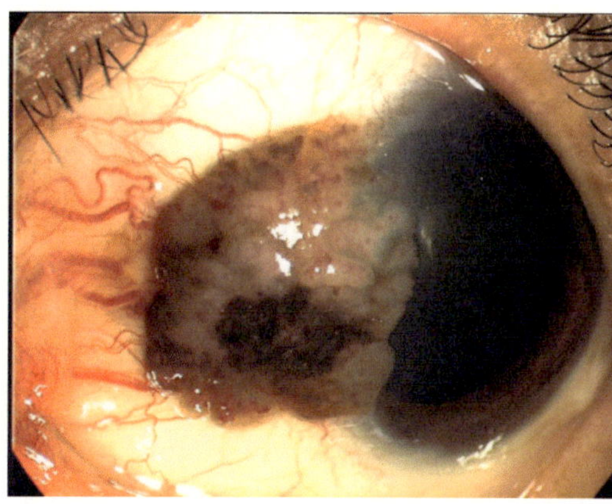

Fig. 6. Conjunctival-corneal intraepithelial neoplasia presents as a nodular mass with papillomatous pattern and hyperpigmentation (note feeder vessels are present).

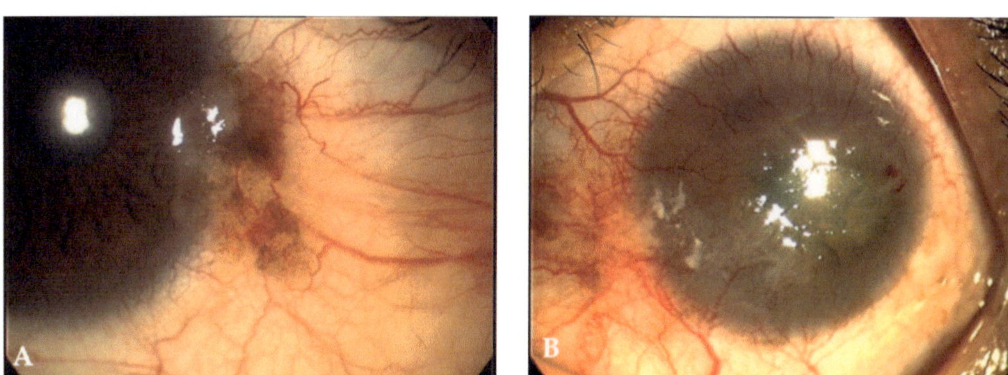

Fig. 7. Bilateral conjunctival-corneal intraepithelial neoplasia in an HIV-infected patient. A. Pigmented lesion with fibrovascular fond arising at the limbus. B. Diffused, flat lesion involving 360 degrees of the limbus (note central corneal epithelia defect is present in the photograph).

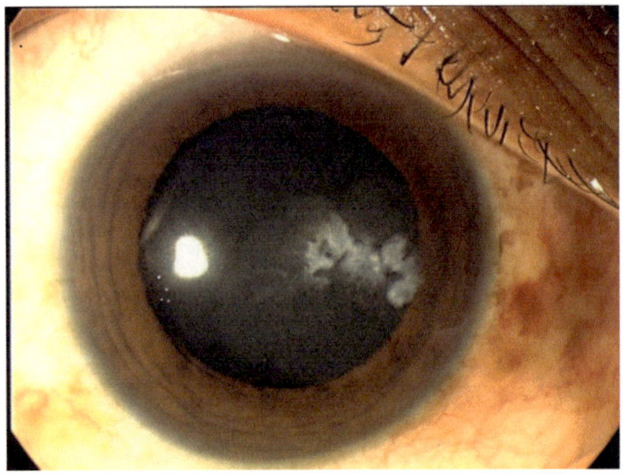

Fig. 8. Corneal intraepithelial neoplasia is present as a flat grayish mass with a fimbriated border and surface keratinization.

3.3 Squamous cell carcinoma

Squamous cell carcinoma is the final stage of this tumor where dysplastic epithelial invade beyond the basement membrane to the conjunctival substantia propia or corneal stroma. Clinically, invasive squamous cell carcinoma is generally larger and more elevated than CIN. (Fig.9) In practice, it may not be possible to distinguish invasive squamous cell carcinoma from intraepithelial lesion or carcinoma in-situ by using clinical features alone. However, an advanced lesion or mass that is immobile and fix to the globe should be suspected as an invasive lesion. A long term neglected mass or incomplete excised mass can invade through the globe or orbit. (Fig.10)

Local invasion is the most prevalent mechanism of tumor spread. Intraocular invasion may be associated with iritis, glaucoma, retinal detachment, or rupture of the globe. Metastases are rare, and the first site of extraocular involvement is regional lymph nodes.

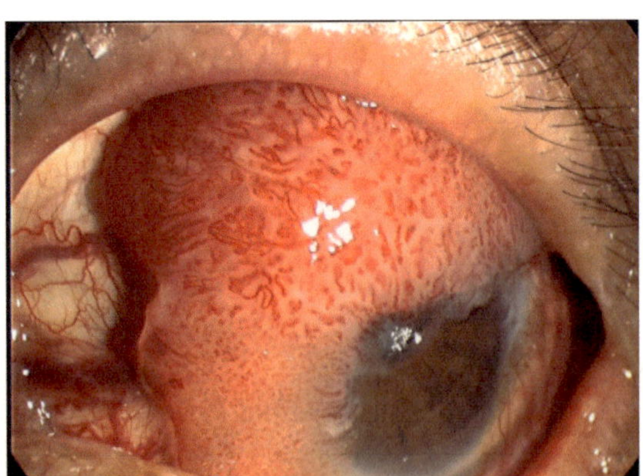

Fig. 9. Invasive squamous cell carcinoma involves two quadrants of conjunctiva and cornea (note papillary vascular pattern present on the mass with feeder vessels).

A rare variant of conjunctival squamous cell carcinoma is the mucoepidermoid carcinoma. Clinically, this tumor occurs in older patients and has a yellow globular cystic component due to the presence of abundant mucous-secreting cells within cysts. It tends to be more aggressive than the standard squamous cell carcinoma, thus deserves wider excision and closer follow-up. The spindle cell variant of squamous cell carcinoma is likewise aggressive. (Shields et al. 2007)

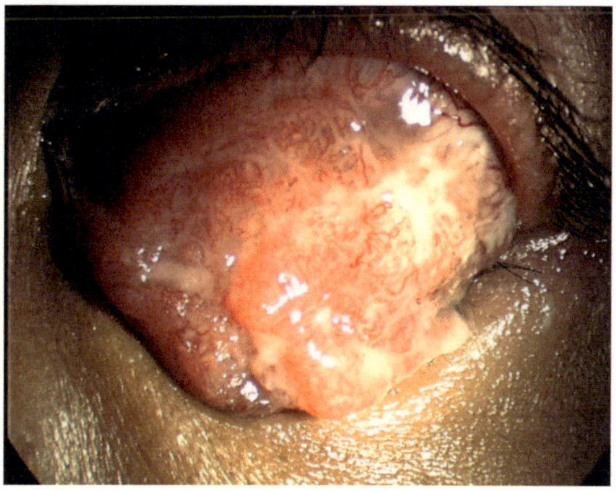

Fig. 10. An advanced squamous cell carcinoma involves the entire cornea and conjunctival surface with protrusions of the mass onto the lower eyelid.

4. Diagnosis and investigations

There are several points to cover before reaching diagnostic and management planning for OSSN, including clinical and pathologic findings, as well as the extension and complications of the tumors.

- Clinical feature of the lesion: morphology, size, site, surface, feeder vessels, and exact anatomical location whether it is conjunctival (move with conjunctiva when applying topical anesthesia with cotton tip applicator) or scleral involvement (fixed to the globe).
- Assessment of extension of the lesions
    - Intraocular invasion: perform gonioscopy to assess the invasion angle of the tumor. (Fig.11) Dilated fundus examination should be done to assess the intraocular invasion. In cases with media opacity, B-scan ultrasonography is helpful to assess sclera and intraocular spread.
    - Orbital invasion: by using CT scans or MRI scans, the accuracy and extension of the mass can accurately assess for the orbital or anterior eye involvement.
    - Regional lymph node spread: it is critical to assess the regional lymph nodes (preauricular, submandibular and cervical lymph nodes) as part of the clinical examination.

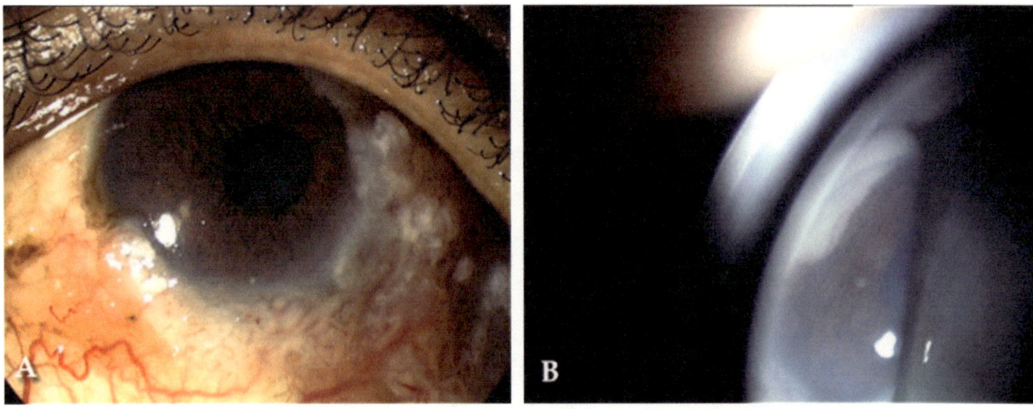

Fig. 11. Squamous cell carcinoma A. Diffused mass involves more than two quadrants of the limbus. B. Gonioscopic findings in the same eye show angle invasion by the mass.

- Pathologic diagnosis

  Since clinical appearance alone may not differentiate intraepithelial from invasive lesions, the gold standard for definite diagnosis is tissue histology, which can be performed by incisional or excisional biopsy. For relatively small tumors (≤ 4 clock hours of limbal involvement or ≤ 15 mm basal diameter), excisional biopsy is generally preferred to incisional biopsy. Larger lesions can be approached by wedge or punch biopsy. Incisional biopsy is also appropriate for conditions that are ideally treated with topical chemotherapy, or other treatments, such as radiation.

4.1 Histology

Histologic features of OSSN can be classified according to the presence of dysplastic cells originating in the basal cell layers which extend toward the surface. There are various patterns of dysplastic changes, ranging from the small squamous cells with increased nuclear-to-cytoplasmic (N/C) ratio, large squamous cells with hyperchromatic nuclei, and spindle cells bearing oval-shaped nuclei. The dysplastic cells contain abnormal nuclei either with nuclear pleomorphism or anisonucleosis. In addition, mitotic figures are increased and gradually pushed upward to the surface along with the degree of dysplasia. Many mitotic figures are abnormal. The histologic terms used to describe the OSSN include(Font et al. 2006):

- *Dysplasia*: dysplastic epithelial lesions of the conjunctiva and cornea divides into three grades based on the thickness of intraepithelial involvement. Koilocytes are rarely identified but suggestive for HPV infection when encountered. The thickness of involvement can be estimated using Periodic acid-Schiff (PAS) stain to demonstrate the presence of glycogen in non-neoplastic superficial squamous cells. Moreover, proliferating cell nuclear antigen (PCNA), Ki-67 and p53 immunostaining as well as argyrophillic nucleolar organizer region (AgNOR) staining may be useful for grading the dysplastic lesions as well as for correlation with clinical morphologic findings. (Aoki et al. 1998) Grading of dysplasia is described as:
  - Mild - less than a third thickness of the epithelium is occupied by atypical cells.(Fig.12A)

- Moderate - within three quarters thickness of the epithelium is occupied by atypical cells.
- Severe – nearly full thickness of the epithelium is occupied by atypical cells.(Fig.12B)

- *Carcinoma in situ*: full-thickness epithelial neoplasia with loss of the normal surface layer. (Fig.12C) Arborizarion of the proliferating blood vessels and extension of connective tissue along the neoplastic area may mimic the sessile papilloma.(Pizzarello & Jakobiec 1978)
- *Invasive squamous cell carcinoma*: the entire thickness of the epithelium has been replaced by the dysplastic cells and the basement membrane of the basal epithelial layer has been breached due to invasion of dysplastic cells into the substantia propia. Formation of cancer cell nests and single cancer cells with bizarre nuclei in the stroma is definitive of invasive carcinoma.(Tunc et al. 1999) (Fig.12D)

4.2 Cytology

Ocular surface cytology can be performed by two major techniques:first is exfoliative cytology by using spatula scrapings or a cytobrush to collect the sample, and second is impression cytology by using the collecting devices to collect the sample by contact with the surface of the lesions. The cytologic features of OSSN have been reviewed by several authors.(Lee & Hirst 1995)

- *Dysplasia*: Squamous cells with enlarged nuclei bearing fine to coarse granulation of the nuclear chromatins, irregular nuclear borders, scanty cytoplasm. The background is clean.
- *Carcinoma in situ*: Variable numbers of dysplastic cells with an admixture of intact and well preserved malignant cells. They are variable in size with scanty cytoplasm, usually < 1 nuclear diameter in width. The enlarged nuclei displays neoplastic features of hyperchromatism, irregular nuclear membrane thickening, or crusting of nuclear membranes. The other nuclear features include abnormal clearing or condensation of nuclear chromatins and large acidophilic nucleoli. However, background of the smear is clean.
- *Invasive squamous cell carcinoma*: Cytologic features of the SCC have been graded into two groups.
  - Grade 1-2: Marked cytologic aberration with bizarre malignant cell features including tadpole cells with cytolplasmic tails, fiber or spindle cells, hyperkeratinized cells with opaque refractile red or orange cytoplasm, and malignant nuclei.
  - Grade 3-4: Large or small cancer cells with scanty cytoplasm. Nonkeratinized cells maybe partially destructed cells, or complete loss of cytoplasm bearing large to huge pleomorphic nuclei. With deeper invasion and ulceration, tumor "diathesis" background- necrotic tumor cells, debris, blood, and leukocyte exudates are more prominent.

The advantages of cytology are a simple technique in diagnosis and follow-up after treatment in OSSN, particularly for detection of recurrences. However, some problems have been reported in exfoliative cytology techniques which may include a degree of uncomfort for the patient, problems with drying artifacts, problems with cellular overlap (difficult to interpret the specimens reliably) and non-localized lesions.

Impression cytology (IC) is a technique for collecting the superficial layers of the ocular surface by applying collecting devices. Commonly used are cellulose acetate filter paper with a pore size ranging from 0.025 - 0.45 micron or other materials (nitrocellulose filters, Biopore membranes, or polyether sulfone filters)(Calonge et al. 2004) so that cells adhere to the surface of the device and can be removed and processed further for analysis by a diversity of methods. IC represents a simple and non-invasive technique for both diagnosis and follow-up after treatment of several disorders of the ocular surface. The main advantages are that it allows relatively easy collection of epithelial samples with minimal

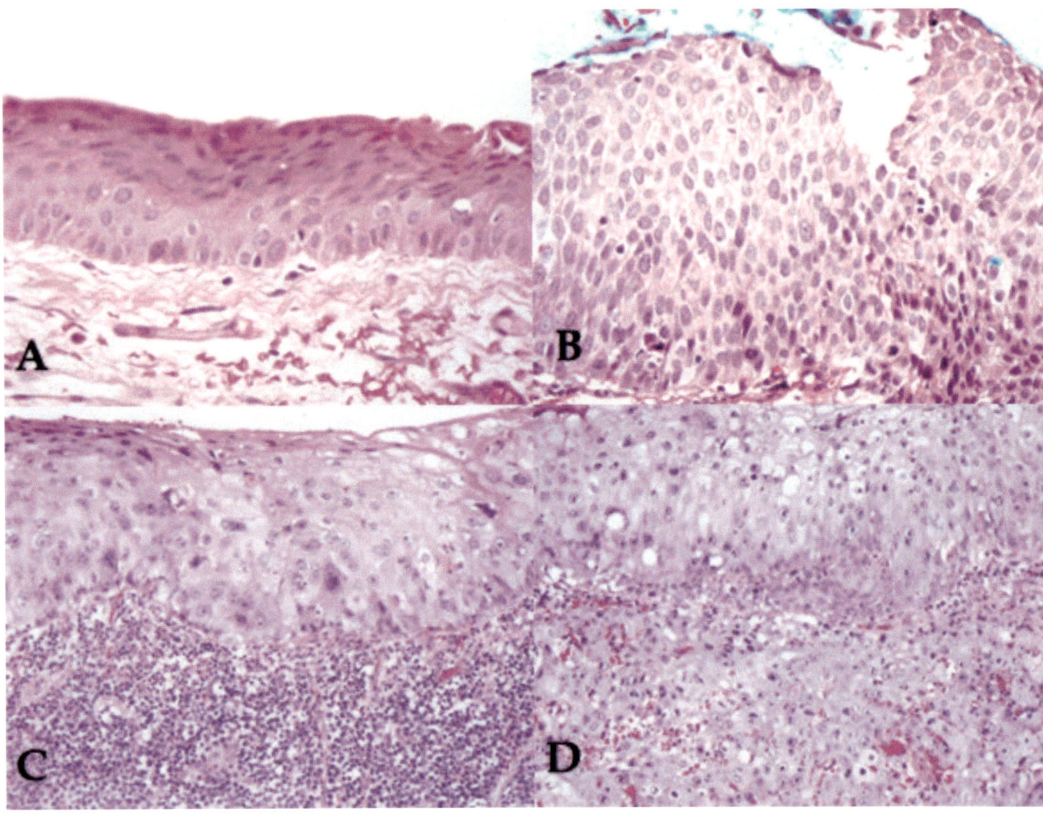

Fig. 12. Histologic features. A. Mild dysplasia; the basal cells are disordered with increased nuclear sizes and coarse nuclear chromatin. B. Severe dysplasia; the epithelial cells are varied in shapes and sizes with large pleomorphic nuclei. The surface cells are flattened with pyknotic nuclei. C. Carcinoma in situ: the entire thickness of the epithelium is composed of dysplastic cells bearing pleomorphic nuclei. Note the inflammatory reaction in the stroma. D. Invasive squamous cell carcinoma; the invasive nest in the stroma is composed of bizarre cells similar to those in the epithelium. The nuclei are plemorphic with thick nuclear membranes and prominent nucleoli (Hematoxylin and Eosin stain. Original magnification X40)

discomfort to the patient, can be performed on an outpatient basis, and allows more precise localization of the area being studied. In addition, a cell to cell relationship can be assessed, which allows one to see cells the way they exist in vivo.

Successful results of IC in diagnosis of OSSN in histologic-confirmed cases have been reported, with positive results of 77% - 80% of the cases.(Nolan et al. 1994; Tole et al. 2001) One study of ocular surface tumors found that IC had a positive and negative predictive value of 97.4% and 53.9%, respectively, when compared to histology.(Tananuvat et al. 2008) The limitations of IC are that, first, IC may be less sensitive for cases with keratotic lesions, because keratotic lesions are common in OSSN (68%) compared with a much lower incidence in cervical cancer. Second, IC may not distinguish carcinoma in situ from minimally invasive disease, because only the superficial cells are collected in the IC method. Therefore, a tissue biopsy remains necessary in cases with negative cytology.

At present, no cytologic criteria have been identified that reliably differentiate invasive carcinoma from in situ in IC samples. Squamous cell abnormalities may be classified into 4 groups, using a modification of the Bethesda system in cervical cytology(Solomon et al. 2002): (1) atypical squamous cells (ASC) (Fig.13 B); (2) low grade squamous intraepithelial lesions (LSIL), which encompass squamous papilloma and mild dysplasia(Fig.13 C); (3) high grade squamous intraepithelial lesions (HSIL), which encompass moderate to severe dysplasia and carcinoma in situ (CIS) (Fig.13 D-E); and (4) squamous cell carcinoma (SCC).(Fig.13 F) One series of OSSN found that SCC from cytology had a highest rate of correlation(91.7%) with histology followed by HSILs (45.5%), ASCs(42.9%),normal epithelia (33%), and LSILs (21.4%), respectively.(Tananuvat et al. 2008) Barros and coworkers used a scoring index modified from the Bethesda system which revealed a predictive index score of ≥4.5 represented the best cut-off point for diagnosis of SCC by using IC with a sensitivity of 95%, specificity of 93%, positive predictive value of 95%, and a negative predictive value of 93%.(Barros et al. 2009) However, the skill and the experience of cytologist are necessary for interpretation of the IC specimens.

4.3 Immunohistochemical analysis: Ki-67 proliferative index

Ki-67 nuclear antigen is expressed in all phases of the cell cycle, except the G0 phase. Ki-67 immunohistochemical analysis has been applied in the histopathologic diagnosis of malignant tumors. In normal cervical squamous mucosa, Ki-67 positive cells are found mainly in the parabasal layer. In cervical squamous intraepithelial lesions (SILs), the number of Ki-67 positive cells increased as the cell grading went from normal to low grade SIL(LSIL) to high grade SIL(HSIL). Similar findings have been reported in case of conjunctival SCC and intraepithelial neoplasia. One study compared tissue specimens obtained from SCC, CIN, and non-CIN (pterygium) lesions, revealed that Ki-67 proliferative index (Ki-67 PI) was significantly higher in SCC and CIN than in pterygium.(Ohara et al. 2004) In another study, the Ki-67 PI of CINs accounted for 20-48% which was significantly higher than non-CIN lesions (8-12%) and normal conjunctivae (8-12%). This study also showed that there was no statistical significance of P53-positive cells in CIN lesion compared to non-CIN lesions and normal conjunctiva due to the wide standard deviations. (Kuo et al. 2006) Therefore, Ki-67 PI may serve as a meaningful diagnostic marker for OSSN.

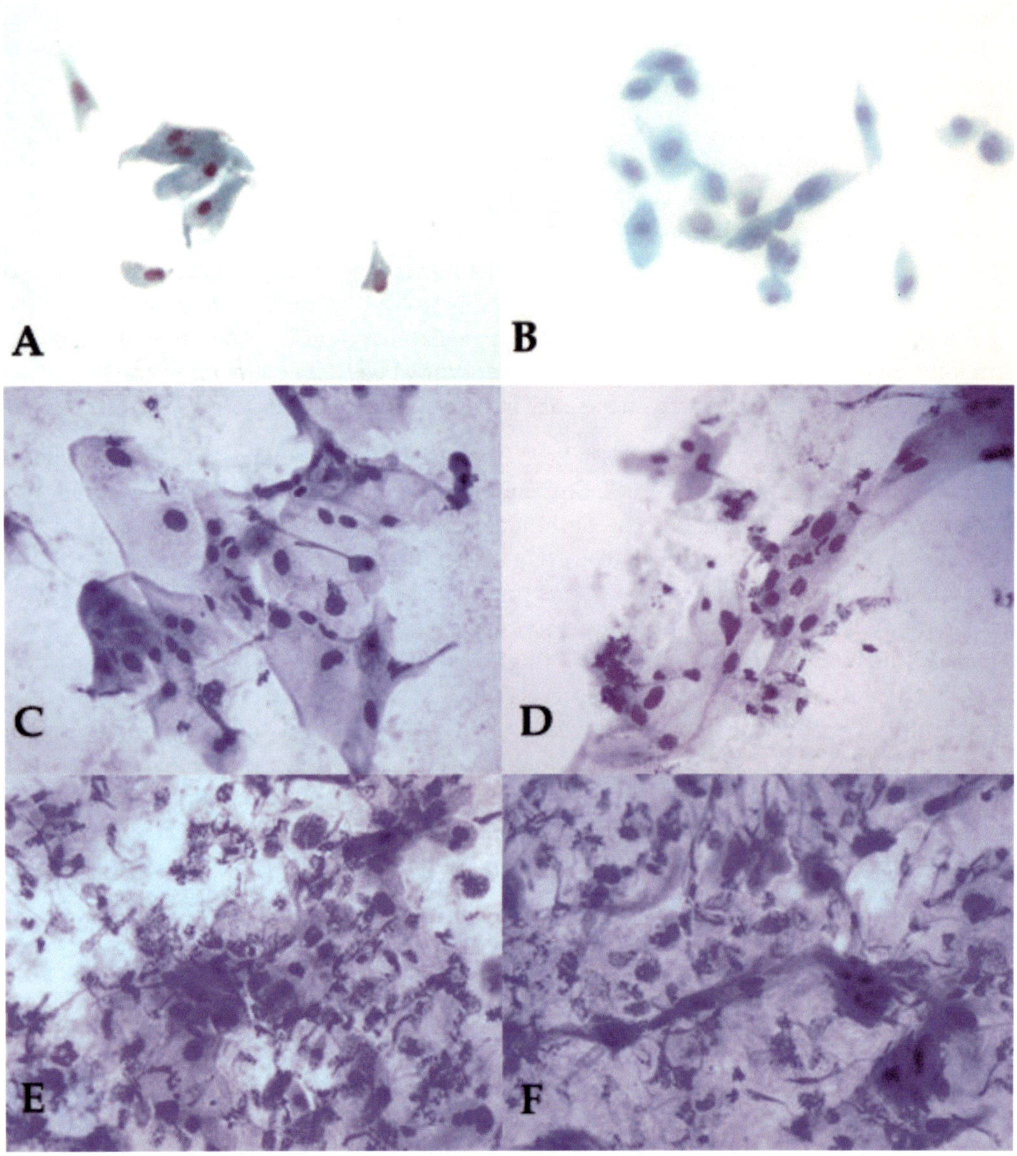

Fig. 13. Cytologic features from impression cytology specimens. A. Normal squamous cells with small nuclei and fine keratohyaline granules. B. Atypical cells with increased nuclear-to-cytoplasmic (N/C)ratio and glassy cytoplasm. C. Low grade corneal intraepithelial lesion; the dysplastic cells are varied in sizes with increased N/C ratio. They are similar to basal cells. Large polygonal squamous cells with small nuclei are also included. D. High grade corneal intraepithelial lesion; the nuclei are pleomorphic with coarse nuclear chromatins. E. High grade corneal intraepithelial lesion with inflammatory exudates on the background. The dysplastic cells cluster together with pleomorphic nuclei. F. Squamous cell carcinoma. The small and spindle cancer cells are aggregated together with the inflammatory background. Nuclear details are hardly noted as the cells overlap one another. (Papanicolaou stain. Original magnification X40)

4.4 Other investigation tools

Recently, in vivo confocal microscopy has proved useful as a noninvasive technique to investigate various ocular surface lesions including OSSN. Two studies found that confocal microscopic findings highly correlated with histologic features in CIN, thus provided real-time monitoring of the condition during treatment. (Alomar et al. 2011; Parrozzani et al. 2011)When compared to histology, however, there were some limitations. First, confocal microscopy provides en face images of cells compared to cross-sectional images from tissue histology. Second, fixation process required for histology results in shrinkage of tissue, therefore, morphometric comparison between living and fixed tissue have to be viewed in this context. Third, it is difficult to obtain in vivo confocal microscopic images and histologic images from exactly the same site of the tissue being examined.

The ultra high resolution (UHR) optical coherence tomography (OCT), a novel diagnostic technique for assessment of anterior eye segment lesions, was used for diagnosis and follow up after treatment of conjunctival-corneal intraepithelial neoplasia (CCIN) in a prospective case series. The UHR OCT images correlated well with the histologic specimens obtained from incisional biopsy before treatment. The UHR OCT was able to detect residual disease that was clinically invisible. The limitation of this machine was its capability to detect microinvasive lesions because the resolution of the current UHR OCT is approximately 2 micron, thus could not detect intracellular features. (Shousha et al. 2011)

Differential diagnosis

Because of the noninvasive nature of OSSN, the diagnosis is often missed or delayed. The patients' symptoms are sometimes treated as chronic conjunctivitis. Other conditions that are commonly mistaken include pterygium, pingecular, corneal pannus, viral keratoconjunctivitis, and corneal dystrophy.

5. Management

5.1 Conjunctival papilloma

Many conjunctival papilloma regress spontaneously. A pedunculated papilloma that is small, cosmetically acceptable and asymptomatic may be observed, although it may take months to years for spontaneous resolution. Larger and more peduculated lesions are generally symptomatic and of poor cosmetic acceptance, thus surgery adjunct with cryotherapy is recommended. A sessile papilloma must be observed closely. If there is any evidence of dysplastic change, excision with cryotherapy should be preformed.

Complete excision without manipulation of the tumor (no touch technique) is a crucial part of the surgical excision to minimize the risk of the virus spreading to uninvolved healthy conjunctiva. Double freeze-thaw cryotherapy is applied to the remaining conjunctiva to prevent tumor recurrence. An incomplete excision can stimulate growth and lead to a recurrence of the lesion and a worse cosmetic outcome. (Fig.14) Topical interferon- alpha 2b (Schechter et al. 2002; Kothari et al. 2009) and mitomycin C(Hawkins et al. 1999; Yuen et al. 2002) have been employed in the treatment of conjunctival papilloma. Immunomodulating agents such as oral cimetidine have led to regression of viral related papilloma. (Chang & Huang 2006)

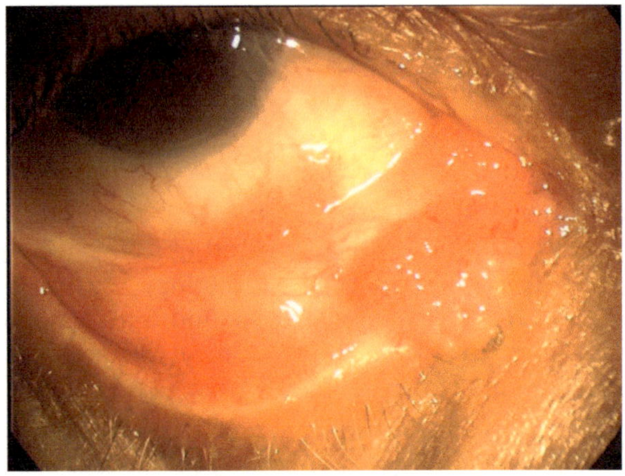

Fig. 14. Multifocal recurrence conjunctival papillomas involving lower palpebral conjunctiva, fornix, canruncle, and lower punctum after two previous excisions.

5.2 Preinvasive and invasive squamous neoplasia

5.2.1 Surgery

The management of OSSN varies with the extent of the lesion. The most accepted method of OSSN remains complete surgical excision. However, residual tumor cells left at the bordering tissue can induce tumor recurrence. Adjuvant therapies such as cryotherapy, alcohol abrasion, or topical agents are used in order to absolutely eradicate tumor cells from the ocular surface. Thus, the main treatment strategy is complete excision of the tumor with a wide surgical free margin followed by double freeze-thaw cryotherapy at the conjunctival margin and alcohol epitheliectomy for the corneal component. In case the tumor is adherent to the globe, a thin lamella of underlying sclera should be removed.

In order to decrease the chance of tumor recurrence, the standard surgical technique should be emphasized in all cases. The "no touch" technique purposed by Shield et al (Shields et al. 1997) is a widely accepted surgical approach as the conjunctival components, along with Tenon's fascia, should be excised with minimal manipulation of the tumor because cells from these friable tumors can seed into adjacent tissue. In addition, the surgery should be performed using microscopic techniques and the operative field should be left dry until after the tumor is completely removed to minimize spreading of tumor cells. Cryotherapy is thought to act through its direct destructive effects on cells, as well as the obliteration of microcirculation in the areas treated, resulting in ischemic infraction of the abnormal tissue. This is performed by freezing the surrounding bulbar conjunctiva as it is lifted away from the sclera using the cryoprobe. When the ice ball reaches the size of 4-5 mm, it is allowed to thaw and the cycle repeated. The complications that may occur from misuse of this technique or when the globe is accidentally frozen include cataract, uveitis, sclera and corneal thinning, and phthisis bulbi.

In cases of advanced tumors, the large conjunctival defect created by excision , particularly those over 4 clock hours, often require tissue replacement from a transpositional conjunctival flap, a free conjunctival autograft from the opposite eye, buccal mucosa graft, or amniotic membrane transplantation.

However, OSSN can be diffused or multifocal, with borders that are difficult to detect clinically, and there is also a chance for skipped areas from histopathologic examination. Reported recurrence rate after surgical treatment is significant (range between 15%-52%). (Lee & Hirst 1995; Tabin et al. 1997; Sudesh et al. 2000; McKelvie et al. 2002) Incomplete excision with positive surgical margins has been identified as a major risk factor for recurrence. (McKelvie et al. 2002) The more severe grades of OSSN appear to recur at higher rates. With adjunctive cryotherapy, the recurrent rate appears to be reduced (from 28.5% and 50% after simple excision, to 7.7% and 16.6% after excision with cryotherapy in primary and recurrence OSSN, respectively). (Sudesh et al. 2000)

The drawbacks of surgical treatment are complications resulted from the healing process, particularly in advanced lesions, including tissue granulation, symblepharon, pseudopterygium, diplopia from tissue shortening, blepharoptosis, limbal stem cell deficiency, and other complications. These surgical problems instigate further investigation into safer, alternative treatments.

5.2.2 Chemotherapy

Due to the relatively high rate of recurrence after surgical excision, various topical treatments have been advocated as a sole therapy for OSSN. Topical therapy offers a nonsurgical method for treating the entire ocular surface with less dependence on defining the tumor margin, potentially eliminating subclinical lesions. Topical treatment can offer a high drug concentration, avoiding systemic side effects. Furthermore, the increased cost, stress, pain, and trauma associated with surgical procedures are avoided. Topical medications have been used effectively for treating this condition comprised of mitomycin C (MMC), 5-fluorouracil (5-FU), and interferon, with MMC used most commonly by a group of external disease specialists. (Stone et al. 2005) These agents have been used as a sole therapy or a surgical adjuvant (preoperatively, intraoperatively, and postoperatively) for treatment of OSSN.

Mitomycin C

Mitomycin C (MMC) is an ankylating antibiotic that binds to DNA during all phases of the cell cycle leading to irreversible cross-linking and inhibition of nucleotide synthesis. When applied to conjunctival surfaces as a surgical adjunct, MMC has been shown to inhibit fibroblast cell migration, decrease extracellular matrix production, and to induce apoptosis in Tenon's capsule fibroblast. It is well known that chronic tissue effects from topical MMC administration can persist for many years after cessation of the treatment, thereby mimicking the effect of ionizing radiation. (McKelvie & Daniell 2001)

MMC has been widely used in glaucoma and pterygium surgery for its anti-fibrotic effect on subconjunctival fibroblast. The use of MMC for treatment of OSSN was first described in 1994.(Frucht-Pery & Rozenman 1994) Since then several case series using different concentrations and durations have been published. Common protocol ranges from topical MMC 0.02%-0.04% given four times a day to the affected eye for 7 to 28 days.(Fig.15) One case series demonstrated that even a smaller concentration of 0.002% of MMC was effective in treatment of primary and recurrent OSSN. (Prabhasawat et al. 2005) Several studies (similar to those used in fractionation of radiation in treatment of systemic cancers) preferred a cycle of 7 days in alternate weeks (1 week on and 1 week off) to allow cells of the ocular surface to recover/repair. (McKelvie & Daniell 2001; Shields & Shields 2004) One randomized control trial found that MMC 0.04% eye drops used 4 times a day for 3 weeks was effective and caused early resolution of noninvasive OSSN. A relative resolution rate in MMC versus placebo was 40.87 and the mean time for tumor resolution in this study was 121 days, and there was no serious complication in midterm follow-up. (Hirst 2007) MMC has also been used as a surgical adjunct for OSSN: preoperative, to decrease the size of the extensive lesions before surgical excision (chemoreduction), intraoperative, and postoperative to decrease recurrences.(Kemp et al. 2002; Chen et al. 2004; Gupta & Muecke 2010)

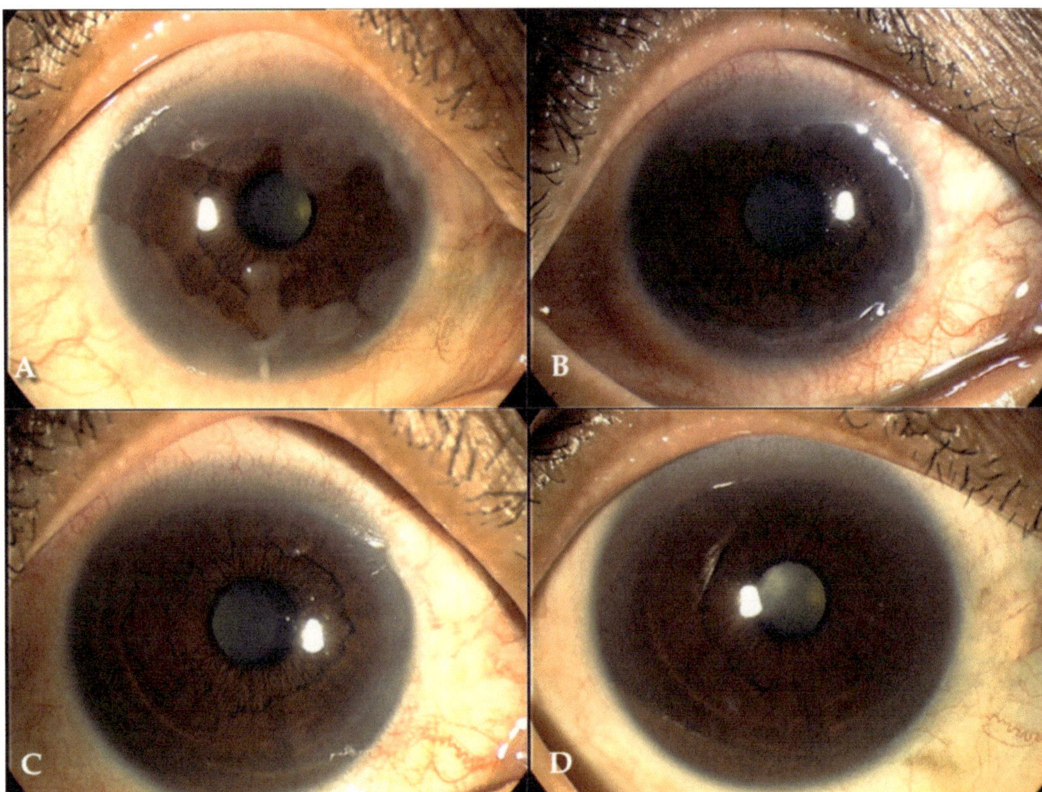

Fig. 15. Severe corneal intraepithelial neoplasia treated with mitomycin C 0.02% four times daily, alternating weeks: A. Appearance before treatment; B. Lesion partially resolved two months after treatment ; C. Completely resolved mass three months after treatment; D. Cornea is clear without recurrence eight years later.

Reported complications of MMC in treatment of OSSN included conjunctival hyperemia, punctuated epithelial erosion, and keratoconjunctivitis. A large retrospective series (n= 100 eyes) of ocular surface tumors treated with topical MMC 0.04% revealed that allergic reaction and punctual stenosis were two common complications. (Khong & Muecke 2006) Some of these side effects can be managed by stopping the medication and adding topical steroid three to four times daily. No significant changes were found on corneal endothelial cells after treatment with topical MMC 0.04% in a cyclic manner. (Panda et al. 2008)

However, MMC was found to have deleterious effects on endothelium cells after pterygium surgery, thus its judicious use and long term follow-up are mandatory.(Bahar et al. 2009) Even though common side effects related to topical MMC are self-limited, limbal stem cell deficiency appeared to be a significant long-term complication. (Dudney & Malecha 2004; Russell et al. 2011) Mckelvie and coworker reported the effects of MMC in treatments of OSSN on impression cytology; MMC appeared to produce cell death by apoptosis and necrosis. Cellular changes related to MMC mimic those caused by radiation-cytolmegaly, nucleomegaly, and vacuolation. These changes may persist at least 8 months after cessation of MMC therapy. (McKelvie & Daniell 2001) MMC-induced long term cytologic changes on the ocular surface have been demonstrated in another study. (Dogru et al. 2003) Serious complications of MMC such as scleromalacia, corneal perforation, cataract, glaucoma, and anterior uveitis have been reported in pterygium treatment and should be of concern if this agent is used in an open conjunctival wound or used excessively.(Rubinfeld et al. 1992)(Fig.16)

When MMC is prescribed as a treatment for OSSN, certain precaution should be taken. Patients and their families are advised to carefully handle the medication. Pregnant women and young children should avoid direct contact with the medication. Patients should be instructed to close their eyes for at least 5 minutes after instillation of MMC or punctal plugs are placed in both superior and inferior puncta to avoid nasolacrimal and systemic absorption of the drug. Since MMC is a chemotherapeutic agent, all residual bottles should be returned to the pharmacy for proper disposal.

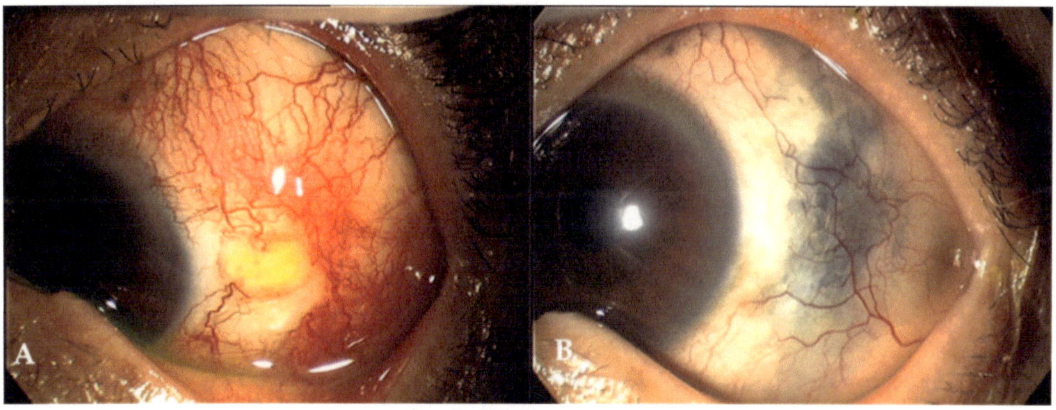

Fig. 16. A. Scleritis in eye with conjunctival intraepithelial neoplasia after excisional biopsy and postoperative mitomycin C. B. Scleral thinning in the same eye one year later after scleritis resolved.

5-Fluorouracil

Similar to MMC, topical 5-fluorouracil (5-FU) has been used to inhibit subconjunctival fibroblasts in glaucoma surgery. 5-FU is an antimetabolite used to treat many epithelial cancers because of its rapid action on rapidly proliferating cells. It acts by the inhibition of thymidylate synthetase during the S phase of the cell cycle, preventing DNA and RNA synthesis in rapidly dividing cells because of a lack of thymidine. Pulse 1% topical 5-FU in cycle of 4 days "on" followed by 30 days "off" until resolution of the lesion was a well-tolerated and effective method in treatment of OSSN, alone or as an adjunct to excision or debulking therapy. (Yeatts et al. 2000; Al-Barrag et al.; Parrozzani et al.; Rudkin & Muecke) Local side effects associated with topical 5-FU, such as lid toxicity, superficial keratitis, epiphora, and corneal epithelial defect have been reported. (Rudkin & Muecke 2011) By using confocal microscopy, there was no long-term corneal toxicity associated with 1% topical 5-FU compared to the controlled eye. (Parrozzani et al. 2011)The advantages of this agent are its few side effects, plus the medication is inexpensive, easy to handle by both medical personnel, as well as the patients.

Interferon

Interferons (IFN) are a group of proteins that bind to surface receptors of target cells, triggering a cascade of intracellular antiviral and antitumor activities. Systemic interefon-alpha has been used in treatment of hairy cell leukemia, condyloma acuminate, Karposi's sarcoma in AIDS, and hepatitis (both B and C). Recombinant topical IFNα-2b (1 million IU/ml) 4 times a day has been used effectively in treatment of primary OSSN. (Sturges et al. 2008) The antiviral effects of IFNα-2b may explain why it may be less effective as a primary treatment for lesions not linked to HPV infections. Topical IFNα-2b has been used effectively in management of recurrent or recalcitrant lesions where surgical excision or MMC have failed. (Holcombe & Lee 2006) This agent is well tolerated and does not markedly damage the limbal stem cells. Subconjunctival/perilesional IFN-α-2b (1-3 million IU/ml) has also been used effectively for treatment of both primary and recurrent OSSN. (Nemet et al. 2006; Karp et al. 2010) Topical instillation of IFN appears to be associated with few side effects, such as follicular conjunctivitis and conjunctival injections, which appeared to completely resolve after cessation of the medication. (Schechter et al. 2008) There was a report of corneal epithelial microcyst after topical administration interferon identical to that which had been reported with systemic interferon therapy. (Aldave & Nguyen 2007) Subconjunctival IFNα-2b has been associated with transient fever and myalgias , similar to systemic applications.

Topical chemotherapeutic agents have demonstrated acceptable efficacy in treatment of OSSN. Comparison of these three drugs for treatment of noninvasive OSSN reveals that MMC is the most effective (88%), followed by 5-FU(87%), and IFNα-2b (80%). MMC has the highest rate of side effects, perhaps because MMC is the most frequently used topical agent. IFNα-2b is the least toxic, however, it is the costliest of the three agents. (Sepulveda et al. 2010) The relative indications of using topical treatments in OSSN are: 1) >2 quadrants conjunctival involvement, 2) > 180 degree limbal involvement, 3) extension into the clear cornea involving the papillary axis, 4) positive margin after excision, and 5) patient unable to undergo surgery. (Sepulveda et al. 2010) However, some clinicians prefer surgical excision as an initial treatment of invasive lesions if the extension is less than 6 clock hours of involvement, because this provides confirmation of the diagnosis with little cosmetic disfigurement if properly performed.(Shields et al. 2002) When topical agents are considered as a treatment regimen of OSSN, they should be used with caution as long-term effects on the ocular surface of the eye, as well as the adjacent eyelids and nasolacrimal drainage system, have not yet been completely defined.

Other treatment modalities in management of OSSN include plaque brachytherapy with Iodine-125 (Walsh-Conway & Conway 2009), beta-radiation therapy, gamma radiation, and immunotherapy with dinitrochlorobenzene (DNCB). (Lee & Hirst 1995) Aggressive treatments such as enucleation or exenteration are considered in cases with ocular or orbital invasion. (Shields & Shields 2004)

6. Clinical course

OSSN is a slow growing tumor; however in neglected cases it can invade the globe and orbit and may lead to death. It has a potential for recurrence after treatment. In a series of OSSN, both intraepithelial and invasive lesions, it was found that sclera involvement occurred in 37%, orbital invasion 11%, and no metastasis or death was related to the tumors. (Tunc et al. 1999) In a series of 26 conjunctival SCC, intraocular invasion occurred in 11% of the patients, corneal or sclera involvement 30%, and orbital invasion 15%. Exenteration was required in 23% of cases, and 8% died of metastatic diseases. (McKelvie et al. 2002) Predicting factors related to significantly increased tumor recurrence include old age, large diameter lesions, high proliferation index (Ki-67 score), and positive surgical margin. (McKelvie et al. 2002)

A long-term study of CCIN also found that the recurrence rate after surgery was higher in cases with positive surgical margins than those with free margins (56% versus 33%). Timing for recurrence ranged from 33 days to 11.5 years after primary treatment, and those with incomplete excision recurred earlier than those with free margins. (Tabin et al. 1997) The slow growth of recurrent tumors and evidence of late recurrence 10 years after surgery warranted the need to have annual patient follow-ups for the remainder of their lives.

OSSN in immunosuppressed individuals seem to have an aggressive course in contrast to a relatively benign clinical course in classic OSSN.(Masanganise & Magava 2001; Gichuhi & Irlam 2007) The tumors often grow rapidly and have a tendency to invade the globe or orbit. This problem is exacerbated by poor health care facilities, and patient compliance, which are often present in HIV endemic areas. Management with standard approaches with these patients is often associated with higher rates of recurrence and intraocular or orbital invasion. Thus, treatment regimens may need a wide excision with a histological analysis of the margin, as well as other adjuncts such as cryotherapy, topical chemotherapeutic agents to prevent local recurrence, intraocular or orbital invasion, and metastasis. In addition, it is crucial for every HIV patient to have a detailed eye examination at presentation and maintain a close follow-up to detect recurrent disease early in its course.

7. Conclusion

OSSN is a spectrum of diseases ranging from simple dysplasia to invasive carcinoma. This lesion is considered a low grade malignancy, but its invasive counterpart can spread to the globe or orbit. It is the most common ocular surface tumor and its incidence varies in different geographic locations. The main risk factor is UV-B exposure as its incidence increases in areas close to the equator. Other important risk factors are the human papilloma virus and human immunodeficiency virus. However, it is unclear whether host factors (e.g. genetic factors and HIV-related immune impairment) or characteristics of the ocular surface epithelia may also be part of the etiopathogenesis of OSSN. Symptoms range from none at all to severe pain or visual loss. Clinically, these tumors most commonly arise in the interpalpebral area, particularly at the limbal region. Early diagnosis and management decrease the risk of locally aggressive and can improve the patients' prognosis for local control and preservation of vision. In clinical practice, OSSN is generally evaluated by tissue histology. The developments of pre-operative diagnostic techniques such as impression cytology are of value in diagnosis and follow-up after treatment. Surgical excision adjunct with cryotherapy combined with alcohol abrasion in cases of corneal involvement are the main treatment strategy. Recurrence rates are higher for more severe grades of OSSN and have been related to the adequate of surgical margins at the initial excision. The standard management care of OSSN appears to shift toward topical chemotherapy such as MMC, 5 FU, and interferon as a sole therapy, or a surgical adjunct, particularly in diffused or un-operable cases. These alternative treatments continue to evolve despite a paucity of long term results in published literature. Invasive disease may cause intraocular or orbital involvement with eye loss, and occasionally may lead to death. Recurrence after initial treatment is variable and warrants life-long follow-up in all case of OSSN.

8. References

Al-Barrag, A.; Al-Shaer,M.; Al-Matary,N. & Al-Hamdani, M. (2010). 5-Fluorouracil for the treatment of intraepithelial neoplasia and squamous cell carcinoma of the conjunctiva, and cornea. *Clin Ophthalmol*, vol. 4, (July,2010), pp 801-8, ISSN 1177-5483 (Electronic)

Aldave, AJ. & Nguyen, A. (2007). Ocular surface toxicity associated with topical interferon alpha-2b. *Br J Ophthalmol*, vol. 91, No.8, (Aug,2007), pp 1087-8, ISSN 0007-1161

Alomar, TS.; Nubile, M. ; Lowe, J. & Dua, HS. (2011). Corneal intraepithelial neoplasia: in vivo confocal microscopic study with histopathologic correlation. *Am J Ophthalmol*, vol. 151, No.2, (Feb,2011), pp 238-47, ISSN 1879-1891 (Electronic)

Aoki, S.; Kubo, E.; Nakamura, S.; Tsuzuki, A.; Tsuzuki, S.; Takahashi, Y. & Akagi, Y. (1998). Possible prognostic markers in conjunctival dysplasia and squamous cell carcinoma. *Jpn J Ophthalmol*, vol. 42, No.4, (Jul-Aug,1998), pp 256-61, ISSN 0021-5155

Ateenyi-Agaba, C.; Dai, M.; Le Calvez, F.; Katongole-Mbidde, E.; Smet, A.; Tommasino, M.; Franceschi, S.; Hainaut, P. & Weiderpass, E. (2004). TP53 mutations in squamous-cell carcinomas of the conjunctiva: evidence for UV-induced mutagenesis. *Mutagenesis*, vol. 19, No.5, (Sep,2004), pp 399-401, ISSN 0267-8357

Bahar, I.; Kaiserman, I.; Lange, AP.; Slomovic, A.; Levinger, E.; Sansanayudh, W. & Slomovic, AR. (2009). The effect of mitomycin C on corneal endothelium in pterygium surgery. *Am J Ophthalmol*, vol. 147, No.3, (Mar,2009), pp 447-452 e1, ISSN 1879-1891 (Electronic)

Barros, JN.; Lowen, MS.; Ballalai,PL.; Mascaro, VL.; Gomes, JA. & Martins, MC. (2009). Predictive index to differentiate invasive squamous cell carcinoma from preinvasive ocular surface lesions by impression cytology. *Br J Ophthalmol*, vol. 93, No.2, (Feb,2009), pp 209-14, ISSN 1468-2079 (Electronic)

Calonge, M.; Diebold, Y.; Saez, V.; Enriquez de Salamanca, A.; Garcia-Vazquez, C.; Corrales, RM. & Herreras, JM. (2004). Impression cytology of the ocular surface: a review. *Exp Eye Res*, vol. 78, No.3, (Mar,2004), pp 457-72, ISSN 0014-4835

Cha, SB.; Shields, CL.; Shields, JA.; Eagel, Jr., RC.; De Potter, P. & Talansky, M. (1993). Massive precorneal extension of squamous cell carcinoma of the conjunctiva. *Cornea*, vol. 12, No.6, (Nov,1993), pp 537-40, ISSN 0277-3740

Chang, SW. & Huang, ZL. (2006). Oral cimetidine adjuvant therapy for recalcitrant, diffuse conjunctival papillomatosis. *Cornea,* vol. 25, No.6, (Jul,2006), pp 687-90, ISSN 0277-3740

Chen, C.; Louis, D.; Dodd, T. & Muecke, J. (2004). Mitomycin C as an adjunct in the treatment of localised ocular surface squamous neoplasia. *Br J Ophthalmol,* vol. 88, No.1, (Jan, 2004), pp 17-8, ISSN 0007-1161

Chidzonga, MM.; Mahomva,L.; Makunike-Mutasa, R. & Masanganise, R. (2009). Xeroderma pigmentosum: a retrospective case series in Zimbabwe. *J Oral Maxillofac Surg,* vol. 67, No.1, (Jan, 2009), pp 22-31, ISSN 1531-5053 (Electronic)

Dogru, M.; Erturk, H.; Shimazaki,J.; Tsubota, K. & Gul, M. (2003). Tear function and ocular surface changes with topical mitomycin (MMC) treatment for primary corneal intraepithelial neoplasia. *Cornea,* vol. 22, No.7, (Oct,2003), pp 627-39, ISSN 0277-3740

Dudney, BW. & Malecha, MA. (2004). Limbal stem cell deficiency following topical mitomycin C treatment of conjunctival-corneal intraepithelial neoplasia. *Am J Ophthalmol,* vol. 137, No.5, (May,2004), pp 950-1, ISSN 0002-9394

Eng, HL.; Lin, TM.; Chen, SY.; Wu, SM. & Chen, WJ. (2002). Failure to detect human papillomavirus DNA in malignant epithelial neoplasms of conjunctiva by polymerase chain reaction. *Am J Clin Pathol,* vol. 117, No.3, (Mar,2002), pp 429-36, ISSN 0002-9173

English, DR.; Armstrong, BK.; Kricker, A. & Fleming, C. (1997). Sunlight and cancer. *Cancer Causes Control,* vol. 8, No.3, (May,1997), pp 271-83, ISSN 0957-5243

Font, RL.; Croxatto, JO. & Rao, NA. (2006). Tumors of the conjunctiva and caruncle. In: *Tumors of the eye and ocular adnexa.* SG Silverberg, pp. 7-10, American Registry of Pathology,ISBN 1-881041-99-9, Washington DC

Frucht-Pery, J. & Rozenman, Y. (1994). Mitomycin C therapy for corneal intraepithelial neoplasia. *Am J Ophthalmol,* vol. 117, No.2, (Feb,1994), pp 164-8, ISSN 0002-9394

Gichuhi, S. & Irlam, JJ. (2007). Interventions for squamous cell carcinoma of the conjunctiva in HIV-infected individuals. *Cochrane Database Syst Rev,* vol.18, No.2,(April,2007), pp CD005643, ISSN 1469-493X (Electronic)

Guech-Ongey, M.; Engels, EA.; Goedert,JJ.; Biggar, RJ. & Mbulaiteye, SM. (2008). Elevated risk for squamous cell carcinoma of the conjunctiva among adults with AIDS in the United States. *Int J Cancer,* vol. 122, No.11, (Jun ,2008), pp 2590-3, ISSN 1097-0215 (Electronic)

Guex-Crosier, Y. & Herbort, CP. (1993). Presumed corneal intraepithelial neoplasia associated with contact lens wear and intense ultraviolet light exposure. *Br J Ophthalmol,* vol. 77, No.3, (Mar,1993), pp 191-2, ISSN 0007-1161

Gupta, A. & Muecke, J. (2010). Treatment of ocular surface squamous neoplasia with Mitomycin C. *Br J Ophthalmol,* vol. 94, No.5, (May,2010), pp 555-8, ISSN 1468-2079 (Electronic)

Guthoff, R.; Marx, A. & Stroebel, P. (2009). No evidence for a pathogenic role of human papillomavirus infection in ocular surface squamous neoplasia in Germany. *Curr Eye Res,* vol. 34, No.8, (Aug,2009), pp 666-71, ISSN 1460-2202 (Electronic)

Hawkins, AS.; Yu, J.; Hamming, NA. & Rubenstein, JB. (1999). Treatment of recurrent conjunctival papillomatosis with mitomycin C. *Am J Ophthalmol,* vol. 128, No.5, (Nov,1999), pp 638-40, ISSN 0002-9394

Hirst, LW. (2007). Randomized controlled trial of topical mitomycin C for ocular surface squamous neoplasia: early resolution. *Ophthalmology*, vol. 114, No.5, (May,2007), pp 976-82, ISSN 1549-4713 (Electronic)

Hirst, LW.; Axelsen, RA. & Schwab, I. (2009). Pterygium and associated ocular surface squamous neoplasia. *Arch Ophthalmol*, vol. 127, No.1, (Jan,2009), pp 31-2, ISSN 1538-3601 (Electronic)

Holcombe, DJ. & Lee, GA. (2006). Topical interferon alfa-2b for the treatment of recalcitrant ocular surface squamous neoplasia. *Am J Ophthalmol*, vol. 142, No.4, (Oct,2006), pp 568-71, ISSN 0002-9394

Jain, RK.; Mehta, R. & Badve, S. (2010). Conjunctival squamous cell carcinoma due to ocular prostheses: a case report and review of literature. *Pathol Oncol Res*, vol. 16, No.4, (Dec,2010), pp 609-12, ISSN 1532-2807 (Electronic)

Jeng, BH.; Holland, GN.; Lowder, CY.; Deegan, 3rd, WF.; Raizman, MB. & Meisler, DM. (2007). Anterior segment and external ocular disorders associated with human immunodeficiency virus disease. *Surv Ophthalmol*, vol. 52, No.4, (Jul-Aug,2007), pp 329-68, ISSN 0039-6257

Karp, CL.; Galor, A.; Chhabra, S.; Barnes, SD. & Alfonso, EC. (2010). Subconjunctival/perilesional recombinant interferon alpha2b for ocular surface squamous neoplasia: a 10-year review. *Ophthalmology*, vol. 117, No.12, (Dec,2010), pp 2241-6, ISSN 1549-4713 (Electronic)

Karp, CL.; Scott, IU.; Chang, TS. & Pflugfelder, SC. (1996). Conjunctival intraepithelial neoplasia. A possible marker for human immunodeficiency virus infection? *Arch Ophthalmol*, vol. 114, No.3, (Mar,1996), pp 257-61, ISSN 0003-9950

Kemp, EG.; Harnett, AN. & Chatterjee, S. (2002). Preoperative topical and intraoperative local mitomycin C adjuvant therapy in the management of ocular surface neoplasias. *Br J Ophthalmol*, vol. 86, No.1, (Jan,2002), pp 31-4, ISSN 0007-1161

Khong, JJ. & Muecke, J. (2006). Complications of mitomycin C therapy in 100 eyes with ocular surface neoplasia. *Br J Ophthalmol*, vol. 90, No.7, (Jul,2006), pp 819-22, ISSN 0007-1161

Kothari, M.; Mody, K. & Chatterjee, D. (2009). Resolution of recurrent conjunctival papilloma after topical and intralesional interferon alpha2b with partial excision in a child. *J AAPOS*, vol. 13, No.5, (Oct,2009), pp 523-5, ISSN 1528-3933 (Electronic)

Kraemer, KH.; Lee, MM. & Scotto, J. (1987). Xeroderma pigmentosum. Cutaneous, ocular, and neurologic abnormalities in 830 published cases. *Arch Dermatol*, vol. 123, No.2, (Feb,1987), pp 241-50, ISSN 0003-987X

Kuo, KT.; Chang, HC.; Hsiao, CH. & Lin, MC. (2006). Increased Ki-67 proliferative index and absence of P16INK4 in CIN-HPV related pathogenic pathways different from cervical squamous intraepithelial lesion. *Br J Ophthalmol*, vol. 90, No.7, (Jul,2006), pp 894-9, ISSN 0007-1161

Lee, GA. & Hirst, LW. (1995). Ocular surface squamous neoplasia. *Surv Ophthalmol*, vol. 39, No.6, (May-Jun,1995), pp 429-50, ISSN 0039-6257

Lee, GA.; Williams, G.; Hirst, LW. & Green, AC. (1994). Risk factors in the development of ocular surface epithelial dysplasia. *Ophthalmology*, vol. 101, No.2, (Feb,1994), pp 360-4, ISSN 0161-6420

Manderwad, GP.; Kannabiran, C.; Honavar, SG. & Vemuganti, GK. (2009). Lack of association of high-risk human papillomavirus in ocular surface squamous neoplasia in India. *Arch Pathol Lab Med*, vol. 133, No.8, (Aug,2009), pp 1246-50, ISSN 1543-2165 (Electronic)

Masanganise, R. & Magava, A. (2001). Orbital exenterations and squamous cell carcinoma of the conjunctiva at Sekuru Kaguvi Eye Unit, Zimbabwe. *Cent Afr J Med*, vol. 47, No.8, (Aug,2001), pp 196-9, ISSN 0008-9176

McKelvie, PA. & Daniell, M. (2001). Impression cytology following mitomycin C therapy for ocular surface squamous neoplasia. *Br J Ophthalmol*, vol. 85, No.9, (Sep,2001), pp 1115-9, ISSN 0007-1161

McKelvie, PA.; Daniell, M.; McNab, A.; Loughnan, M. & Santamaria, JD. (2002). Squamous cell carcinoma of the conjunctiva: a series of 26 cases. *Br J Ophthalmol*, vol. 86, No.2, (Feb,2002), pp 168-73, ISSN 0007-1161

Nakamura, Y.; Mashima, Y.; Kameyama, K.; Mukai, M. & Oguchi, Y. (1997). Detection of human papillomavirus infection in squamous tumours of the conjunctiva and lacrimal sac by immunohistochemistry, in situ hybridisation, and polymerase chain reaction. *Br J Ophthalmol*, vol. 81, No.4, (Apr,1997), pp 308-13, ISSN 0007-1161

Napora, C.; Cohen, EJ.; Genvert, GI.; Presson, AC.; Arentsen, JJ.; Eagle, RC. & Laibson, PR. (1990). Factors associated with conjunctival intraepithelial neoplasia: a case control study. *Ophthalmic Surg*, vol. 21, No.1, (Jan,1990), pp 27-30, ISSN 0022-023X

Nemet, AY.; Sharma, V. & Benger, R. (2006). Interferon alpha 2b treatment for residual ocular surface squamous neoplasia unresponsive to excision, cryotherapy and mitomycin-C. *Clin Experiment Ophthalmol*, vol. 34, No.4, (May-Jun,2006), pp 375-7, ISSN 1442-6404

Newton, R.; Ferlay, J.; Reeves, G.; Beral , V.& Parkin, DM. (1996). Effect of ambient solar ultraviolet radiation on incidence of squamous-cell carcinoma of the eye. *Lancet*, vol. 347, No.9013, (May ,1996), pp 1450-1, ISSN 0140-6736

Newton, R.; Ziegler, J.; Ateenyi-Agaba, C.; Bousarghin, L.; Casabonne, D.; Beral, V.; Mbidde, E.; Carpenter,L.; Reeves,G.; Parkin, DM.; Wabinga, H.; Mbulaiteye,S.; Jaffe,H.; Bourboulia,D.; Boshoff,C.; Touze, A. & Coursaget, P. (2002). The epidemiology of conjunctival squamous cell carcinoma in Uganda. *Br J Cancer*, vol. 87, No.3, (Jul ,2002), pp 301-8, ISSN 0007-0920

Ng, J.; Coroneo, MT.; Wakefield, D. & Di Girolamo, N. (2008). Ultraviolet radiation and the role of matrix metalloproteinases in the pathogenesis of ocular surface squamous neoplasia. *Invest Ophthalmol Vis Sci*, vol. 49, No.12, (Dec,2008), pp 5295-306, ISSN 1552-5783 (Electronic)

Nolan, GR.; Hirst, LW.; Wright, RG. & Bancroft, BJ. (1994). Application of impression cytology to the diagnosis of conjunctival neoplasms. *Diagn Cytopathol*, vol. 11, (1994), pp 246-249, ISSN 8755-1039

Ohara, M.; Sotozono, C.; Tsuchihashi, Y. & Kinoshita, S. (2004). Ki-67 labeling index as a marker of malignancy in ocular surface neoplasms. *Jpn J Ophthalmol*, vol. 48, No.6, (Nov-Dec,2004), pp 524-9, ISSN 0021-5155

Panda, A.; Pe'er, J.; Aggarwal, A.; Das, H.; Kumar, A. & Mohan, S. (2008). Effect of topical mitomycin C on corneal endothelium. *Am J Ophthalmol*, vol. 145, No.4, (Apr,2008), pp 635-638, ISSN 0002-9394

Parrozzani, R.; Lazzarini, D.; Alemany-Rubio, E.; Urban, F. & Midena, E. (2011). Topical 1% 5-fluorouracil in ocular surface squamous neoplasia: a long-term safety study. *Br J Ophthalmol*, vol. 95, No.3, (Mar,2011), pp 355-9, ISSN 1468-2079 (Electronic)

Parrozzani, R.; Lazzarini, D.; Dario, A. & Midena, E. (2011). In vivo confocal microscopy of ocular surface squamous neoplasia. *Eye (Lond)*, vol. 25, No.4, (Apr,2011), pp 455-60, ISSN 1476-5454 (Electronic)

Pizzarello, L. & Jakobiec, FA. (1978). Bowen's disease of the conjunctiva: a misnomer. In: *Ocular and adnexal tumors.* FA Jakobiec, pp. 553-71, Aesculapius Pub,ISBN 9780912684154, Birmingham

Porges, Y. & Groisman, GM. (2003). Prevalence of HIV with conjunctival squamous cell neoplasia in an African provincial hospital. *Cornea*, vol. 22, No.1, (Jan,2003), pp 1-4, ISSN 0277-3740

Prabhasawat, P.; Tarinvorakup, P.; Tesavibul,N.; Uiprasertkul, M.; Kosrirukvongs, P.; Booranapong, W. & Srivannaboon, S. (2005). Topical 0.002% mitomycin C for the treatment of conjunctival-corneal intraepithelial neoplasia and squamous cell carcinoma. *Cornea*, vol. 24, No.4, (May,2005), pp 443-8, ISSN 0277-3740

Ramasubramanian, A.; Shields, CL.; Sinha, N. & Shields, JA. (2010). Ocular surface squamous neoplasia after corneal graft. *Am J Ophthalmol*, vol. 149, No.1, (Jan,2010), pp 62-5, ISSN 1879-1891 (Electronic)

Rubinfeld, RS.; Pfister,RR.; Stein,RM.; Foster,CS.; Martin, NF.; Stoleru, S.; Talley, AR. & Speaker, MG. (1992). Serious complications of topical mitomycin-C after pterygium surgery. *Ophthalmology*, vol. 99, No.11, (Nov,1992), pp 1647-54, ISSN 0161-6420

Rudkin, AK. & Muecke, JS. (2011). Adjuvant 5-fluorouracil in the treatment of localised ocular surface squamous neoplasia. *Br J Ophthalmol*, vol. 95, No.7, (Jul,2011), pp 947-50, ISSN 1468-2079 (Electronic)

Russell, HC.; Chadha,V.; Lockington, D. & Kemp, EG. (2011). Topical mitomycin C chemotherapy in the management of ocular surface neoplasia: a 10-year review of treatment outcomes and complications. *Br J Ophthalmol*, vol. 94, No.10, (Oct,2011), pp 1316-21, ISSN 1468-2079 (Electronic)

Schechter, BA.; Koreishi, AF.; Karp, CL. & Feuer, W. (2008). Long-term follow-up of conjunctival and corneal intraepithelial neoplasia treated with topical interferon alfa-2b. *Ophthalmology*, vol. 115, No.8, (Aug,2008), pp 1291-6, 1296 e1, ISSN 1549-4713 (Electronic)

Schechter, BA.; Rand, WJ.; Velazquez, GE.; Williams , WD.& Starasoler, L. (2002). Treatment of conjunctival papillomata with topical interferon Alfa-2b. *Am J Ophthalmol*, vol. 134, No.2, (Aug,2002), pp 268-70, ISSN 0002-9394

Scott, IU.; Karp, CL. & Nuovo, GJ. (2002). Human papillomavirus 16 and 18 expression in conjunctival intraepithelial neoplasia. *Ophthalmology*, vol. 109, No.3, (Mar,2002), pp 542-7, ISSN 0161-6420

Sen, S.; Sharma, A. & Panda, A. (2007). Immunohistochemical localization of human papilloma virus in conjunctival neoplasias: a retrospective study. *Indian J Ophthalmol*, vol. 55, No.5 (Sep-Oct,2007), pp 361-3, ISSN 0301-4738

Sepulveda, R.; Pe'er, J.; Midena, E.; Seregard, S.; Dua, HS. & Singh, AD. (2010). Topical chemotherapy for ocular surface squamous neoplasia: current status. *Br J Ophthalmol*, vol. 94, No.5, (May,2010), pp 532-5, ISSN 1468-2079 (Electronic)

Shelil, AE.; Shields,CL.; Shields , JA.& Eagle, Jr., RC. (2003). Aggressive conjunctival squamous cell carcinoma in a patient following liver transplantation. *Arch Ophthalmol*, vol. 121, No.2, (Feb,2003), pp 280-2, ISSN 0003-9950

Shields, CL.; Demirci, H.; Karatza, E. & Shields, JA. (2004). Clinical survey of 1643 melanocytic and nonmelanocytic conjunctival tumors. *Ophthalmology*, vol. 111, No.9, (Sep,2004), pp 1747-54, ISSN 1549-4713 (Electronic)

Shields, CL.; Manchandia, A.; Subbiah, R.; Eagle, Jr., RC. & Shields, JA. (2008). Pigmented squamous cell carcinoma in situ of the conjunctiva in 5 cases. *Ophthalmology*, vol. 115, No.10, (Oct,2008), pp 1673-8, ISSN 1549-4713 (Electronic)

Shields, CL.; Naseripour, M. & Shields, JA. (2002). Topical mitomycin C for extensive, recurrent conjunctival-corneal squamous cell carcinoma. *Am J Ophthalmol*, vol. 133, No.5, (May,2002), pp 601-6, ISSN 0002-9394

Shields, CL. & Shields, JA. (2004). Tumors of the conjunctiva and cornea. *Surv Ophthalmol*, vol. 49, No.1, (Jan-Feb,2004), pp 3-24, ISSN 0039-6257

Shields, JA.; Shields , CL.& De Potter, P. (1997). Surgical management of conjunctival tumors. The 1994 Lynn B. McMahan Lecture. *Arch Ophthalmol*, vol. 115, No.6, (Jun,1997), pp 808-15, ISSN 0003-9950

Shields, JA.; Eagle, RC.; Marr, BP.; Shields, CL.; Grossniklaus, HE. & Stulting, RD. (2007). Invasive spindle cell carcinoma of the conjunctiva managed by full-thickness eye wall resection. *Cornea*, vol. 26, No.8, (Sep,2007), pp 1014-6, ISSN 0277-3740

Shome, D.; Honavar, SG.; Manderwad, GP. & Vemuganti, GK. (2006). Ocular surface squamous neoplasia in a renal transplant recipient on immunosuppressive therapy. *Eye (Lond)*, vol. 20, No.12,(Dec,2006), pp 1413-4, ISSN 0950-222X

Shousha, MA.; Karp,CL.; Perez, VL.; Hoffmann, R.; Ventura,R.; Chang, V.; Dubovy, SR. & Wang, J. (2011). Diagnosis and Management of Conjunctival and Corneal Intraepithelial Neoplasia Using Ultra High-Resolution Optical Coherence Tomography. *Ophthalmology*, vol.118, No. 8 (August,2011), pp 1531-7, ISSN 1549-4713 (Electronic)

Simbiri, KO.; Murakami, M.; Feldman, M.; Steenhoff, AP.; Nkomazana, O.; Bisson, G. & Robertson, ES. (2010). Multiple oncogenic viruses identified in Ocular surface squamous neoplasia in HIV-1 patients. *Infect Agent Cancer*, vol. 5, (Mar,2010), pp 6, ISSN 1750-9378 (Electronic)

Sjo, NC.; von Buchwald, C.; Cassonnet, P.; Norrild,B.; Prause, JU.; Vinding, T. & Heegaard, S. (2007). Human papillomavirus in normal conjunctival tissue and in conjunctival papilloma: types and frequencies in a large series. *Br J Ophthalmol*, vol. 91, No.8, (Aug,2007), pp 1014-5, ISSN 0007-1161

Solomon, D.; Davey, D.; Kurman, R.; Moriarty,A.; O'Connor, D.; Prey,M.; Raab, S.; Sherman, M.; Wilbur, D.; Wright, Jr.,T. & Young, N. (2002). The 2001 Bethesda System: terminology for reporting results of cervical cytology. *JAMA*, vol. 287, No.16, (Apr ,2002), pp 2114-9, ISSN 0098-7484

Spitzer, MS.; Batumba, NH.; Chirambo, T.; Bartz-Schmidt, KU.; Kayange, P.; Kalua, K. & Szurman, P. (2008). Ocular surface squamous neoplasia as the first apparent manifestation of HIV infection in Malawi. *Clin Experiment Ophthalmol*, vol. 36, No.5, (Jul,2008), pp 422-5, ISSN 1442-9071 (Electronic)

Stone, DU.; Butt, AL. & Chodosh, J. (2005). Ocular surface squamous neoplasia: a standard of care survey. *Cornea*, vol. 24, No.3, (Apr,2005), pp 297-300, ISSN 0277-3740

Sturges, A.; Butt, AL.; Lai, JE. & Chodosh, J. (2008). Topical interferon or surgical excision for the management of primary ocular surface squamous neoplasia. *Ophthalmology*, vol. 115, No.8, (Aug,2008), pp 1297-302, 1302 e1, ISSN 1549-4713 (Electronic)

Sudesh, S.; Rapuano, CJ.; Cohen,EJ.; Eagle, Jr.,RC. & Laibson, PR. (2000). Surgical management of ocular surface squamous neoplasms: the experience from a cornea center. *Cornea*, vol. 19, No.3, (May,2000), pp 278-83, ISSN 0277-3740

Sun, EC.; Fears, TR. & Goedert, JJ. (1997). Epidemiology of squamous cell conjunctival cancer. *Cancer Epidemiol Biomarkers Prev*, vol. 6, No.2, (Feb,1997), pp 73-7, ISSN 1055-9965

Tabin, G.; Levin, S.; Snibson, G.; Loughnan, M. & Taylor, H. (1997). Late recurrences and the necessity for long-term follow-up in corneal and conjunctival intraepithelial neoplasia. *Ophthalmology*, vol. 104, No.3, (Mar,1997), pp 485-92, ISSN 0161-6420

Tananuvat, N.; Lertprasertsuk, N.; Mahanupap, P. & Noppanakeepong, P. (2008). Role of impression cytology in diagnosis of ocular surface neoplasia. *Cornea*, vol. 27, No.3, (Apr,2008), pp 269-74, ISSN 0277-3740

Taylor, HR.; West, S.; Munoz,B.; Rosenthal, FS.; Bressler, SB. & Bressler, NM. (1992). The long-term effects of visible light on the eye. *Arch Ophthalmol*, vol. 110, No.1, (Jan,1992), pp 99-104, ISSN 0003-9950

Tole, DM.; McKelvie, PA. & Daniell, M. (2001). Reliability of impression cytology for the diagnosis of ocular surface squamous neoplasia employing the Biopore membrane. *Br J Ophthalmol*, vol. 85, No.2, (Feb,2001), pp 154-8, ISSN 0007-1161

Tulvatana, W.; Bhattarakosol,P.; Sansopha,L.; Sipiyarak,W.; Kowitdamrong, E.; Paisuntornsug, T. & Karnsawai, S. (2003). Risk factors for conjunctival squamous cell neoplasia: a matched case-control study. *Br J Ophthalmol*, vol. 87, No.4, (Apr,2003), pp 396-8, ISSN 0007-1161

Tunc, M.; Char, DH.; Crawford, B & Miller, T. (1999). Intraepithelial and invasive squamous cell carcinoma of the conjunctiva: analysis of 60 cases. *Br J Ophthalmol*, vol. 83, No.1, (Jan,1999), pp 98-103, ISSN 0007-1161

Verma, V.; Shen, D.; Sieving, PC. & Chan, CC. (2008). The role of infectious agents in the etiology of ocular adnexal neoplasia. *Surv Ophthalmol*, vol. 53, No.4 (Jul-Aug,2008), pp 312-31, ISSN 0039-6257

Waddell, KM.; Lewallen, S.; Lucas, SB.; Atenyi-Agaba, C.; Herrington, CS. & Liomba, G. (1996). Carcinoma of the conjunctiva and HIV infection in Uganda and Malawi. *Br J Ophthalmol*, vol. 80, No.6, (Jun,1996), pp 503-8, ISSN 0007-1161

Walsh-Conway, N. & Conway, RM. (2009). Plaque brachytherapy for the management of ocular surface malignancies with corneoscleral invasion. *Clin Experiment Ophthalmol*, vol. 37, No.6, (Aug,2009), pp 577-83, ISSN 1442-9071 (Electronic)

Yeatts, RP.; Engelbrecht, NE.; Curry, CD.; Ford, JG. & Walter, KA. (2000). 5-Fluorouracil for the treatment of intraepithelial neoplasia of the conjunctiva and cornea. *Ophthalmology*, vol. 107, No.12, (Dec,2000), pp 2190-5, ISSN 0161-6420

Yuen, HK.; Yeung, EF.; Chan, NR.; Chi, SC. & Lam, DS. (2002). The use of postoperative topical mitomycin C in the treatment of recurrent conjunctival papilloma. *Cornea*, vol. 21, No.8, (Nov,2002), pp 838-9, ISSN 0277-3740

3

Excess Fibroblast Growth Factor-7 (FGF-7) Activates β-Catenin and Leads to Ocular Surface Squamous Neoplasia in Mice

Chia-Yang Liu and Winston W.-Y. Kao
Edith J. Crawley Vision Research Center/Department of Ophthalmology, College of Medicine/University of Cincinnati. Cincinnati OH USA

1. Ocular surface squamous neoplasia

Human ocular surface squamous neoplasia (OSSN) is the most common ocular surface pre-cancerous and cancerous lesion previously known by various names such as conjunctival intraepithelial neoplasia, corneal intraepithelial neoplasia (CIN), or both together (CCIN) (Grossniklaus et al., 1987). Clinically, OSSN manifests in different grades ranging from simple dysplasia to squamous cell carcinoma (Grossniklaus et al., 1987). Because of the high incidence of OSSN in the limbal area, where the corneal epithelial stem cells are located, the limbal transition zone/stem cell theory has been proposed for the development of CIN by Lee and Hirst (Lee and Hirst, 1995). Tseng and co-investigators have suggested that the slow cycling limbal stem cells may become hyper-proliferative by stimulations such as alterations in this anatomic site influenced by other factors, e.g., carcinogens, irradiation (eg, UVB), and the phorbol ester tumor promoter, 12-O-tetradecanoylphorbol 13-acetate (TPA) (Tseng, 1989), which can cause abnormal proliferation of the conjunctival and corneal epithelium and lead to the formation of CIN. Nevertheless, the etiology and pathogenesis of CIN and ocular surface carcinoma remain elusive. To date, there is no appropriate animal model available to study the molecular and cellular mechanisms of this disease. Therefore, the availability of such animal model will not only aid to understand the pathogenesis but also yield a more effective treatment for OSSN.

2. Generation *Krt12^{rtTA}/tet-O-FGF-7* bi-transgenic mice and induction of FGF-7 overexpression by doxycycline

It has been well documented that the mouse *Krt12* gene expression is restricted to the differentiated corneal epithelium (Liu et al. 1993, 1994). To generate a corneal epithelium-specific and Dox-inducible transgenic driver mouse line, we have genetically introduced ("knock-in") an ires-rtTA (internal ribosome entry site-reverse tetracycline transactivator) cDNA into the 3′-untranslated region of themouse *Krt12* gene locus via conventional gene-targeting techniques (Chikama et al., 2005). The resulting transgenic mouse line was designated as *Krt12^{rtTA}*, in which like K12 expression pattern, the rtTA is constitutively and specifically expressed by the corneal epithelium. The *Krt12^{rtTA}* mouse line was then crossed with the *tetO-FGF-7* mouse line (a gift from Dr. Jeffrey Whitsett, Cincinnati Children's Hospital Medical Center, Tichelaar et al., 2000) to generate the *Krt12$^{rtTA/rtTA}$/tet-O-FGF-7* bi-transgenic mouse strain. To induce FGF-7 expression, mice were injected once intra-peritoneally with Dox (80 µg/g body weight; Clontech Laboratories) dissolved in PBS (pH 7.4) at a concentration of 10 mg/ml and fed Dox-chow (1 g/Kg chow, Bioserv, Frenchtown, NJ). Control animals were fed regular chow. As shown in Figure 1, FGF-7 over-expression can be induced by doxycycline (Dox) induction and results in a phenotype resembling OSSN (Chikama et al., 2008). This bi-transgenic mouse line may serve as an animal model for understanding the relationship between signaling pathway and the pathological progression of this disease.

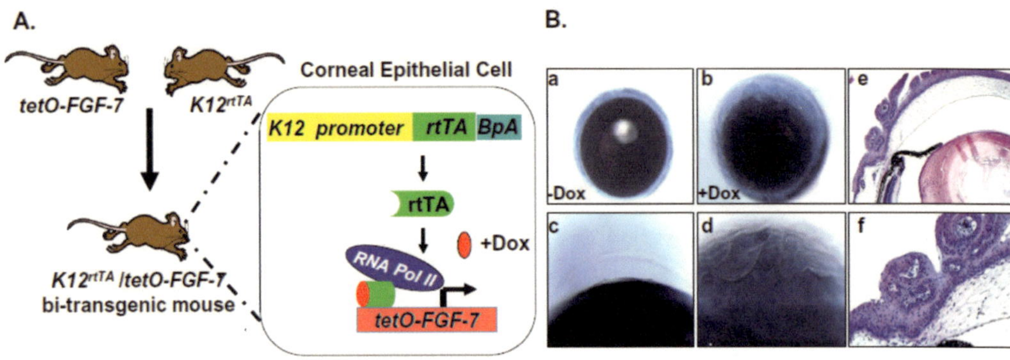

Fig. 1. **Over-expression of FGF-7 resulted in OSSN in Cornea.** A). Diagram showing that corneal epithelium-specific induction of FGF-7 by Dox in *Krt12^{rtTA}/rtTA/tetO-FGF-7* bi-transgenic mice. B) *K12^{rtTA} /tetO-FGF-7* bi-transgenic mice exposed to Dox through mother fed doxycycline chow in the dam since post-nantal day1 (P1) showed corneal intra-epithelial neoplasia at P21 (Bb, Bd) compared to age-matched non-induced mice (Ba, Bc). Papilloma-like epithelial lesion with mesenchymal invasion was found mainly in the peripheral/limbal region (Be, Bf).

3. FGF-7 over-expression and ocular surface carcinogenesis

FGF-7 is a potent mitogen for epithelial cells (Panos et al., 1993; Rubin et al., 1989). The pattern of expression of FGF-7 and its receptor suggest that FGF-7 serves as a paracrine produced by mesenchymal cells in modulating epithelial cells during embryonic development and the maintenance of homeostasis in adults (Finch et al., 1995). FGF-7 enhances epithelial cell proliferation in various organs (Finch et al., 1989, Rubin et al., 1995). Interestingly, aberrant up-regulation of FGF-7 has been reported to be associated with many human neoplastic tumors of epithelial cell origin (Cho et al., 2007; Manavi et al., 2007; Hishikawa et al., 2004; Mehta et al., 2000; Kovacs et al., 2006; Niu et al., 2007). Human papilloma virus 16 (HPV16) and long-term UV irradiation are the major risk factors for corneal intraepithelial neoplasia (Napora et al., 1990). Interestingly, it has been demonstrated that FGF-7 level within the cancer lesion was elevated throughout the progression of multi-stage epidermal carcinogenesis in *K14-HPV16* transgenic mice (Arbeit et al., 1996; Pietras et al., 2008). It has been reported that the exposure to UVB irradiation can induce a rapid intracellular production of ROS (reactive oxidative stress), which in turn is capable of triggering phosphorylation and activation of the FGF-7 receptor, FGFR2-IIIb, similar to those induced by FGF-7 (Marchese et al., 2003). These results lead to our hypothesis that aberrant activation of FGF-7 signaling pathway(s) may be accountable for tumorigenesis derived from limbal stem cells that undergo oncogenic transformation by insults such as long-term UVB exposure and/or infection of HPV etc, which exhibit the characteristic phenotypes of OSSN (Scott et al., 2002; Karp et al., 1996; Kiire et al., 2006). The FGF-7/FGFR signaling is likely the hub that integrates the input through UVB and HPV with the genesis and formation of OSSN (Figure 2). This may explain why excess FGF-7 caused OSSN phenotype in the Dox-treated *Krt12$^{rtTA/rtTA}$/tet-O-FGF-7* bi-transgenic mouse model (Chikama et al., 2008).

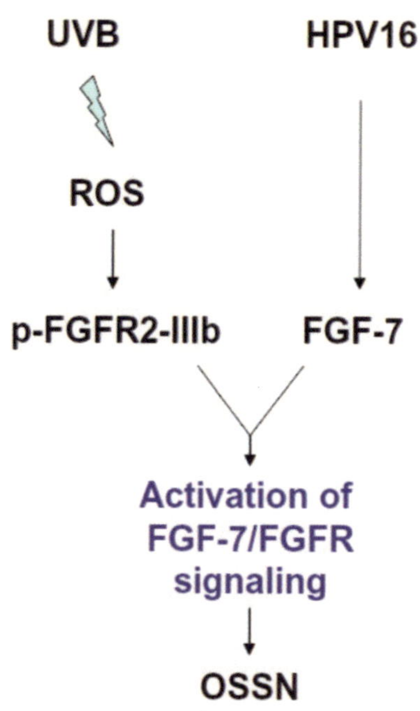

Fig. 2. Hypothetical schema showing that FGF-7/FGFR2 signaling can be activated by UVB and/or HPV type 16, two major risk factors for human OSSN. HPV16 transgene was known to be able to up-regulate FGF-7 (Artbeit et al., 1996). On the other hand, UVB can induced intracellular ROS which in turn phosphorylated and activated FGFR2-IIIb (Marchese et al., 2003).

The precise spatio-temporal expression of FGF-7 is important for ocular surface tissue morphogenesis. FGF-7 are secreted by mesenchymal cells, which bind with high affinity to the same FGF receptor 2 (FGFR2-IIIb) isoform expressed mainly by the epithelial cells (Igarashi et al., 1998). In cornea, expression of FGF-7 and its cognate receptor FGFR2-IIIb is higher in limbal stroma and epithelium, respectively, than in the central cornea, implicating that FGF-7 may promote limbal stem cell proliferation and participate in modulation of corneal epithelium renewal and homeostasis (Li and Tseng, 1996, 1997). However, excess FGF-7 are capable of altering epithelial fates during embryonic development. For example, over-expression of FGF-7 driven by αA-crystalline promoter, which is activated in mouse lens at E11.5, resulted in the suppression of cornea-type epithelial differentiation and the induction of ectopic lacrimal gland formation in the corneas of the transgenic mice (Makarenkova et al., 2000; Govindarajan et al., 2000; Lovicu et al., 1999). In order to understand such an influence at a later stage when epithelial cells have undergone corneal type epithelial differentiation, we developed a *Krt12^rtTA/rtTA^/tetO-FGF-7* bi-transgenic mouse line in which over-expression of FGF-7 by Dox induction caused squamous cell carcinoma of the cornea resembling OSSN in human (Chikama et al., 2008). Less is known, however, about the signaling pathways by which FGF-7 mediates control of corneal epithelial cell proliferation.

4. FGF signaling pathway and its action in mammalian cells

FGF signaling, which is involved in the control of cell proliferation, differentiation, migration, survival and polarity, is transduced through FGF receptors (FGFR). FGFR1, FGFR2, FGFR3 and FGFR4 are FGF receptors, consisting of an extracellular immunoglobulin-like (Ig-like) domain and a cytoplasmic tyrosine kinase domain (Lee et al., 1989; Dionne et al., 1990; Partanen et al., 1990, 1991; Powers et al., 2000; Katoh and Katoh, 2003). FGF receptor isoforms with distinct ligand affinity are generated by alternative splicing of mutually exclusive exons in the latter half of the third Ig-like domain. FGF dimers associated with heparan sulfate proteoglycan bind to FGF receptors to induce receptor dimerization and receptor auto-phosphorylation. FGF signals are transduced via multiple signaling pathways such as the mitogen-activated protein kinases (MAPK), the phospholipase-C gamma (PLCγ), and the PI3K-PKB/AKT (Eswarakumar et al., 2005; Dailey et al., 2005; Katoh and Katoh, 2006; Kouhara et al., 1997; Ong et al., 2000) (Figure 3). A key component of FGF signaling is the docking protein called FGFR substrate 2 (FRS2) which is phosphorylated on tyrosine residues upon FGF stimulation. FRS2 consists of N-terminal myristylation signal, phosphotyrosine binding (PTB) domain and C-terminal region with multiple Src homology-2 (SH2) binding sites. FRS2 is recruited to the auto-phosphorylated FGF receptors through the interaction with phospho-tyrosine residues. FRS2, bound to auto-phosphorylated FGFRs, is tyrosine phosphorylated in the C-terminal region, which in turns recruits growth factor receptor-bound protein 2 (GRB2) and a SH2-containing tyrosine phosphatase, SHP2. In most cell types, FRS2-GRB2-SHP2 signaling complex recruits the guanine nucleotide exchange factor, Son of sevenless (SOS), which activates Ras and downstream effectors of MAPK (Figure 3, highlighted in grey). The MAPKs which include ERKs, p38, and Jun N-terminal kinases (JNKs) regulate the activity of downstream kinases or transcription factors. Although MAPK family shares many structural similarities, the ERK1/2 kinases are generally considered responsible for the mitogenic response, while the p38 and JNK are usually associated with inflammatory or stress-responses (Johnson et al., 2002).

Alternatively upon FGF stimulation, FRS2-SHP2-GRB2 complex may recruit GRB2-associated binding protein 1 (GAB1) to activate PI3K (Figure 3, highlighted in yellow), which phosphorylates PIP2 to generate phosphatidylinositol-3,4,5-triphosphate (PIP3) (Ong et al., 2002; Cantley, 2002). PIP3 induces the translocation of PKB/AKT to plasma membrane, where PKB/AKT is phosphorylated and activated by phosphoinositide-dependent kinase (PDK) (Luo et al., 2003). The ability of FGFs to protect cells from apoptosis is primarily due to the activation of the PKB/AKT survival pathway, a PI3K dependent activation of PDK, leads to the activation of PKB/AKT which in turn attenuates the activity and/or suppression of pro-apoptotic factors (Schlessinger, 2000 Schlessinger. PKB/AKT phosphorylates a variety of substrates, such as glycogen synthase kinase (GSK-3β), forkhead transcription factor (FKHR), FOXO1 (Burgering and Medema, 2003). It is of interest to note that inhibition of GSK-3β via phosphorylation its Ser-9 by activated PKB/AKT and provides additional anti-apoptotic protection (Jope and Johnson, 2004) and possibly the accumulation and nuclear translocation of β-catenin. Furthermore, a wide variety of agents, e.g., SB-216763, SB-415286, and LiCl, is known to attenuate GSK-3β activities via phosphorylation at Ser-9 by PKB/AKT and allow the accumulation and nuclear translocation of transcription factor β-catenin (Frame and Cohen, 2000).

FGF signal also activates phosphatidyl inositol (Pt Ins) hydrolysis, release of intracellular calcium and activation of protein kinase C (PKC) via recruitment of the SH2 domain of PLCγ to the FGFR. Activated PLCγ hydrolyzes Pt Ins [4,5] P2 to form diacylglygerol (DAG) and Ins [1,4,5] P3 which stimulates calcium release and activation of calcium/calmodulin dependent protein kinases (Figure 3, highlighted in blue). The loss of this pathway does notappear to impair the proliferative response (Mohammadi et al., 1992). It remains unknown which individual aforementioned signaling pathways and/or their combination is responsible for the patho-physiology of OSSN caused by excess FGF-7 in our *Krt12*$^{rtTA/rtTA}$*/tet-O-FGF-7* mice.

5. Cross-talk between FGF and Wnt pathways may be mediated by common target proteins

It has been shown that FGF and Wnt signaling pathways crosstalk takes place during a variety of cellular processes, such as embryogenesis (Loebel et al., 2003; McGrew et al., 1997; Tickle, 1995; Ng, 2002; Villanueva et al., 2002; Gunhaga et al., 2003; Shackleford et al., 1993) and carcinogenesis (MacArthur et al., 1995; Katoh, 2002; McWhirter, 1997, 1999; Kirikoshi et al., 2000; Shimokawa et al., 2003; Chamorro et al., 2005; Katoh and Katoh, 2005). A key event in the canonical Wnt pathway is the activation of β-catenin that subsequently regulates transcription of specific target genes that modulate cell fate, proliferation, migration, and apoptosis. In the absence of Wnt signals, cytosolic β-catenin is phosphorylated by GSK-3β, which targets β-catenin for proteasome-mediated degradation. However, in the presence of a Wnt signal, GSK-3β is inactivated by phosphorylation, and results in accumulation and nuclear translocation of stable β-catenin that binds DNA elements of members of the lymphoid enhancer factor/T-cell factor (LEF/TCF) family of transcription factors. Thus, it activates transcription of Wnt-target genes (Moon et al., 2002) (Figure 4). β-catenin also functions at the cell membrane where, as a component of the adherent junction, it links cadherin to the cytoskeleton (Kemler et al., 1993).

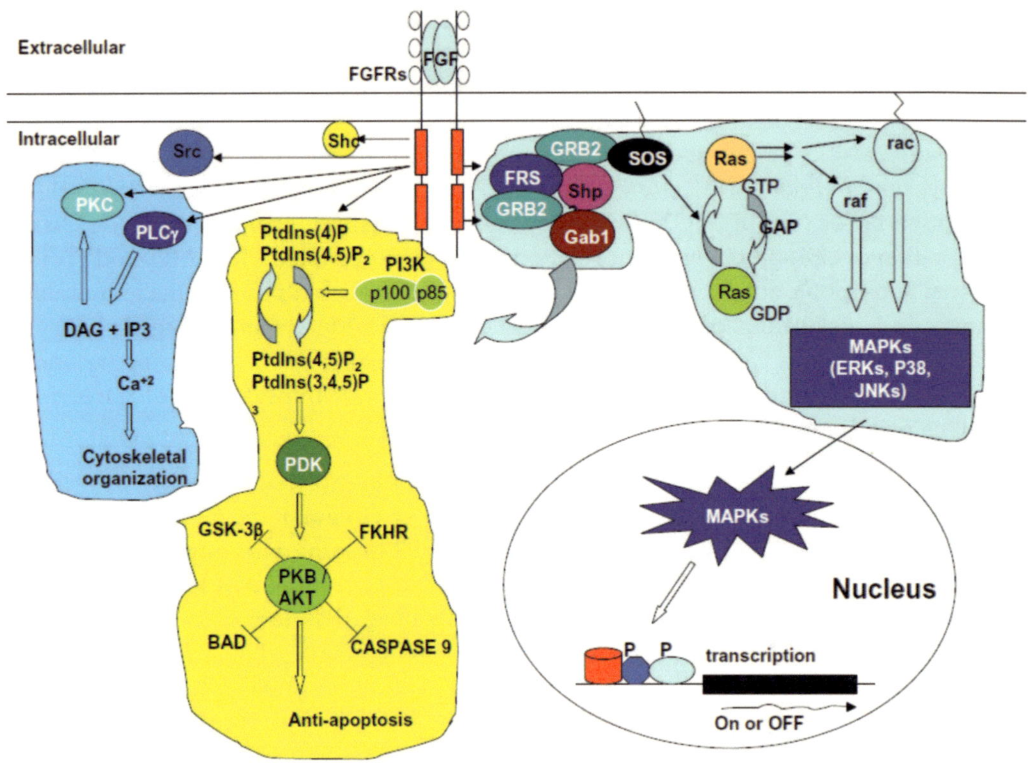

Fig. 3. **FGF signal transduction pathways.** Activated FGFRs (red rectangles) stimulate PLCγ pathway (blue highlight), the PI3K/PKB-AKT pathway (yellow highlight), and the FRS2-Ras-MAP kinase pathway (grey highlight). The activated MAP kinases (ERKs, p38, or JNKs) are translocated to the nucleus where they phosphorylate (P) transcription factors, thereby regulating target genes. In some cell types, FGF signaling also phosphorylates the Shc and Src proteins. Abbreviations: PKB/AKT, protein kinase b; DAG, diacyl glycerol; ERKs, Extracellular signal-regulated kinases; FKHR, forkhead homolog 1; FRS2, Fibroblast growth factor receptor substrate 2; GAP, GTPase-activating protein; Gab1, Grb2-associated binding protein 1; GRB2, Growth factor receptor-bound protein 2; GSK-3β, Glycogen synthase kinase 3β;MAPK, Mitogen-activated protein kinase; JNKs, Jun N-terminal Kinases; PDK, 3-phosophoinositide-dependent protein kinase;PI3K, Phosphoinositide 3-kinase; PKC, protein kinase C; PLCγ: phospholipase C gamma; Rac, Ras-related C3 botulinum toxin substrate; Shp2, Src homology 2-containing tyrosine phosphatase; SOS, Son of sevenless, guanine nucleotide exchange factor.

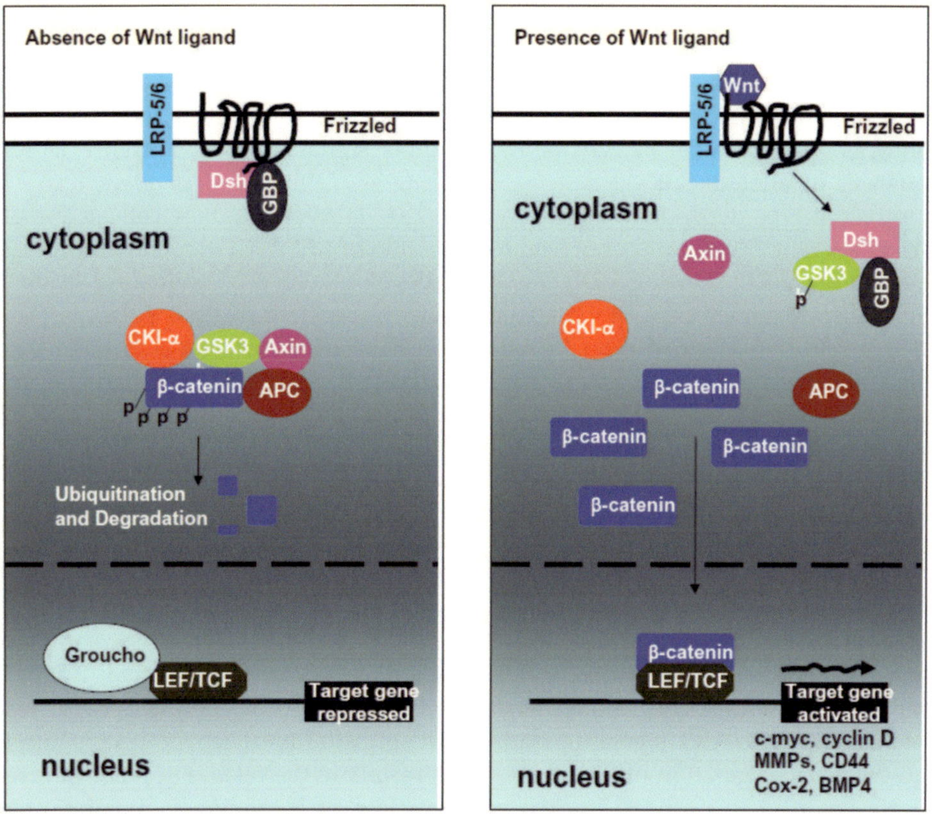

Fig. 4. **Graphical depiction of the schema of the canonical Wnt signaling pathway.** (Left panel) In the absence of Wnt ligand, LEF/TCF transcription factors are inert due to their association with a repressor (groucho protein) on their nuclear DNA binding sites. Beta-catenin, which is needed for release of the repressor protein, is captured by a degradation complex containing casein kinase I alpha (CKI-α), GSK-3β, Axin, and adenomatosis polyposis coli (APC) before it can enter the nucleus and is phosphorylated by GSK-3β and subsequently ubiquitinylated and degraded by the proteasome (Right panel). When Wnt ligand binds to its receptors, Frizzled and LRP5/6, dishevelled (Dsh) protein becomes activated. Repression of GSK-3β by an alternative complex containing Dsh and GSK-3β binding protein (GBP) releases β-catenin from the aforementioned degradation complex. Unbound β-catenin enters the nucleus to complex with LEF/TCF, displacing groucho and enabling formation of an active transcription complex.

A possible candidate that can mediate both Wnt and FGF signalings is GSK-3β, which can also be phosphorylated by PKB/AKT besides Dishevelled protein (Jope and Johnson, 2004). Evidence for this assertion has been provided during FGF-2 treatment of neuronal cells, which increases GSK-3β phosphorylation and nuclear localization of β-catenin. Over-expression of β-catenin maintains neural progenitor cells in a proliferative state in the presence of FGF-2, but enhances neuronal differentiation in the absence of FGF-2, suggesting that FGF signaling regulates neural progenitor cell proliferation and also affects lineage commitment during neural differentiation, in part, via β-catenin signaling (Israsena et al., 2004). Similarly, in neural cells, the neuroprotective effects of FGF-1 may utilize GSK-3β inactivation via activation of the PI3K-PKB/AKT cascade (Hashimoto et al., 2002). In addition, FGF-2-treated human endothelial cells show an increase in nuclear β-catenin by a reduction in GSK-3β activity (Holnthoner et al., 2002). Although GSK-3β has been shown to be a phosphorylation target of FGF as well as other signaling pathways such as IGF, the consequences of altered GSK-3β activity on β-catenin/LEF/TCF-dependent transcription seems to be cell-type dependent. For example in 293 embryonic kidney cells, IGF-mediated phosphorylation of GSK-3β does not lead to induction of LEF/TCF-dependent transcription (Playford et al., 2000). During early Xenopus development, FGF signaling leads to the inhibition of endogenous GSK-3β via a PKB/AKT independent p90RSK pathway (Torres et al., 1999). p90RSK over-expression increases the level of membrane-associated β-catenin without fluctuation in nuclear levels. The fact that both FGF and Wnt signaling target a common protein implicates that the assignment of particular proteins such as GSK-3β to a specific "pathway" is arbitrary since their activity can be influenced by a number of different routes. Furthermore, since proteins such as GSK-3β are targeted by several signal transduction pathways, they have the potential to act as molecular switches between these pathways, and thus serve as nodal points for pathway cross-talk (Figure 5). In addition, GSK-3β also binds to and phosphorylates the SNAIL transcriptional repressor, inducing its cytoplasmic translocation and degradation (Zhou et al., 2004). SNAIL represses E-cadherin transcription, a key tight junction molecule which establishes and maintains cell-cell adhesion (Batlle et al., 2000; Katoh and Katoh, 2005; Thiery and Sleeman, 2006). Taken together, these data support a model whereby the inhibition of GSK-3β activity via FGF-dependent PI3K-PKB/AKT signaling leads to an epithelial-mesenchymal transition (EMT) through the down-regulation of E-cadherin. This results in the release of β-catenin from the E-cadherin complex to promote nuclear accumulation of β-catenin. It remains unknown which aforementioned pathway is employed or in combination in the corneal epithelium elicited by excess FGF-7. Further investigation should lead to a clear mechanistic event of FGF-7 signaling in corneal epithelium and tumor formation.

6. Nuclear accumulation of the β-catenin protein in tumors

In human cancers, exon 3 of the *CTNNB*1 gene, which encodes β-catenin, is a mutational "hot spot" for gain-of-function isoforms. This exon encodes the critical Ser/Thr residues, which are sites for priming by casein kinase1 (CK1) (Ser 45) and phosphorylation by GSK-3β (Ser 33, 37 and Thr 41). As a result, this β-transducin repeat-containing protein (β-TrCP) recognition site marks β-catenin for degradation. Therefore mutations within this exon increase the stability and nuclear accumulation of the β-catenin protein. Indeed, somatic mutations in *CTNNB*1 gene are strongly associated with a wide variety of human tumors including colorectal carcinoma, desmoid tumor, endometrial carcinoma, hepatocellular carcinoma, hepatoblastoma, intestinal carcinoma gastric, medulloblastoma, melanoma, ovarian carcinoma, pancreatic carcinoma, pilomatricoma, prostate carcinoma, squamous cell carcinoma of the head and neck, thyroid carcinoma, and Wilms' tumor (Polakis, 2000). To test the hypothesis that β-catenin accumulation in corneal epithelial cell nucleus plays a pivotal role in mediating FGF-7 signaling networks leading to the formation of corneal neoplasia in *Krt12$^{rtTA/rtTA}$/tetO-FGF-7* bi-transgenic mice induced by Dox, we have crossed *K12$^{rtTA/rtTA}$/tetO-FGF-7/tetO-Cre* mice with two different floxed *Ctnnb*1 mouse strains for the analysis the role of β-catenin in corneal intraepithelial neoplasia model. In the first mouse line, loxP sites flank an essential part (exon 2 through exon 6) of the *Ctnnb1*gene (*Ctnnb1*$^{loxEx2-6}$) (Brault et al., 2001). Upon Cre-mediated recombination, the region containing exon 2 to 6 of the *Ctnnb1* gene is deleted. This deletion causes a frame shift and premature termination of β-catenin translation. As a result, no β-catenin gene-product is produced from this allele. Interestingly, *K12*$^{rtTA/rtTA}$*/tetO-FGF-7/tetO-Cre/Ctnnb1*$^{loxEx2-6/loxEx2-6}$ tetra-transgenic mice treated with Dox from P7 to P21 (i.e., short term induction for 14 days) failed to develop corneal epithelial hyperplasia, suggesting that this phenotype caused by excess FGF-7 is dependent on β-catenin (Chia-Yang Liu et al., in preparation for publication).

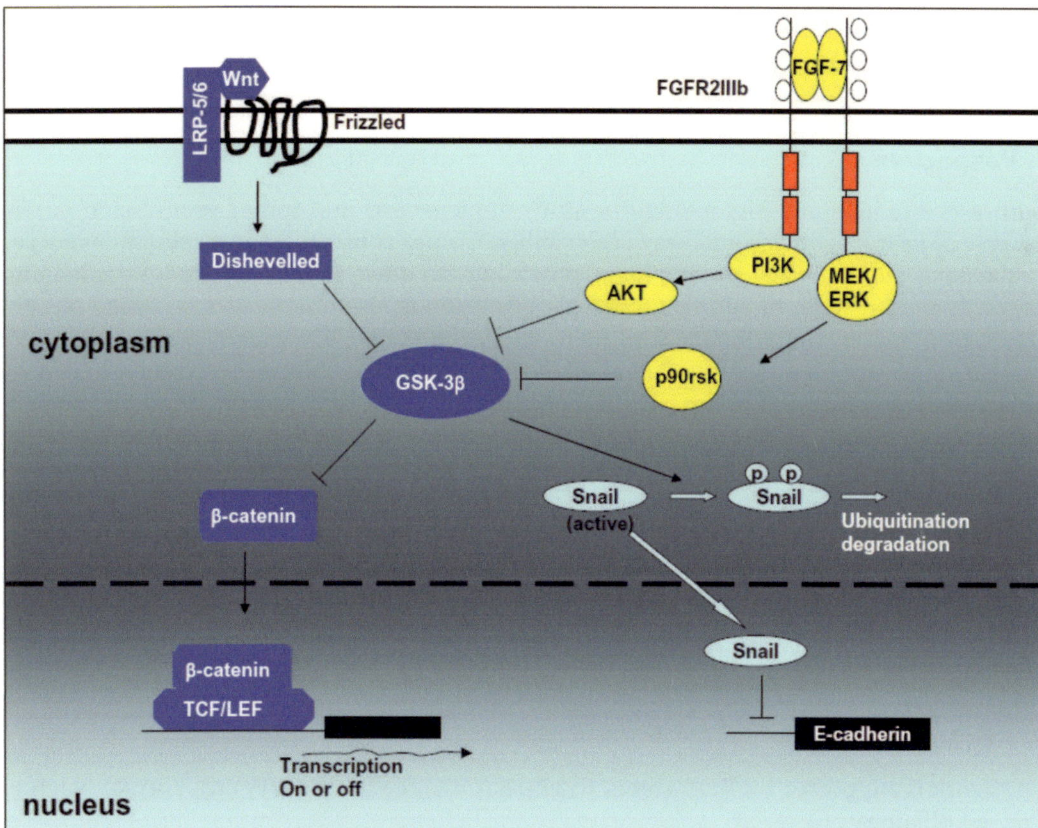

Fig. 5. **Cross-talk between FGF and Wnt pathways.** Elements of the FGF (yellow and red) and Wnt/β-catenin (blue) pathways are shown. Depicted is how activation of the FGF receptor on the cell membrane can lead to activation of β-catenin through different mechanisms. In some cell types, activation by FGF of either PI3K/AKT or MAP kinase/p90 ribosomal S6 kinase (p90rsk) can promote GSK-3β phosphorylation, which is associated with translocation of β-catenin to the nucleus. Inhibition of GSK-3b by Wnt, PI3K/AKt, or MAPK pathways suppressed the phosphorylation of Snail (green) and thus induces the nuclear localization and protein stabilization of Snail, which suppress E-cadherin and lead to cell migration.

In the second mouse line, loxP sites flank only exon 3 of the *Ctnnb1*gene (*Ctnnb1^{floxedEx3}*) (Harada et al., 1999). Upon Cre-mediated recombination, exon 3 of the β-catenin gene is deleted. Exon 2 is spliced in frame to exon 4 and thus a mutant protein designated as ΔE3 β-catenin is produced. However, this mutant protein lacks its phosphorylation sites which are necessary for the subsequent ubiquitinylation and degradation of β-catenin. Therefore, this allele (*Ctnnb1^{floxedEx3}*) encodes a more stable, constitutively dominant active β-catenin protein mimicking the canonical Wnt signaling pathway. Indeed, Dox-treated *K12$^{rtTA/wt}$/tetO-Cre/Ctnnb1$^{floxedEx3/Wt}$* tri-transgenic heterozygous mice all exhibited corneal epithelial hyperplasia at different developmental stages from P1 to P30. Moreover, X-gal positive cells completely correlated with the hyperplastic transformation and stromal invasion in the cornea of Dox-induced *Krt12$^{rtTA/wt}$/tetO-Cre/Ctnnb1$^{floxedEx3/Wt}$/TOPgal* quadruple transgenic heterozygous mice (Zhang et al., 2010). These results strongly indicate that regulation of β-catenin signaling plays a pivotal role in the maintenance of normal corneal epithelial homeostasis.

7. Pespective

Cornea is a unique and idea model for study angiogenesis and tumor progression *in vivo* because of its transparency and easy accessibility. Cornea consists of three cellular layers i.e., epithelium, stroma, and endothelium providing an idea model to study epithelium-mesenchym transition. In addition, corneal epithelium is also unique as a stratified but not keratinized epithelium, which allows us to study the epithelial metaplasia. Human OSSN consists of a spectrum of dysplasia and/or neoplasia which is relatively common in clinical ophthalmology practice. Primary surgical excision and various adjunctive therapies such as mitomycin-C (MMC), 5-fluorouracil (5-FU), or interferon alpha-2b (INF-α2b) remain as the mainstay of treatment but the recurrence rate is high. To improve the clinical outcome of OSSN treatment, agents aiming at the down regulation of signal transducing molecules that modulate β-catenin are required. It is anticipated that signal transduction molecule(s), e.g., ERK→p90RSK→GSK-3β→β-catenin and/or PI3K→PKB/AKT→GSK-3β→β-catenin, which could mediate FGF-7 signaling networks responsible for the formation of corneal epithelial neoplasia will aid in the design of novel regimens for the treatment of human OSSN and other human cancers.

8. Acknowledgment

This work is supported by RO1 grants EY12486 (CYL), EY13755 (WWYK), and Research to Prevent Blindness

9. References

Arbeit, J.M., Olson, D.C. & Hanahan, D. (1996). Upregulation of fibroblast growth factors and their receptors during multi-stage epidermal carcinogenesis in K14-HPV16 transgenic mice. Oncogene; 13:1847-1857

Batlle, E., Sancho, E., Franci, C., Dominguez, D., Monfar, M., Baulida, J. & Garcia, De Herreros A. (2000) The transcription factor snail is a repressor of *E-cadherin* gene expression in epithelial tumour cells. Nat Cell Biol; 2:84-89.

Brault, V., Moore, R., Kutsch, S., Ishibashi, M., Rowitch, D.H., McMahon, A.P., Sommer, L., Boussadia, O. & Kemler, R. (2001) Inactivation of the beta-catenin gene by Wnt1-Cre-mediated deletion results in dramatic brain malformation and failure of craniofacial development. Development; 128:1253-1264.

Burgering, B.M. & Medema, R.H. (2003) Decisions on life and death: FOXO Forkhead transcription factors are in command when PKB/Akt is off duty. J Leukoc Biol ; 73:689-701.

Chamorro, M.N., Schwartz, D.R., Vonica, A., Brivanlou, A.H., Cho, K.R. & Varmus, H.E. (2005) FGF20 and DKK1 are transcriptional target of b-catenin and FGF20 is implicated in cancer and development. EMBO J; 24:73-84.

Cantley, L.C. (2002) The phosphoinositide 3-kinase pathway. Science; 296:1655-1657.

Chikama, T., Hayashi, Y., Liu, C.Y., Terai, N., Terai, K., Kao, C.W., Wang, L., Hayashi, M., Nishida, T., Sanford, P., Doestchman, T. & Kao W. (2005) Characterization of tetracycline-inducible double transgenic Krt12rtTA/+/tet-O-LacZ mice. Invest Ophthalmol Vis Sci. 46:1966-1972.

Chikama, T., Liu, C.Y., Meij, J.T.A., Hayashi, Y., Wang, I.J., Liu, Y., Nishida, T. & Kao, W.W.Y. (2008) Excess FGF-7 in corneal epithelium causes corneal intraepithelial neoplasia in young mice and epithelium hyperplasia in adult mice. Am J of Pathol; 172:638-649.

Cho, K., Ishiwata, T., Uchida, E., Nakazawa, N., Korc, M., Naito, Z. & Tajiri, T. (2007) Enhanced expression of keratinocyte growth factor and its receptor correlates with venous invasion in pancreatic cancer. Am J Pathol.; 170:1964-1974.

Dailey, L., Ambrosetti, D., Mansukhani, A. & Basilico, C. (2005) Mechanisms underlying differential responses to FGF signaling. Cytokine Growth Factor Rev; 16:233-247.

Dionne, C.A., Crumley, G., Bellot, F., Kaplow, J.M., Searfoss, G., Ruta, M., Burgess, W.H., Jaye, M. & Schlessinger, J. (1990) Cloning and expression of two distinct high-affinity receptors cross-reacting with acidic and basic fibroblast growth factors. EMBO J; 9:2685-2692.

Eswarakumar, V.P., Lax, I. & Schlessinger, J. (2005) Cellular signaling by fibroblast growth factor receptors. Cytokine Growth Factor Rev; 16:139-149.

Finch, P.W., Rubin, J.S., Miki, T. & Ron, D. & Aaronson, S.A. (1989) Human KGF is FGF-related with properties of a paracrine effector of epithelial cell growth. Science; 245:752-755.

Finch, P.W., Cunha, G.R., Rubin, J.S., Wong, J. & Ron, D. (1995) Pattern of keratinocyte growth factor and keratinocyte growth factor receptor expression during mouse fetal development suggests a role in mediating morphogenetic mesenchymal-epithelial interactions. Dev Dyn; 203:223-240.

Frame, S. & Cohen P. (2000) GSK3 takes centre stage more than 20 years after its discovery. Biochem J; 359:1-16.

Govindarajan, V., Ito, M., Makarenkova, H.P., Lang, R.A. & Overbeek, P.A. (2000) Endogenous and ectopic gland induction by FGF-10. Dev. Biol.; 225:188-200.

Grossniklaus, H.E., Green, W.R., Lukenback, M. & Chan, C.C. (1987) Conjunctival lesions in adults: a clinical and histopathologic review. Cornea; 6:78-116.

Gunhaga, L., Marklund, M., Sjodal, M., Hsieh, J.C., Jessell, T.M. & Edlund, T. (2003) Specification of dorsal telencephalic character by sequential Wnt and FGF signaling. Nat Neurosci; 6:701-707.

Harada, N., Tamai, Y., Ishikawa, T., Sauer, B., Takaku, K., Oshima, M. & Taketo, M.M. (1999) Intestinal polyposis in mice with a dominant stable mutation of the beta-catenin gene. EMBO J.; 18:5931-5942.

Hashimoto, M., Sagara, Y., Langford, D., Everall, I.P., Mallory, M., Everson, A., Digicaylioglu, M. & Masliah, E. (2002) Fibroblast growth factor 1 regulates signaling via the glycogen synthase kinase-3beta pathway. Implications for neuroprotection. J Biol Chem; 277:32985-32991.

Hishikawa, Y., Tamaru, N., Ejima, K., Hayashi, T. & Koji, T. (2004) Expression of keratinocyte growth factor and its receptor in human breast cancer: its inhibitory role in the induction of apoptosis possibly through the over-expression of Bcl-2. Arch Histol Cytol.; 67:455-464.

Holnthoner, W., Pillinger, M., Groger, M., Wolff, K., Ashton, A.W., Albanese, C., Neumeister, P., Pestell, R.G. & Petzelbauer, P. (2002) Fibroblast growth factor-2 induces Lef/Tcf-dependent transcription in human endothelial cells. J Biol Chem; 277:45847-45853.

Igarashi, M., Finch, P.W. & Aaronson, S.A. (1998) Characterization of recombinant human fibroblast growth factor (FGF)-10 reveals functional similarities with keratinocyte growth factor (FGF-7). J Biol Chem.; 273:13230-13235.

Israsena, N., Hu, M., Fu, W., Kan, L. & Kessler, J,A. (2004) The presence of FGF2 signaling determines whether beta-catenin exerts effects on proliferation or neuronal differentiation of neural stem cells. Dev Biol; 268:220-231.

Johnson, G.L. & Lapadat, R. (2002) Mitogen-activated protein kinase pathways mediated by ERK, JNK, and p38 protein kinases. Science; 298:1911-1912.

Jope, R.S. & Johnson, G.V.W. (2004) The glamour and gloom of glycogen synthase kinase-3. Trends Biochem Sci; 29:95-102

Karp, C.L., Scott, I.U., Chang, T.S. & Pflugfelder, S.C. (1996) Conjunctival intraepithelial neoplasia. A possible marker for human immunodeficiency virus infection? Arch Ophthalmol.;114:257-261.

Katoh, M. & Katoh, M. (2003) *FGFR2* and *WDR11* are neighboring oncogene and tumor suppressor gene on human chromosome *10q26*. Int J Oncol;22:1155-1159.

Katoh, M. (2002) WNT and FGF gene clusters. Int J Oncol ; 21:1269-1273.

Katoh, M. & Katoh, M. (2005) Comparative genomics on FGF20 orthologs. Oncol Rep; 14:287-290.

Katoh, M. & Katoh, M. Comparative genomics on *SNAI1*, *SNAI2*, and *SNAI3* orthologs. Oncol Rep;14:1083-1086.

Katoh, M. & Katoh, M. (2005) Comparative genomics on FGF8, FGF17, and FGF18 orthologs. In J Mol Med; 16:493-496.

Katoh, M. & Katoh, M. (2005) Comparative genomics on FGF16 orthologs. Int J Mol Med; 16:959-963.

Katoh, M. & Katoh, M. (2006) FGF signaling network in the gastrointestinal tract. Int J Oncol; 29:163-168.

Kemler, R. (1993) From cadherins to catenins: cytoplasmic protein interactions and regulation of cell adhesion. Trends Genet; 9:317-321.

Kiire, C.A. & Dhillon, B. (2006) The aetiology and associations of conjunctival intraepithelial neoplasia. Br J Ophthalmol.; 90:109-113.

Kirikoshi, H., Sagara, N., Saitoh, T., Tanaka, K., Sekihara, H., Shiokawa, K. & Katoh, M. (2000) Molecular cloning and characterization of human FGF20 on chromosome 8p21.3-p22. Biochem Biophys Res Commun; 274:337-343.

Kouhara, H., Hadari, Y.R., Spivak-Kroizman, T., Schilling, J., Bar-Sagi, D., Lax, I. & Schlessinger, J. (1997) A lipid-anchored Grb2-binding protein that links FGF-receptor activation to the Ras/MAPK signaling pathway. Cell ; 89:693-702.

Kovacs, D., Cota, C., Cardinali, G., Aspite, N., Bolasco, G., Amantea, A., Torrisi, M.R. & Picardo, M. (2006) Expression of keratinocyte growth factor and its receptor in clear cell acanthoma. Exp Dermatol.; 15:762-768.

Lee, F.S., Lane, T.F., Kuo, A., Shackleford, G.M. & Leder, P. (1995) Insertional mutagenesis identifies a member of the Wnt gene family as a candidate oncogene in the mammary epithelium of int-2/Fgf-3 transgenic mice. Proc Natl Acad Sci USA; 92:2268-2272.

Lee, G.A. & Hirst, L.W. (1995) Ocular surface squamous neoplasia. Surv Ophthalmol; 39:429-450.

Lee, P.L., Johnson, D.E., Cousens, L.S., Fried, V.A. & Williams, L.T. (1989) Purification and complementary DNA cloning of a receptor for basic fibroblast growth factor. Science; 245:57-60.

Li, D.Q. & Tseng, S.C. (1996) Differential regulation of cytokine and receptor transcript expression in human corneal and limbal fibroblasts by epidermal growth factor, transforming growth factor-alpha, platelet-derived growth factor B, and interleukin-1 beta. Invest Ophthalmol Vis Sci; 37:2068-2080.

Li, D.Q. & Tseng, S.C. (1997) Differential regulation of keratinocyte growth factor and hepatocyte growth factor/scatter factor by different cytokines in human corneal and limbal fibroblasts. J Cell Physiol; 172:361-372.

Liu, C.Y., Zhu, G., Westerhausen-Larson, A., Converse, R.L., Kao, C.W.C., Sun, T.T. & Kao, W.W.Y. (1993) Cornea-specific expression of K12 keratin during mouse development. Curr Eye Res.; 12:963-974.

Liu, C.Y., Zhu, G., Converse, R.L., Kao, C.W.C., Nakamura, H., Tseng, S.C.G., Mui, M.M., Seyer, J., Justice, M.J., Stech, M.E., Hansen, G.M. & Kao, W.W.Y. (1994) Characterization and chromosomal localization of the cornea- specific murine keratin gene Krt1.12. J Biol Chem.; 269:24627-24636.

Loebel, D.A., Watson, C.M., DeYoung, R.A. & Tam, P.P. (2003) Lineage choice and differentiation in mouse embryos and embryonic stem cells. Dev Biol; 264:1-14.

Lovicu, F.J., Kao, W.W. & Overbeek, P.A . (1999) Ectopic gland induction by lens-specific expression of keratinocyte growth factor (FGF-7) in transgenic mice. Mech. Dev; 88:43-53.

Luo, J., Manning, B.D. & Cantley, L.C. (2003) Targeting the PI3K-Akt pathway in human cancer: Rationale and promise. Cancer Cell; 4:257-262.

MacArthur, C.A., Shankar, D.B. & Shackleford, G.M. (1995) Fgf-8, activated by proviral insertion, cooperates with the Wnt-1 transgene in murine mammary tumorigenesis. J Virol ; 69:2501-2507.

Makarenkova, H.P., Ito, M., Govindarajan, V., Faber, S.C., Sun, L., McMahon, G., Overbeek, P.A. & Lang, R.A. (2000) FGF10 is an inducer and Pax6 a competence factor for lacrimal gland development. Development; 127:2563-2572.

Manavi, M., Hudelist, G., Fink-Retter, A., Gschwandtler-Kaulich, D., Pischinger, K. & Czerwenka, K. (2007) Gene profiling in Pap-cell smears of high-risk human papillomavirus-positive squamous cervical carcinoma. Gynecol Oncol.; 105:418-426.

Marchese, C., Maresca, V., Cardinali, G., Belleudi, F., Ceccarelli, S., Bellocci, M., Frati, L., Torrisi, M.R. & Picardo, M. (2003) UVB-induced activation and internalization of keratinocyte growth factor receptor. Oncogene; 22:2422-24231.

McGrew, L.L., Hoppler, S. & Moon, R.T. (1997) Wnt and FGF pathways cooperatively pattern antero-posterior neural ectoderm in Xenopus. Mech Dev; 69:105-114.

McWhirter, J.R., Goulding, M., Weiner, J.A., Chun, J. & Murre, C. (1997) A novel fibroblast growth factor gene expressed in the developing nervous system is a downstream target of the chimeric homeodomain oncoprotein E2A-Pbx1. Development; 124:3221-3232.

McWhirter, J.R., Neuteboom, S.T., Wancewicz, E.V., Monia, B.P., Downing, J.R. & Murre, C. (1999) Oncogenic homeodomain transcription factor E2A-Pbx1 activates a novel WNT gene in pre-B acute lymphoblastoid leukemia. Proc Natl Acad Sci USA; 96:11464-11469.

Mehta, P.B., Robson, C.N., Neal, D.E. & Leung, H.Y. (2000) Serum keratinocyte growth factor measurement in patients with prostate cancer. J Urol; 164:2151-2155.

Mohammadi, M., Dionnem, C.A., Li, W., Li, N., Spivak, T. & Honegger, A.M. (1992) Point mutation in FGF receptor eliminates phosphatidylinositol hydrolysis without affecting mitogenesis. Nature; 358:681-684.

Moon, R.T., Bowerman, B., Boutros, M. & Perrimon, N. (2002) The promise and perils of Wnt signaling through beta-catenin. Science; 296:1644-1646.

Napora, C., Cohen, E.J., Genvert, G.I., Presson, A.C., Arentsen, J.J., Eagle, R.C. & Laibson, P.R. (1990) Factors associated with conjunctival intraepithelial neoplasia: a case control study. Ophthalmic Surg.; 21:27-30.

Ng, J.K., Kawakami, Y., Buscher, D., Raya, A., Itoh, T., Koth, C.M., Rodriguez, Esteban. C., Rodriguez-Leon, J., Garrity, D.M., Fishman, M.C., Izpisua Belmonte, J.C. (2002) The limb identity gene Tbx5 promotes limb initiation by interacting with Wnt2b and Fgf10. Development; 129:5161-5170.

Niu, J., Chang, Z., Peng, B., Xia, Q., Lu, W., Huang, P., Tsao, M.S. & Chiao, P.J. (2007) Keratinocyte growth factor/fibroblast growth factor-7-regulated cell migration and invasion through activation of NF-kappaB transcription factors. J Biol Chem.; 282:6001-6011.

Ong, S.H., Guy, G.R., Hadari, Y.R., Laks, S., Gotoh, N., Schlessinger, J. & Lax, I. (2000) FRS2 proteins recruit intracellular signaling pathways by binding to diverse targets on fibroblast growth factor and nerve growth factor receptors. Mol Cell Biol; 20:979-989.

Ong, S.H., Hadari, Y.R., Gotoh, N., Guy, G.R. & Schlessinger, J. & Lax, I. (2001) Stimulation of phosphatidylinositol 3-kinase by fibroblast growth factor receptors is mediated by coordinated recruitment of multiple docking proteins. Proc Natl Acad Sci USA; 98:6074-6079.

Panos, R.J., Rubin, J.S., Csaky, K.G., Aaronson, S.A. & Mason, R.J. (1993) Keratinocyte growth factor and hepatocyte growth factor/scatter factor are heparin-binding growth factors for alveolar type II cells in fibroblast-conditioned medium. J Clin Invest; 92:969-977

Partanen, J., Makela, T.P., Alitalo, R., Lehvaslaiho, H. & Alitalo, K. (1990) Putative tyrosine kinases expressed in K-562 human leukemia cells. Proc Natl Acad Sci USA; 87:8913-8917.

Partanen, J., Makela, T.P., Eerola, E., Korhonen, J., Hirvonen, H., Claesson-Welsh, L. & Alitalo, K. (1991) FGFR-4, a novel acidic fibroblast growth factor receptor with a distinct expression pattern. EMBO J; 10:1347-354.

Pietras, K., Pahler, J., Bergers, G. &, Hanahan, D. (2008) Functions of paracrine PDGF signaling in the proangiogenic tumor stroma revealed by pharmacological targeting. PLoS Med.; 5:e19

Playford, M.P., Bicknell, D., Bodmer, W.F. & Macaulay, V.M. (2000) Insulin-like growth factor 1 regulates the location, stability, and transcriptional activity of beta-catenin. Proc Natl Acad Sci USA; 97:12103-12108.

Polakis, P. (2000) Wnt signaling and cancer. Genes Dev. 2000; 14:1837-1851.

Powers, C.J., McLeskey, S.W. & Wellstein, A. (2000) Fibroblast growth factors, their receptors and signaling. Endocr Relat Cancer; 7:165-197.

Rubin, J.S., Osada, H., Finch, P.W., Taylor, W.G., Rudikoff, S. & Aaronson, S.A. (1989) Purification and characterization of a newly identified growth factor specific for epithelial cells. Proc Natl Acad Sci USA; 86:802-806.

Rubin, J.S., Bottaro, D.P., Chedid, M., Miki, T., Ron, D., Cheon, G., Taylor, W.G., Fortney, E., Sakata, H., Finch, P.W. & LaRochelle, W.J. (1995) Keratinocyte growth factor. Cell Biol. Intern.; 19:399-411.

Schlessinger, J. (2000) Cell signaling by receptor tyrosine kinases. Cell; 103:211-225.

Scott, I.U., Karp, C.L. & Nuovo, G.J. (2000) Human papillomavirus 16 and 18 expression in conjunctival intraepithelial neoplasia. Ophthalmology.; 109:542-547.

Shackleford, G.M., MacArthur, C.A., Kwan, H.C. & Varmus, H.E. (1993) Mouse mammary tumor virus infection accelerates mammary carcinogenesis in Wnt-1 transgenic mice by insertional activation of int-2/Fgf-3 and Hst/Fgf-4. Proc Natl Acad Sci USA; 90:740-744.

Shimokawa, T., Furukawa ,Y., Sakai, M., Li, M., Miwa, N., Lin, Y.M. & Nakamura, Y. (2003) Involvement of the FGF18 gene in colorectal carcinogenesis, as a novel downstream target of the β-catenin/T-cell factor complex. Cancer Res; 63:6116-6120.

Thiery, J.P. & Sleeman, J.P. (2006) Complex networks orchestrate epithelial-mesenchymal transitions. Nat Rev Mol Cell Biol ; 7:131-142.

Tichelaar, J., Lu, W.W. & Whitsett, J.A. (2000) Conditional expression of fibroblast growth factor-7 in the developing and mature lung, J. Biol. Chem. 275: 11858-11864.

Tickle, C. (1995) Vertebrate limb development. Curr Opin Genet Dev; 5:478-484.

Torres, M.A., Eldar-Finkelman. H., Krebs, E.G. & Moon, R.T. (1999) Regulation of ribosomal S6 protein kinase-p90(rsk), glycogen synthase kinase 3, and beta-catenin in early Xenopus development. Mol Cell Biol; 19:1427-1437.

Tseng, S.C.G. (1989) Concept and application of limbal stem cells. Eye; 3:141-157.

Villanueva, S., Glavic, A., Ruiz, P. & Mayor, R. (2002) Posteriorization by FGF, Wnt, and retinoic acid is required for neural crest induction. Dev Biol; 241:289-301.

Zhang, Y., Call, M.K., Yeh, L.K., Liu, H., Kochel, T., Wang, I.J., Chu, P.H., Taketo, M.M., Jester, J.V., Kao, W.W. & Liu, C.Y. (2010) Aberrant expression of a beta-catenin gain-of-function mutant induces hyperplastic transformation in the mouse cornea. J Cell Sci.; 123:1285-1294.

Zhou, B.P., Deng, J., Xia, W., Xu, J., Li, Y.M., Gunduz, M. & Hung, M.C. (2004) Dual regulation of Snail by GSK-3b-mediated phosphorylation in control of epithelial - mesenchymal transition. Nat Cell Biol; 6:931-940.

4

Conjunctival Intraepithelial Neoplasia – Clinical Presentation, Diagnosis and Treatment Possibilities

Valentín Huerva[1] and Francisco J. Ascaso[2]
[1]Department of Ophthalmology, Universitary Hospital "Arnau de Vilanova" and IRB, Lleida
[2]Department of Ophthalmology, "Lozano Blesa" University Clinic Hospital, Zaragoza, Spain

1. Introduction

Conjunctival tumors are one of the most frequent tumors of the eye and adnexa. They comprise a large variety of conditions, from benign lesions such as papilloma to malignant lesions such as epidermoid carcinoma or melanoma which may threaten visual function and patient´s life if not diagnosed early. Although conjunctival tumors may arise from any type of the conjunctival cells, epithelial and melanocytic are the most frequent origins. Epithelial tumors account for a third to half of all tumors, with a higher prevalence in countries with larger actinic exposure. Aproximately 40% of the tumors have an epithelial origin and 64.5 % of them were pre-cancerous lesions (Saornil et al, 2009). The clinical differentiation between pre-cancerous benign and malign lesions is difficult, requiring a biopsy for a definitive diagnosis.

Squamous neoplasia of the conjunctiva /cornea is a rare malignancy of conjunctival limbal stem cells, and the management of this malignancy may affect the ultimate outcome. The clinical distinction of squamous conjunctival neoplasia from other amelanocytic conjunctival tumors is based on certain clinical features of the tumor, and its correct management requires an understanding of normal anatomy and histology of the cornea and conjunctiva, as well as knowledge of the principles of tumor management.

Conjunctiva is a thin and flexible mucous membrane that extends from the internal surface of the eyelids to the fornix and anterior ocular surface up to the corneoscleral limbus. Histologically, conjunctiva is similar to other mucous membranes and comprises a non-keratinized stratified epithelium having two or more layers over the stroma formed by fibrovascular connective tissue containing vessels, nervous and lymphatic tissue. Basal layer of epithelium comprises melanocytes which produces melanine and inject it in the surrounding cells. Throughout the length of epithelium we can observe cup-shaped cells in charge of producing the mucoid component of the lacrimal film. These cells are called *goblet cells*.

1.1 Definition of Ocular Surface Squamous Neoplasias (OSSN)

Squamous cell neoplasia may occur as a localized lesion confined to the surface epithelium (conjunctival intraepithelial neoplasia) or as a more invasive squamous cell carcinoma that has broken through the basement membrane and invaded the underlying stroma (Shields & Shields, 2004).

Currently, the accepted term for the localized variety is conjunctival intraepithelial neoplasia (CIN). However, other authors prefer the terms dysplasia (mild, moderate, or severe) and carcinoma-in-situ. Where there are no longer normal surface cells then the process may be termed carcinoma-in-situ. Those cases where the cornea is invaded by the process are usually called conjunctiva-cornea intraepithelial neoplasia (CCIN). Squamous neoplasia constitutes the most frequent primary malignancy of the ocular surface.

1.1.1 Conjuntival Intraepithelial Neoplasia (CIN)

CIN is confined to the epithelium by definition. The term CIN was suggested in 1978, according with the general pathologic classification of intraepithelial tumors developed for cervical intraepithelial neoplasia (Pizzarello & Jakobiec, 1978). CIN includes previous terms referred to this epithelial neoplasia such as: Bowen´s disease, Bowenoid epithelioma, intraepithelial epithelioma, intraepithelioma, dysplasia and carcinoma in situ (CIS).

Subjective symptoms referred by the patients include: foreign body sensation, redness, irritation, and a growth on the ocular surface (Giaconi & Karp, 2003).

Clinically, CIN appears as a fleshy, sessile or minimally elevated lesion usually at limbus in the interpalpebral fissure and less commonly in the forniceal or tarsal conjunctiva (Shields & Shields, 2004). The limbal lesion may extend for a variable distance into the epithelium of the adjacent cornea. A white plaque (leukoplakia) may occur on the surface of the lesion due to secondary hyperkeratosis.

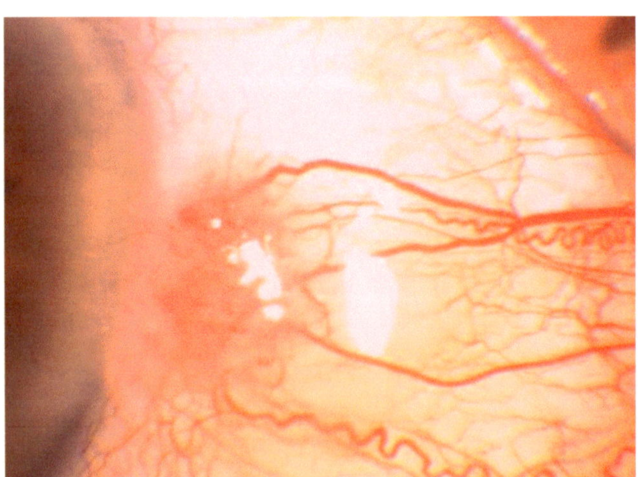

Fig. 1. Conjunctival intraepithelial neoplasia showing corneal invasion.

1.1.2 Squamous Cell Carcinoma (SCC)

Squamous cell carcinoma is characterized by an extension of abnormal epithelial cells through the basement membrane to gain access to the conjunctival stroma (Shields & Shields, 2004). Clinically, invasive squamous cell carcinoma is similar to CIN; however, it may be larger and more elevated than CIN. Even though the cells of invasive squamous cell carcinoma gain access to the blood vessels and lymphatic channels, regional and distant metastases are both rather uncommon. Clinically it is very difficult to distinguish between CIN and SCC (Erie et al, 1986). In many occasions it is necessary to perform a biopsy.

1.2 Incidence

OSSN accounts for only 5% of all ocular malignancies (Lee & Hirts, 1995). CIN is the most common conjunctival malignancy (Grossniklaus et al, 1987). CIN occurred more commonly in pale-skinned groups than in more pigmented people, with an increased incidence in males (75%) vs females (25%), and a mean age of 60 years (Grossniklaus et al, 1987). OSSN associated with human immunodeficiency virus (HIV) is seen at younger ages (average 35 years), usually not in a bulbar location, and is more aggressive from a clinical point of view. Its incidence can vary from 0.13 to 1.9/100.000 inhabitants (Lee & Hirts, 1995), (Giaconi & Karpp, 2003), (Saornil et al, 2009). OSSN incidence varies geographically, increasing with closer distance to the equator. For example, Uganda has 1.2 cases/100.000 persons/year compared to the United Kingdom with less than 0.02 cases/100.000 persons/year. This might suggest a role of ultraviolet light exposure in the etiology of these tumors. US data indicate an incidence of 0.03/100.000 people/year, with a 6-fold increase in association with HIV infection (Sun et al, 1997), (Verma et al, 2008). The lesions are more common in males and elderly, with the majority occurring at the limbus. In Africa the incidence is changing. The tumor is more common, aggressive, more frequent in young persons, especially women (Ateenyi-Agaba, 1995). This is relationed with the coexistence of pandemic AIDS and exposition to the human papillomavirus (HPV) and ultraviolet radiations. Africa has the highest prevalence of HPV infection in the world (with more than 25 % of women from 15 to 74 years affected), followed by South America (14.3%), Asia (8.7%) and Europe (5.2%) (Clifford, 2005). A study in the Kampala Cancer Registry in Uganda showed an increase from 6 cases of OSSN/1.000.000 persons per year between 1970 and 1988 to 35 cases/1.000.000 persons per year in 1992 (Ateenyi-Agaba, 1995). In Australia, a study found that 78.5% of affected people were male with a mean age of 60 years (Lee & Hirst, 1997). Similarly, another study in United Kingdom showed that the 77% were male, being 69% of them older than 60 years (McKelvie et al, 2002). Nevertheless, a study in Zimbabwe found that a 70% of patients were young women with a mean age of 35 years (Pola et al, 2003), while in South Africa mean age was 37 years (Mahomed & Chetty, 2002). A study in Tanzania showed that the 45.8% of 168 conjunctival biopsies were OSSN (Poole, 1999).

2. Etiologic factors for CIN

To date, CIN etiology remains unclear. The most probably explanation may be multifactorial causes. There are many known factors which may contribute to the development of these neoplasias.

The first one is the age, with an average of 60 years (Lee & Hirst, 1995). However, it ranges from 4 to 90 years. The second factor attributed is the UV light exposure (Lee et al, 1994). This justify a higher prevalence of CIN in the ecuatorial areas, as we have previously commented. The exposition to the petroleum products, heavy cigarrete smoking, light hair and ocular pigmentation have also been associated (Napora et al, 1990).

Younger patients affected by Xeroderma pigmentosum (Herle et al, 1991) and HIV may show a higher incidence (Karp et al, 1996). The majority of CIN cases reported in Africa are HIV-positive: 71% in Uganda, 86% in Malawi (Waddell, et al 1996), 70.6% in South Africa (Mahomed & Chetty 2002) and 92.3% in Zimbabwe (Porges & Groisman 2003). On the other hand, the prevalence of CIN in a HIV-positive population in Kenya was 7.8% (Chisi et al, 2006). These findings suggest that CIN is a marker for HIV infection. OSSN in HIV/AIDS patients presents at a younger age (35-40 years old) than in HIV-negative patients (Timm et al, 2004). Additionally, malignancy seems to be more aggressive in HIV/AIDS patients (Kaimbo 1998). It is unclear whether immunosuppression or HIV itself plays a role in this pathogenesis. Although it has been speculated about the role of HIV in conjunctival squamous cell carcinoma in immunosuppression and activation of oncogenic viruses such as HPV in the conjunctiva, thus far only oral and anogenital HPV has been shown to occur more frequently in HIV-positive patients (Verma et al, 2008). Immunosuppression itself may contribute to the carcinogenesis. Several studies have also demonstrated an association between immunosupression secondary to HIV infection and increased risk of cervical intraepithelial neoplasia (Palefsky, 1991).

The role of HPV remains also unclear in the etiology of CIN. It has been proved the causal relationship between HPV type 16 and 18 and uterine cervical carcinoma (Scott el al, 2002), (Giaconi & Karp, 2003), (Verma et al, 2008). However, multiple studies worldwide have failed to document an unequivocal association of HPV with conjunctival squamous cell carcinoma (Tuppurainen, 1992), (Eng et al, 2002). A small study of CIN has demonstrated mRNA from the *E6* region of HPV, which signals actively transcribed virus (Scott et al 2002). Furthermore, this study in United States demonstrated the lack of such mRNA from normal conjunctivas, whereas African case series have revealed a high prevalence of HPV DNA in clinically normal conjunctivas for HPV 6 and 11, but not HPV 16 and 18 were found (Verma et al, 2008). In controversy HPV types 16 and 18 may be detected in CIN, in non neoplasic lesions and in apparently healthy conjunctiva (Karcioglu & Issa, 1997). Another study in Thailand concluded that solar elastosis is more frequently founded in OSSN cases that in controls, and HPV DNA was not found in any of the specimens (Tulvatana et al, 2003). HPV 5 and 8 were the most common in nearly half of OSSN in a series recently reported in Uganda (Ateenyi-Agaba, et al 2010). The frequency was the same in infected VIH than in non infected VIH. HPV 5 is not reported in caucasian CIN. HPV 16 and 18 may considerer as disease of sexual transmission whereas HPV 5 may appear by other possible vias. It has been shown in cervical cancer that the high risk variants HPV 16 and HPV 18 lead to carcinogenesis by inactivating tumor suppressor gene products *p53* and *Rb* in the host with the viral oncoproteins E6 and E7, respectively (Verma et al, 2008). Furthermore, integration of viral sequences into the host genome leads to the constitutive expression of E6/E7 in transformed cervical cells. HPV 5 show highest downregulation of basal interleukin-8 secretion in primary human keratinocytes. This may weaken the response to UV-induced damage and consecutively mutations. Given the conflicting association studies, it appears that UV-B radiation plays a much greater role than HPV in the etiology of CIN (Verma et al, 2008).

3. Clinical presentation of CIN

The clinical presentation of CIN may be variable. There are many different pictures on the ocular surface that constitute a CIN. The subjective symptoms may be also variable in intensivity. Appart from the presence of a growth or mass in their ocular suface, patients may complain no symptoms. Size, color and growth may be variable in each case. The presence of a red eye make, sometimes, that the patient was treated as a conjunctivitis. Foreing body sensation, redness, or irritation may be referred many times. CIN is characterized by a slowly progressive course with low malignant potential. In general, two forms of CIN have been described: nodular (or well localized) and diffuse. The diffuse type is less common and very difficult to diagnose in early stages. This situation may be similar to a chronic conjunctivitis and its surgical treatment may result complicated because clinical borders of the lesion may be indistinguishable (Lee & Hirst, 1995), (Giaconi & Karp, 2003).

The typical location of this slow-growing lesion is the interpalpebral limbus, but it may also arise in the forniceal and palpebral conjunctiva. Limbal lesions may spread onto the cornea. The abnormal corneal epithelium has a frosted appearance with fringed borders and usually demonstrates diffuse punctate staining. Flat or elevated, the lesion may appear relatively translucent, gelatinous, or pearly white. Secondary hyperkeratosis over the surface of the lesion may give rise to a white plaque-like appearance clinically named leukoplakia. Often, there are surrounding corkscrew-like vascular tufts. Pigmentation may be seen and the lesion may be clinically misdiagnosed as melanoma (Shields et al, 2008).

The percentages of CIN that develops into SCC have not been reported in the literature. In cases of SCC the tumor may reach to eye globe, the orbit and cranial extension, with vision loss due to a enucleation or exenteration (Lopez-Garcia et al, 2000). Up to 4% rates of metastasis to cervical lymph nodes have been reported, while metastases to distance are less common (Bhattacharyya et al, 1997). There is not a particular simptomatology for every macroscopic form of CIN. Some of the characteristic forms of presentation of precancerous and malignant lesions are described:

3.1 Precancerous lesions: Actinic keratosis and conjunctival keratotic plaque

Both lesions, impossible to differentitate clinically, consist in a white plaque on the limbal or bulbar conjunctiva, in the exposed interpalpebral conjunctiva. They have a low grade of proliferation and very few possibilities to convert into CIN or SCC. Definitive diagnosis consisted in the histological study (Mauriello el al 1996), (Shields et al, 2004).

3.2 Leucoplakic lesions

Leucoplakia (white plaque) consist in a conjuctival lesion, generally at the limbus, which may be round or irregular. A process of keratosis is involved (Shields & Shields, 2008). These lesion may also extend onto the cornea. Likewise, leukoplakic lesions may appear onto a very diffuse CIN (Huerva et al, 2006). Extensive leukoplakia should raise suspiction of invasive SCC (Shields & Shields, 2008).

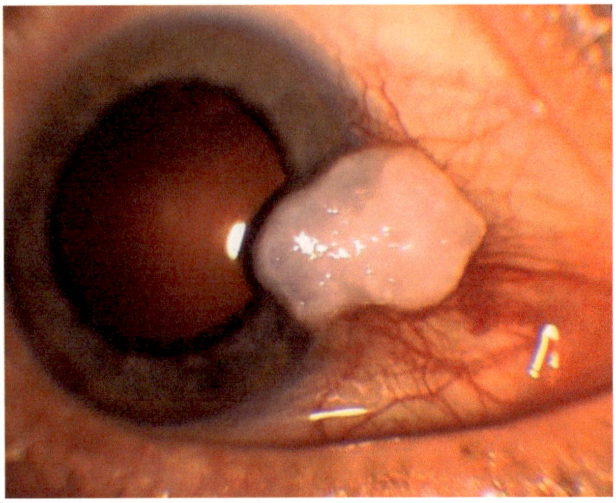

Fig. 2. Leukoplakic CIN, occuping conjunctiva, limbus and cornea at the interpalpebral fissure. Histopatology showed complete dysplasia of the epithelium.

3.3 Papillomatous lesions

CIN may developed simulating a sessile papilloma. The lesion consist in a fleshy red appearance owing numerous fine vascular channels that ramify throughtout the stroma beneath the epithelial surface of the lesion (Shields & Shields, 2008). The presence of displasic epithelial cells helps to the differential diagnosis between papilloma and CIN. In rare occasions papillomas may developed into a CIN.

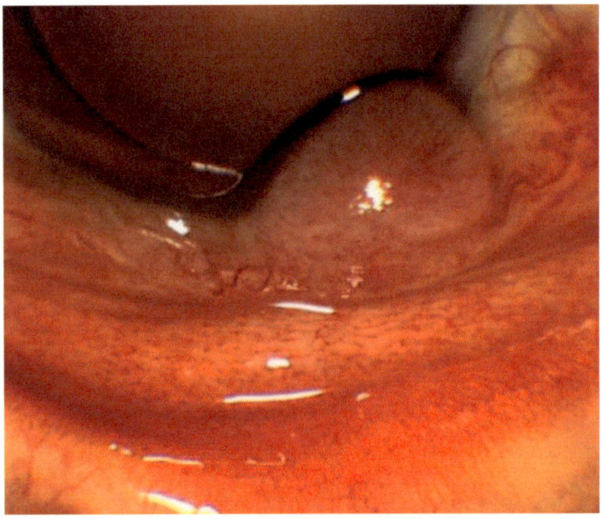

Fig. 3. CIN with papillomatous appearance at the exposed interpalpebral fissure affecting the limbus.

3.4 Fleshly lesions

Clinically, CIN appears as a fleshy, sessile, or minimally elevated lesion usually at the limbus in the interpalpebral fissure and less commonly in the forniceal or palpebral conjunctiva. The size of extension may be variable in each case. The presence of redness may simulate an inflammation. Extensive cases consist in a red gelatinous mass with vascular dilatations that may invade superior and nasal bulbar conjunctiva, including the caruncula, inferior conjuctiva and fornix invading tarsal conjunctiva and even corneal extension. Plaques of leukoplakia may also be present. (Erie et al, 1986), (Shields & Shields, 2004), (Huerva et al, 2006).

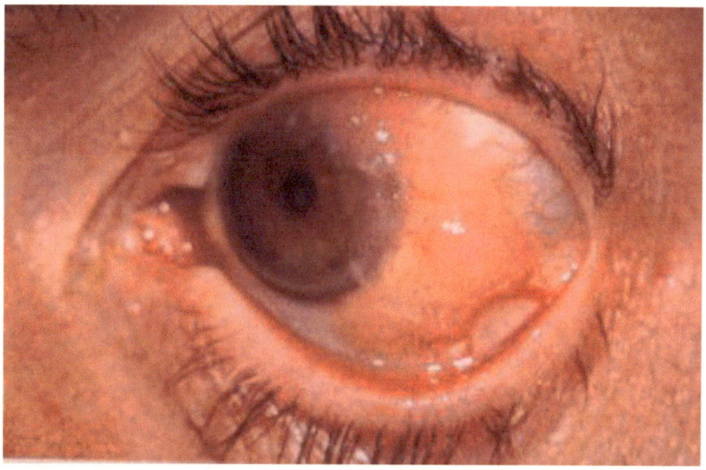

Fig. 4. Fleshy nodular gelatinous mass involving bulbar conjunctiva and limbus.

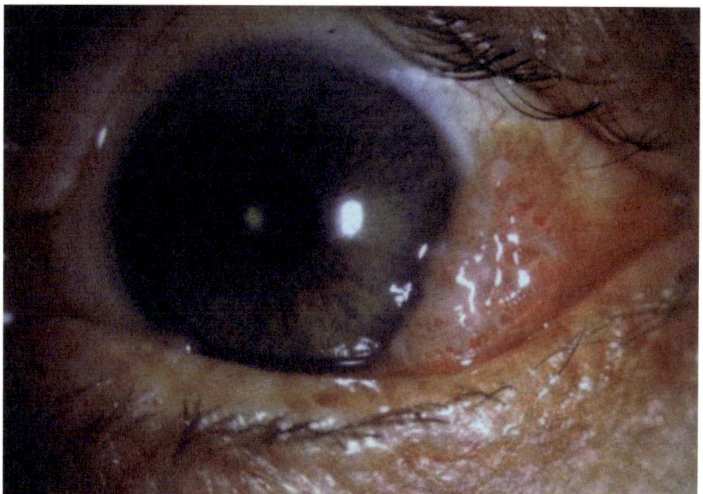

Fig. 5. Fleshy nodular mass at the interpalpebral bulbar conjunctiva.

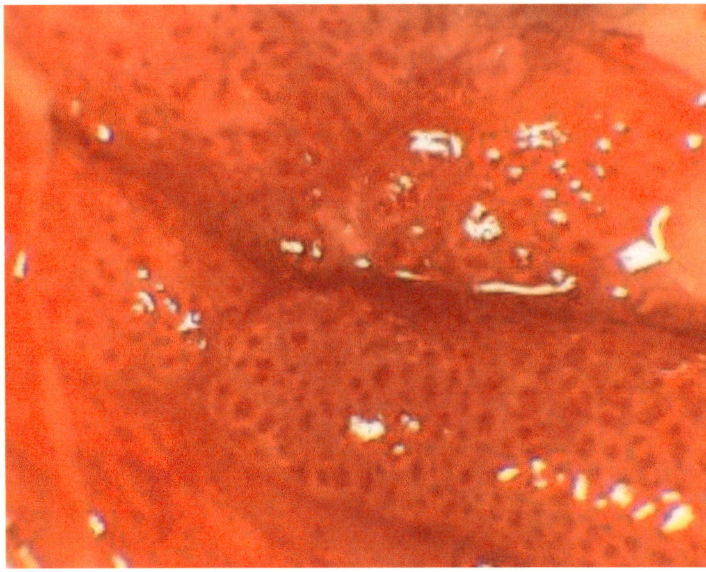

Fig. 6. Fleshy diffuse CIN affecting the inferior fornix resembling a chronic conjunctivitis.

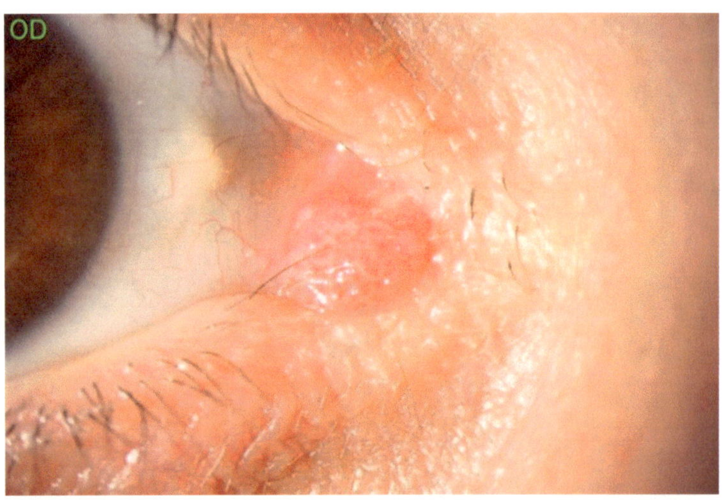

Fig. 7. Nodular fleshy CIN at the caruncle.

3.5 Corneal invasion (Conjunctiva-Cornea Intraepithelial Neoplasia) (CCIN)

This condition is called when the fleshy or papillomatous CIN lesions invading the superficial cornea. The lesions are well documented at the limbus occuping different degrees. Generally, in the extensive cases the cornea may be invaded (Huerva et al, 2006). The form of invasion may be variable: nodular, frothy vascular irregular extension and pedunculated and may simulate other conjunctival lesions as a pterigium or pannus (Shields & Shields, 2008).

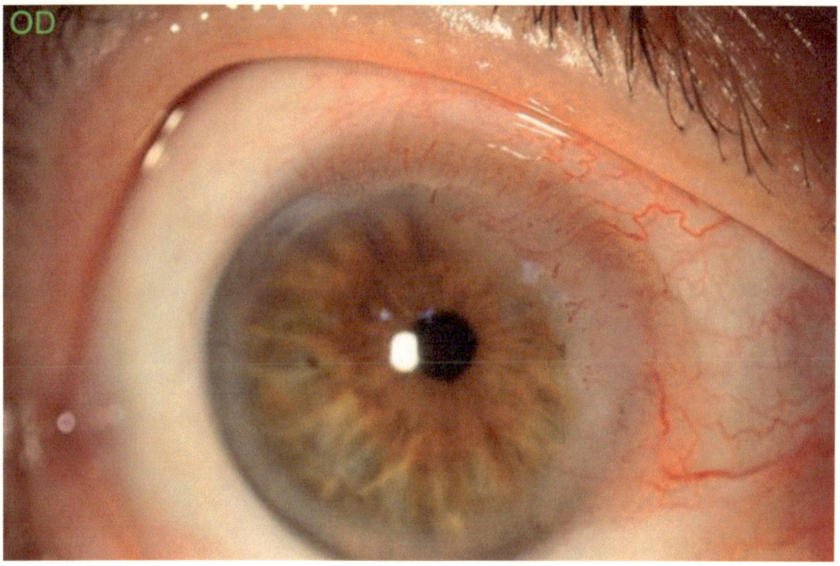

Fig. 8. CCIN: dysplasia in 180 degrees at the corneoscleral limbus resembling a corneal pannus.

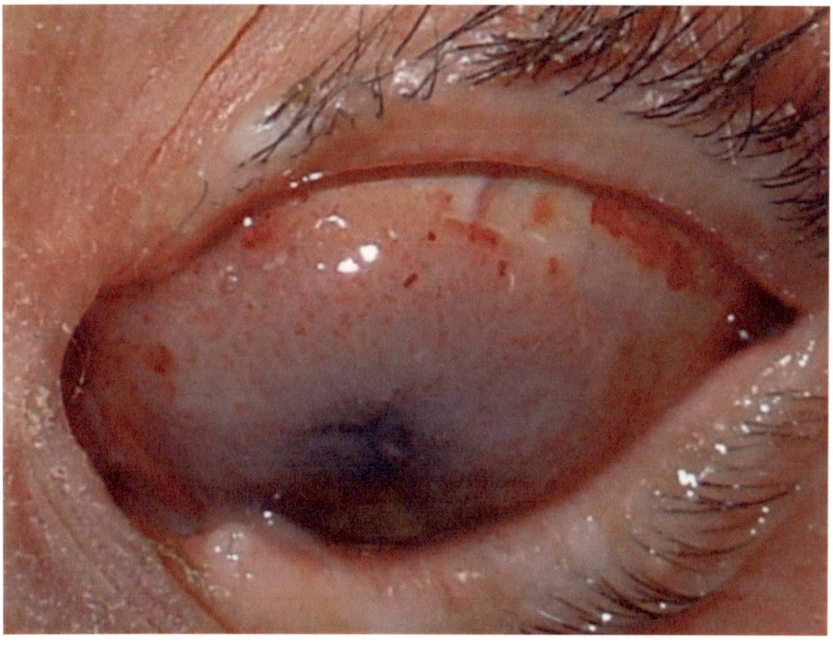

Fig. 9. CCIN. The tumor invade almost 3/4 size of the corneal surface.

3.6 Squamous cell carcinoma

Clinical presentation of invasive SCC is the same that the CIN. As the CIN, it is frequently observed at the interpalpebral region. Definitive diagnosis is only histopathologic (Shileds & Shields, 2008).

There are some different histological types with very aggressive potential effect. Mucoepidermoid or adenoid SSC has an epidermal component and variable quantities of mucin. It often presents with inflammatory signs (Mauriello et al, 1997). Spindle cell SCC is composed by pleomorphic spindle cells. Both are very aggressive with high potential of ocular invasion and distant metastases (Shields & Shields, 2008).

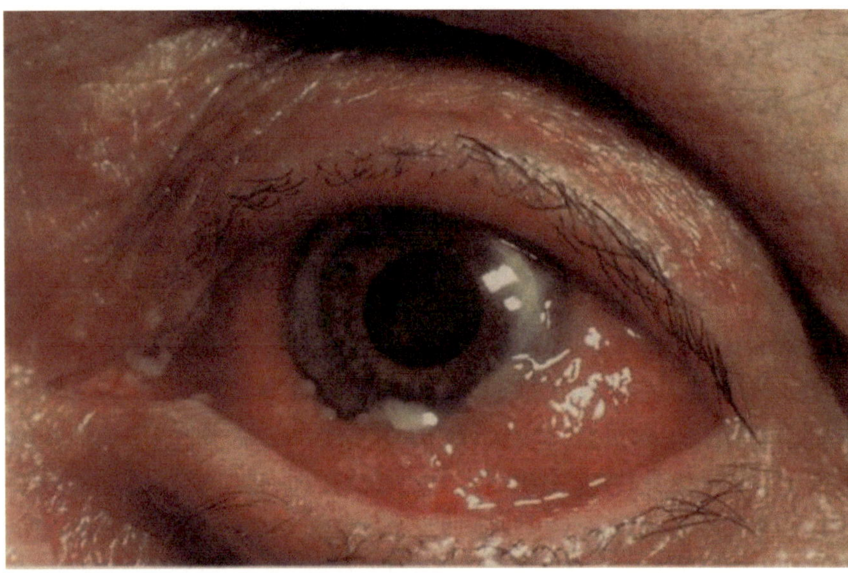

Fig. 10. Diffuse SCC involving the whole bulbar conjunctiva. Leukoplakic plaques are also present. Chronic conjunctivitis may be misdiagnosed. It clinically resembles a diffuse CIN. For definitive diagnosis a incisional biopsy is necessary.

4. Diferential diagnosis

Clinical differentiation between CIN and other limbal lesions is based on characteristic clinical features (Erie et at, 1986). However, it is generally admitted that the grade of dysplasia cannot be consistently determined on clinical inspection alone (Lee & Hirts, 1995). The main differential diagnoses for localized CIN include pinguecula, pterygium and squamous papilloma. The differential diagnosis of conjuctival amelanotic tumors includes CIN, invasive SCC, malignant melanoma and a variety of benign described entities, which include squamous papilloma, solar elastosis and epithelial hyperplasia, keratosis or reactive atypia. Conjunctival pseudoepitheliomatous hyperplasia, keratoacantoma, and conjunctival hereditary benign intraepithelial dyskeratosis may be also considered in CIN diferential diagnosis (Shields & Shields, 2008). In these cases the hyperkeratosis and inflammatory cells are present in the histologic samples. Solar elastosis is a pathognomonic sign in the pathological diagnosis of degenerative diseases of the conjunctiva such as pingueculae and pterygium. In a study, the clinical diagnosis of OSSN may be accurate in 89.5% of the cases (Tulwatana et al, 2003). Solar elastosis was found in 53.3% of OSSN cases compared to 3.3% of matched controls. Solar elastosis has also been identified as a risk factor for OSSN (Tulwatana et al, 2003). On this basis, the clinical diagnosis alone cannot distinguish benign conjuntival limbal tumors from OSSN or reliably exclude, albeit an uncommon diagnosis, amelanotic malignant melanoma. The difficulty in distinguishing clinically between pterygium and CIN was illustrated in a histopathological review of 533 cases of pterygium, in which 9.8% were shown to have evidence of dysplasia (Hirst et al, 2009). The capacity of a clinician to distinguish between grades of CIN, or between CIN and invasive SCC, is also limited (Rudkin et al, 2011). Clinical diagnosis of CIN may be increased by the use of exfoliation or impression cytology. However, histopathology of the excised tumor is the only reliable diagnostic method and it is generally accepted to be the most appropriate approach to lesions presumed to be CIN. The main hazard of clinical misdiagnosis of an excised benign limbal lesion is exposing the patient to unnecessary surgery. For an experienced ocular oncologist, the misdiagnosis of localized limbal OSSN occurs in 10.5% of cases (Rudkin et al, 2011).

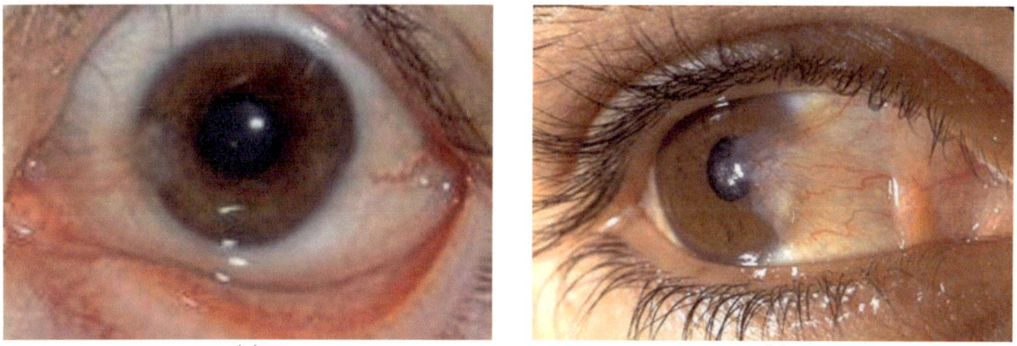

(a) (b)

Fig. 11. Images of Pterigium (a,b) with corneal invasion may resembling in some a cases a CIN. On the other hand in already of 10 % of the cases may show epithelial conjuntival atypia.

5. Impression cytology in diagnosis of CIN

The management of ocular surface neoplasia depends on the ability to distinguish between benign, preinvasive, and invasive lesions. However, follow-up of suspicious lesions by repeated biopsies may cause complications such as scarring, lid deformity, limbal deficiency, and patient discomfort.

As it has been described, the clinical appearance of the lesion may be suggestive of CIN. However, a tissue biopsy is necessary to confirm the diagnosis. Because many patients with primary or recurrent CIN may be treated with topical chemotherapy without surgical excision of the lesion, impression cytology has been used to confirm the diagnosis without performing histological evaluation of the excisional biopsy. Impression cytology is a simple technique for removing one to three superficial layers of the epithelium by applying collecting devices, either cellulose acetate filter papers or Biopore membrane device. Rates of positivity between 77 and 80% have been reported (Nolan et al, 1994), (Tole et al, 2001). The disadvantage is that the superficial nature of the sample, which sometimes only contains keratinized cells, may be falsely negative. Cytological assessment does not provide enough information regarding the deepest structure of the lesion, in particular, evidence of invasion. Abundance of surface keratin may make sampling inaccurate. Another limitation is that impression cytology may not distinguish in situ from minimally invasive disease, because only superficial cells are collected in the method. However, high-grade dysplasia in OSSN cytology findings have a high correlation with histology findings, and the presence of abundance dysplastic cells in cytology suggest preinvasive or invasive disease in subsequent histology (Tananuvat et al, 2008). Although impression cytology have a high sensitivity for the diagnosis of ocular surface squamous neoplasia, including CIN, there are still cases in which impression cytology yields false negative results. The keratotic surface of the lesion or the presence of dysplastic cells deep within the epithelium are the reason for these false negative results. Repeated consecutive applications of the collecting filter paper to the surface of CIN by approaching the deeper epithelium may result in higher sensitivity of the technique to confirm the diagnosis (Kheirkhah et al, 2011). For the diagnosis of CIN, the second and third applications of impression citology may be significantly more sensitive than the first application. Consecutive repeated applications of the filter paper resulted in a significant higher sensitivity due to access to deeper epithelium. Keratinizing CIN lesions may result in a false negative impression cytology test due to the small number of cells present in the sample. It seems that keratinization leads to more false negative results at first application and repeated sampling in this population of CIN cases is more likely to result in subsequent positive due to the progressive elimination of the keratotic material.

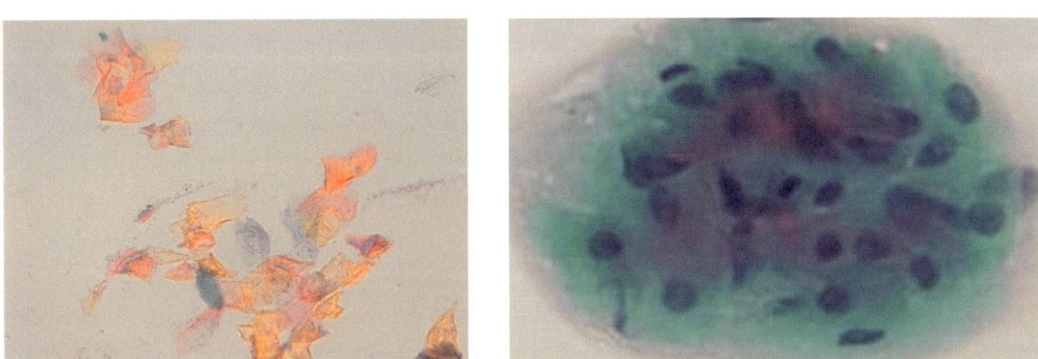

(a) (b)

Fig. 12. Impression cytology from a CIN. Papanicolaou staining. A. False negative for CIN, squamous superficial keratinized material (a). Atypical dysplasic squamous cells from a CIN. Some pleomorphic and hiperchromatic nuclei (b).

In conclusion, repeated consecutive applications of impression citology will lead to a more significant sensitivity for diagnosis in eyes with CIN, thereby obviating the need for excisional biopsy. An additional advantage of impression cytology is the preservation of limbal stem cells, which are located in the basal layer of the limbal epithelium and are responsible for renewal of corneal epithelium throughout life. In most cases of OSSN, the lesions affect predominantly the limbus and have a tendency to recur. Moreover, the technique may be used in the follow-up of patients after treatment to determine the recurrence of the disease, as well as the effects of treatment such as topical chemotherapy.

6. Histopathological findings

The definitive term of CIN or SCC corresponds to the histologic study. When the abnormal conjunctival epithelial cellular proliferation involves only partially the epithelium thickness is classified as mild CIN, a condition also called mild or moderate dysplasia. When it affects full thickness epithelium it is called severe CIN, a condition also called severe dysplasia. In these cases there may be an intact surface layer of cells. Where there are no longer normal surface cells then the process is termed carcinoma-in-situ. Histopathologically, mild CIN (dysplasia) is characterized by a partial thickness replacement of the surface epithelium by abnormal epithelial cells which lack of normal maturation. Severe CIN (severe dysplasia) is characterized by a nearly full-thickness replacement of the epithelium by similar cells. Carcinoma-in-situ represents full thickness replacement by abnormal epithelial cells (Shields & Shields, 2004). Squamous cell carcinoma is an extension of abnormal epithelial cells through the basement membrane to gain access to the conjunctival stroma and have grown in sheets or cords into the stromal tissue. A rare variant of squamous cell carcinoma of the conjunctiva is the mucoepidermoid carcinoma wich presents abundant mucous-secretory cells within cysts. Another rare variety is the spindle cell variant of squamous cell carcinoma that is likewise aggressive. Histopathologically, invasive squamous cell carcinoma is characterized by malignant squamous cell that have violated the basement membrane

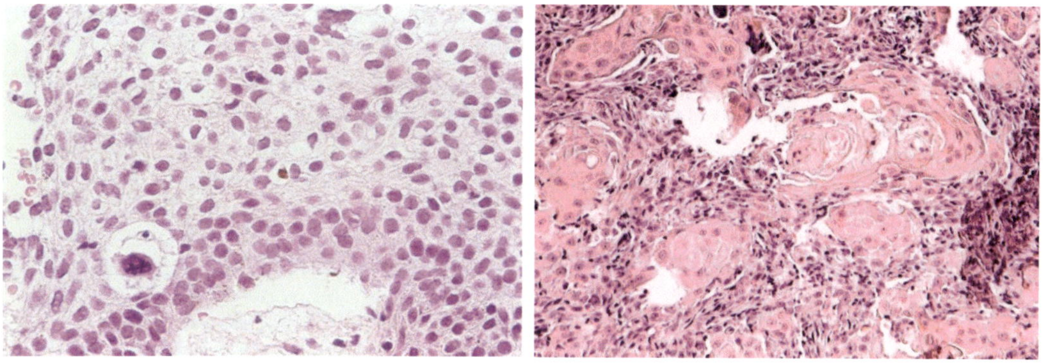

(a) (b)

Fig. 13. Histological specimens. (a): CIN Grade 3. Total replacement of the epithelium by displasic cells. Hematoxilin-eosin x 40. (b): SCC, Displasic cell islets of squamous cells after invading the basement membrane, presence of keratosic perls. Hematoxilin-eosin x 10.

(Shields & Shields, 2004). According to the definition, CIN may be classified in four stages (Kheirkhah et al, 2011):

- ***CIN grade I:*** mild dysplasia limited to the basal one third of the thickness of the corneal or conjunctival epithelium.
- ***CIN grade II:*** moderate dysplasia confined to the basal two thirds of the corneal or conjunctival epithelium.
- ***CIN grade III:*** or SCC in situ: severe dysplasia that may involve the entire thickness of the corneal or conjunctival epithelium without invading the basement membrane.
- ***Invasive SCC:*** severe dysplasia with invasion through the basement membrane.

7. Human Papilloma Virus (HPV) detection

As it has been described in the chapter of etiologic factors, the presence of HPV in cases of CIN remains controversial. DNA of HPV may be detectable by in situ hybridization. HPV types 16 and 18, commonly detectable, in uterine cervix may also be detectable in CIN. However, in non neoplasic lesions and in apparently healthy conjunctiva it may also be detectable (Karcioglu & Issa, 1997). In African case series there is a high prevalence of DNA HPV 6 and 11, but not HPV 16 and 18 (Verma et al, 2008). On the other hand, in a series reported recently in Uganda, HPV 5 and 8 were the most common in nearly half of OSSN (Ateenyi-Agaba, et al, 2010). We have detected the presence of DNA HPV type 11. It is possible that different HPV associated to other risk factors may contribute to the development of CIN.

The presence of DNA HPV is not strictly necessary in the diagnosis of CIN. However, when it is possible its determination may clarify the role of these different types of virus in the development of CIN.

8. Staging for conjunctival intraepithelial neoplasia

CIN constitutes a localized malignant situation that, in absence of treatment, may growth progressively with possible transformation into SCC. It develops rarely metastases at distance or produces ocular, orbital or intraccraneal invasion. The clinical TNM classification of the conjunctival carcinoma is as follows (McGowan, 2009) :

Clinical classification (TNM):

Primary tumor (T)

TX Primary tumor cannot be assessed

T0 No evidence of primary tumor

Tis Carcinoma *in situ*

T1 Tumor 5 mm or less in greatest dimension

T2 Tumor more than 5 mm. in greatest dimension, without invasion of adjacent structures

T3 Tumor invades adjacent structures (excluding the orbit)

T4 Tumor invades the orbit with or without further extension

T4a Tumor invades orbital soft tissues, without bone invasion

T4b Tumor invades bone

T4c Tumor invades adjacent paranasal sinuses

T4d Tumor invades brain

Regional lymph nodes (N)

NX Regional lymph nodes cannot be assessed

N0 No regional lymph node metastasis

N1 Regional lymph node metastasis

Distant metastasis (M)

MX Distant metastasis cannot be assessed

M0 No distant metastasis

M1 Distant metastasis

According to this classification with the difference of clinical appearance, the cases of CIN may be: Tis, T1 or T2, N0 and M0.

9. Treatment

The management of CIN or SCC of the conjunctiva varies with the extent or recurrence of the lesion.

9.1 Surgical treatment

While the extent of the lesion determines the management of lesions in the limbal area involves alcohol epitheliectomy for the corneal component and partial lamellar scleroconjunctivectomy, with wide margins (4-5 mm) for the conjunctival component followed by freeze-thaw cryotherapy to the remaining adjacent bulbar conjunctiva (The no touch technique) (Shields & Shields, 2004). In some cases, microscopically controlled excision (Mohs surgery) may be performed at the time of surgery to ensure tumor free margins (Buus et al, 1994). Those tumors in the forniceal region can be managed by wide local resection and cryotherapy. Following surgical excision, large conjunctival defects may be successfully reconstructed with transpositional conjunctival flaps, free conjunctival grafts, oral mucosal grafts, and amniotic membrane grafts (Gündüz et al, 2006). In all cases, the full conjunctival component along with the underlying Tenon's fascia should be excised using the "no touch technique". A thin lamella of underlying sclera should be removed, in the limbal región, when the tumor is adherent to the globe. Intraoperative mitomycine-C (MMC) application has also been combined with excision of ocular surface neoplasia to prevent postoperative recurrences (Siganos et al, 2002). However, studies show a 53%

recurrence rate in pathologic studies which revealed involved margins and a 5% recurrence rate when clear margins are confirmed (Erie et al, 1986). In extensive lesions, surgical excision is difficult, and additional procedures have been employed. Extensive resections in very extensive CIN may produce a limbal stem deficiency (Huerva et al, 2006). Adjuvant radiation has the potential complications of cataracts, scleral necrosis, corneal rupture, scarring of the cornea and conjunctiva, moderate to severe conjunctivitis, and loss of eyelashes (Giaconi & Karp, 2003). For those patients with extensive tumors or those tumors that are recurrent, treatment with topical mitomycin C, 5-fluorouracil, or interferon alfa 2b have been employed.

9.2 Topical chemoteraphy

Topical chemotherapy has a number of advantages over surgical approach. It enables to treat the entire ocular surface and is not dependent upon surgical margins. Primary treatment with a chemotherapeutic agent avoids potential complications of surgery, which can include scarring of the conjunctiva and cornea, limbal stem cell failure and incomplete excision of the lesion. Topical chemotherapics may be preferred over surgery by some patients, and when the patient refuse surgery, topical chemotherapics have been successfully used as primary treatment.

9.2.1 Topical mitomycin C (MMC)

For tumors with extensive involvement, where surgical removal bears significant risks for postoperative problems, topical MMC should have been considered for a long time. Topical MMC 0.02% or 0.04% 4 times daily in 7 to 14-day for two cycles (Shields & Shields, 2004) have been successfully employed for preoperative chemoreduction and to manage recurrent and residual tumors following surgical resection (Shields et al, 2002), (Frucht-Pery et al, 2002), (Shields et al,2005). MMC had been effectively used to treat primary CIN, with reported success rates between 85% (Wilson et al, 1997) and 100% (Frucht-Pery & Rozenmam, 1994), (Ramos-Lopez et al, 2004). Another large study has shown topical MMC to be an efficient treatment of most, but not all cases, of CIN. Tumor regrowth occurred in approximately 17% of cases (Frucht-Pery et al,1997). To avoid possible complications, the lacrimal punctal occlusion is mandatory during topical treatment. Chemoreduction with MMC cycles reduced the tumor size, especially in the surrounding thinner portions, and allowed for a subsequent limited surgical excision in all cases (Shields et al, 2005). Possible complications with topical MMC include superficial punctate epitheliopathy (Shields & Shields, 2004), conjunctival hyperemia, pain, allergy, corneal-scleral, melting disturbance of tear film stability, goblet cell loss, squamous metaplasia and limbal stem cells depletion (Frucht-Pery & Rozenmam, 1994), (Wilson et al, 1997), (Dogru et al, 2003), (Dudney & Malecha, 2004), (Khong & Muecke, 2006). Edema and endothelial apoptosis have been observed in experimental models (Chang, 2004). MMC toxicity seems to be dose dependent, occurring with the repetition of treatment cycles. Chemoreduction with topical MMC, followed by interferon alfa 2b (1 million IU/mL) 4 times daily, is an effective treatment in extensive CIN cases where surgical resection with safety margins is infeasible and corneal extension resection and the repetitive cycles of MMC adjunctive could cause a depletion of limbal stem cells and other commented side effects on the ocular surface (Huerva et al,

2006). In a follow-up of 18 months, topical Cyclosporine A (0,05%) combined with topical low dose of MMC (0,01%) four times a day for 12 weeks after positive margins following surgical excision showed no recurrence of the tumor (Tunc & Erbilen, 2006). In these cases Cyclosporine A has been employed by the antineovascular effect on the ocular surface.

9.2.2 5-Fluoracil (5-FU)

Other treatment options in the management of CIN include 5-fluorouracil (5-FU). However, compared with MCC, the experience with this alternative treatment is limited. Topical 1% 5-FU drops used 4 times daily for 2 to 4 days for each cycle and repeated at 30 to 45 day intervals have been reported. Following initial treatment, 4 patients were disease-free with a mean follow-up of 18.5 months. Of the 3 patients with tumor recurrence, 2 remained tumor-free following additional topical 5-FU treatment and 1 patient had a persistent tumor despite additional treatment with 5-FU and became tumor-free following treatment with topical MMC (Yeatts et al, 2000). No adverse reactions to pulsed treatment were reported. Another study using topical 1% 5-FU drops 4 times daily for 4 weeks in 8 eyes with recurrent, incompletely excised, and untreated conjunctival OSSN showed complete clinical regression at 3 months in all cases. OSSN recurred in 1 patient at 6 months but this was successfully treated with another course of 5-FU (Midena et al, 2000). Transient toxic keratoconjunctivitis that was noticeable with this treatment. Short-term complications include lid toxicity in 52% of patients, keratopathy in 11% and epiphora in 5% (Rudkin et al, 2010).

9.2.3 Interferon (INF) alpha 2b

Topical MMC and 5-fluorouracil have been used to reduce recurrence rates when used as an adjunct to surgical escisión and as a primary treatment; however, their use can be associated with marked ocular surface toxicity. Topical (1.000.000 IU/ ml/ four times a day) or subconjuctival INF alfa 2b (3 million IU/ml/ weekly) have been employed to treat CIN. In general, topical INF alpha-2b is well tolerated. Subconjunctival administration presents more side effects as flu-like symptoms (fatigue, fever, myalgias, malaise) and mild liver disturbances (Huerva & Mangues, 2008). Local conjunctival injection and follicular conjunctivitis are the most frequently reported side effects (Schechter et al, 2002) after topical administration. Redness and increase of CIN volume without ocular discomfort have been reported in a case (Huerva el al, 2007). Fine, diffuse, clear epithelial microcysts in the cornea after instillation of topical interferon a-2b have recently documented in other case (Aldave & Nguyen, 2007).

Topical INF alpha 2-b, sometimes combined with subconjunctival INF alpha 2-b, seems to be effective as primary treatment for CIN, in recurrent cases, and also in retreatment after recurrence when INF has been used previously for a short period of time (Huerva & Mangues, 2008). Approximately, 9% of CIN treated with subconjunctival and/or topical INF alpha 2b showed recurrences, and 33 % of them were successfully retreated with topical IFN alpha 2b (Huerva & Magues, 2008). Another one (16,6%) achieved complete remission after intraperioperative MMC (Hawkins et al, 1999). For INF alpha 2b topical treatment, the average time to complete tumor response is 11 weeks (range 2-59). For INF alpha 2b subconjunctival and topical treatment, the average time to complete tumor response is 5.5 weeks (range 2-12), (Huerva & Mangues, 2008). Previous studies found the same observation (Karp et al, 2001). The time to clinical resolution using topical INF alpha 2-b was longer (11.6 weeks) that the combined intralesional and topical interferon (4.5 weeks), but that INF alpha 2b treatment involved fewer side effects. In general, it seems that the disadvantage with topical treatment is the long duration. We must emphasize the importance of long term follow-up for CIN patients because recurrences can occur anywhere from 33 days to 11.5 years (Tabin et al, 1997), although most recurrent CIN occurs within 2 years of initial excision (Schechter et al, 2005).

Many surgeons add adjunctive topical therapy to their surgical regimens for larger lesions (Stone el al, 2005). However, all sizes of lesions could be treated with topical INF alpha as the primary treatment because it is an effective, non-invasive treatment alternative to surgery that increases quality of life with low costs (Huerva et al, 2006), (Huerva et al, 2007), (Huerva et al, 2009). Actually, no clear consensus on the best way to manage the disorder has been established, because long-term, well designed studies are still needed. However, two recent studies have addressed the above questions and confirmed the effectiveness of this topical therapy for CIN. The first study (Schechter, et al, 2008) demonstrated total resolution of the tumor in 96.4% of cases treated with INF alfa 2b with a mean follow-up of 42.4 months. The second study (Sturges et al, 2008) demonstrated that topical treatment with INF and surgical excision have the same effectiveness as primary treatment for CIN for a mean follow-up of 35.6 months. The authors concluded that topical IFN alfa-2b and aggressive surgical excision can be considered equally effective as first choice for treating CIN. Topical INF alfa-2b has some advantages over conventional excision, including the reduction of risk to loose limbar stem cells secondary to surgical trauma and, thus, compromising the integrity of the ocular surface. This therapeutic mode can be recommended particularly for patients who reject any type of surgery, or mentally retarded patients in whom surgery is complicated as well as extended cases where an aggressive excision could cause the loss of limbar stem cells (Huerva, 2008).

Topical INF or subconjunctival INF remains a controversial issue. A recent report (Karp et al, 2010) concluded that subconjunctival 0.5 ml injection of 3 million IU IFN alfa 2b is a viable medical alternative for the treatment of ocular surface squamous neoplasia (OSSN) with a mean duration of follow-up of 55 months. The authors state that the advantages of perilesional INF alfa 2b injection include more rapid tumor resolution, ensured compliance, and perhaps more direct delivery to the tumor site when compared with topical INF drops. However, some patients may be apprehensive about receiving injections around the eye and may prefer eyedrops. A single weekly injection of INF may have better compliance than 4 eye-drops per day dosing for a mean of three months in many patients. Direct delivery to the tumor site may occur in well-localized lesions, while annular lesions or multifocal disease requires injection over the entire involved area, increasing the risk of conjunctival hemorrhage. By contrast, topical therapy is delivered to the entire ocular surface and has very good success rates. Topical therapy could be recommended for patients who reject any surgical procedure or those who are apprehensive about injections.

Weekly subconjunctival Pegilated INF alpha 2b might be an alternative in resistant cases of CIN or recurrent conjunctival papillomatosis avoiding a mutilating surgery (Tseng, 2009), (Karp et al, 2010).

9.2.4 Other treatment possibilities

Other treatment options in the management of conjuctival OSSN include topical retinoids, cidofovir and photodynamic therapy (PDT). Topical unguent of trans-reinoic acid (0,01%) showed complete resolution of CIN in 20% of cases, whereas 40% showed only partial response (Espana el al, 2003). This treatment may be then only adjuvant to surgery

Regression of diffuse conjunctival CIN was demonstrated following a 6 week course of topical cidofovir eyedrops (2.5 mg/ml) with later residual lesion after surgical excision (Sherman et al, 2002).

Following PDT, using verteporfin, a complete clinical CIN regression, supported with angiographic evidence, has been reported at 1 month, without any recurrence for a mean follow-up of 8.6 months (Barbazetto et al, 2004). Likewise, histopathological evidence showing tumor regression following treatment with PDT in a patient with in situ CIN has been reported (Sears et al, 2008).

10. References

Aldave AJ, Nguyen A. Ocular surface toxicity associated with topical interferon a-2b. Br J Ophthalmol 2007;91: 1087-88.

Ateenyi-Agaba C. Conjunctival squamous cell carcinoma associated with HIV infection in Kampala, Uganda. Lancet 1995; 345: 695-96.

Ateenyi-Agaba C, Franceschi S, wabwire-Mangen F et al. Human papillomavirus infection and squmaus cell carcinoma of the conjunctiva. Br J Cancer 2010; 102: 262-67.

Bahattacharyya N, Wenokur RK, Rubin PA. Metastasis of squamous cell carcinoma of the conjunctiva. Case report and review of the literature. Am J Otolaryngol 1997; 18: 217-19.

Barbazetto IA, Lee TC, Abramson DH. Treatment of conjunctival squamous cell carcinoma with photodynamic therapy. *Am J Ophthalmol* 2004; 138: 183-89.

Buus DR, Tse DT, Folberg R, Buuns DR. Microscopically controlled excision of conjunctival squamous cell carcinoma. *Am J Ophthalmol* 1994; 117: 97-102.

Chang SW. Early corneal edema following topical application of mitomycin-C. J Cataract Refract Surg 2004; 30: 1742-50.

Chisi SK, Kollmann MKH, Karimurio J. Conjunctival squamous cell carcinoma in patients with Human Immunodeficiency Virus infection seen at two hospitals in Kenya. East African Med J 2006; 83: 267-70.

Clifford GM, Gallus S, Herrero R, Munoz N, Snijders PJF, Vaccarella S, et al. Worldwide distribution of human papillomavirus types in cytologically normal women in the International Agency for Research on Cancer HPV prevalence surveys: a pooled analysis. Lancet 2005; 366: 991-98.

Dogru M, Erturk H, Shimazaki J, Tsubota K, Gul M. Tear function and ocular surface changes with topical mitomycin (MMC) treatment for primary corneal intraephitelial neoplasia. Cornea 2003; 22: 627-39.

Dudney BW, Malecha MA. Limbal stem cell deficiency following topical mitomycin C treatment of conjunctival-corneal intraephitelial neoplasia. Am J Ophthalmol 2004; 137: 950-51.

Eng HL, Lin TM, Chen SY, et al. Failure to detect human papillomavirus DNA in malignant epithelial neoplasms of conjunctiva by polymerase chain reaction. Am J Clin Pathol 2002;117: 429–36.

Erie JC, Campbell RJ, Leisegang TJ. Conjunctival and corneal intraepithelial and invasive neoplasia. Ophtalmology 1986; 93:176-83.

Espana EM, Chodosh J, Mateo AJ, Di Pascuale MA, Tseng SC. Topical retinoids as a noninvasive treatment of conjunctival intraepithelial neoplasia. Microcirugía Ocular 2003, nº4: 1-7.

Frucht-Pery J, Rozenmam Y. Mitomycin C therapy for corneal intraepithelial neoplasia. Am J Ophthalmol 1994; 117: 164-68.

Frucht-Pery J, Sugar J, Baum J et al. Mitomycin C treatment for conjunctival-corneal intraepithelial neoplasia: a multicenter experience. Ophthalmology 1997; 104: 2085-93.

Frucht-Pery J, Rozenman Y, Pe'er J. Topical mitomycin-C for partially excised conjunctival squamous cell carcinoma. Ophthalmology 2002; 109: 548-52.

Giaconi JA, Karp CL. Current treatment options for conjunctival and corneal intraepithelial neoplasia. Ocul Surf 2003;1: 66-73.

Grossniklaus HE, Green WR, Luckenbach M, Chan CC. Conjunctival lesions in adults. A clinical and histopathologic review. Cornea 1987; 6:78-116.

Gündüz K, Uçakhan OO, Kanpolat A, Günalp I. Nonpreserved human amniotic membrane transplantation for conjunctival reconstruction after excision of extensive ocular surface neoplasia. *Eye* 2006; 20: 351-57.

Hawkins AS, Yu J, Hamming NA, Rubenstein JB. Treatment of recurrent conjunctival papillomatosis with mytomycin C. Am J Ophthalmol 1999; 128:638-40.

Herle RW, Durso F, Metzler JP, Varsa EW. Epibulbar squmaous cell carcinomas in brothers with xeroderma pigmantosa. J Pediatr Ophthalmol Strabismus 1991; 28. 350-53.

Hirst LW, Axelsen RA, Schwab I. Pterygium and associated ocular surface squamous neoplasia. Arch Ophthalmol 2009; 127: 31-2.

Huerva V, Mateo AJ, Mangues I, Jurjo C. Short-term mitomycin C followed by long-term interferon alpha 2β for conjunctiva-cornea intraepithelial neoplasia. Cornea 2006; 25:1220-23.

Huerva V, Sánchez MC, Mangues I. Tumor-volume increase at beginning of primary treatment with topical interferon alpha 2-beta in a case of conjunctiva-cornea intraepithelial neoplasia. J Ocul Pharmacol Ther 2007;23:143-45.

Huerva V, Mangues I. Treatment of conjunctival squamous neoplasias with interferon alpha 2b. J Fr Ophtalmol 2008; 31: 317-25.

Huerva V. Topical interferon alfa-2b or surgical excision for primary treatment of conjunctiva-cornea intraepithelial neoplasia. Arch Soc Esp Oftalmol 2009; 84: 5-6

Huerva V, Mangues I, Schoenenberger JA. Interferon alpha 2b eyedrops as treatment of conjunctival intraepithelial neoplasia. Farm Hosp 2009; 33: 335-36.

Kaimbo WA, Kaimbo D, Parys-Van Ginderdeuren R, Missotten L. Conjunctival squamous cell carcinoma and intraepithelial neoplasia in AIDS patients in Congo Kinshasa. Bull Soc Belge Ophtalmol 1998; 268: 135–41.

Karcioglu ZA, Issa TM. Human papillomavirus in neoplastic and non-neoplastic conditions of the external eye. Br J Ophthalmol 1997; 81: 595-598.

Karp CL, Scott IU, Chang TS, Pflugfelder SC. Conjunctival intraepithelial neoplasia: a possible marker for human immunodeficiency virus infection ?. Arch Ophthalmol 1996; 114: 257-61.

Karp CL, Moor JK, Rosa RH Jr. Treatment of conjunctival and corneal intraepithelial neoplasia with topical interpferon alpha-2b. Ophthalmology 2001; 108: 1093-98.

Karp CL, Galor A, Chhabra S, Barnes SD, Alfonso EC. Subconjunctival/Perilesional recombinant interferon α2b for ocular surface squamous neoplasia. Ophthalmology 2010; 117: 2241-46.

Karp CL, Galor A, Lee Y, Yoo SH. Pegylated interferon alpha 2b for treatment of ocular surface squamous neoplasia: a pilot study. Ocul Immunol Inflamm 2010;18:254-60.

Kheirkhah A, Mahbod M, Farzbod F, Zavareh MK, Behrouz MJ, Hashemi H. Repeated applications of impression cytology to increase sensitivity for diagnosis of conjunctival intraepithelial neoplasia. Br J Ophthalmol. 2011 Apr 15. [Epub ahead of print].

Khong JJ, Muecke J. Complications of mitomycin C therapy in 100 eyes with ocular surface neoplasia. Br J Ophthalmol 2006; 90: 819-22.

Lee GA, Hirst LW. Ocular surface squamous neoplasia. Surv Ophthalmol 1995;39: 429-50.

Lee GA, Williams G, Hirst LW, Green AC. Risk factors in the development of ocular surface epithelial dysplasia. Ophthalmology 1994; 101: 360-64.

Lee GA, Hirst LW. Retrospective study of ocular surface squamous neoplasia. Austr New Zealand J Ophthalmol 1997; 25: 269-76.

López García JS, Elosúa de Juan I, González Morales ML, de Pablo Martín C, Alvarez Lledo J, Martínez Garchitorena J. Squamous cell carcinoma of the conjunctiva with orbital invasion. Arch Soc Esp Oftalmol. 2000;75: 637-41.

Mahomed A, Chetty R. Human immunodeficiency virus infection, Bcl-2, p53 protein, and Ki-67 analysis in ocular surface squamous neoplasia. Arch Ophthalmol 2002; 12: 554-8.

Mauriello JA Jr, Napolitano J, McLean IW. Actinic keratosis and dysplasia of the conjunctiva: a clinicopatological study of 45 cases. Can J Ophthalnmol 1996; 30: 312-16.

Mauriello JA, Abdelsalam A, McLean IW. Adenoid aquamous carcinoma of the conjunctiva – a clinicapathological study of 14 cases. Br J Ophthalmol 1997; 81: 1001-05.

McGowan HD. Squamous Neoplasia of the Conjunctiva: The New TNM Classification by the American Joint Committee on Cancer (AJCC). Ophthalmology Rounds 2009; 7 (1) : 130-38E.

McKelvie PA, Daniell M, McNab A, Loughnan M, Santamaria JD. Squamous cell carcinoma of the conjunctiva: a series of 26 cases. British J Ophthalmol 2002; 86: 168-73.

Midena E, Angeli CD, Valenti M, de Belvis V, Boccato P. Treatment of conjunctival squamous cell carcinoma with topical 5-fluorouracil. Br J Ophthalmol 2000; 84: 68-72.

Napora C, Cohen EJ, Genvert GI, et al. Factors associated with conjunctival intraepithelial neoplasia: a case control study. Ophthalmic Surg 1990; 21: 27-30.

Nolan GR, Hirst LW, Wright RG, et al. Application of impression cytology to the diagnosis of conjunctival neoplasms. Diagn Cytopathol 1994;11: 246–49.

Palefsky JM. Human papillomavirus- associated anogenital neoplasia and other solid tumors in human immunodeficiency virus-infected individuals. Curr Opin Oncol 1991; 3. 881- 85.

Pizzarello ID, Jakobiec FA (1978). Bowen´s disease of the conjunctiva: a misnorner, In: *Ocular and adnexal tumors,* Jakobiec FA (ed), pp. (553-571), Al. Aesculapius, Birmingham.

Pola EC, Masanganise R, Rusakaniko S. The trend of ocular surface squamous neoplasia among ocular surface tumour biopsies submitted for histology from Sekuru Kaguvi Eye Unit, Harare between 1996 and 2000. Central African Journal of Medicine 2003 ;49:1-4.

Poole TR. Conjunctival squamous cell carcinoma in Tanzania. British J Ophthalmol 1999; 83: 177-9.

Porges Y, Groisman GM. Prevalence of HIV with conjunctival squamous cell neoplasia in an African provincial hospital. Cornea 2003;22: 1-4.

Ramos-Lopez JF, Martinez-Costa R, Cisneros-Lanuza AL, et. al. Treatment of conjunctival intraephitelial neoplasia with topical mitomycin C 0,02%. Arch Soc Esp Oftalmol 2004; 79: 375-78.

Rudkin AK, Dodd T, Muecke JS. The differential diagnosis of localised amelanotic limbal lesions: a review of 162 consecutive excisions. Br J Ophthalmol. 2011; 95: 350-54.

Schechter BA, Schrier A, Nagler RS, Smith EF, Velasquez GE. Regression of presumed primary conjunctival and corneal intraepithelial neoplasia with topical interferon alpha-2b. Cornea 2002; 21: 6-11.

Schechter BA, Nagler RS, Schrier A. Recurrent intraepithelial neoplasia treatment. Ophthalmology 2005, 112:1319.

Schechter BA, Koreishi AF, Karp CL, Feuer W. Long-term follow-up of conjunctival and corneal intraepithelial neoplasia treated with topical interferon alfa-2b. Ophthalmology 2008; 115: 1291-296.

Saornil MA, Becerra E, Méndez MC, Blanco G. Conjunctival tumors. Arch Soc Esp Oftalmol. 2009; 84: 7-22.

Scott IU, Karp CL, Nuovo GJ. Human papillomavirus 16 and 18 expression in conjunctival intraepithelial neoplasia. Ophthalmology 2002;109: 542–7.

Sears KS, Rundle PR, Mudhar HS, Rennie IG. The effects of photodynamic therapy on conjunctival in situ squamous cell carcinoma--a review of the histopathology. Br J Ophthalmol 2008; 92: 716-17.

Sherman MD, Feldman KA, Farahmand SM, Margolis TP. Treatment of conjunctival squamous cell carcinoma with topical cidofovir. Am J Ophthalmol 2002; 134: 432-33.

Shields CL, Naseripour M, Shields JA: Topical mitomycin C for extensive, recurrent conjunctival-corneal squamous cell carcinoma. Am J Ophthalmol 2002; 133: 601–06.

Shields CL, Shields JA. Tumors of the conjunctiva and cornea. Surv Ophthalmol 2004; 49: 3-24.

Shields CL, Demicri H, Karatza E, et al. Clinical survey of 1643 melanocytic and nonmelanocytic tumors of the conjunctiva. Ophthalmology 2004; 111: 1747-54.

Shields CL, Demirci H, Marr BP, et al. Chemoreduction with topical Mytomycin C prior to resection of extensive squamous cell carcinoma of the conjuntiva. Arch Ophthalmol 2005; 123: 109-13.

Shields CL, Manchandia A, Subbiah R, Eagle RC Jr, Shields JA. Pigmented squamous cell carcinoma in situ of the conjunctiva in 5 cases. Ophthalmology 2008; 115: 1673-78.

Shields JA, Shields CL. (2008). Eyelid, Conjunctival, and Orbital Tumors. Wolters Kluwer, Lippincott, Williams & Wilkins, Philadelphia.

Siganos CS, Kozobolis VP, Christodoulakis EV. The intraoperative use of mitomycin-C in excision of ocular surface neoplasia with or without limbal autograft transplantation. Cornea.2002; 21:12-16.

Stone DU, Butt AL, Chodosh J. Ocular surface squamous neoplasia. Cornea 2005; 24:297-300.

Sturges A, Butt AL, Lai JE, Chodosh J. Topical interferon or surgical excision for the management of primary ocular surface squamous neoplasia. Ophthalmology 2008; 115: 1297-1302.

Sun EC, Fears TR, Goedert JJ. Epidemiology of squamous cell conjunctival cancer. Cancer Epidemiol Biomarkers Prev. 1997;6: 73-77.

Tabin G, Levin S, Snibson G, Loughnan M, Taylor H. Late recurrences and the necessity for long-term follow-up in corneal and conjunctival intraepithelial neoplasia. Ophthalmology 1997; 104:485-92.

Tananuvat N, Lertprasertsuk N, Mahanupap P, Noppanakeepong P. Role of Impression Cytology in Diagnosis of Ocular Surface Neoplasia. Cornea 2008; 27: 269–74.

Timm A, Stropahl G, Schittowski M, et al. Association of malignant tumors of the conjunctiva and HIV infection in Kinshasa (D.R. Congo). First results. Ophthalmologe 2004; 101:1011–16.

Tole D, MecKelvie P, Daniell M. Reliability of impression cytology for the diagnosis of ocular surface squamous neoplasia employing the Biopore membrane. Br J Ophthalmol. 2001;85: 154–58.

Tseng SH. Conjuctival papilloma. Ophthalmology 2009; 116: 1013.

Tulwatana W, Bhattarakosol P, Sansopha L, et al. Risk factors for conjunctival squamous cell neoplasia: a matched case-control study. Br J Ohthalmol 2003; 87: 396-98.

Tunc M, Erbilen E. Topical Cyclosporine-A combined with Mitomycin C for conjunctival and corneal squamous cell carcinoma. Am J Ophthalmol 2006; 142: 673-75.

Tuppurainen K, Raninen A, Kosunen O, et al. Squamous cell carcinoma of the conjunctiva. Failure to demonstrate HPV DNA by in situ hybridization and polymerase chain reaction. Acta Ophthalmol (Copenh) 1992; 70: 248–54.

Verma V, Defan, S, Sieving P, Chan CC. The role of infectious agents in the etiology of ocular adnexal neoplasia. Surv Ophthalmol. 2008; 53: 312-331.

Waddell KM, Lewallen S, Lucas SB, Atenyi-Agaba C, Herrington CS, Liomba G. Carcinoma of the conjunctiva and HIV infection in Uganda and Malawi.. Br J Ophthalmol 1996;80: 503-8.

Wilson MW, Hungerford JL, George SM, Madreperla SA. Topical Mitomycin C for the treatment of conjunctival and corneal epithelial dysplasia and neoplasia. Am J Ophthalmol 1997; 124: 303-11.

Yeatts RP, Engelbrecht NE, Curry CD, Ford JG, Walter KA. 5-Fluorouracil for the treatment of intraepithelial neoplasia of the conjunctiva and cornea. Ophthalmology 2000; 107:2190-95.

Part 3

Intraepithelial Neoplasia of Breast

5

Intraepithelial Neoplasia of Breast

Simonetta Monti and Andres Del Castillo
Senology Division, European Institute of Oncology, Milan, Italy

1. Introduction

The early proliferative lesions of the breast have taken on greater significance as a result of mammographic screening and the use of even more sensitive imaging technologies. The intraductal proliferative lesions of the breast are a group of cytologically and architecturally diverse proliferations, typically originating from the terminal duct-lobular unit and confined to the mammary duct-lobular system. In this chapter we considere the most important of these lesions, lobular carcinoma in situ and ductal carcinoma in situ.

Lobular Carcinoma in situ

Foote and Stewart (Foote & Stewart, 1941) first described lobular carcinoma in situ (LCIS) in detail in 1941, emphasizing the morphologic similarity of LCIS cells to those of invasive lobular carcinoma. The multicentricity and high frequency of bilaterality of LCIS were recognized early on. LCIS generally occurs in younger women, and microcalcifications are not a feature (in contrast to the high frequency of microcalcifications seen with ductal proliferative lesions). Microscopically, LCIS is usually characterized by a solid, occlusive proliferation of loosely cohesive uniform cells, some of which may contain intracytoplasmic lumens. The incidence of LCIS is otherwise benign breast biopsy is reported as between 0,5% and 3,8%

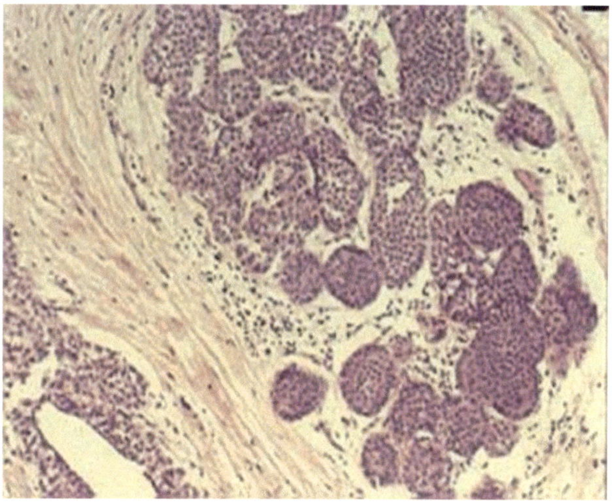

Fig. 1. Lobular carcinoma in situ

Ductal carcinoma in situ

Ductal carcinoma in situ is a heterogeneous group of lesions with diverse malignant potential and range of treatment options. It was infrequently diagnosed in the past, when it accounted for only 1% to 5% of all breast cancers. It usually presented as a palpable lesion, Paget disease, or bloody nipple discharge (Intra et al. 2003). The clinical presentation of Ductal Carcinoma In Situ shifted from a palpable lesion in the pre-mammographic era to a non-palpable lesion detected on the basis of mammographic microcalcifications or density (Tavassoli, 2008).

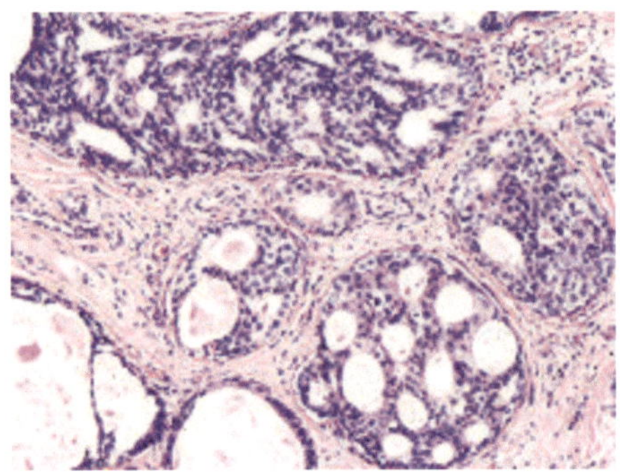

Fig. 2. Ductal carcinoma in situ

2. New classification

As mammographic screening became widespread, the frequency of diagnosis of intraepithelial proliferative lesions increased markedly, highlighting deficiencies in their classification as well a lack of data on natural history, and making clinical management a challenge. The new classification of these entities (DCIS and LCIS), principally due to Tavassoli (Tavassoli et al. 2003), was based on the concept of intraepithelial neoplasia

Ductal intra-epithelial neoplasia (DIN) terminology	Conventional terminology
Low-risk DIN	Intraductal hyper-plasia (IDH)
Flat DIN 1	Flat epithelial atypia
DIN 1	<2 mm: atypical duc-tal hyperplasia (ADH)
	>2 mm: ductal carcinoma in situ, low grade (DCIS, grade 1)
DIN 2	Ductal carcinoma in situ, intermediate grade (DCIS, grade 2)
DIN 3	Ductal carcinoma in situ, high grade (DCIS, grade 3)

Table 1. DIN translational table (Tavassoli FA 1997)

developed for cervix, vagina, vulva, prostate and pancreas. It does not use the term "cancer" diminishing the likelihood of overtreatment, and perhaps reduces also the level of anxiety and emotional stress a patient feels when told she has a cancer, even if it is only in situ.

3. Diagnosis and treatment

3.1 Diagnosis

The role of clinical examination in the ongoing surveillance of women with these high risk lesions is limited. While many DINs are detected through microcalcifications at mammography, the detection of LIN can be occasionally occur after a biopsy, for example in plastic surgery a histological evaluation of tissue excised in a breast reduction. In this case there is therefore a clear indication for meticulous assessment of both breasts ongoing surveillance of the breast at a relatively short interval. So standard core biopsy (14-18 gauge) is probably the most prevalent method for initial diagnosis of LIN. In the case of DIN it is diagnosed primarily via mammography plus ultrasound followed by stereotactic needle biopsy. However, new techniques such as magnetic resonance imaging (MRI) and analysis of ductal cytology aim to improve DIN detection (Sickles, 1983).

The use of breast MRI for patients with DIN is not yet established. MRI may be more sensitive for DIN detection than mammography but can lack specificity. The potential benefits of MRI include fewer re-excisions after BCS, decreased local recurrence rates after excision, and earlier detection and treatment of contralateral breast cancer (Leonard & Swain, 2004).

At present, therefore, mammography plus ultrasound and SCNB remain the standard diagnostic approaches for DIN (Leonard & Swain 2004).

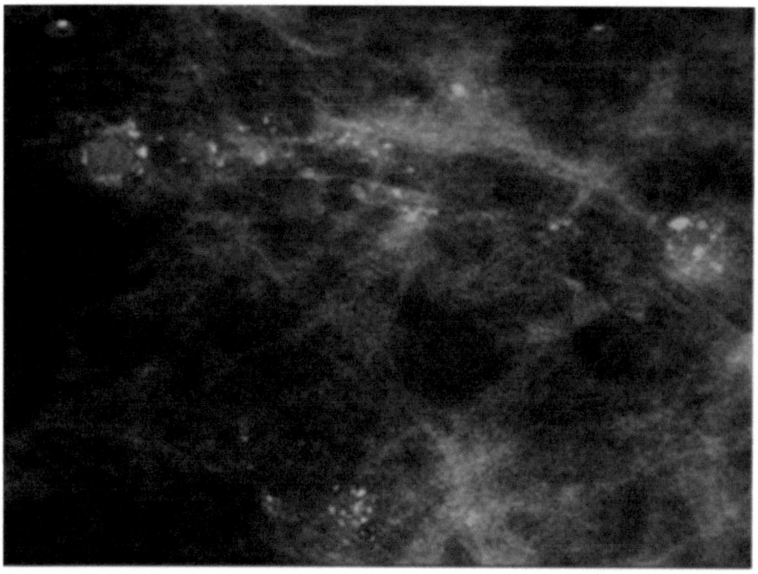

Fig. 3. A typical mammographic view of DIN

3.2 Treatment

Where the surgical biopsy reveals LIN , the margins of excision are paramount in determining further treatment. If the margins are clear, that is, the lesion appears to have been completely excised, no further treatment is required. Where surgical excision reveals a high risk lesion with an involved surgical margin or margins, re-excision should be considered. The goal of course is complete excision, but it must be recognized that LIN can be very extensive, sometimes occupying an entire quadrant or more of the breast. If a generous diagnostic excision suggests this, usually because several margins are involved, it may be clear that a substantially wider excision would have an adverse cosmetic outcome. In such cases observation and surveillance as detailed may be the preferred option. But the patient will be fully informed of the risk of subsequent cancer and involved in this decision. So, while for the LIN management is not yet clear the standard of treatment and in some institutions the decision is made on an individual, case by case basis, for DIN.

The standard of care consists of (a) breast conservative surgery (BCS) (mastectomy is still indicated in large lesions - masses or microcalcifications), axillary dissection is not indicated because of the low prevalence of nodal metastases and the significant morbidity associated with lymph node dissection (b) radiotherapy (RT) after conservative surgery, and (c) medical treatment in estrogen receptor-positive patients (Tavassoli ,2008; Farante et al. 2010; Cox et al. 2001; Intra et al.2003).

Surgical treatment

The main goal of surgical treatment for women with DIN is BCS plus RT, particularly for those patients with small solid masses, mammographically detected lesions, or limited microcalcification areas (Fisher et al. 1991; Schwartz et al. 2000; Silverstein et al. 1992).

However, mastectomy is still indicated in DIN patients with multicentricity, diffuse microcalcification, large palpable masses, when there is an inability to obtain negative margins as well other contraindications to breast conservation or a personal preference for mastectomy (Farante et al. 2010). At present, mastectomy is performed in about 30% of DIN patients, BCS without RT in about 30% of DIN patients, and BCS followed by RT in about 40% of DIN patients (Guerrieri-Gonzaga et al. 2009; Schmidt et al. 2006; Kuerer et al. 2008).

One important issue in breast cancer surgery is that of surgical margins, mainly in DIN patients, since these lesions are typically vague masses, which often cannot be adequately seen or felt and, thus, the pathological sampling of margins is fairly random (Fisher at al. 1999; Allred 2005). The current treatment of positive or focally involved margins in DIN patients is re-excision (Farante et al. 2010).

There is considerable debate regarding whether width of a negative margin is (width of a margin negative for tumor cells) associated with a decreased risk of recurrence, and classification of the margins makes summary statements difficult. About 10 years ago, the "Consensus on DCIS of Philadelphia" and Silverstein et al. proposed 10 mm of width margin as a limit of oncological safety (Schwartz et al. 2000). Since then other authors have proposed progressively smaller measures, down to 1 mm (Mansell, 2003).

Another important topic in DIN patients is the management of the axilla. Before the sentinel lymph node biopsy (SLNB) era, axillary dissection (AD) was a part of the standard surgical treatment for these patients (Farante et al. 2010). SLNB is recommended for patients with invasive breast cancer to determine prognosis and to guide adjuvant treatment decisions. In general, SLNB is not recommended for patients with a final or definitive diagnosis of DIN because the preinvasive cells do not metastasize (Virnig et al. 2010).

So not only is AD not necessary, neither should SLNB always be required because of the low prevalence of metastatic involvement, so an SLN biopsy should not be considered a standard procedure in the treatment of all patients with DCIS. The sole criteria for proposing SLN biopsy in DIN should be when there exists any uncertainty regarding the presence of invasive foci at definitive histology (Intra et al. 2008).

Major cancer centers agree that SLNB should be performed (a) always when mastectomy is performed (Cody 2007; Yi et al. 2008; Intra et al. 2007). (b)with large lesions (masses or micro-calcifications) and G3 tumors. (Cody 2007; Julian et. al 2007) and (c) after performing core or mammotome biopsies.

In cases of DIN patients with a positive SLNB, AD should not be immediately performed except for only those cases that present mammary invasion on final pathologic evaluation (Farante et al. 2010).

Radiation therapy

External RT

The standard course of current external RT after BCS for DIN, delivers a total dose of 50 Gy in daily fractions of 1.8/2 Gy without boost (Farante et al. 2010). The role of RT in DIN patients with conservative treatment has been mainly defined by four randomized trials (Bryan et al. 2003; Bijker et al. 2006; Houghton et al. 2003; Emdin et al. 2006). Additional radio-therapy reduced the LR rate by about 50%, with no effect on survival. The controversy is, instead, related if all DIN patients have to undergo RT. According to the 2009 St Gallen Consensus (Goldhirsch et al. 2009) RT could be avoided in elderly patients and in those with G1 DIN and clearly negative margins.

At the IEO in Milan, RT is not administered to DIN patients with G1 or G2 without comedo-necrosis. On the other hand, at least four significant papers from the Saint Gallen Consensus (Goldhirsch et al. 2009), the ECOG trial (Hughes et al. 2009), the Newport Consensus Conference III (Silverstein et al. 2009) and from the National Consensus Cancer Network (National Comprehensive cancer Network, 2009), suggested that some DIN patient sub-groups (i.e., G1 or G2 tumors without comedo-necrosis, and other low-risksub-groups) could not be candidates to receive RT after BCS.

4. Biomarkers

To guide such optimal treatment, histological classification is not sufficient and additional biological factors are being investigated for their ability to predict outcome for individual patients with intraepitalial neoplasia of the breast. As the molecular and genetic understanding of breast cancer has increased, new biological characteristics have been identified as prognostic indicators, as new adjuvant treatments have been developed. This has resulted in an increasingly personalized approach to breast cancer treatment that takes into account the diverse biological characteristics of the individual and their disease. A biomarker is an objectively measured feature that indicates a normal biological response, a pathogenic process, or the likelihood of response to a pharmacologic therapy. In oncology, biomarkers may be used to detect or stage disease, monitor response to therapy, and predict outcome (Madu & Lu 2010). A biomarker may be DNA, RNA, or a protein, measured directly in tissue, serum or other body fluids. An optimal biomarker for intraepithelial neoplasias of the breast would provide information additional to that provided by factors such as grade, lesion size, age and margin status (already established as related to the risk of local recurrence) so as to make it possible to predict which cases are unlikely to ever progress to invasive breast cancer and thus would require no further treatment after lesion removal, and also to predict which cases should receive local excision or mastectomy, or would benefit from adjuvant RT (Barker et al. 2003).

4.1 Estrogen receptors (ER)

Estrogens play a central role in the growth and differentiation of normal breast epithelium, stimulating cell proliferation and regulating the expression of genes, including that coding for the progesterone receptor (PgR) (Henderson et al. 1998; Peterson et al. 1987). In the normal pre-menopausal breast, ER-positive cells are luminal cells constituting about 7% of the total epithelial cell population (Peterson et al. 1987). They seem to secrete factors which influence, in paracrine manner, the proliferation of adjacent ER-negative cells (Peterson et al. 1987; Clarke et al. 1997). ER positivity and proliferation activity (as measured by Ki-67) are almost mutually exclusive in normal breast epithelium (Clarke et al. 1997). The proportion of ER-positive cells increases with age to reach a plateau after menopause (Shoker et al. 1999)

High ER expression in normal epithelium is a risk factor for breast cancer, conferring a 3-fold increase in risk compared to minimal expression (Khan et al. 1998). ER positivity together with KI-67 expression, may correlate with progression to more severe lesions in non-atypical epithelial hyperplasia (Iqbal et al. 2001). It has also been suggested that an increased percentage of ER-positive cells in adjacent normal lobules is associated with increased risk of invasive breast cancer rather than ER-positivity within the non-atypical epithelial hyperplasia *per se* (Gobbi et al. 2005)

In other benign breast lesions, such as sclerosing adenosis, radial scar, papilloma, fibroadenoma, and phylloides tumor, the percentage of ER-positive cells is higher than in normal breast tissue (Shoker et al. 2000). Similarly, ER-alpha expression is significantly elevated in hyperplastic enlarged lobular units (HELU), which are the earliest histologically identifiable lesions with premalignant potential. By contrast, intense ER-alpha staining in enlarged lobular units with columnar alteration (ELUCA) seems associated with reduced risk of subsequent invasive carcinoma (McLaren et al. 2005).

Unlike in normal breast, in ADH (atypical ductal hyperplasia), LN (lobular neoplasia) and DCIS (ductal carcinoma in situ), ER-positive cells are surrounded by contiguous cells which are also characterized by ER-positivity (Clarke et al. 1997). Furthermore, in DCIS, cells that are both ER-positive and Ki-67-positive are a characteristic finding (Shoker et al. 2000). In general, non-comedo carcinomas more frequently exhibit ER positivity (Bose et al. 1996; Page et al. 1982).

The expression of ER-beta by breast epithelium is the inverse of that of ER-alpha, declining progressively from normal breast tissue to ADH, DCIS, and IDC (Intraductal Carcinoma)

(Roger at al. 2001; Shaaban et al. 2003). According to a recent article, a high ER-alpha/ER-beta ratio in non-atypical epithelial hyperplasia predicts progression to carcinoma (Shaaban et al. 2005). For the optimal envisagement of the ER network, it should be kept in mind that important regulators exist, such as hsp-27 (O'Neill et al. 2004) or AIB1 (Hudelist et al. 2003), exhibiting more intense expression in breast cancer.

4.2 Progesterone receptors (PgR)

As is the case with ER levels, PgR levels are elevated in early premalignant breast lesions (Lee et al. 2006) and PgR expression decreases with progression to malignancy (Ariga et al. 2001). In DCIS, PgR positivity is associated with ER positivity and lack of comedo necrosis (Barnes et al. 2005; Claus et al. 2001). Studies on the relation of PgR expression to tumor grade (Barnes et al. 2005; Ringberg et al. 2001, Rody et al. 2004; Lebrecht et al. 2002) and recurrence rate (Kepple et al. 2006; Provenzano et al. 2003) have provided contrasting results (reviewed in Provenzano et al. 2003). In ductal carcinoma, PgR expression has been associated with histological grade, but not with lymph node involvement, tumor size, or prognosis (Ariga et al. 2001). Data on PgR expression in lobular neoplasia is scarce but it seems to be expressed in most cases (Fadare et al. 2006; Fisher et al. 1996).

The ratio of PgR-A to PgR-B appears important. In normal breast tissue and non-atypical hyperplasia, PgR-A and PgR-B are expressed in approximately equal quantities, but at an early stage of progression, one receptor (usually PgR-A in advanced lesions) predominates (Mote et al. 2002). In vitro studies indicate that PgR-A exerts modulating effects on cell morphology and adhesion (McGowan et al. 1999; Grahal et al. 2005). In the normal tissue of BRCA mutation carriers, PgR-B is absent (Mote et al. 2004).

4.3 HER2

HER2 or human epidermal growth factor receptor 2 (c-ErbB-2) is a tyrosine kinase receptor and oncoprotein encoded by the ERBB2 gene on chromosome 17q. Alterations in ERBB2 expression are important in malignant transformation (De Potter et al. 1989; Ross et al. 1999). Some studies have found that HER2 was not overexpressed in benign proliferative breast disease or ADH (Gusterson et al. 1988; Heffelfinger et al. 2000) while another used fluorescence in situ hybridization to demonstrate that the extent of HER2 amplification increased with progression to invasive carcinoma (Xu et al. 2002). Patients with benign breast lesions showing low levels of HER2 amplification were found in one study to have a two-fold increased risk of developing breast cancer (Stark et al. 2000); however another study found that HER2 overexpression in benign lesions was not a significant risk factor for developing cancer (Rohan et al. 1998).

A quarter of LCIS cases have been found to be HER2 positive, irrespective of the coexistence of an invasive component (Mohsin et al. 2005). Occasional positivity has also been found in pleomorphic ductal-lobular carcinomas in situ (Sneige et al. 2002).

As far as the role of HER2 in DCIS is concerned, HER2 immunoreactivity has been primarily associated with DCIS of higher grade, in the absence or presence (Tsuda et al. 1998) of IDC , and with comedo type (Albonico et al. 1996). Interestingly, given the association of higher grade with HER2 amplification, the latter has been regarded as an independent prognostic factor (Tsuda et al. 1993). Allred et al (Allred et al. 1992) documented that the percentage of

HER2 immunoreactivity is significantly higher in DCIS than IDC: one of the possible explanations proposed by the authors was that HER2 may be more important for the initiation than the progression of breast cancer, or that HER2 may be downregulated during breast cancer progression.

4.4 P53

P53 is a tumour suppressor gene located on 17p. p53 protein mediates its tumor suppressor functions via the transcriptional regulation or repression of a variety of genes (Toledo et al. 2006; Vogelstein et al. 2000) and is an important component of breast cancer pathophysiology (Gasco et al. 2002). Regarding the role of p53 as a risk factor in benign breast lesions, there data is controversial: the immunohistochemical detection of p53 in benign breast lesions has been associated with elevated cancer risk (Rohan et al. 1998), although there are studies with conflicting results (Younes et al. 1995).

Considering the various types of lesions in the continuum between benign lesions and breast cancer, various studies have assessed the role of p53. In epithelial hyperplasia without atypia, p53 mutations have not been detected (Done et al. 1998). In ADH, the presence and role of p53 mutations is still an open field: p53 mutations were initially not documented (Chitemerere et al. 1996); subsequently studies pointing to p53 mutations appeared (Kang et al. 2001), and, more recently, the presence of mutated p53 in ADH has been demonstrated with the use of laser capture microdissection microscope, single-stranded conformational polymorphism (SSCP) and sequencing (Keohavong et al. 2004). Regarding LN, there is scarcity of data: in two studies, no p53 immunoreactivity was demonstrated in LN lesions (Siziopikou et al. 1996; Sapino et al. 2000), whereas a more recent study on LCIS reported p53 immunoreactivity in one fifth of cases (Mohson et al. 2005).

p53 mutations/accumulation are present in a significant percentage of DCIS cases (Lebeau et al. 2003; Poller et al. 1993), especially in the comedo type (O'Malley et al. 1994). However, the clinical significance of p53 accumulation remains still elusive; although it has been found to influence the proliferation rate (Rudas et al. 1997), a recent study showed that it does not affect the proliferation rate of the DCIS lesion *per se* (Lebeau et al. 2003). Is worth noting that the coexistence of DCIS with IDC is not associated with a different degree of p53 immunostaining (Myonlas et al. 2005).

4.5 Ki-67

Ki-67 is a cell cycle-associated nuclear protein, which is expressed in all cycle phases, with the exception of G0 and early G1, and reacts with MIB-1 antibody (Gerdes et al. 1984). Protein Ki-67 is extensively used as a proliferative index and is linked with malignancy, even in FNA (fine needle aspiration) specimens (Midulla et al. 2002). Moreover, its intrinsic association with apoptosis (bcl-2 status, see below) and p53 expression (see above) seems to be of importance in the diagnosis and prognosis of precursors and pre-invasive breast lesions: low Ki-67 expression/bcl-2 positivity and p53 negativity are a trait of ADH and, subsequently, well-differentiated carcinomas. Conversely, high Ki-67 expression/bcl-2 negativity within the lobules implicate lesions with a potential of poorly differentiated carcinoma (Viacava P et al. 1999). As mentioned above, also in the context of non-atypical hyperplasia, high Ki-67 and ER-alpha expression seem to predict progression to cancer (Ariga et al. 2001; Shaaban et al. 2002).

Interestingly enough, a clinical application of Ki-67 expression intensity seems to emerge. In non-atypical ductal hyperplasia, lesions with high Ki-67 expression can be clinically detected scintimammographically, since high (99m)Tc-(V)**DMSA** uptake seems to be their characteristic feature. According to the authors, this could prove useful in identifying women with benign but high-risk breast disease (Papantoniou et al. 2006).

4.6 Bcl-2

The bcl-2 gene is located on 18q. Bcl-2 protein, and belongs to a family of proteins playing a central role in the regulation of apoptosis (reviewed in van Delft et al. 2006; Reed et al. 1994; Hockenbery et al. 1994) and other pathways (reviewed by Kim (Kim, 2005)). With respect to the overall role of apoptosis in breast cancer pathogenesis, there seems to be an intriguing pattern incorporating the proliferation of the lesion. Growth imbalance in favour of proliferation seems crucial in the transition from normal epithelium to hyperplasia and later, from pre-invasive lesions to IDC. Conversely, apoptosis becomes more important at an intermediate stage: in the transition from hyperplasia to preinvasive lesions, the imbalance is in favour of apoptosis (Bai et al. 2001). Bcl-2 is present in the whole spectrum of breast lesions: predominantly in benign lesions, ADH, LN, and well-differentiated DCIS (Sizioupikou et al. 1996; Kapucuoglu et al. 1997; Meteoglu et al. 2005). More specifically, there is a gradual increase in the extent of apoptosis (Bai et al. 2001; Mustonen et al. 1997) and a parallel decrease in bcl-2 expression in benign/precursors/preinvasive/invasive lesions as they become histologically more aggressive (Mustonen et al. 1997) . Bcl-2 positivity tends to coincide with p53 negativity in normal breast tissue, non-atypical ductal hyperplasia, ADH, LN and in the majority of the DCIS (Sizioupikou et al. 1996). The role of Bcl-2 expression as a risk factor for breast cancer is described above, together with Ki-67 (see above).

4.7 Vascular endothelial growth factor (VEGF) and angiogenesis

VEGF is a potent angiogenic growth factor, commonly involved in tumor-induced angiogenesis, with a putative therapeutic significance in the context of breast cancer (Lebeau et al. 2003). Interestingly, VEGF gene polymorphisms have been associated with modified breast cancer risk in various populations (Jacobs et al. 2006)

Viacava et al (Viacava et al. 2004) have thoroughly examined the angiogenesis in precursor and preinvasive lesions. Increased vascularization is present in all preinvasive lesions and increases with lesion severity. In ductal lesions, angiogenesis is more intense in poorly/intermediately differentiated intraductal carcinomas than in non-atypical ductal hyperplasia and ADH. Similarly, LCIS, showing microvascular density similar to that of poorly/intermediately differentiated intraductal carcinoma, is more vascularized than ALH. In the same study, VEGF expression in normal glandular structures was lower than in lesions, with the highest levels found in ductal lesions. Interestingly, no correlation was found between VEGF expression and the degree of vascularization in that study. On the other hand, Hieken TJ et al. suggested **that VEGF** expression may help predict the biologic aggressiveness of DCIS (Hieken et al. 2001). Additionally, in the context of DCIS, Vogl et al provide evidence to support the idea that VEGF expression is not regulated by the HER2 pathway (Vogl et al. 2005).

4.8 E-cadherin

E-cadherin, a tumor suppressor gene located on 17q, has been implicated especially in lobular breast cancer molecular pathogenesis (Berx et al. 1995). In clinical practice, immunohistochemistry for E-cadherin is a helpful marker for differential diagnosis, since most cases of low-grade DCIS exhibit E-cadherin positivity, whereas LN is almost always E-cadherin negative (Bratthauer et al. 2002, reviewed in Lerwill et al. 2004 and Putti et al. 2005). This implies that E-cadherin disruption is an early event, prior to progression, in lobular carcinogenesis (Vos et al. 1997; Mastracci et al. 2005); more specifically, DNA alterations accompanying the loss of protein expression pertain to LCIS but not to ALH (Mastracci et al. 2005). As expected according to the above, only few studies have focused on E-cadherin in ductal lesions. In the context of DCIS, hypermethylation of E-cadherin 5' **CpG** islands has been demonstrated (Nass et al. 2000) , and, at the protein level, E-cadherin has been linked to better differentiation (Gupta et al. 1997). Moreover, mutational analysis of E-cadherin provided evidence to support that DCIS is the precursor of invasive ductal carcinoma in cases where LCIS coexists (Rieger-Christ et al. 2001).

4.9 TGF-beta

The transforming growth factor-beta (TGF-β) pathway has ambivalent importance in the pathogenesis of breast cancer (reviewed in Wakefield et al. 2001). Serum **TGF-**beta levels do not differ between patients with breast cancer, DCIS and benign lesions (Lebrecht et al. 2004); however, TGF-beta expression becomes more accentuated in IDC, compared with DCIS (Walker et al. 1992). Surprisingly enough, an interesting study recently showed that loss of TGF-beta-RII expression in epithelial cells of hyperplasia without atypia is associated with increased risk of IDC (Gobbi et al. 1999). No reports exist on ADH and LN, to our knowledge.

4.10 P16 (INK4a)

p16 is an inhibitor of cyclin-dependent kinases 4 and 6 (reviewed in Rocco & Sidransky 2001). With respect to the role of p16, controversial results exist. According to some authors, aberrant methylation of p16 is not demonstrated in benign conditions, epithelial hyperplasia and intraductal papillomas, but is restricted in cancerous epithelium (Lehmann et al. 2004). Conversely, another study showed that IDC demonstrates hypomethylation of p16 and hyperactivity of the p16 gene (enhanced expression of p16 mRNA), contrary to the hypermethylated, inactive state in the normal epithelium (Van Zee et al. 1998). Independently, Di Vinci et al. distinguish between p16 hypermethylation and p16 protein overexpression; the former seems not to be specifically associated with malignancy and to occur both in benign and malignant lesions, whereas the latter, together with cytoplasmic sequestration, is a feature of breast carcinoma (Di Vinci et al. 2005). In the context of such controversy, no studies exist with respect to p16 as a risk factor, with the exception of a study in Poland envisaging p16 as a low penetrance breast cancer susceptibility gene (Debniak et al. 2005)

4.11 p27(Kip1)

The p27 gene encodes for an inhibitor of the cyclin - CDK (cyclin-dependent kinase) active complex. Although numerous studies exist with respect to the role of p27 in breast cancer (reviewed in Colozza et al. 2005; Alkarain et al. 2004 and Musgrove et al. 2004), there is a lack of data regarding precursors, pre-invasive lesions and other predisposing conditions. p27 expression has been documented in DCIS, but its clinicopathological significance is still uncertain (Oh et al. 2001).

4.12 P21 (Waf1)

p21 is a cell cycle regulator, implicated in a variety of pathways (Dotto 2000). p21 immunoreactivity has been detected both in benign and malignant epithelium, and thus its role is hard to interpret (Krogerus et al. 2000). Studies focusing especially on ADH or LN do not exist. As far as DCIS is concerned, p21 positivity has been independently associated with clinical recurrence (Provenzano et al. 2003) . On the other hand, Oh YL et al. found a significant correlation between positive p21 immunoreactivity (67.3% of the cases) and well-differentiated histologic grade, non-comedo type, ER-positive and p53-negativity. According to these authors, DCIS with p21+/p53- is likely to be the non-comedo type (Oh et al. 2001).

4.13 14-3-3 sigma

Umbricht and coworkers identified 14-3-3 sigma as a gene whose expression is lost in breast carcinomas, primarily by methylation-mediated silencing. Importantly, the hypermethylation of the locus was absent in hyperplasia without atypia, but was detectable with increasing frequency as the breast lesions progressed from atypical hyperplasia to DCIS, and finally to invasive carcinoma (Umbricht et al. 2001); interestingly, methylated alleles existed in the periductal stromal breast tissue. Subsequently, a parallel, stepwise reduction at the 14-3-3 sigma protein level was documented (Simooka et al. 2004).

Despite the emerging role of 14-3-3 sigma in breast carcinogenesis, to date no studies exist assessing its role as a risk factor for breast cancer development.

5. Genetic events

Complex and heterogeneous sets of genetic alterations are involved in the etiology of breast cancer. However, some of these genetic events occur more often early, or late, in carcinogenesis. Rather, breast cancer to be viewed as the result of accumulation of various major and minor genetic events in a fairly, random order, which is referred to as the "bingo principle" analogous to winning the "prize" (in this case cancer) in this popular game. With the establishment of new global genetic screening techniques such as comparative genomic hybridization (CGH), a pattern of genetic alterations has emerged. More recently other methods have been used for the characterization of pre-invasive breast lesions, such as cDNA microarray and proteonomics analysis. Numerous studies have documented differences in the copy number, sequence and expression level of specific genes in cohorts of invasive breast carcinomas, but relatively little is known of the events that mediate the transition of normal human breast epithelial cells to premalignant and early tumorigenic states. Non neoplastic breast tissue often harbors genetic changes that can be important to understanding the local breast environment within which cancer develops. In fact, most pre invasive lesions of the breast are thought to derive from the transition zone between the duct and the functional unit of the breast, the lobule, which is composed of acini that are lined by an outer myoepithelial layer and a inner luminal or glandular layer containing a putative stem or progenitor cell component, which gives rise to the above- mentioned cells. These cells have recently been described and characterized in more detail. It is noteworthy that many characteristics of these cells are shared in mouse and human cells. At present, the relationship between these cells and breast cancer specific stem cells is unclear. However, these cells can serve as a tool to explain the presence of monoclonal patches within a breast lobule or parts of the ductal tree. In addition, the description of non-recurrent genetic changes within the morphologically normal breast tissue, requiring a large subset of affected cells, favors the idea of long living cells as targets of the initial starting of the genetic cascade towards an overt malignancy. The finding of genetic changes within morphologically normal beast tissue is nowadays not only associated with an increased local recurrence risk, but also exerts a tremendous influence on the validity of progression models of breast cancer and especially the relationship toward proposed precursor lesions.

A recent study (Hannafon, et al. 2011) hypothesized that micro RNA expression might be dysregulated prior to invasive breast carcinoma. This study provides the first report of a microRNA expression profile in normal breast epithelium and the first integrated analysis of microRNA and microRNA expression in paired samples of histologically normal epithelia and preinvasive breast cancer. They further demonstrated, by modulating the expression of several microRNA samples, that the expression of their predicted target genes is affected. Taken together, these findings support their hypothesis that changes in microRNA expression in early breast cancer may control many of the parallel changes in gene expression in this stage. This work also implicates the loss of the tumor suppressor miR-125b and the gain of the oncogenic miRNA miR-182 and miR-183 as major contributors to early breast cancer development. Additionally this study has revealed novel candidate markers of preinvasive breast cancer, which could contribute to the identification of new diagnostic and therapeutic targets.

Another study (Kretschmer et al., 2011) has identified, using transgenic mouse model of DCIS (mice were transgenic for the WAP-SV40 early genome region, so that expression of the SV40 oncogene is activated by lactation) and identified seven genes that are significantly up regulated in DCIS: DEPDC1, NUSAP1, EXO1,RRM2,FOXM1,MUC1 and SPP1. A similar upregulation of homologues of these murine genes was observed in human DCIS samples.So, comparing murine markers for the DCIS of the mammary gland with genes up-regulated in human DCIS samples it is possible to identify a set of genes which might allow early detection of DCIS and invasive carcinoma in the future.

Cichon and her co-workers (Cichon et al., 2010) identified alterations in stromal cell function that may be critical for disease progression from benign disease to invasive cancer: key functions of myoepithelial cells that maintain tissue structure are lost, while tissue fibroblasts become activated to produce proteases that degrade the extracellular matrix and trigger the invasive cellular phenotype. Gene expression profiling of stromal alterations associated with disease progression has also identified key transcriptional changes that occur early in disease development. This study suggests approaches to identify processes that control earlier stages of disease progression.

Future studies aimed at studying post-translational modifications of histone proteins of the different stages of breast cancer promise to shed new light on the epigenetic regulatory control of gene expression during tumorigenesis (Fiegl et al., 2006).

6. Conclusions

Intraepithelial neoplasias of the breast are non-obligate precursor lesions with an increased risk of invasive carcinoma. The evolution to invasive carcinoma may not however be linear and may involve multiple pathways. Genomic instability drives tumorigenic process in invasive carcinoma and premalignant breast lesions and might promote the accumulation of genetic alterations in apparently normal tissue before histological abnormalities are detectable. Evidence suggests that genomic changes in breast parenchyma affect the behavior of epithelial cells and, ultimately, might affect tumor growth and progression. Inherent instability in genes that maintain genomic integrity, as well as exogenous chemical and environmental pollutants, have been implicated in breast cancer development. Although molecular mechanisms of tumorigenesis are unclear at present, carcinogenetic agents could contribute to field of genomic instability localized to specific areas of the breast. The use of molecular profiling technologies to identify distinct features that predict the future behavior of invasive disease is well documented. However, the application of such approaches to the identification of molecular predictors of clinical behavior of normal breast tissue and pre-invasive disease has been hampered by several problems. First, because pre-invasive disease is frequently microscopic in size, all of the tissue is processed through the use of standard pathological formalin fixed paraffin embedded (FFPE) processes and utilized for clinical diagnostic purposes. Second, standard FFPE processes pose a significant technical challenge for high throughput array CGH and gene expression microarray profiling. Third, and most importantly, large clinical cohorts and clinical trials of pre-invasive disease with well-annotated clinical samples and long (10-20 years) clinical follow up are lacking. Understanding the functional importance of genomic instability in early carcinogenesis is important for improving diagnostic and treatment strategies (Ellsworth et al., 2004)

7. Future directions

Despite many molecular studies, breast carcinogenesis is still not well understood. Our knowledge of the genetic and molecular biology of intraepithelial breast lesions is increasing at a remarkably rapid rate. In addition, more and more data are now available on the morphology and immunophenotype of the different precursor lesions, allowing the pathologists to recognize them. Epidemiologic studies have yielded information on the progression risk of several lesions. Future studies are likely to identify markers at a very early stage indeed that can play a role in the development of these precursor lesions from normal breast tissue. Clearly, prospective studies based on larger patient cohorts representing the whole spectrum of breast cancer are needed before the full power of gene expression profiling will be realized in clinical medicine. Results from studies so far are encouraging for the future.

8. References

Albonico, G., Querzoli, P., Ferretti, S., Magri, E. & Nenci, I. (1996)., Biophenotypes of breast carcinoma in situ defined by image analysis of biological parameters., *Pathology, Research & Practice*, vol. 192, no. 2, pp. 117-123.

Alkarain, A., Jordan, R. & Slingerland, J. (2004). p27 deregulation in breast cancer: prognostic significance and implications for therapy, *Journal of Mammary Gland Biology & Neoplasia*, vol. 9, no. 1, pp. 67-80.

Allred, D.C., Clark, G.M., Molina, R., Tandon, A.K., Schnitt, S.J., Gilchrist, K.W., Osborne, C.K., Tormey, D.C. & McGuire, W.L. (1992). Overexpression of HER-2/neu and its relationship with other prognostic factors change during the progression of in situ to invasive breast cancer., *Human pathology*, vol. 23, no. 9, pp. 974-979.

Allred, DC (2005). Ductal carcinoma in situ of the breast: pathologic and biologic perspectives. American Society of Clinical Oncology 2005 educational book 41st annual meeting, May 13–17, pp 75–79.

Ariga, N., Suzuki, T., Moriya, T., Kimura, M., Inoue, T., Ohuchi, N. & Sasano, H. (2001). Progesterone receptor A and B isoforms in the human breast and its disorders., *Japanese Journal of Cancer Research*, vol. 92, no. 3, pp. 302-308.

Aubele, M., Werner, M. & Hofler, H. (2002). Genetic alterations in presumptive precursor lesions of breast carcinomas, *Analytical Cellular Pathology*, vol. 24, no. 2-3, pp. 69-76.

Bai, M., Agnantis, N.J., Kamina, S., Demou, A., Zagorianakou, P., Katsaraki, A. & Kanavaros, P. (2001). In vivo cell kinetics in breast carcinogenesis., *Breast Cancer Research*, vol. 3, no. 4, pp. 276-283.

Barker, P.E. (2003). Cancer biomarker validation: standards and process: roles for the National Institute of Standards and Technology (NIST), *Annals of the New York Academy of Sciences*, vol. 983, pp. 142-150.

Barnes, N.L., Boland, G.P., Davenport, A., Knox, W.F. & Bundred, N.J. (2005). Relationship between hormone receptor status and tumour size, grade and comedo necrosis in ductal carcinoma in situ., *British Journal of Surgery*, vol. 92, no. 4, pp. 429-434.

Berx, G., Cleton-Jansen, A.M., Nollet, F., de Leeuw, W.J., van de Vijver, M., Cornelisse, C. & van Roy, F. (1995). E-cadherin is a tumour/invasion suppressor gene mutated in human lobular breast cancers., *EMBO Journal*, vol. 14, no. 24, pp. 6107-6115.

Bjurstam, N., Bjorneld, L., Warwick, J., Sala, E., Duffy, S.W., Nystrom, L., Walker, N., Cahlin, E., Eriksson, O., Hafstrom, L.O., Lingaas, H., Mattsson, J., Persson, S., Rudenstam, C.M., Salander, H., Save-Soderbergh, J. & Wahlin, T. (2003). The Gothenburg Breast Screening Trial., *Cancer*, vol. 97, no. 10, pp. 2387-2396.

Bose, S., Lesser, M.L., Norton, L. & Rosen, P.P. (1996). Immunophenotype of intraductal carcinoma., *Archives of Pathology & Laboratory Medicine*, vol. 120, no. 1, pp. 81-85.

Bratthauer, G.L., Moinfar, F., Stamatakos, M.D., Mezzetti, T.P., Shekitka, K.M., Man, Y.G. & Tavassoli, F.A. (2002). Combined E-cadherin and high molecular weight cytokeratin immunoprofile differentiates lobular, ductal, and hybrid mammary intraepithelial neoplasias., *Human pathology*, vol. 33, no. 6, pp. 620-627.

Bryan J., Land S., Allred C et al. (2003). DCIS: evidence from randomized trials. Proceedings of the 8th international conference March 12–15, 2003, St Gallen, Switzerland. Breast 12(Suppl. 1):S9 (S24) Breast Cancer Research and Treatment 123.

Buchberger, W., DeKoekkoek-Doll, P., Springer, P., Obrist, P. & Dunser, M. (1999). Incidental findings on sonography of the breast: clinical significance and diagnostic workup., *AJR.American Journal of Roentgenology,* vol. 173, no. 4, pp. 921-927.

Buchberger, W., Niehoff, A., Obrist, P., DeKoekkoek-Doll, P. & Dunser, M. (2000). Clinically and mammographically occult breast lesions: detection and classification with high-resolution sonography., *Seminars in Ultrasound, CT & MR,* vol. 21, no. 4, pp. 325-336.

Burbank, F. (1997). Stereotactic breast biopsy of atypical ductal hyperplasia and ductal carcinoma in situ lesions: improved accuracy with directional, vacuum-assisted biopsy., *Radiology,* vol. 202, no. 3, pp. 843-847.

Burstein, H.J., Polyak, K., Wong, J.S., Lester, S.C. & Kaelin, C.M. (2004). Ductal carcinoma in situ of the breast, *New England Journal of Medicine,* vol. 350, no. 14, pp. 1430-1441.

Chitemerere, M., Andersen, T.I., Holm, R., Karlsen, F., Borresen, A.L. & Nesland, J.M. (1996). TP53 alterations in atypical ductal hyperplasia and ductal carcinoma in situ of the breast., *Breast Cancer Research & Treatment,* vol. 41, no. 2, pp. 103-109.

Cichon, M.A., Degnim A.C, Visscher DW, Radisky DC. (2010). Microenvironmental influences that drive progression from benign breast disease to invasive breast cancer. *Journal of Mammary Gland Biology and Neoplasia,* vol. 15, no. 4, pp. 389-397.

Clarke, R.B., Howell, A., Potten, C.S. & Anderson, E. 1997, Dissociation between steroid receptor expression and cell proliferation in the human breast., *Cancer research,* vol. 57, no. 22, pp. 4987-4991.

Claus, E.B., Chu, P., Howe, C.L., Davison, T.L., Stern, D.F., Carter, D. & DiGiovanna, M.P. (2001). Pathobiologic findings in DCIS of the breast: morphologic features, angiogenesis, HER-2/neu and hormone receptors., *Experimental & Molecular Pathology,* vol. 70, no. 3, pp. 303-316.

Cody, H.S.,3rd (2007). Sentinel lymph node biopsy for breast cancer: indications, contraindications, and new directions., *Journal of surgical oncology,* vol. 95, no. 6, pp. 440-442.

Colozza, M., Azambuja, E., Cardoso, F., Sotiriou, C., Larsimont, D. & Piccart, M.J. (2005). Proliferative markers as prognostic and predictive tools in early breast cancer: where are we now?, *Annals of Oncology,* vol. 16, no. 11, pp. 1723-1739.

Cornfield, D.B., Palazzo, J.P., Schwartz, G.F., Goonewardene, S.A., Kovatich, A.J., Chervoneva, I., Hyslop, T. & Schwarting, R. (2004). The prognostic significance of multiple morphologic features and biologic markers in ductal carcinoma in situ of the breast: a study of a large cohort of patients treated with surgery alone., *Cancer,* vol. 100, no. 11, pp. 2317-2327.

Cox, C.E., Nguyen, K., Gray, R.J., Salud, C., Ku, N.N., Dupont, E., Hutson, L., Peltz, E., Whitehead, G., Reintgen, D. & Cantor, A. (2001). Importance of lymphatic mapping in ductal carcinoma in situ (DCIS): why map DCIS?., *American Surgeon,* vol. 67, no. 6, pp. 513-519.

De Potter, C.R., Van Daele, S., Van de Vijver, M.J., Pauwels, C., Maertens, G., De Boever, J., Vandekerckhove, D. & Roels, H. (1989). The expression of the neu oncogene product in breast lesions and in normal fetal and adult human tissues., *Histopathology,* vol. 15, no. 4, pp. 351-362.

Debniak, T., Gorski, B., Huzarski, T., Byrski, T., Cybulski, C., Mackiewicz, A., Gozdecka-Grodecka, S., Gronwald, J., Kowalska, E., Haus, O., Grzybowska, E., Stawicka, M., Swiec, M., Urbanski, K., Niepsuj, S., Wasko, B., Gozdz, S., Wandzel, P., Szczylik, C., Surdyka, D., Rozmiarek, A., Zambrano, O., Posmyk, M., Narod, S.A. & Lubinski, J. (2005). A common variant of CDKN2A (p16) predisposes to breast cancer., *Journal of medical genetics,* vol. 42, no. 10, pp. 763-765.

Dershaw, D.D., Abramson, A. & Kinne, D.W. (1989). Ductal carcinoma in situ: mammographic findings and clinical implications., *Radiology,* vol. 170, no. 2, pp. 411-415.

Di Vinci, A., Perdelli, L., Banelli, B., Salvi, S., Casciano, I., Gelvi, I., Allemanni, G., Margallo, E., Gatteschi, B. & Romani, M. (2005). p16(INK4a) promoter methylation and protein expression in breast fibroadenoma and carcinoma., *International Journal of Cancer,* vol. 114, no. 3, pp. 414-421.

Done, S.J., Arneson, N.C., Ozcelik, H., Redston, M. & Andrulis, I.L. (1998). p53 mutations in mammary ductal carcinoma in situ but not in epithelial hyperplasias., *Cancer research,* vol. 58, no. 4, pp. 785-789.

Dooley, W.C., Ljung, B.M., Veronesi, U., Cazzaniga, M., Elledge, R.M., O'Shaughnessy, J.A., Kuerer, H.M., Hung, D.T., Khan, S.A., Phillips, R.F., Ganz, P.A., Euhus, D.M., Esserman, L.J., Haffty, B.G., King, B.L., Kelley, M.C., Anderson, M.M., Schmit, P.J., Clark, R.R., Kass, F.C., Anderson, B.O., Troyan, S.L., Arias, R.D., Quiring, J.N., Love, S.M., Page, D.L. & King, E.B. (2001). Ductal lavage for detection of cellular atypia in women at high risk for breast cancer., *Journal of the National Cancer Institute,* vol. 93, no. 21, pp. 1624-1632.

Dotto, G.P. (2000). p21(WAF1/Cip1): more than a break to the cell cycle?, *Biochimica et biophysica acta,* vol. 1471, no. 1, pp. M43-56.

Edorh, A., Leroux, A., N'sossani, B., Parache, R.M. & Rihn, B. (1999). Detection by immunohistochemistry of c-erbB2 oncoprotein in breast carcinomas and benign mammary lesions., *Cellular & Molecular Biology,* vol. 45, no. 6, pp. 831-840

Ellsworth, D.L., Ellsworth R.E., Liebman M.N., Hooke J.A., & Shriver C. D. (2004). Genomic instability in histologically normal breast tissues: implications for carcinogenesis., *Lancet Oncology,* vol.5, no.12, pp.753-8

Emdin, S.O., Granstrand, B., Ringberg, A., Sandelin, K., Arnesson, L.G., Nordgren, H., Anderson, H., Garmo, H., Holmberg, L., Wallgren, A. & Swedish Breast Cancer, G. (2006). SweDCIS: Radiotherapy after sector resection for ductal carcinoma in situ of the breast. Results of a randomised trial in a population offered mammography screening., *Acta Oncologica,* vol. 45, no. 5, pp. 536-543.

EORTC Breast Cancer Cooperative, G., EORTC Radiotherapy, G., Bijker, N., Meijnen, P., Peterse, J.L., Bogaerts, J., Van Hoorebeeck, I., Julien, J.P., Gennaro, M., Rouanet, P., Avril, A., Fentiman, I.S., Bartelink, H. & Rutgers, E.J. (2006). Breast-conserving treatment with or without radiotherapy in ductal carcinoma-in-situ: ten-year results of European Organisation for Research and Treatment of Cancer randomized phase III trial 10853--a study by the EORTC Breast Cancer Cooperative Group and EORTC Radiotherapy Group., *Journal of Clinical Oncology,* vol. 24, no. 21, pp. 3381-3387.

Ernster, V.L., Ballard-Barbash, R., Barlow, W.E., Zheng, Y., Weaver, D.L., Cutter, G., Yankaskas, B.C., Rosenberg, R., Carney, P.A., Kerlikowske, K., Taplin, S.H., Urban, N. & Geller, B.M. (2002). Detection of ductal carcinoma in situ in women undergoing screening mammography., *Journal of the National Cancer Institute,* vol. 94, no. 20, pp. 1546-1554.

Fabian, C.J., Kimler, B.F., Zalles, C.M., Klemp, J.R., Kamel, S., Zeiger, S. & Mayo, M.S. (2000). Short-term breast cancer prediction by random periareolar fine-needle aspiration cytology and the Gail risk model., *Journal of the National Cancer Institute,* vol. 92, no. 15, pp. 1217-1227.

Fadare, O., Dadmanesh, F., Alvarado-Cabrero, I., Snyder, R., Stephen Mitchell, J., Tot, T., Wang, S.A., Ghofrani, M., Eusebi, V., Martel, M. & Tavassoli, F.A. (2006). Lobular intraepithelial neoplasia [lobular carcinoma in situ] with comedo-type necrosis: A clinicopathologic study of 18 cases., *American Journal of Surgical Pathology,* vol. 30, no. 11, pp. 1445-1453.

Farante, G., Zurrida, S., Galimberti, V., Veronesi, P., Curigliano, G., Luini, A., Goldhirsch, A. & Veronesi, U. (2011). The management of ductal intraepithelial neoplasia (DIN): open controversies and guidelines of the Istituto Europeo di Oncologia (IEO), Milan, Italy, *Breast Cancer Research & Treatment,* vol. 128, no. 2, pp. 369-378.

Fiegl H., Millinger S., Goebel G., Müller-Holzner E., Marth C., Laird PW., & Widschwendter M.(2006). Breast cancer DNA methylation profiles in cancer cells and tumor stroma: association with HER-2/neu status in primary breast cancer., *Cancer Research,* vol. 66, no. 1, pp. 29-33.

Fisher, B., Land, S., Mamounas, E., Dignam, J., Fisher, E.R. & Wolmark, N. (2001). Prevention of invasive breast cancer in women with ductal carcinoma in situ: an update of the National Surgical Adjuvant Breast and Bowel Project experience., *Seminars in oncology,* vol. 28, no. 4, pp. 400-418.

Fisher, E.R., Costantino, J., Fisher, B., Palekar, A.S., Paik, S.M., Suarez, C.M. & Wolmark, N. (1996). Pathologic findings from the National Surgical Adjuvant Breast Project (NSABP) Protocol B-17. Five-year observations concerning lobular carcinoma in situ., *Cancer,* vol. 78, no. 7, pp. 1403-1416.

Fisher, E.R., Dignam, J., Tan-Chiu, E., Costantino, J., Fisher, B., Paik, S. & Wolmark, N. (1999). Pathologic findings from the National Surgical Adjuvant Breast Project (NSABP) eight-year update of Protocol B-17: intraductal carcinoma., *Cancer,* vol. 86, no. 3, pp. 429-438.

Fisher, E.R., Leeming, R., Anderson, S., Redmond, C. & Fisher, B. (1991). Conservative management of intraductal carcinoma (DCIS) of the breast. Collaborating NSABP investigators., *Journal of surgical oncology,* vol. 47, no. 3, pp. 139-147.

Foote, F.W. & Stewart, F,W. (1941). Lobular carcinoma in situ. A rare form of mammary cancer. *American Journal of Pathology,* vol. 17, pp. 491-496.

Frisell, J., Lidbrink, E., Hellstrom, L. & Rutqvist, L.E. (1997). Followup after 11 years--update of mortality results in the Stockholm mammographic screening trial., *Breast Cancer Research & Treatment,* vol. 45, no. 3, pp. 263-270.

Gasco, M., Shami, S. & Crook, T. (2002). The p53 pathway in breast cancer, *Breast Cancer Research,* vol. 4, no. 2, pp. 70-76.

Gerdes, J., Lemke, H., Baisch, H., Wacker, H.H., Schwab, U. & Stein, H. (1984). Cell cycle analysis of a cell proliferation-associated human nuclear antigen defined by the monoclonal antibody Ki-67., *Journal of Immunology,* vol. 133, no. 4, pp. 1710-1715.

Gobbi, H., Dupont, W.D., Parl, F.F., Schuyler, P.A., Plummer, W.D., Olson, S.J. & Page, D.L. (2005). Breast cancer risk associated with estrogen receptor expression in epithelial hyperplasia lacking atypia and adjacent lobular units., *International Journal of Cancer,* vol. 113, no. 5, pp. 857-859.

Gobbi, H., Dupont, W.D., Simpson, J.F., Plummer, W.D.,Jr, Schuyler, P.A., Olson, S.J., Arteaga, C.L. & Page, D.L. (1999). Transforming growth factor-beta and breast cancer risk in women with mammary epithelial hyperplasia., *Journal of the National Cancer Institute,* vol. 91, no. 24, pp. 2096-2101.

Goldhirsch, A., Ingle, J.N., Gelber, R.D., Coates, A.S., Thurlimann, B., Senn, H.J. & Panel, m. (2009). Thresholds for therapies: highlights of the St Gallen International Expert Consensus on the primary therapy of early breast cancer 2009, *Annals of Oncology,* vol. 20, no. 8, pp. 1319-1329.

Graham, J.D., Yager, M.L., Hill, H.D., Byth, K., O'Neill, G.M. & Clarke, C.L. (2005). Altered progesterone receptor isoform expression remodels progestin responsiveness of breast cancer cells., *Molecular Endocrinology,* vol. 19, no. 11, pp. 2713-2735.

Guerrieri-Gonzaga, A., Botteri, E., Rotmensz, N., Bassi, F., Intra, M., Serrano, D., Renne, G., Luini, A., Cazzaniga, M., Goldhirsch, A., Colleoni, M., Viale, G., Ivaldi, G., Bagnardi, V., Lazzeroni, M., Decensi, A., Veronesi, U. & Bonanni, B. (2009). Ductal intraepithelial neoplasia: postsurgical outcome for 1,267 women cared for in one single institution over 10 years., *Oncologist,* vol. 14, no. 3, pp. 201-212.

Gupta, S.K., Douglas-Jones, A.G., Jasani, B., Morgan, J.M., Pignatelli, M. & Mansel, R.E. (1997). E-cadherin (E-cad) expression in duct carcinoma in situ (DCIS) of the breast., *Virchows Archiv,* vol. 430, no. 1, pp. 23-28.

Gusterson, B.A., Machin, L.G., Gullick, W.J., Gibbs, N.M., Powles, T.J., Elliott, C., Ashley, S., Monaghan, P. & Harrison, S. (1988). c-erbB-2 expression in benign and malignant breast disease., *British journal of cancer,* vol. 58, no. 4, pp. 453-457.

Hannafon, B.N., Sebastiani, P., de Las Morenas, A., Lu, J.,& Rosenberg, C.L. (2011). Expression of microRNA and their gene targets are dysregulated in preinvasive breast cancer. *Breast Cancer Research & Treatment,* vol. 13, no. 2 , pp. R24

Heffelfinger, S.C., Yassin, R., Miller, M.A. & Lower, E.E. (2000). Cyclin D1, retinoblastoma, p53, and Her2/neu protein expression in preinvasive breast pathologies: correlation with vascularity., *Pathobiology,* vol. 68, no. 3, pp. 129-136.

Henderson, B.E., Ross, R. & Bernstein, L. (1988). Estrogens as a cause of human cancer: the Richard and Linda Rosenthal Foundation award lecture, *Cancer research,* vol. 48, no. 2, pp. 246-253.

Hieken, T.J., Farolan, M., D'Alessandro, S. & Velasco, J.M. (2001). Predicting the biologic behavior of ductal carcinoma in situ: an analysis of molecular markers., *Surgery,* vol. 130, no. 4, pp. 593-600.

Hockenbery, D.M. (1994). bcl-2 in cancer, development and apoptosis, *Journal of Cell Science - Supplement,* vol. 18, pp. 51-55.

Holland, R., Peterse, J.L., Millis, R.R., Eusebi, V., Faverly, D., van de Vijver, M.J. & Zafrani, B. (1994). Ductal carcinoma in situ: a proposal for a new classification, *Seminars in diagnostic pathology,* vol. 11, no. 3, pp. 167-180.

Houghton, J. George, W.D. Cuzick, J. Duggan, C. Fentiman, IS. Spittle, M. UK Coordinating Committee on Cancer Research. Ductal Carcinoma in situ Working Party. DCIS trialists in the UK, Australia,and New Zealand (2003). Radiotherapy and tamoxifen in women with completely excised ductal carcinoma in situ of the breast in the UK, Australia, and New Zealand: randomised controlled trial., *Lancet,* vol. 362, no. 9378, pp. 95-102.

Hudelist, G., Czerwenka, K., Kubista, E., Marton, E., Pischinger, K. & Singer, C.F. (2003). Expression of sex steroid receptors and their co-factors in normal and malignant breast tissue: AIB1 is a carcinoma-specific co-activator., *Breast Cancer Research & Treatment,* vol. 78, no. 2, pp. 193-204.

Hughes, L.L., Wang, M., Page, D.L., Gray, R., Solin, L.J., Davidson, N.E., Lowen, M.A., Ingle, J.N., Recht, A. & Wood, W.C. (2009). Local excision alone without irradiation for ductal carcinoma in situ of the breast: a trial of the Eastern Cooperative Oncology Group., *Journal of Clinical Oncology,* vol. 27, no. 32, pp. 5319-5324.

Hwang, E.S., Kinkel, K., Esserman, L.J., Lu, Y., Weidner, N. & Hylton, N.M. (2003). Magnetic resonance imaging in patients diagnosed with ductal carcinoma-in-situ: value in the diagnosis of residual disease, occult invasion, and multicentricity., *Annals of Surgical Oncology,* vol. 10, no. 4, pp. 381-388.

Ikeda, D.M. & Andersson, I. (1989). Ductal carcinoma in situ: atypical mammographic appearances., *Radiology,* vol. 172, no. 3, pp. 661-666.

Intra, M., Rotmensz, N., Mattar, D., Gentilini, O.D., Vento, A., Veronesi, P., Colleoni, M., De Cicco, C., Cassano, E., Luini, A. & Veronesi, U. (2007). Unnecessary axillary node dissections in the sentinel lymph node era., *European journal of cancer,* vol. 43, no. 18, pp. 2664-2668.

Intra, M., Rotmensz, N., Veronesi, P., Colleoni, M., Iodice, S., Paganelli, G., Viale, G. & Veronesi, U. (2008). Sentinel node biopsy is not a standard procedure in ductal carcinoma in situ of the breast: the experience of the European institute of oncology on 854 patients in 10 years., *Annals of Surgery,* vol. 247, no. 2, pp. 315-319.

Intra, M., Veronesi, P., Mazzarol, G., Galimberti, V., Luini, A., Sacchini, V., Trifiro, G., Gentilini, O., Pruneri, G., Naninato, P., Torres, F., Paganelli, G., Viale, G. & Veronesi, U. (2003). Axillary sentinel lymph node biopsy in patients with pure ductal carcinoma in situ of the breast., *Archives of Surgery,* vol. 138, no. 3, pp. 309-313.

Iqbal, M., Davies, M.P., Shoker, B.S., Jarvis, C., Sibson, D.R. & Sloane, J.P. (2001). Subgroups of non-atypical hyperplasia of breast defined by proliferation of oestrogen receptor-positive cells., *Journal of Pathology,* vol. 193, no. 3, pp. 333-338.

Jacobs, E.J., Feigelson, H.S., Bain, E.B., Brady, K.A., Rodriguez, C., Stevens, V.L., Patel, A.V., Thun, M.J. & Calle, E.E. (2006). Polymorphisms in the vascular endothelial growth factor gene and breast cancer in the Cancer Prevention Study II cohort., *Breast Cancer Research,* vol. 8, no. 2, pp. R22.

Julian, T.B., Land, S.R., Fourchotte, V., Haile, S.R., Fisher, E.R., Mamounas, E.P., Costantino, J.P. & Wolmark, N. (2007). Is sentinel node biopsy necessary in conservatively treated DCIS?, *Annals of Surgical Oncology,* vol. 14, no. 8, pp. 2202-2208.

Kang, J.H., Kim, S.J., Noh, D.Y., Choe, K.J., Lee, E.S. & Kang, H.S. (2001). The timing and characterization of p53 mutations in progression from atypical ductal hyperplasia to invasive lesions in the breast cancer., *Journal of Molecular Medicine,* vol. 79, no. 11, pp. 648-655.

Kapucuoglu, N., Losi, L. & Eusebi, V. (1997). Immunohistochemical localization of Bcl-2 and Bax proteins in in situ and invasive duct breast carcinomas., *Virchows Archiv,* vol. 430, no. 1, pp. 17-22.

Keohavong, P., Gao, W.M., Mady, H.H., Kanbour-Shakir, A. & Melhem, M.F. (2004). Analysis of p53 mutations in cells taken from paraffin-embedded tissue sections of ductal carcinoma in situ and atypical ductal hyperplasia of the breast., *Cancer letters,* vol. 212, no. 1, pp. 121-130.

Kepple, J., Henry-Tillman, R.S., Klimberg, V.S., Layeeque, R., Siegel, E., Westbrook, K. & Korourian, S. (2006). The receptor expression pattern in ductal carcinoma in situ predicts recurrence., *American Journal of Surgery,* vol. 192, no. 1, pp. 68-71.

Kerlikowske, K., Molinaro, A., Cha, I., Ljung, B.M., Ernster, V.L., Stewart, K., Chew, K., Moore, D.H. 2nd & Waldman, F. (2003). Characteristics associated with recurrence among women with ductal carcinoma in situ treated by lumpectomy., *Journal of the National Cancer Institute,* vol. 95, no. 22, pp. 1692-1702.

Khan, S.A., Rogers, M.A., Khurana, K.K., Meguid, M.M. & Numann, P.J. (1998). Estrogen receptor expression in benign breast epithelium and breast cancer risk., *Journal of the National Cancer Institute,* vol. 90, no. 1, pp. 37-42.

Kim, R. (2005). Unknotting the roles of Bcl-2 and Bcl-xL in cell death, *Biochemical & Biophysical Research Communications,* vol. 333, no. 2, pp. 336-343.

Krassenstein, R., Sauter, E., Dulaimi, E., Battagli, C., Ehya, H., Klein-Szanto, A. & Cairns, P. (2004). Detection of breast cancer in nipple aspirate fluid by CpG island hypermethylation., *Clinical Cancer Research,* vol. 10, no. 1 Pt 1, pp. 28-32.

Kretschmer ,C., Sterner-Kock, A., Siedentopf, F., Schoenegg, W., Schlag, P.M., & Kemmner, W., (2011). Identification of early molecular markers for breast cancer. *Molecular Cancer*. vol.10, no.1, pp. 15.

Krishnamurthy, S., Sneige, N., Thompson, P.A., Marcy, S.M., Singletary, S.E., Cristofanilli, M., Hunt, K.K. & Kuerer, H.M. (2003). Nipple aspirate fluid cytology in breast carcinoma., *Cancer,* vol. 99, no. 2, pp. 97-104.

Krogerus L.A., Leivonen M. & Häastö A.L. (2000). Expression patterns of biologic markers in small breast cancers and preneoplastic breast lesions. *Breast,* vol.9, no.5, pp.281-285.

Kuerer, H.M., Albarracin, C.T., Yang, W.T., Cardiff, R.D., Brewster, A.M., Symmans, W.F., Hylton, N.M., Middleton, L.P., Krishnamurthy, S., Perkins, G.H., Babiera, G., Edgerton, M.E., Czerniecki, B.J., Arun, B.K. & Hortobagyi, G.N. (2009). Ductal carcinoma in situ: state of the science and roadmap to advance the field, *Journal of Clinical Oncology,* vol. 27, no. 2, pp. 279-288.

Lagios, M.D. (1990). Duct carcinoma in situ. Pathology and treatment., *Surgical Clinics of North America,* vol. 70, no. 4, pp. 853-871.

Lebeau, A., Unholzer, A., Amann, G., Kronawitter, M., Bauerfeind, I., Sendelhofert, A., Iff, A. & Lohrs, U. (2003). EGFR, HER-2/neu, cyclin D1, p21 and p53 in correlation to cell proliferation and steroid hormone receptor status in ductal carcinoma in situ of the breast., *Breast Cancer Research & Treatment,* vol. 79, no. 2, pp. 187-198.

Lebrecht, A., Buchmann, J., Hefler, L., Lampe, D. & Koelbl, H. (2002). Histological category and expression of hormone receptors in ductal carcinoma in situ of the breast., *Anticancer Research,* vol. 22, no. 3, pp. 1909-1911.

Lebrecht, A., Grimm, C., Euller, G., Ludwig, E., Ulbrich, E., Lantzsch, T., Hefler, L. & Koelbl, H. (2004). Transforming growth factor beta 1 serum levels in patients with preinvasive and invasive lesions of the breast., *International Journal of Biological Markers,* vol. 19, no. 3, pp. 236-239.

Lee, C.H., Carter, D., Philpotts, L.E., Couce, M.E., Horvath, L.J., Lange, R.C. & Tocino, I. (2000). Ductal carcinoma in situ diagnosed with stereotactic core needle biopsy: can invasion be predicted?., *Radiology,* vol. 217, no. 2, pp. 466-470.

Lee, S., Mohsin, S.K., Mao, S., Hilsenbeck, S.G., Medina, D. & Allred, D.C. (2006). Hormones, receptors, and growth in hyperplastic enlarged lobular units: early potential precursors of breast cancer., *Breast Cancer Research,* vol. 8, no. 1, pp. R6.

Lehman, C.D., Gatsonis, C., Kuhl, C.K., Hendrick, R.E., Pisano, E.D., Hanna, L., Peacock, S., Smazal, S.F., Maki, D.D., Julian, T.B., DePeri, E.R., Bluemke, D.A., Schnall, M.D. & ACRIN Trial 6667 Investigators, G. (2007). MRI evaluation of the contralateral breast in women with recently diagnosed breast cancer., *New England Journal of Medicine,* vol. 356, no. 13, pp. 1295-1303.

Leonard, G.D. & Swain, S.M. (2004). Ductal carcinoma in situ, complexities and challenges, *Journal of the National Cancer Institute,* vol. 96, no. 12, pp. 906-920.

Lerwill, M.F. (2004). Current practical applications of diagnostic immunohistochemistry in breast pathology, *American Journal of Surgical Pathology,* vol. 28, no. 8, pp. 1076-1091.

Li, C.I., Malone, K.E., Saltzman, B.S. & Daling, J.R. (2006). Risk of invasive breast carcinoma among women diagnosed with ductal carcinoma in situ and lobular carcinoma in situ, 1988-2001., *Cancer,* vol. 106, no. 10, pp. 2104-2112.

Madu, C.O. & Lu, Y. (2010). Novel diagnostic biomarkers for prostate cancer., *Journal of Cancer,* vol. 1, pp. 150-177.

Mansel, R.E. (2003). Ductal carcinoma in situ: surgery and radiotherapy., *Breast,* vol. 12, no. 6, pp. 447-450.

Mastracci, T.L., Tjan, S., Bane, A.L., O'Malley, F.P. & Andrulis, I.L. (2005). E-cadherin alterations in atypical lobular hyperplasia and lobular carcinoma in situ of the breast., *Modern Pathology,* vol. 18, no. 6, pp. 741-751.

McGowan, E.M. & Clarke, C.L. (1999). Effect of overexpression of progesterone receptor A on endogenous progestin-sensitive endpoints in breast cancer cells., *Molecular Endocrinology,* vol. 13, no. 10, pp. 1657-1671.

McLaren, B.K., Gobbi, H., Schuyler, P.A., Olson, S.J., Parl, F.F., Dupont, W.D. & Page, D.L. (2005). Immunohistochemical expression of estrogen receptor in enlarged lobular units with columnar alteration in benign breast biopsies: a nested case-control study., *American Journal of Surgical Pathology,* vol. 29, no. 1, pp. 105-108.

Megha, T., Ferrari, F., Benvenuto, A., Bellan, C., Lalinga, A.V., Lazzi, S., Bartolommei, S., Cevenini, G., Leoncini, L. & Tosi, P. (2002). p53 mutation in breast cancer. Correlation with cell kinetics and cell of origin., *Journal of clinical pathology,* vol. 55, no. 6, pp. 461-466.

Menell, J.H., Morris, E.A., Dershaw, D.D., Abramson, A.F., Brogi, E. & Liberman, L. (2005). Determination of the presence and extent of pure ductal carcinoma in situ by mammography and magnetic resonance imaging., *Breast Journal,* vol. 11, no. 6, pp. 382-390.

Meteoglu, I., Dikicioglu, E., Erkus, M., Culhaci, N., Kacar, F., Ozkara, E. & Uyar, M. (2005). Breast carcinogenesis. Transition from hyperplasia to invasive lesions., *Saudi medical journal,* vol. 26, no. 12, pp. 1889-1896.

Midulla, C., Pisani, T., De Iorio, P., Cenci, M., Divizia, E., Nofroni, I. & Vecchione, A. (2002). Cytological analysis and immunocytochemical expression of Ki67 and Bcl-2 in breast proliferative lesions., *Anticancer Research,* vol. 22, no. 2B, pp. 1341-1345.

Miller, A.B., To, T., Baines, C.J. & Wall, C. (2002). The Canadian National Breast Screening Study-1: breast cancer mortality after 11 to 16 years of follow-up. A randomized screening trial of mammography in women age 40 to 49 years, *Annals of Internal Medicine,* vol. 137, no. 5 Part 1, pp. 305-312.

Miller, A.B., To, T., Baines, C.J. & Wall, C. (2000). Canadian National Breast Screening Study-2: 13-year results of a randomized trial in women aged 50-59 years., *Journal of the National Cancer Institute,* vol. 92, no. 18, pp. 1490-1499.

Mohsin, S.K., O'Connell, P., Allred, D.C. & Libby, A.L. (2005). Biomarker profile and genetic abnormalities in lobular carcinoma in situ., *Breast Cancer Research & Treatment,* vol. 90, no. 3, pp. 249-256.

Morrow, M., Strom, E.A., Bassett, L.W., Dershaw, D.D., Fowble, B., Harris, J.R., O'Malley, F., Schnitt, S.J., Singletary, S.E., Winchester, D.P., American College of, S., College of American, P., Society of Surgical, O. & American College of, R. (2002). Standard for the management of ductal carcinoma in situ of the breast (DCIS), *CA: a Cancer Journal for Clinicians,* vol. 52, no. 5, pp. 256-276.

Mote, P.A., Bartow, S., Tran, N. & Clarke, C.L. (2002). Loss of co-ordinate expression of progesterone receptors A and B is an early event in breast carcinogenesis., *Breast Cancer Research & Treatment,* vol. 72, no. 2, pp. 163-172.

Mote, P.A., Leary, J.A., Avery, K.A., Sandelin, K., Chenevix-Trench, G., Kirk, J.A., Clarke, C.L. & kConFab, I. (2004). Germ-line mutations in BRCA1 or BRCA2 in the normal breast are associated with altered expression of estrogen-responsive proteins and the predominance of progesterone receptor A., *Genes, chromosomes & cancer,* vol. 39, no. 3, pp. 236-248.

Musgrove, E.A., Davison, E.A. & Ormandy, C.J. (2004). Role of the CDK inhibitor p27 (Kip1) in mammary development and carcinogenesis: insights from knockout mice, *Journal of Mammary Gland Biology & Neoplasia,* vol. 9, no. 1, pp. 55-66.

Mustonen, M., Raunio, H., Paakko, P. & Soini, Y. (1997). The extent of apoptosis is inversely associated with bcl-2 expression in premalignant and malignant breast lesions., *Histopathology,* vol. 31, no. 4, pp. 347-354.

Mylonas, I., Makovitzky, J., Jeschke, U., Briese, V., Friese, K. & Gerber, B. (2005). Expression of Her2/neu, steroid receptors (ER and PR), Ki67 and p53 in invasive mammary ductal carcinoma associated with ductal carcinoma In Situ (DCIS) Versus invasive breast cancer alone., *Anticancer Research,* vol. 25, no. 3A, pp. 1719-1723.

Nass, S.J., Herman, J.G., Gabrielson, E., Iversen, P.W., Parl, F.F., Davidson, N.E. & Graff, J.R. (2000). Aberrant methylation of the estrogen receptor and E-cadherin 5' CpG islands increases with malignant progression in human breast cancer., *Cancer research,* vol. 60, no. 16, pp. 4346-4348.

National Comprehensive Cancer Network (NCCN) Guidelines for Treatment of Cancer by Site: Breast Cancer. (2009). Available from http://www.nccn.org/professionals/physician_gls/breast.pdf

Nofech-Mozes, S., Spayne, J., Rakovitch, E. & Hanna, W. (2005). Prognostic and predictive molecular markers in DCIS: a review, *Advances in Anatomic Pathology,* vol. 12, no. 5, pp. 256-264.

Nystrom, L., Andersson, I., Bjurstam, N., Frisell, J., Nordenskjold, B. & Rutqvist, L.E. (2002). Long-term effects of mammography screening: updated overview of the Swedish randomised trials, *Lancet,* vol. 359, no. 9310, pp. 909-919.

Oh, Y.L., Choi, J.S., Song, S.Y., Ko, Y.H., Han, B.K., Nam, S.J. & Yang, J.H. (2001). Expression of p21Waf1, p27Kip1 and cyclin D1 proteins in breast ductal carcinoma in situ: Relation with clinicopathologic characteristics and with p53 expression and estrogen receptor status., *Pathology international,* vol. 51, no. 2, pp. 94-99.

O'Malley, F.P., Vnencak-Jones, C.L., Dupont, W.D., Parl, F., Manning, S. & Page, D.L. (1994). p53 mutations are confined to the comedo type ductal carcinoma in situ of the breast. Immunohistochemical and sequencing data., *Laboratory Investigation,* vol. 71, no. 1, pp. 67-72.

O'Neill, P.A., Shaaban, A.M., West, C.R., Dodson, A., Jarvis, C., Moore, P., Davies, M.P., Sibson, D.R. & Foster, C.S. (2004). Increased risk of malignant progression in benign proliferating breast lesions defined by expression of heat shock protein 27., *British journal of cancer,* vol. 90, no. 1, pp. 182-188.

Orel, S.G., Mendonca, M.H., Reynolds, C., Schnall, M.D., Solin, L.J. & Sullivan, D.C. (1997). MR imaging of ductal carcinoma in situ., *Radiology,* vol. 202, no. 2, pp. 413-420.

Page, D.L., Dupont, W.D., Rogers, L.W. & Landenberger, M. (1982). Intraductal carcinoma of the breast: follow-up after biopsy only., *Cancer,* vol. 49, no. 4, pp. 751-758.

Papantoniou, V., Tsiouris, S., Koutsikos, J., Sotiropoulou, M., Mainta, E., Lazaris, D., Valsamaki, P., Melissinou, M., Zerva, C. & Antsaklis, A. (2006). Scintimammographic detection of usual ductal breast hyperplasia with increased proliferation rate at risk for malignancy., *Nuclear medicine communications,* vol. 27, no. 11, pp. 911-917.

Parker, S.H., Burbank, F., Jackman, R.J., Aucreman, C.J., Cardenosa, G., Cink, T.M., Coscia, J.L.,Jr, Eklund, G.W., Evans, W.P.,3rd & Garver, P.R. (1994). Percutaneous large-core breast biopsy: a multi-institutional study., *Radiology,* vol. 193, no. 2, pp. 359-364.

Petersen, O.W., Hoyer, P.E. & van Deurs, B. (1987). Frequency and distribution of estrogen receptor-positive cells in normal, nonlactating human breast tissue., *Cancer research,* vol. 47, no. 21, pp. 5748-5751.

Poller, D.N., Roberts, E.C., Bell, J.A., Elston, C.W., Blamey, R.W. & Ellis, I.O. (1993). p53 protein expression in mammary ductal carcinoma in situ: relationship to immunohistochemical expression of estrogen receptor and c-erbB-2 protein., *Human pathology,* vol. 24, no. 5, pp. 463-468.

Provenzano, E., Hopper, J.L., Giles, G.G., Marr, G., Venter, D.J. & Armes, J.E. (2003). Biological markers that predict clinical recurrence in ductal carcinoma in situ of the breast., *European journal of cancer,* vol. 39, no. 5, pp. 622-630.

Putti, T.C., Pinder, S.E., Elston, C.W., Lee, A.H. & Ellis, I.O. (2005). Breast pathology practice: most common problems in a consultation service, *Histopathology,* vol. 47, no. 5, pp. 445-457.

Reed, J.C. (1994). Bcl-2 and the regulation of programmed cell death, *Journal of Cell Biology,* vol. 124, no. 1-2, pp. 1-6.

Rieger-Christ, K.M., Pezza, J.A., Dugan, J.M., Braasch, J.W., Hughes, K.S. & Summerhayes, I.C. (2001). Disparate E-cadherin mutations in LCIS and associated invasive breast carcinomas., *Molecular Pathology,* vol. 54, no. 2, pp. 91-97.

Ringberg, A., Anagnostaki, L., Anderson, H., Idvall, I., Ferno, M. & South Sweden Breast Cancer, G. (2001). Cell biological factors in ductal carcinoma in situ (DCIS) of the breast-relationship to ipsilateral local recurrence and histopathological characteristics., *European journal of cancer,* vol. 37, no. 12, pp. 1514-1522.

Roberts, M.M., Alexander, F.E., Anderson, T.J., Forrest, A.P., Hepburn, W., Huggins, A., Kirkpatrick, A.E., Lamb, J., Lutz, W. & Muir, B.B. (1984). The Edinburgh randomised trial of screening for breast cancer: description of method., *British journal of cancer,* vol. 50, no. 1, pp. 1-6.

Rocco, J.W. & Sidransky, D. (2001). p16(MTS-1/CDKN2/INK4a) in cancer progression, *Experimental cell research,* vol. 264, no. 1, pp. 42-55.

Rody, A., Diallo, R., Poremba, C., Speich, R., Wuelfing, P., Kissler, S., Solbach, C., Kiesel, L. & Jackisch, C. (2004). Estrogen receptor alpha and beta, progesterone receptor, pS2 and HER-2/neu expression delineate different subgroups in ductal carcinoma in situ of the breast., *Oncology reports,* vol. 12, no. 4, pp. 695-699.

Roger, P., Sahla, M.E., Makela, S., Gustafsson, J.A., Baldet, P. & Rochefort, H. (2001). Decreased expression of estrogen receptor beta protein in proliferative preinvasive mammary tumors., *Cancer research,* vol. 61, no. 6, pp. 2537-2541.

Rohan, T.E., Hartwick, W., Miller, A.B. & Kandel, R.A. (1998). Immunohistochemical detection of c-erbB-2 and p53 in benign breast disease and breast cancer risk., *Journal of the National Cancer Institute,* vol. 90, no. 17, pp. 1262-1269.

Ross, J.S. & Fletcher, J.A. (1999). HER-2/neu (c-erb-B2) gene and protein in breast cancer, *American Journal of Clinical Pathology,* vol. 112, no. 1 Suppl 1, pp. S53-67.

Rudas, M., Neumayer, R., Gnant, M.F., Mittelbock, M., Jakesz, R. & Reiner, A. (1997). p53 protein expression, cell proliferation and steroid hormone receptors in ductal and lobular in situ carcinomas of the breast., *European journal of cancer,* vol. 33, no. 1, pp. 39-44.

Santamaria, G., Velasco, M., Farrus, B., Zanon, G. & Fernandez, P.L. (2008). Preoperative MRI of pure intraductal breast carcinoma--a valuable adjunct to mammography in assessing cancer extent., *Breast,* vol. 17, no. 2, pp. 186-194.

Sapino, A., Frigerio, A., Peterse, J.L., Arisio, R., Coluccia, C. & Bussolati, G. (2000). Mammographically detected in situ lobular carcinomas of the breast., *Virchows Archiv,* vol. 436, no. 5, pp. 421-430.

Schnitt, S.J., Silen, W., Sadowsky, N.L., Connolly, J.L. & Harris, J.R. (1988). Ductal carcinoma in situ (intraductal carcinoma) of the breast, *New England Journal of Medicine,* vol. 318, no. 14, pp. 898-903.

Schoonjans, J.M. & Brem, R.F. (2000). Sonographic appearance of ductal carcinoma in situ diagnosed with ultrasonographically guided large core needle biopsy: correlation with mammographic and pathologic findings., *Journal of Ultrasound in Medicine,* vol. 19, no. 7, pp. 449-457.

Schwartz, G.F., Solin, L.J., Olivotto, I.A., Ernster, V.L. & Pressman, P.I. (2000). Consensus Conference on the Treatment of In Situ Ductal Carcinoma of the Breast, April 22-25, 1999, *Cancer,* vol. 88, no. 4, pp. 946-954.

Shaaban, A.M., Jarvis, C., Moore, F., West, C., Dodson, A. & Foster, C.S. (2005). Prognostic significance of estrogen receptor Beta in epithelial hyperplasia of usual type with known outcome., *American Journal of Surgical Pathology,* vol. 29, no. 12, pp. 1593-1599.

Shaaban, A.M., O'Neill, P.A., Davies, M.P., Sibson, R., West, C.R., Smith, P.H. & Foster, C.S. (2003). Declining estrogen receptor-beta expression defines malignant progression of human breast neoplasia., *American Journal of Surgical Pathology,* vol. 27, no. 12, pp. 1502-1512.

Shaaban, A.M., Sloane, J.P., West, C.R. & Foster, C.S. (2002). Breast cancer risk in usual ductal hyperplasia is defined by estrogen receptor-alpha and Ki-67 expression., *American Journal of Pathology,* vol. 160, no. 2, pp. 597-604.

Shapiro, S. (1997). Periodic screening for breast cancer: the HIP Randomized Controlled Trial. Health Insurance Plan., *Journal of the National Cancer Institute,* vol. Monographs, no. 22, pp. 27-30.

Shoker, B.S., Jarvis, C., Clarke, R.B., Anderson, E., Hewlett, J., Davies, M.P., Sibson, D.R. & Sloane, J.P. (1999). Estrogen receptor-positive proliferating cells in the normal and precancerous breast., *American Journal of Pathology,* vol. 155, no. 6, pp. 1811-1815.

Shoker, B.S., Jarvis, C., Clarke, R.B., Anderson, E., Munro, C., Davies, M.P., Sibson, D.R. & Sloane, J.P. (2000). Abnormal regulation of the oestrogen receptor in benign breast lesions., *Journal of clinical pathology,* vol. 53, no. 10, pp. 778-783.

Sickles E.A. (1983). Sonographic detectability of breast calcifications., *Proceedings of SPIE,* vol. 419, pp. 51-52

Silverstein, M.J., Cohlan, B.F., Gierson, E.D., Furmanski, M., Gamagami, P., Colburn, W.J., Lewinsky, B.S. & Waisman, J.R. (1992). Duct carcinoma in situ: 227 cases without microinvasion., *European journal of cancer,* vol. 28, no. 2-3, pp. 630-634.

Silverstein, M.J., Recht, A., Lagios, M.D., Bleiweiss, I.J., Blumencranz, P.W., Gizienski, T., Harms, S.E., Harness, J., Jackman, R.J., Klimberg, V.S., Kuske, R., Levine, G.M., Linver, M.N., Rafferty, E.A., Rugo, H., Schilling, K., Tripathy, D., Vicini, F.A., Whitworth, P.W. & Willey, S.C. (2009). Special report: Consensus conference III. Image-detected breast cancer: state-of-the-art diagnosis and treatment, *Journal of the American College of Surgeons,* vol. 209, no. 4, pp. 504-520.

Simooka, H., Oyama, T., Sano, T., Horiguchi, J. & Nakajima, T. (2004). Immunohistochemical analysis of 14-3-3 sigma and related proteins in hyperplastic and neoplastic breast lesions, with particular reference to early carcinogenesis., *Pathology international,* vol. 54, no. 8, pp. 595-602.

Siziopikou, K.P., Prioleau, J.E., Harris, J.R. & Schnitt, S.J. (1996). bcl-2 expression in the spectrum of preinvasive breast lesions., *Cancer,* vol. 77, no. 3, pp. 499-506.

Slanetz, P.J., Giardino, A.A., Oyama, T., Koerner, F.C., Halpern, E.F., Moore, R.H. & Kopans, D.B. (2001). Mammographic appearance of ductal carcinoma in situ does not reliably predict histologic subtype., *Breast Journal,* vol. 7, no. 6, pp. 417-421.

Smith, G.L., Smith, B.D. & Haffty, B.G. (2006). Rationalization and regionalization of treatment for ductal carcinoma in situ of the breast., *International journal of radiation oncology, biology, physics,* vol. 65, no. 5, pp. 1397-1403.

Sneige, N., Wang, J., Baker, B.A., Krishnamurthy, S. & Middleton, L.P. (2002). Clinical, histopathologic, and biologic features of pleomorphic lobular (ductal-lobular) carcinoma in situ of the breast: a report of 24 cases., *Modern Pathology,* vol. 15, no. 10, pp. 1044-1050.

Stark, A., Hulka, B.S., Joens, S., Novotny, D., Thor, A.D., Wold, L.E., Schell, M.J., Melton, L.J.,3rd, Liu, E.T. & Conway, K. (2000). HER-2/neu amplification in benign breast disease and the risk of subsequent breast cancer., *Journal of Clinical Oncology,* vol. 18, no. 2, pp. 267-274.

Stomper, P.C., Connolly, J.L., Meyer, J.E. & Harris, J.R. (1989). Clinically occult ductal carcinoma in situ detected with mammography: analysis of 100 cases with radiologic-pathologic correlation., *Radiology,* vol. 172, no. 1, pp. 235-241.

Tabar, L., Vitak, B., Chen, H.H., Duffy, S.W., Yen, M.F., Chiang, C.F., Krusemo, U.B., Tot, T. & Smith, R.A. (2000). The Swedish Two-County Trial twenty years later. Updated mortality results and new insights from long-term follow-up., *Radiologic clinics of North America,* vol. 38, no. 4, pp. 625-651.

Tavassoli, F.A. (2008). Lobular and ductal intraepithelial neoplasia, *Pathologe,* vol. 29, no. Suppl 2, pp. 107-111.

Tavassoli, F.A., Hoeffler H, Rosai J et al. 2003 Intraductal proliferative lesions In: Tavassoli F.A,, Devilee P (eds) World Health Organization Classification of Tumors: Pathology and genetics of Tumor of the breast and the female genital organs IARC Press, Lyon pp 65-66

Toledo, F. & Wahl, G.M. (2006). Regulating the p53 pathway: in vitro hypotheses, in vivo veritas, *Nature Reviews.Cancer,* vol. 6, no. 12, pp. 909-923.

Tsuda, H. & Hirohashi, S. (1998). Multiple developmental pathways of highly aggressive breast cancers disclosed by comparison of histological grades and c-erbB-2 expression patterns in both the non-invasive and invasive portions., *Pathology international,* vol. 48, no. 7, pp. 518-525.

Tsuda, H., Iwaya, K., Fukutomi, T. & Hirohashi, S. (1993). p53 mutations and c-erbB-2 amplification in intraductal and invasive breast carcinomas of high histologic grade., *Japanese Journal of Cancer Research,* vol. 84, no. 4, pp. 394-401.

Umbricht, C.B., Evron, E., Gabrielson, E., Ferguson, A., Marks, J. & Sukumar, S. (2001). Hypermethylation of 14-3-3 sigma (stratifin) is an early event in breast cancer., *Oncogene,* vol. 20, no. 26, pp. 3348-3353.

van Delft, M.F. & Huang, D.C. (2006). How the Bcl-2 family of proteins interact to regulate apoptosis, *Cell research,* vol. 16, no. 2, pp. 203-213.

Van Zee, K.J., Calvano, J.E. & Bisogna, M. (1998). Hypomethylation and increased gene expression of p16INK4a in primary and metastatic breast carcinoma as compared to normal breast tissue., *Oncogene,* vol. 16, no. 21, pp. 2723-2727.

Viacava, P., Naccarato, A.G. & Bevilacqua, G. (1999). Different proliferative patterns characterize different preinvasive breast lesions., *Journal of Pathology,* vol. 188, no. 3, pp. 245-251.

Viacava, P., Naccarato, A.G., Bocci, G., Fanelli, G., Aretini, P., Lonobile, A., Evangelista, G., Montruccoli, G. & Bevilacqua, G. (2004). Angiogenesis and VEGF expression in pre-invasive lesions of the human breast., *Journal of Pathology,* vol. 204, no. 2, pp. 140-146.

Virnig, B.A., Tuttle, T.M., Shamliyan, T. & Kane, R.L. (2010). Ductal carcinoma in situ of the breast: a systematic review of incidence, treatment, and outcomes, *Journal of the National Cancer Institute,* vol. 102, no. 3, pp. 170-178.

Vogelstein, B., Lane, D. & Levine, A.J. (2000). Surfing the p53 network., *Nature,* vol. 408, no. 6810, pp. 307-310.

Vogl, G., Dietze, O. & Hauser-Kronberger, C. (2005). Angiogenic potential of ductal carcinoma in situ (DCIS) of human breast., *Histopathology,* vol. 47, no. 6, pp. 617-624.

Vos, C.B., Cleton-Jansen, A.M., Berx, G., de Leeuw, W.J., ter Haar, N.T., van Roy, F., Cornelisse, C.J., Peterse, J.L. & van de Vijver, M.J. (1997). E-cadherin inactivation in lobular carcinoma in situ of the breast: an early event in tumorigenesis., *British journal of cancer,* vol. 76, no. 9, pp. 1131-1133.

Wakefield, L.M., Piek, E. & Bottinger, E.P. (2001). TGF-beta signaling in mammary gland development and tumorigenesis, *Journal of Mammary Gland Biology & Neoplasia,* vol. 6, no. 1, pp. 67-82.

Walker, R.A. & Dearing, S.J. (1992). Transforming growth factor beta 1 in ductal carcinoma in situ and invasive carcinomas of the breast., *European journal of cancer,* vol. 28, no. 2-3, pp. 641-644.

Warren, J.L., Weaver, D.L., Bocklage, T., Key, C.R., Platz, C.E., Cronin, K.A., Ballard-Barbash, R., Willey, S.C. & Harlan, L.C. (2005). The frequency of ipsilateral second tumors after breast-conserving surgery for DCIS: a population based analysis., *Cancer,* vol. 104, no. 9, pp. 1840-1848.

Winchester, D.P. & Strom, E.A. (1998). Standards for diagnosis and management of ductal carcinoma in situ (DCIS) of the breast. American College of Radiology. American

College of Surgeons. College of American Pathologists. Society of Surgical Oncology, *CA: a Cancer Journal for Clinicians,* vol. 48, no. 2, pp. 108-128.

Wrensch, M.R., Petrakis, N.L., Miike, R., King, E.B., Chew, K., Neuhaus, J., Lee, M.M. & Rhys, M. (2001). Breast cancer risk in women with abnormal cytology in nipple aspirates of breast fluid., *Journal of the National Cancer Institute,* vol. 93, no. 23, pp. 1791-1798.

Xu, R., Perle, M.A., Inghirami, G., Chan, W., Delgado, Y. & Feiner, H. (2002). Amplification of Her-2/neu gene in Her-2/neu-overexpressing and -nonexpressing breast carcinomas and their synchronous benign, premalignant, and metastatic lesions detected by FISH in archival material., *Modern Pathology,* vol. 15, no. 2, pp. 116-124.

Yi, M., Krishnamurthy, S., Kuerer, H.M., Meric-Bernstam, F., Bedrosian, I., Ross, M.I., Ames, F.C., Lucci, A., Hwang, R.F. & Hunt, K.K. (2008). Role of primary tumor characteristics in predicting positive sentinel lymph nodes in patients with ductal carcinoma in situ or microinvasive breast cancer., *American Journal of Surgery,* vol. 196, no. 1, pp. 81-87.

Younes, M., Lebovitz, R.M., Bommer, K.E., Cagle, P.T., Morton, D., Khan, S. & Laucirica, R. (1995). p53 accumulation in benign breast biopsy specimens., *Human pathology,* vol. 26, no. 2, pp. 155-158.

Part 4

Intraepithelial Neoplasia of Prostate

6

Prostate Cancer Precursor Diseases

A.G. Papatsoris, C. Kostopoulos, V. Migdalis and M. Chrisofos
2nd Department of Urology, School of Medicine, University of Athens, Sismanoglio General Hospital, Athens, Greece

1. Introduction

Prostate cancer remains the most common non-cutaneous malignancy in the Western world and is the second leading cause of cancer death in males, after lung cancer (Nelson et al., 2003; Papatsoris & Anagnostopoulos, 2009). Based on experimental and preclinical findings, novel anti-prostate cancer strategies have been developed (Papatsoris & Papavassiliou, 2001; Papatsoris et al., 2005). However, the causes of prostate cancer, prostatic carcinogenesis, and the histological changes preceding and leading to the initiation of prostate cancer have yet to be elucidated. Several research groups are trying to solve the puzzle of prostatic carcinogenesis by focusing within the morphological continuum between benign glands at one end and premalignant lesions and invasive disease at the other (Vis & Van Der Kwast, 2001). In parallel, clinicians are frequently confronted with morphological features on the prostate needle biopsy that, although negative for cancer, raise suspicion of concomitant malignancy.

2. Definition of prostate cancer precursor lesions

There are several criteria that should be met in order to consider a prostatic lesion as premalignant (Vis & Van Der Kwast, 2001). An epidemiological relationship must be revealed, the precursor lesion should present at an earlier age than the cancer, and clear morphological similarities (e.g. cellular, histological, and architectural) should be present. Also, premalignant lesions should be close to their presumed malignant equivalents. The prostate has a greater frequency, severity, and extent of premalignant lesions in comparison with other organs. The definitive proof of a relationship between a premalignant lesion and malignancy is the clinical evidence of progression into invasive prostate cancer.

The earliest report on premalignant prostatic lesions dates back to 1926 (Orteil, 1926). In 1965, *McNeal* described lesions with possible premalignant features in prostatic epithelium (McNeal, 1965). In 1986, *McNeal and Bostwick* described the first criteria for the diagnosis of "intraductal neoplasia" which was classified into three grades (McNeal & Bostwick, 1986). In 1987, *Bostwick and Brawer* introduced the term "PIN" - prostatic intraepithelial neoplasia (Bostwick & Brawer, 1987). At an international conference in 1989, the term "PIN" was accepted as a replacement for various other terms (e.g. intraductal hyperplasia, hyperplasia with malignant change, large acinar atypical hyperplasia, marked atypia, ductal-acinar dysplasia). Initially, PIN was categorized into three grades with regard to architectural and cytological characteristics, taking into account that the alterations cover a continuum. However, in 1989, at the aforementioned workshop on premalignant prostatic lesions, the classification was altered to low-grade (formerly grade I) and high-grade (formerly grades II and III) PIN - LGPIN and HGPIN, respectively (Bostwick, 1989).

Conventional histopathology examination is used to differentiate precursor lesions of prostate cancer. Benign glands show a continuous basal cell layer, while in prostate cancer the basal cell layer is immunohistochemically absent. Immunostaining for p63 (a p53 homologue) was shown to be useful as a basal cell-specific marker (Signoretti et al., 2000; Shah, 2004). It is frequently used in addition to 34βE12 immunostaining in difficult diagnostic cases, where the main advantage of p63 over 34βE12 is that there is less variable staining.

A wide range of "atypical" epithelial proliferative processes with a variety of names, often with confusing and overlapping terminology, has been described. Several morphological lesions have been proposed that may act as potential precursor lesions of prostate cancer. These are the morphologically distinct entities of focal atrophy or post-atrophic hyperplasia (PAH), atypical adenomatous hyperplasia (AAH) or adenosis, and PIN.

3. Prostatic atrophy and PAH

Focal prostatic atrophy reportedly is present in up to 85% of prostates at autopsy (Amin, 1999; Billis, 1998). It should be distinguished from diffuse atrophy, as the latter is not considered premalignant. A role for focal atrophy in the pathogenesis of PIN and/or prostate cancer was proposed by Franks, over 50 years ago (Franks, 1954). *De Marzo* observed that focal atrophic lesions showed an increased proliferative activity of luminal cells and a decreased frequency of apoptosis (DeMarzo et al., 1999). Concerning the classification of focal prostatic atrophy, although there are distinct histologic variants, the terminology is currently non-standardized and no formal classification has been tested for interobserver reliability. According to the current classification focal atrophy lesions were categorized into 4 distinct subtypes as follows: (i) simple atrophy, (ii) simple atrophy with cyst formation, (iii) postatrophic hyperplasia and (iv) partial atrophy (De Marzo et al., 2006).

Simple atrophy consists of atrophic cells lining acini with relatively normal caliber that lack papillary fronds, where the number of glands per unit area does not appear to be increased relative to normal tissue. (De Marzo et al., 2006). Simple atrophy demonstrates strong basal cell-specific antikeratin immunoreactivity (Bostwick, 1996). Simple atrophy with cyst formation is a subtype of simple atrophy. Two general patterns are now encompassed: those containing very large diameter glands (> 1 mm) and those containing smaller, rounded glands. The amount of cytoplasm at times may be so attenuated as to be nearly invisible. When there is significant cytoplasm in the luminal cell, it tends to be clear. Atrophy with cyst formation tends to have less inflammation than the other sub-types (De Marzo et al., 2006). In sclerotic atrophy, the stroma is more extensively sclerosed, resulting in a wider separation of the acinar elements; these continue to have the cytological features described above (DeMarzo et al., 1999; De Marzo et al., 2006). Post-Atrophic Hyperplasia (PAH) consists of acini that are smaller, round and appear in a lobular distribution, often surrounding a somewhat dilated duct with an apparent increase in the number of small glands compared to normal tissue. Some authors tend to refer to some of these lesions as "lobular atrophy" or "lobular hyperplasia" (De Marzo et al., 2006). In lobular atrophy, the lesion is circumscribed with a central duct surrounded by small acini (Grignon & Sakr, 1996). The acini frequently have ectatic lumens and are lined by a flattened epithelium having scant cytoplasm and hyperchromatic nuclei with inconspicuous nucleoli. Basal cells are present but are difficult to recognize; however, they are readily identified with immunohistochemical stains for 34βE12 cytokeratin. The stroma is sclerotic and compressed, particularly around the central duct.

PAH, which may closely mimic the histology of prostate cancer, may represent a diagnostic pitfall (Bostwick, 1996). Recent studies have reported that the frequency of PAH in radical prostatectomy specimens was remarkably similar to that in cystoprostatectomy specimens, implying that the simultaneous finding of PAH with prostate cancer is coincidental (Amin, 1999; Grignon & Sak, 1996). PAH develops in a background of lobular or sclerotic atrophy and so retains many features of these lesions (Anton et al., 1999; Cheville & Bostwick, 1995; Grignon & Sakr, 1996). In PAH, there is an apparent secondary proliferation of small acini. The secretory cells have more abundant pale or clear cytoplasm than in usual atrophy, though generally not as much as in adenocarcinoma or AAH. The nuclei also become less hyperchromatic, and small chromocenters or nucleoli may be seen. The double cell layer is maintained and can be confirmed with basal cell-specific anticytokeratin antibodies. Despite the observation that focal atrophic lesions and PAH consist of flattened and dispersed acini, immunostaining with 34βE12 cytokeratin is almost always positive and continuous, as it is for benign epithelial glands (Anton et al., 1999; Cheville & Bostwick, 1995).

4. AAH and sclerosing adenosis

The prevalence of AAH in transurethral prostatectomy (TURP) specimens without cancer ranges from 1.6% to 7.3% (Gaudi & Epstein, 1994). In biopsy specimens, the prevalence is lower, for example 0.8% in one series (Gaudin & Epstein, 1995). The increase in frequency of AAH in needle biopsies is presumably related to ultrasound-guided biopsy of the transition zone. AAH can be diagnosed throughout the prostate, but it is most often located in the transition zone of the prostate in intimate association with benign nodular hyperplasia (Bostwick & Qian, 1995). It can also be found near the apex and in the periurethral area (Bostwick, 1996). In AAH, the basal cell layer is discontinuous and fragmented on 34βE12 cytokeratin immunostaining (Cheng et al., 1998).

There is considerable morphologic evidence suggesting that AAH is associated with low-grade adenocarcinoma arising in the transition zone (Cheville & Bostwick, 1995). AAH, a putative precursor of transition zone adenocarcinoma, has common features with low-grade adenocarcinoma and may cause problems in differential diagnosis, especially in the needle biopsy setting (Srigley, 2004). AAH is a lesion characterized by a proliferation of small acinar structures that mimics adenocarcinoma because of histological similarities (Grignon & Sakr, 1996). At low magnification, the lesion is circumscribed, although the small acini may show some infiltrative features. These acini are seen in association with a usually hyperplastic nodule and are most often at the periphery of the nodule. The nuclei tend to be uniform and round with inconspicuous or small nucleoli. There is limited data that AAH has a proliferation rate higher than hyperplasia but lower than adenocarcinoma (Bostwick & Qian, 1995; Cheng et al., 1998; Grignon & Sakr, 1996). AAH is diploid, as are most examples of low-grade adenocarcinoma, while a few markers (blood group antigens, peanut agglutinin) show similar patterns of expression in AAH and adenocarcinoma (Grignon & Sakr, 1996). Recent cytogenetic analyses have detected abnormalities of chromosome 8 in a very small proportion (4–7%) of AAH cases (Bostwick & Qian, 1995; Cheng et al., 1998).

Sclerosing adenosis is a circumscribed proliferation of small acinar structures in a cellular spindled sclerotic stroma (Grignon & Sakr, 1996; Srigley, 2004). The acini range from irregular in shape to small, round, and uniform. Usually, there is thickening of the tubular basement membrane, a valuable diagnostic clue (Grignon & Sakr, 1996). Nucleoli are generally inconspicuous but can be prominent in a few cells, while the lumens can contain basophilic mucin or crystalloids (Grignon & Sakr, 1996). Sclerosing adenosis is usually an incidental finding in about 2% of transurethral resection of the prostate (TURP) or radical prostatectomy specimens, (Bostwick et al., 2008; Grignon et al., 1992; Cheng & Bostwick, 2010; Sakamoto et al, 1991) and rarely is present in needle biopsy specimens (Cheng & Bostwick 2010; Srigley, 2004). Sclerosing adenosis may simulate adenocarcinoma and accounts for up to 10% of cases overdiagnosed as adenocarcinoma (Berney et al., 2007; Bostwick & Cheng, 1999; Cheng & Bostwick, 2010). Multiple light microscopic and immunohistochemical features separate typical sclerosing adenosis from adenocarcinoma, including: (i) intact basal cell layer, a finding that can be confirmed immunohistochemically with antibodies directed against high-molecular-weight cytokeratin 34βE12, (ii) unique immunophenotype of many of the basal and spinde cells in the stroma, including abundant S100 protein and smooth muscle actin (SMA) reactivity, as well as structural characteristics of myoepithelial cells, (iii) cellular spindle cell stroma, (iv) variably thickened basement membrane and (v) absence of significant cytological atypia. (Bostwick et al., 1994; Collina et al., 1992; Grignon et al., 1992; JonesC et al., 1991; Cheng & Bostwick, 2010; Sakamoto et al. 1991; Young & Clement, 1987 ; Young & Clement, 1990). Sclerosing adenosis differs from AAH by displaying myoepithelial features of the basal cells and an exuberant stroma of fibroblasts and loose ground substance (Bostwick et al., 1994).

5. Lesion Suspicious for Cancer (LSC)

As a result of the limited quantity of tissue sampled in prostate biopsies, there is the probability of finding a lesion that raises diagnostic confusion. There may be lesions suspicious for but not conclusive of malignancy. These lesions are small and have a wide diversity of architectural and morphological features. *Vis* proposed the terminology "prostate biopsy suspicious for malignancy" to classify these lesions (Vis et al., 2001). However, histology reports should be unequivocal and as concise as possible and vague diagnoses should not lead to unnecessary biopsy with its associated morbidities.

The controversial diagnostic term "atypical small acinar proliferation" (ASAP) is no longer considered acceptable. It is not considered a diagnostic entity as it can only be diagnosed on needle biopsies and not in prostatectomy specimens. The term ASAP has been replaced by the term "lesion suspicious for cancer" (LSC), as the prostate lesion lacks sufficient criteria to call it a carcinoma. LSC (fig. 1, 2) has gained acceptance as a legitimate way for pathologists to describe minute foci of small prostatic acini that raise the suspicion of carcinoma but that fail to attain the requisite diagnostic threshold for carcinoma (Fadare et al., 2004).

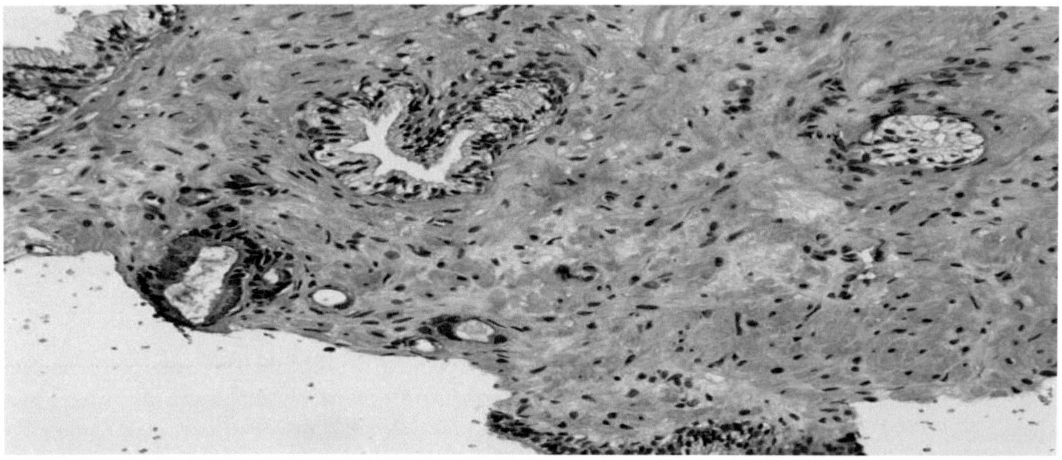

Fig. 1. An accumulation of a few atypical prostatic glands with amphophilic cytoplasm and nuclear enlargement. Compare with benign adjacent glands. This field is consistent with either atypical small prostate gland proliferation or limited prostate adenocarcinoma. (HE × 200)

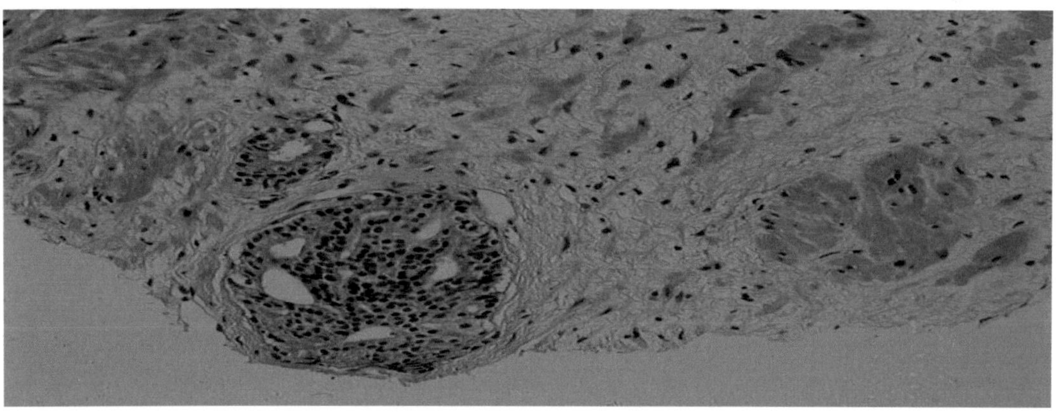

Fig. 2. Atypical cribriform gland at the periphery of a biopsy. Differential diagnosis between HGPIN and cribriform invasive adenocarcinoma may be impossible.

Studies have demonstrated that LSC is diagnosed in 1.5% to 9% of prostatic biopsies and that it predicts definite prostate cancer in about 45% of repeat biopsies (Iczkowski et al., 1997; Iczkowski et al., 1998; Iczkowski & Bostwick, 2000; Iczkowski et al., 2002). Since 1997, there have been efforts to stratify risk in cases of LSC into three categories: likely benign, uncertain, and likely carcinoma (Iczkowski et al., 1997). No single pathologic feature of LSC appeared to increase the likelihood for subsequent cancer (Iczkowski et al., 1998; Iczkowski & Bostwick, 2000; Iczkowski et al., 2002; Scattoni et al., 2005). The mean MIB-1 proliferation index of LSC was significantly higher than in benign prostatic tissue and did not differ from that of low-grade carcinoma.

LSC continues to be associated with a high risk of prostate cancer and requires a repeat biopsy with the extended peripheral zone biopsy scheme (Moore et al., 2005). Sampling should include multiple sites in the prostate, as in 40% of patients; cancer was in different sites from the initial LSC site. The detection rate was lower for patients with a larger prostate than those with a smaller prostate (Scattoni et al., 2005). Hence, patients with LSC should be followed up and undergo repeat biopsy. The role of radical prostatectomy for LSC is not clear, although *Brausi* advocated that prostatectomy could be the treatment of choice in young men with LSC (Brausi et al., 2004).

6. PIN

6.1 Epidemiology of PIN

Epidemiological studies have demonstrated the presence of PIN in men as early as the fourth decade of life and showed that the incidence and extent of PIN increased with age (Sakr et al., 1993). It has been postulated that PIN pre-dates the onset of prostate cancer by 5–10 years (Sakr et al., 1993). In several autopsy and surgical series, PIN was identified in 60% to 90% of prostates harboring carcinoma and was often close to its presumed invasive equivalent (Qian et al., 1997). Studies showed that PIN was present in 82% of step-sectioned autopsy prostates with cancers, but in only 43% of benign prostates from patients of similar age (Vis & Van Der Kwast, 2001). *Qian* found that 86% of a series of 195 whole-mount radical prostatectomies contained HGPIN, usually within 2 mm of the cancer (Qian et al., 1997).

In the United States, 1.300.000 prostate biopsies are performed annually to detect 230.000 new cases of prostate cancer (Joniau et al., 2007; Steiner, 2003). There are approximately 115.000 cases of isolated HGPIN diagnosed each year, representing an estimated 9% of prostate biopsies (Steiner, 2003). The incidence of HGPIN in biopsies ranges from 1.5% to 16.5%, with an average of 6% (Bostwick et al., 1995; Epstein, 2002). The different incidence of HGPIN in published studies derives from differences in defining HGPIN and in the number of patients.

The most likely explanation to account for the variation in incidence of PIN is interobserver reproducibility (Sakr, 1995). Those pathologists who use a lower threshold to define prominent nucleoli will have a higher incidence of HGPIN. Other plausible explanations for the variation in reported incidence of HGPIN relate to the fixative used and to differences in sampling. Furthermore, the variations from one institution to another can be attributed to variation in the population study, the indications for biopsy, and the biopsy compliance rates. The site of the prostate biopsied, the number of biopsies taken, and the quality and processing technique of the biopsy cores can also influence the incidence of PIN.

HGPIN starts in young individuals and increases with age in Caucasians and African-Americans, but is more prevalent in the latter (Epstein, 1995; Sakr et al., 1996). HGPIN in African-Americans precedes HGPIN in Caucasians by approximately a decade (Epstein, 1995). A more extensive form of HGPIN with multifocal or diffuse involvement of the glands appears at a younger age in African-Americans in comparison with Caucasians (Sakr et al., 1996). The replication of the association of chromosome 8q24 variants with increased prostate cancer risk in Tobago men and the higher frequency of the risk alleles in controls in populations of African ancestry further strengthens the possible role of this genomic region in the disproportionate higher burden of prostate cancer in men of African ancestry (Sakr et al., 1996). It has also been shown that prostate cancer grows more rapidly in black than in white men and/or earlier transformation from latent to aggressive prostate cancer occurs in black than in white men (Powell et al., 2010).

6.2 Molecular biology of PIN

The development of PIN is characterized by increased expression of several biomarkers that influence the proliferative potential of the dysplastic prostatic cells. Studies of potential biomarkers, such as growth factors, growth factor receptors, oncogene products, glycosylated tumor antigens, and other biomarkers in PIN, are difficult because these lesions are focal.

Unlike the premalignant polyps of the colon, it is difficult to obtain relatively pure preparations of PIN. One approach, to microdissect areas of PIN, is tedious and still may produce results contaminated by surrounding stroma and histologically normal epithelium. In addition, this technique does not allow differentiation of biomarker expression among the various components (basal versus luminal) of the dysplastic gland or duct.For these reasons, immuno - histochemical techniques as well as fluorescence *in situ* hybridization (FISH) is perhaps best suited for the assessment of biomarker expression in PIN.

FISH analysis has demonstrated strong expression of epidermal growth factor receptor (EGFr) mRNA in PIN (Myers & Grizzle, 1996). The c-erbB-2 gene product (p185erbB-2) is a transmembrane receptor that demonstrates significant homology to EGFr. Moderate-to-strong immunoreactivity for p185erbB-2 was noted in the luminal as well as the basal cells of PIN lesions. This immunostaining was frequently equivalent in pattern and intensity to that of adjacent malignant cells. The pattern of expression was typically coarse cytoplasmic immunoreactivity. Increased expression of the growth factor-related receptors p185erbB-2 and p180erbB-3, as well as the product of the *c-met* protooncogene (a transmembrane tyrosine kinase receptor that binds the mitogen hepatocyte growth factor/scatter factor), is frequently detected in the dysplastic luminal cells and in malignant cells of the prostate (Myers & Grizzle, 1996). Mutation of the p53 gene in PIN may precede the development of highly aggressive prostate cancer (Myers & Grizzle, 1996). The expression of the nm-23H1 gene product is strongly expressed in dysplastic and malignant prostatic cells (Myers & Grizzle, 1996).

It has been demonstrated that expression of the proliferative markers Ki-67 and proliferating cell nuclear antigen (PCNA) in PIN is increased as compared to benign prostatic epithelium (Myers & Grizzle, 1996). Increased PCNA expression also has been detected in the nuclei of stromal and endothelial cells adjacent to PIN (Myers & Grizzle, 1996). This may be associated with the observation of a higher density of blood vessels in the vicinity of PIN lesions. In contrast to the enhanced expression of the biomarkers associated with proliferation, decreased expression of prostate specific antigen (PSA), prostate acid phosphatase, and Leu 7 by dysplastic luminal cells is indicative of an impairment of the process of cellular differentiation (Myers & Grizzle, 1996). *Bostwick* demonstrated a decrease in the expression of neuroendocrine markers (neuron-specific enolase, serotonin, chromagranin, and human chorionic gonadotropin) in PIN. Aberrant glycosylation as well as inappropriate expression of glycosylated tumor antigens was demonstrated by enhanced binding of the lectin *Ulex europaeus* and by increased expression of tumor-associated glycoprotein 72 and the Lewis Y antigen (Myers & Grizzle, 1996). Enhanced expression of proteolytic enzymes, such as cathepsin D and the 72-kD form of collagenase IV, by dysplastic cells may represent an integral event in the development of invasive prostate cancer (Boag & Young, 1994). Moderate-to-strong immunoreactivity for fatty acid synthetase was also detected in PIN (Swinnen et al., 2002).

In HGPIN, studies have demonstrated notable loss of the three critical signaling components of the apoptotic action of transforming growth factor-β; that is, the transmembrane receptor II (TβRII), the key cell cycle inhibitor p27Kip1, and the protagonist downstream Smad4 receptor-activated protein (Zeng & Kyprianou, 2005). Quantitative evaluation of the apoptotic index revealed significantly less value in HGPIN when compared with adjacent areas of benign prostatic hyperplasia (Zeng & Kyprianou, 2005). Apoptotic profiling of HGPIN may contribute to a better understanding of factors that play a role in deregulated prostate growth (Zeng & Kyprianou, 2005).

Prostate carcinogenesis is the result of the accumulation of multiple genetic changes. The most frequently found chromosomal anomalies are overexpression on chromosomes 7p, 7q, and 8q, and inactivation on chromosomes 8p, 10q, 13q, 16q, and 18q (Joniau et al., 2005). Inactivation of tumor suppression genes, such as NKX3-1 (8p) and PTEN (10q), and overexpression of oncogenes, such as c-myc (8q), play an important role in PIN and the initiation of prostate cancer (Qian et al 1995). These findings support the multi-step theory in which PIN is considered a precursor lesion of prostate cancer.

6.3 Similarities between PIN and prostate cancer

The frequency and extent of PIN lesions increase with age, and this is similar to the increase in diagnosis of prostate cancer (Joniau et al., 2005). HGPIN is found significantly more frequently in prostates with cancer (McNeal & Bostwick, 1986). PIN is predominantly located in the peripheral zone of the prostate, the area in which most clinically important prostate cancers are found, and PIN, like prostate cancer, is often multifocal (Joniau et al., 2005). In an autopsy study, HGPIN was found in 63% of cases solely in the peripheral zone; in 36%, in the peripheral and transition zone; and in 1%, solely in the transition zone (Haggman et al., 1997). These findings are similar to the zonal distribution of prostate cancer.

Several genotypic and phenotypic studies have indicated that there are remarkable morphological, molecular, and biochemical similarities between PIN and prostate cancer (Vis & Van Der Kwast, 2001). Molecular abnormalities in PIN are mostly intermediate between benign gland and cancer, reflecting an impairment of cell-differentiation and regulatory control (Bostwick, 1999). PIN is characterized by cellular crowding and stratification. There is inequality in cell and nuclear size. Hyperchromatism is frequently seen with an enlarged nucleus, often containing prominent nucleoli lines. These changes are also seen in Gleason grade 1-4 prostate cancer (Bostwick et al., 1998). Biochemically, the cells of PIN show changes in the cytoskeletal proteins, secretory proteins, and nuclei that are shared with established prostate malignancies.

Prostate cancer and HGPIN have similar proliferative and apoptotic indices (Bostwick et al., 1998). Mitotic figures and apoptotic bodies increase progressively from nodular hyperplasia to HGPIN (Bostwick et al., 1998). During the malignant transformation of PIN, the basal cell layer loses its proliferative function, which is transferred to secretory luminal cell types, as demonstrated by Bonkhoff (Bonkhoff, 1996). Moreover, there is a progressive increase in the number of apoptotic bodies from nodular hyperplasia through PIN to prostate cancer (Bostwick et al., 1996). Greater cytoplasmic expression of bcl-2 is observed in PIN and cancer than in benign and hyperplastic epithelium (Bostwick et al., 1996). Two members of the platelet-derived growth factor (PDGF) peptide family, PDGF-A and PDGF-*α*, are up-regulated in PIN and prostate cancer compared with benign prostatic hyperplasia; BPH (Bostwick et al., 1996). Similarly, there is up-regulation of cathepsinD in PIN and prostate cancer; this autocrine mitogen, which has been studied extensively in other organs as a marker of invasion, correlates with tumor grade and DNA ploidy status in prostate cancer (Bostwick et al., 1996).

Histologically, the atypia observed in HGPIN is virtually indistinguishable from that of prostate cancer except that in HGPIN the basal membrane is still intact (Sakr et al., 1999). As HGPIN progresses, the likelihood of basal cell layer disruption increases. In HGPIN, the basal cell layer is disrupted or fragmented as demonstrated by high-molecular-weight cytokeratin immunolabeling. In prostate cancer, there is a complete loss of the basal cell layer. Both in PIN and prostate cancer, collagenase type IV expression is increased compared to normal prostate epithelium; this enzyme is responsible for basal membrane degradation and thus facilitates invasion (Bostwick et al., 1996). PIN and prostate cancer share several nuclear properties, such as amount of DNA, chromatin texture, chromatin distribution, nuclear perimeter, diameter, and nuclear abnormalities (Baretton et al., 1994).

Several genetic changes encountered in prostate cancer cells can be found in PIN lesions (Bostwick et al., 1996). Allelic loss is common in PIN and prostate cancer (Sakr et al., 1999). The frequent 8p12-21 allelic loss commonly found in prostate cancer is also found in microdissected PIN. Other examples of genetic changes found in prostate cancer that already exist in PIN include loss of heterozygosity at 8p22, 12pter-p12, and 10q11.2 and gain of chromosomes 7, 8, 10, and 12. Alterations in oncogene bcl2 expression and RER+ phenotype are similar for PIN and prostate cancer (Baltaci et al., 2000). As in prostate cancer, there is also evidence of aneuploidy and an increase in microinvascular density, both frequently regarded as evidence of aggressiveness in PIN (Montironi et al., 1993).

6.4 LGPIN

In LGPIN (Fig. 3), secretory cells of the lining epithelium proliferate and "pill up" with irregular spaces between them (Bostwick, 2000 ; Newling, 1990). The nuclei are enlarged, vary in size, have normal or slightly increased chromatin content, and possess small or inconspicuous nucleoli (Zeng & Kyprianou, 2005). More prominent nucleoli, when observable, comprise less than 10% of dysplastic cells. The basal cell layer normally surrounding secretory cells of ducts and acini remains intact. In LGPIN, only 0.7% of reported cases reveal evidence of basal cell layer disruption (Newling, 1999).

LGPIN is rather difficult to recognize, as it shares common features with normal and hyperplastic epithelium (Bostwick, 2000; Newling, 1999). The most common issue that may lead in some cases to discrepant diagnoses between LGPIN and HGPIN is the definition of "prominent" with regard to nucleolar enlargement and visibility.

It has been suggested that LGPIN should not be commented on in diagnostic reports (Epstein, 2002). Firstly, pathologists cannot reproducibly distinguish LGPIN from benign prostate tissue (Epstein et al., 1995). Secondly, when LGPIN is diagnosed on needle biopsy, these patients are not at greater risk of having prostate cancer on repeat biopsy (Keetch, 1995).

The distinction between HGPIN and LGPIN is based primarily on the extent of cytological abnormalities (prominence of the nucleoli) and secondarily on the degree of architectural complexity (Goeman et al., 2003; Weinstein & Epstein, 1993). Immunostaining studies of microvessel density may help to differentiate HGPIN from LGPIN (Sinha et al., 2004).

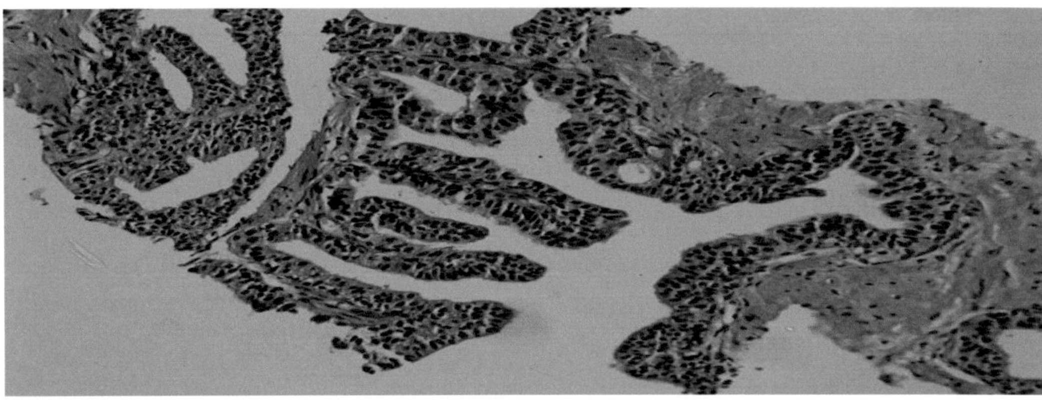

Fig. 3. Papillary structures within a large hyperplastic prostate gland. Minimal nuclear atypia. (HE × 200)

6.5 HGPIN

6.5.1 Why HGPIN?

PIN was initially divided into three different grades (I–III), which now are reduced to the abovementioned LGPIN for PIN I, and HGPIN for PIN II and III. HGPIN includes PIN II and III for two reasons. Firstly, there was a great deal of inter-observer variability in the distinction between PIN II and III (Epstein et al., 1995). Secondly, the finding of PIN II or III on needle biopsy was associated with the same risk of prostate cancer on subsequent biopsy (Weinstein & Epstein, 1993).

6.5.2 Histology of HGPIN

In HGPIN, uniform morphologic abnormalities are detectable (Vis & Van Der Kwast, 2001). Cells have large nuclei of relatively uniform size, and possess prominent nucleoli that are similar to those of cancer cells (fig. 4, 5). Regarding cytological features, the acini and ducts are lined by malignant cells which are uniformly enlarged with an increased nuclear/cytoplasmic ratio, and with less variation in nuclear size in comparison to LGPIN. In HGPIN, at least 10% of cells demonstrate prominent nucleoli similar to those of carcinoma cells, and the majority of cells show coarse clumping of the chromatin which may be accentuated along the nuclear membrane (Vis & Van Der Kwast, 2001). The expanded nuclear chromatin area probably explains the darker "blue" appearance of the lining which characterizes HGPIN at low power microscopic examination. Nuclei toward the centre of the gland tend to have blander cytology than peripherally located nuclei.

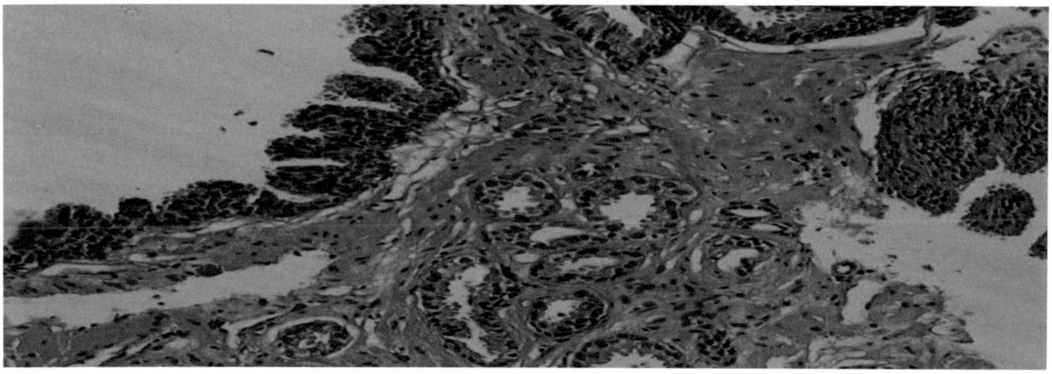

Fig. 4. HGPIN tufted pattern and adjacent carcinoma (with an adequate number of small malignant glands). Small atypical glands are too numerous to represent outpouchings of HGPIN. (HE × 200)

6.5.3 Patterns of HGPIN

There are four architectural patterns of HGPIN: tufting, micropapillary, flat and cribriform, based on the arrangement of the cells within pre-existing ducts or glands (Vis & Van Der Kwast, 2001). Tufting HGPIN is by far the most common pattern (present in 97% of all HGPINs) followed by micropapillary, flat, and cribriform patterns (Yamauchi et al., 2006). In the flat pattern, nuclear atypia is evident without significant architectural changes. In the tufting pattern, nuclei become more pilled up, and undulating mounds of cells are formed. Columns of atypical epithelial cells typically lacking fibrovascular cores characterize the micropapillary pattern. In the cribriform pattern, more complex architectural features, such as a "Roman bridge" and cribriform formation, are encountered.

Patients with HGPIN in only one initial biopsy or a predominant flat/tufting pattern clearly have less risk of cancer being found in subsequent biopsies compared to patients with HGPIN in more than one initial biopsy. Furthermore, a micropapillary and/or cribriform pattern are correlated with a greater risk for development of prostate cancer (Joniau et al., 2005).

Unusual subtypes of HGPIN include PIN with signet-ring morphology and neuroendocrine cells with either Paneth cell-like or small-cell morphology (Bostwick et al., 1993; Vis & Van Der Kwast, 2001). Intraductal HGPIN, in prostates with established cancer, has been associated with high tumor volumes, poorly differentiated tumor components, and a higher progression rate after radical prostatectomy than prostate cancers without these coexisting proliferations (Cohen et al., 2000; McNeal & Bostwick, 1986). Hence, a separate histological entity was proposed, namely, intraductal carcinoma of the prostate, which would be distinguished from HGPIN.

6.5.4 HGPIN and prostate cancer

HGPIN is the most likely precursor of prostatic adenocarcinoma, according to current literature (Dovey et al., 2005; Gaudin et al., 1997; Joniau et al., 2005; Lefkowitz et al., 2002; Pacelli & Bostwick, 1997; Powell et al., 2010; Singh et al., 2009; Vis & Van Der Kwast, 2001). The expression of various biomarkers in HGPIN is either the same as with prostate cancer or intermediate between prostate cancer and benign prostate tissue. The cytological changes are characterized by prominent nucleoli in a substantial proportion (≥5%) of cells, nuclear enlargement and crowding, increased density of cytoplasm, and anisonucleosis (Vis & Van Der Kwast, 2001). Ploidy seems not to discriminate between HGPIN and infiltrating cancer (Baretton et al., 1994). Also, studies reveal consistent down-regulation of epithelial cell adhesion molecules and transmembrane proteins in PIN (Vis & Van Der Kwast, 2001). This is accompanied by up-regulation of enzymes responsible for degradation of the extracellular matrix.

Unlike in prostate cancer, incomplete disruption of the basal cell layer can be shown by 34βE12 cytokeratin immunostaining (Vis & Van Der Kwast, 2001). In HGPIN, more than 50% of abnormal cells are seen to have a disrupted basal cell layer in the acini. Immunohistochemistry is usually not helpful since the lack of a basal cell layer in only a few cribriform or small glands is not sufficient for the diagnosis of cancer. However, in cases where many glands are totally immunonegative for high-molecular-weight cytokeratin, these foci may be diagnostic of cancer. Cases where some of the glands show the expected patchy basal cell layer of PIN and a few, morphologically identical glands are negative for high-molecular-weight keratin should still be diagnosed as HGPIN. In rare cases when sperm can be identified in the glandular lumen, the diagnosis of PIN is favored because only PIN glands are able to communicate with the main prostatic glands that contain sperm; malignant invasive glands cannot retain their continuity with main prostatic glands (Vis & Van Der Kwast, 2001).

In cases of HGPIN with neighboring small atypical glands, the possibility of coexistent invasive carcinoma should be examined (Vis & Van Der Kwast, 2001). When the latter are few, the issue is whether the small glands represent outpouchings or tangential sections of the adjacent HGPIN or whether they represent microinvasive cancer. When these small atypical glands are too many or too crowded to be outpouchings or tangential sections of the HGPIN glands, then the diagnosis of invasive carcinoma can be made (Bostwick et al., 1996).

6.6 Differential diagnosis of PIN

Histologically, PIN can be confused with several benign entities as well as with ductal and acinar adenocarcinoma (fig. 5) of the prostate (Epstein et al., 2002). Benign conditions include prostate central zone hyperplasia, since glands within the central zone at the base of the prostate are complex and large with many papillary infoldings and clear cell cribriform hyperplasia, which consists of crowded cribriform glands with clear cytoplasm (Vis & Van Der Kwast, 2001; Joniau et al., 2005). Both these entities lack significant nuclear atypia. The basal cell layer can display prominent nucleoli but secretory cells can be recognized. Cytologically atypical basal cell hyperplasia usually forms small solid nests of atypical basal cells, mainly in the central zone; these are inconsistent with PIN, which affects medium- or large-sized glands, mainly in the peripheral zone of the prostate (Vis & Van Der Kwast, 2001). In any case, basal cells can be easily identified by immunohistochemistry either with antibodies against high-molecular-weight cytokeratins (cytoplasmic staining pattern) or against p63 (nuclear staining pattern).

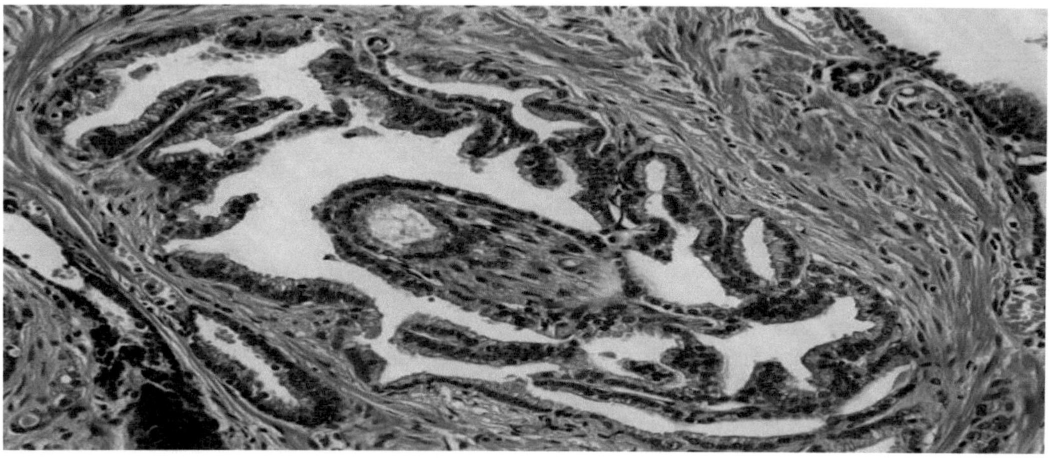

Fig. 5. Complex atypical gland with prominent nucleoli and perineural invasion. Gleason pattern 3 of cribriform adenocarcinoma. Note the coexistent microacinar cancerous pattern on the bottom right. (HE × 200)

With regard to malignant conditions, cribriform acinar adenocarcinoma can be discriminated from cribriform HGPIN when a sufficient number of cribriform glands totally lack basal cells (Vis & Van Der Kwast, 2001). Furthermore, in cribriform carcinoma, sometimes the appearance of foci of back-to-back glands, rather than true cribriform formations, is evident.

Ductal adenocarcinomas of the prostate may demonstrate a patchy basal cell layer (like PIN), but they develop in the transition zone. They may develop true papillary fronts with fibrovascular cores (in contrast to micropapilary PIN). Ductal adenocarcinoma glands are larger, may contain back-to-back glands, may show extensive comedonecrosis, and are usually fragmented in needle biopsy specimens.

Finally, the possibility of intraductal carcinoma (fig. 6) should be considered when multiple cribriform glands with prominent cytological atypia containing comedonecrosis are encountered (Cohen et al., 2000; McNeal & Bostwick, 1986). In these glands, basal cells can be identified, though this lesion should be distinguished from HGPIN since it appears to be a late event in prostate gland carcinogenesis and warrants immediate therapy.

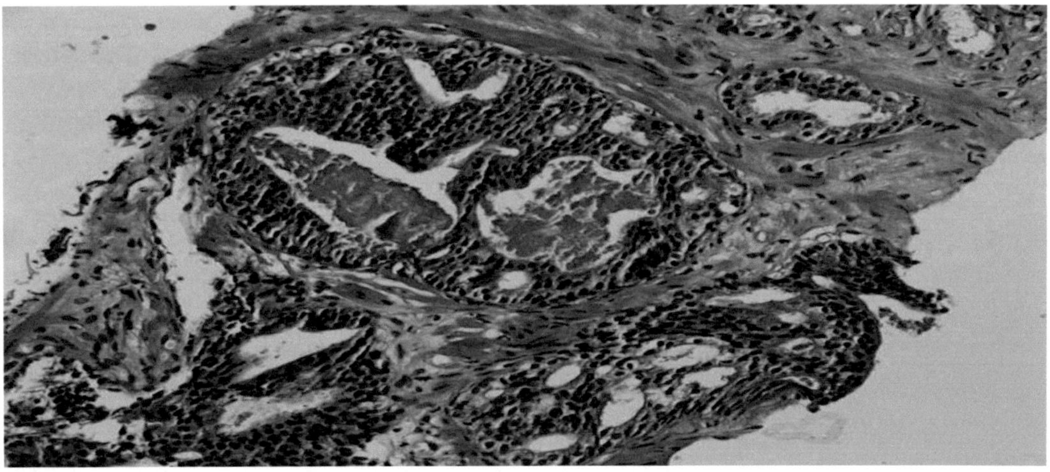

Fig. 6. Many large atypical cribriform glands with extensive comedonecrosis. Retention of basal cell layer remnants would be consistent with intraductal carcinoma rather than HGPIN. (HE × 200)

6.7 Clinical markers of PIN

6.7.1 PSA

PIN lesions do not contribute to an elevation of serum PSA, PSA density, or a decrease in the free-to-total PSA ratio (Alexander et al., 1996; Darson et al., 1999; Ronnett et al., 1993). PIN lesions show less expression of PSA in luminal cells, as determined by immunohistochemistry, than do benign epithelial glands (Ronnett et al., 1993; Alexander et al., 1996). An elevation of PSA should be attributed to the presence of prostate cancer, BPH, or concurrent prostatic inflammation rather than to the presence of PIN.

Immunohistochemical studies show a lower PSA expression in PIN lesions compared to benign tissue and prostate cancer (Darson et al., 1999). PSA produced by PIN lesions follows the route of least resistance and is excreted in the seminal fluid, whereas cancer forms tissue islands without a surrounding basal layer, and PSA diffuses into the blood.

6.7.2 Potential markers

Swinnen demonstrated that fatty acid synthetase immunostaining intensity tended to increase from LGPIN to HGPIN and prostate cancer (Swinnen et al., 2002). This key enzyme in the de novo production of fatty acids enables cancer progression and invasion. Another enzyme, alpha-methylacyl coenzyme A racemase (AMARC), which plays a key role in the beta-oxidation of fatty acids, is rarely expressed in benign prostatic tissue, in contrast to PIN and prostate cancer (Rubin et al., 2002). A statistically significant association of this biomarker with the risk of prostate cancer is yet to be revealed (Hailemariam et al., 2011). A80, a membrane-bound glycoprotein that is related to exocrine differentiation, may be useful in detecting residual and/or recurrent prostate carcinoma after radiation or hormonal therapy (Coogan et al., 2003). Benign glands are generally negative for A80 except for scattered positive cells in about 15% of glandular hyperplasia (Shin et al., 1989). *Coogan* demonstrated that A80 immunostaining in prostate cancer, HGPIN, and LGPIN, in 100%, 92%, and 73% of the examined specimens, respectively (Coogan et al., 2003). Markers including kallikrein-related peptidase 2 (KLK2), early prostate cancer antigen (EPCA), PCA3, hepsin, prostate stem cell antigen are under investigation for the early diagnosis and management of prostate cancer (Darson et al., 1997; Sardana et al., 2008). PCA3 is a prostate specific, non-protein coding RNA that is significantly over expressed in prostate cancer, without any correlation to prostatic volume and/or other prostatic diseases like prostatitis. Recent studies have shown the potential of PCA3, in correlation with other markers, to be used as a prognostic marker for prostate cancer (Bourdoumis et al., 2010).

6.8 Management of PIN

6.8.1 Repeat prostate biopsy

As a consequence of programs for the early detection of prostate cancer, the number of biopsies performed and specimens evaluated has increased substantially. False-positive results may strongly influence a man's quality of life through unnecessary psychological stress, unnecessary treatment, and treatment-associated morbidities. Furthermore, for medico-legal reasons, it is obvious that biopsy false-positive results should be minimized. Currently, the consensus is that the finding of focal atrophy, PAH, AAH, or LGPIN on needle biopsy or in TURP material for BPH should not lead to any diagnostic follow-up (Vis & Van Der Kwast, 2001). However, the finding of HGPIN on needle biopsy indicates a field effect by which the entire prostate is at higher risk of harboring cancer (Langer et al., 1996).

The decisions for diagnostic follow-up in men with PIN should take into account the patient's age, physical status, and co-morbidities. In men developing HGPIN in the eighth decade, knowing that the development of symptomatic prostate cancer will probably occur only after 10 years, a policy of watchful waiting should be recommended.(Ravery V , 2009 ; Vis AN & Van Der Kwast TH , 2001) Men who may not potentially benefit from curative treatment or early hormonal therapy should not undergo follow-up biopsy.

When more extensive repeat biopsy is performed, the likelihood of detecting prostate cancer is increased. If isolated HGPIN is detected in a 12-core biopsy protocol, the cancer incidence in the immediate 12-core repeat biopsy will be only 2% to 3% (Lefkowitz, 2002). In contrast, in repeat biopsies following initial sextant or octant biopsies, the cancer detection rate is 27–30% (Lefkowitz, 2002). However, taking too many biopsies can increase the risk of detecting too many clinically insignificant cancers and can lead to overtreatment (Joniau et al., 2005). Authors have proposed an 8-biopsy regimen, which clearly outperformed the sextant regimen in cancer detection (Joniau et al., 2005; Lefkowitz, 2002).

When follow-up biopsies are performed in men with foci of isolated HGPIN, the site of prostate cancer may not be the same site that raised the suspicion of concurrent carcinoma (Bostwick et al., 1995). The finding of HGPIN after TURP (2.8%-33%) also appears to place men at a higher risk of harboring cancer, although there are few studies on this topic (Gaudin et al., 1997; Pacelli & Bostwick, 1997). It is reasonable to perform needle biopsies on patients, especially younger men, who have HGPIN after TURP.

It has been demonstrated that patients with a flat or tufting HGPIN pattern on initial biopsy clearly have less risk of cancer being found in subsequent biopsy (20%), in comparison with patients with micropapillary or cribriform pattern, who have a relative risk of 70% (Chan & Epstein, 1999). The isolated finding of HGPIN in the cystoprostatectomy specimen has no clinical implications, and the prognosis of the patient is determined by the initial indication (e.g. invasive bladder cancer) for surgery.

The jury is still out concerning the best repeat biopsy strategy following the diagnosis of PIN on initial prostate biopsy. The length of the interval still needs to be established in large prospective studies (Joniau et al., 2005). Repeat biopsy six weeks after the initial biopsy has led to the diagnoses of prostate cancer in 9% of cases with isolated HGPIN (Chan & Epstein, 1999; Ellis & Brawer, 1995; Kronz et al., 2001; O'Dowd et al., 2000). The risk for finding prostate cancer in repeat biopsies seems to increase with the length of the biopsy interval. Age, PSA, and HGPIN were independent predictors for prostate cancer in repeat biopsies, with HGPIN providing the highest risk ratio (Chan & Epstein, 1999; Langer et al., 1996; Sakr et al., 1996). Most urologists recommend follow-up biopsy after 6–12 months, followed by regular PSA monitoring and repeat biopsies as indicated (Shepherd et al., 1996). Men within screening settings who are diagnosed with isolated HGPIN should be followed at regular intervals, and if clinical suspicion persists, the biopsy should be repeated (Ellis & Brawer, 1995; Kronz et al., 2001; Shepherd et al., 1996). The finding of intraductal HGPIN on initial biopsy needs further investigation with repeat biopsy, because this lesion is related to potentially aggressive cancer.

6.8.2 Chemoprevention

Examples of treated premalignant lesions include cervical intraepithelial neoplasia, ductal CIS (carcinoma *in situ*) of the breast, adenomatous polyps of the colon, and Barrett's esophagus (Sporn, 1999). The American Association for Cancer Research designates intraepithelial neoplasia an important target for chemoprevention (O'Shaughnessy et al., 2002). As HGPIN precedes the development of prostate cancer by several years and is easy identifiable, it is a candidate for chemoprevention. Chemoprevention means the administration of drugs or agents aimed at preventing the initiation and progression of cancer. A number of potential preventive agents have been investigated in patients with HG-PIN, including hormones (flutamide, finasteride, leuprolide acetate) and antioxidants such as lycopene, selenium, and catechins. An association beween the E-cadherin/catenin complex and high-grade prostate cancer has been proved and the therapeutic potential of integrin antagonists is being evaluated by ongoing clinical trials with promising results (Drivalos et al., 2011). One of the most promising chemoprevention drugs is the selective oestrogen receptor modulator toremifene citrate (Ravery, 2009). Recognizing the slow growth rate of prostate cancer and the considerable amount of time needed in animal and human studies for adequate follow-up, the noninvasive precursor lesion PIN is a suitable intermediate histological marker to indicate high likelihood of subsequent prostate cancer. HGPIN offers promise as an intermediate endpoint in studies of chemoprevention of prostate cancer (Montironi et al., 1999). Hence, HGPIN is a suitable intermediate histological marker to indicate subsequent likelihood of cancer and it may be worth monitoring young men with a high risk of developing HG-PIN in the future as potential targets for chemoprevention rather than focusing only on chemoprevention in the high-risk HG-PIN patient group (Ravery, 2009).

Anti-androgens (e.g. fluatamide) induce the regression of prostatic epithelium by enhancing apoptosis, suppressing proliferative activity, and inhibiting angiogenesis in BPH, PIN, and prostate cancer (Montironi et al., 1994). PIN is ablated by androgen deprivation therapy, as a result of accelerated apoptosis with subsequent exfoliation of cells into the glandular lumens (Montironi et al., 1994). Studies have documented that angiogenesis in the surrounding stroma of HGPIN glands is severely decreased via suppression of vascular endothelial growth factor (VEGF) production after androgen deprivation therapy (Papatsoris & Papavassiliou, 2001). A marked decrease in the extent and prevalence of HGPIN occurs in patients treated with anti-androgens in comparison to untreated patients (Bostwick & Qian, 1999). It has been suggested that anti-androgens might halt or reverse the process of carcinogenesis and prevent the transition of HGPIN to overt prostate cancer (Bostwick & Qian, 1999; Lieberman et al., 2001; Montironi et al., 1994; van der Kwast et al., 1999). The observed morphological changes (cytoplasmic clearing, prominent glandular atrophy, decreased ratio of glands to stroma) are reversible, and HGPIN lesions recover rapidly. However, it is unclear whether the histopathologic changes of anti-androgen treatment are clinically important (Lieberman et al., 2001; van der Kwast et al., 1999). *Yamauchi* demonstrated that the anti-androgen bicalutamide permitted the persistence of PIN after effective chemoprevention of microscopic prostate cancer in a rat model (Yamauchi et al., 2006). Moreover, there is a risk for amplification of the androgen-receptor (AR) gene in androgen-deficient conditions, as in cases of hormone-refractory prostate cancer (Koivisto et al., 1999). The blockage of 5-alpha reductase with finasteride does not seem to have any effect on the incidence of PIN (Yang et al., 1999). In addition to the above, the role of Ras/mitogen-activated protein kinase (MAPK) in prostate cancer, as well as the therapeutic potential of Ras/map inhibitors are currently under investigation (Papatsoris et al., 2007). Furthermore, it has been demonstrated that men with no evidence of prostate cancer on initial biopsy who were pretreated with finasteride had a significantly greater prostate cancer detection rate at one year than had men in the control group; 30% versus 4% (Cote et al., 1998).

Besides anti-androgens, other drugs (e.g. anti-angiogenics agents) and nutritional supplements (e.g. vitamin D, selenium) have been applied in ongoing chemoprevention trials (Montironi et al., 1994). In a prospective trial evaluating the effects of selenium-vitamin E-isoflavonoid supplement in 100 men with isolated HGPIN in octant biopsies, PSA decreased in a large subgroup (64%). In this subgroup, the overall risk of detecting cancer was 24.5%, compared to 55.6% in a smaller subgroup of patients in whom the PSA continued to rise under supplements (Joniau et al., 2005). *Bettuzzi* administered green tea catechin (GTC) in men with HGPIN and demonstrated that GTC is safe and very effective (Bettuzzi et al., 2006). In particular, after one year, only one prostate cancer was diagnosed among the 30 GTC-treated men (3%), whereas nine cancers were found among the 30 placebo-treated men (30%).

Studies suggest that administration of the nerve-growth factor (NGF) induces a reversion of the androgen-independent / androgen-receptor negative prostate cancer cell lines to a less malignant phenotype, which raises thoughts for a new perspective in prostate cancer therapy (Papatsoris et al., 2007). Moreover, deregulation of the IGF-1/IGF-1-receptor axis has been liked to progression of prostate cancer to androgen independenace and new therapeutic possibilities are currently under research (Papatsoris et al., 2005).

The ideal agent and duration of therapy remains to be defined. The selective alpha-estrogen receptor modulator toremifene was investigated in HGPIN. Studies using the transgenic adenocarcinoma of mouse prostate model (TRAMP) and this anti-estrogen demonstrated a reduction in the incidence of HGPIN and prostate cancer, along with an increase in animal survival (Raghow et al., 2002). The statistically significant reduction in the incidence of prostate cancer and the tolerability profile support toremifene's promise as a chemopreventive agent.

Although small, high-risk population trials will remain the key to the early evaluation of novel chemoprevention agents, large-scale, population-based clinical trials will still be necessary to ensure that valid recommendations are made to men regarding chemoprevention. Until the efficacy of chemopreventive agents is confirmed in well-conducted, randomized, controlled studies, there should be a reluctance to offer chemopreventive agents to men with isolated HGPIN on initial biopsy.

6.8.3 Radical prostatectomy and radiotherapy

HGPIN is sometimes associated with a PSA above normal levels; in other words, in these cases, HGPIN could be regarded as T1c prostate cancer (Newling, 1999). The firm evidence that within six months of the first biopsy showing HGPIN, invasive prostate cancer would be diagnosed in 60% of the cases has made some urologists offer radical prostatectomy to this group of patients (Newling, 1999). Nowadays, radical prostatectomy is not regarded as appropriate therapy for the management of patients with HGPIN (Davidson et al., 1995; Montironi et al., 2002; Newling, 1999). It seems logical that malignant histological changes should be seen before such radical therapy is offered. It has been recently shown that PSA and HGPIN focality at biopsy do not enhance cancer predictivity, thus patients who underwent prostate biopsy with a HGPIN diagnosis do not seem to need any different follow-up rebiopsy strategy than patients with a diagnosis of BPH (Gallo et al., 2008).

The prevalence and extent of PIN lesions decreases significantly after radiation therapy. Following such therapy, PIN retains the typical characteristics of untreated PIN and is readily recognized on histopathology (Cheng et al., 1999). The question remains if recurrence after radiation therapy is due to the growth of incompletely eradicated tumor or progression of incompletely eradicated PIN.

6.8.4 Potential anti-PIN agents

a. **Anti-Angiogenesis Agents**. The changes that occur in HGPIN leading to focal carcinoma include neo-angiogenesis; hence, the use of the anti-angiogenesis agent's thalidomide and platelet growth factor 4 could be important therapeutic interventions (Papatsoris et al., 2005).
b. **Differentiation Factors**. Retinoids and vitamin D analog are known to improve differentiation of epithelial cells, including prostate epithelium.The development of invasiveness, as seen in HGPIN, is characterized by loss of adhesion facility and dedifferentiation with aneuploid nuclear characteristics; these processes may be sensitive to retinoids or vitamin D analogs (Papatsoris et al., 2005; Banach-Petrosky et al, 2006; Kelloff et al., 1999). Gene therapy and immunotherapy are still experimental in prostate cancer and HGPIN. Serial examination of prostate biopsies and subsequent prostatectomy specimens may give an indication of the effectiveness of these agents.

c. **Epigenetic Therapeutics** *(Histone Deacetylase Inhibitors, Hypomethylating Agents).* Epigenetic events, such as histone acetylation/deacetylation and aberrant DNA methylation, represent crucial steps in prostate cancer development, which cause alterations in gene expression (e.g. silencing tumor suppressor genes) without changes in the DNA coding sequence (Kopelovich et al., 2003). Epigenetic changes can be reversed by the use of small molecules, such as histone deacetylase (HDAC) inhibitors and hypomethylating agents. Histones are core protein components of nucleosomes, and their acetylation status regulates gene expression. Deacetylated histones are generally associated with silencing gene expression (Marks et al., 2001). HDAC inhibitors have been shown to induce expression of genes linked to growth inhibition and cellular differentiation. Several phase I trials with these agents are ongoing in patients with prostate cancer and/or PIN (Sandor et al., 2002).

A mechanism to switch off tumor suppressor genes is controlled by a chemical modification known as DNA methylation, a normal cellular process whereby cytosines in the DNA become methylated by the enzyme DNA methyltransferase to give 5-methylcytosine (Kang et al., 2004). However, in cancer cells, the methylation process is deregulated, and many genes, including tumor suppressor genes, become abnormally methylated at cytosine bases. Moreover, it seems that aberrant methylation causes recruitment of HDAC, resulting in a more potent transcriptional inhibition of target genes (Patra et al., 2001). Many studies have demonstrated epigenetic silencing of crucial genes, for example, AR, PTEN, and RARβ, during prostate carcinogenesis (Yamanaka et al., 2003). Novel hypomethylating agents are in various stages of experimental and clinical development.

7. Epilogue

Recurrent chromosomal rearrangements have not been well characterized in prostate cancer (Papatsoris et al., 2007). *Tomlins* used a bioinformatics approach to discover candidate oncogenic chromosomal aberrations on the basis of outlier gene expression, followed by RNA ligase-mediated rapid amplification of cDNA ends and sequencing (Tomlins et al., 2005). The authors identified recurrent gene fusions of the 5-prime untranslated region of TMPRSS2 to two ETS transcription factors, ERG or ETV1, in prostate cancer tissues with outlier expression. By using FISH, they demonstrated that 23 of 29 prostate cancer samples harbored rearrangements in ERG or ETV1. Cell line experiments suggested that the androgen-responsive promoter elements of TMPRSS2 mediate the overexpression of ETS family members in prostate cancer. *Yoshimoto* demonstrated that the occurrence of these genetic events, along with Pten haploinsufficiency, in patients with prostate cancer has a significant clinical impact (Yoshimoto et al., 2008). Most importantly, the identification of ERG as a cooperative initiation event in prostate tumorigenesis suggests that ERG targeted therapies, when feasible, may be effective at preventing the transition between HGPIN and invasive cancer, while pharmacological manipulation of the PTEN/PI3K/AKT pathway may represent a powerful chemopreventive and chemotherapeutic tool in the future (Carver et al., 2009). Surprisingly, the above-mentioned translocation was found in about 70–80% of prostate cancers, but not in HGPIN. Finally, the diagnosis of prostate cancer on needle biopsy has been refined because of the recent discovery of AMARC, which preferentially labels prostate adenocarcinoma (Epstein, 2006). Also, in a recent peer review *Epstein* outlined several recommendations when diagnosing PIN or atypical foci suspicious for carcinoma in needle biopsies (Epstein & Herawi, 2006).

In conclusion, prostate cancer precursor lesions include mainly AAH and PIN (Chrisofos et al., 2007). LSC is not considered a precursor lesion of prostate cancer but shares with PIN the increased risk of diagnosing a definite cancer in subsequent biopsies. LGPIN should not be reported by pathologists due to poor inter-observer reproducibility and a relatively low risk of cancer following re-biopsy. The average incidence of HGPIN or LSC on initial needle biopsy is 6%. Following the diagnosis of HGPIN, the risk of cancer is not statistically higher compared with the risk of cancer following a benign diagnosis. Studies have shown that the risk for cancer after HGPIN diagnosis was not higher than the risk reported after diagnosis of BPH (Gallo et al., 2008). In contrast, the average risk of cancer following a diagnosis of LSC is 40%, and such patients should be re-biopsied within three to six months. Cases diagnosed as LSC have the highest likelihood of being changed upon expert review. Potential markers of prostate cancer precursor lesions include fatty acid synthetase, AMARC, and A80. However, clinical and pathological parameters do not help to stratify which men are at greater risk for a cancer diagnosis. Repeat biopsy should include increased sampling of the initial precursor lesion and adjacent ipsilateral and contralateral sites, with routine sampling of all sextant sites. Radical prostatectomy and radiotherapy are not recommended for the management of patients with HGPIN. Until the efficacy of chemopreventive agents is confirmed in well-conducted, randomized, controlled studies, there should be a reluctance to offer such agents to men with prostate cancer precursor lesion on initial biopsy.

8. References

Alexander EE, Qian J, Wollan PC, Myers R, Bostwick DG. Prostatic intraepithelial neoplasia does not appear to raise serum prostate-specific antigen concentrations. *Urology* 1996; 47: 693–698.

Amin MB, Tamboli P, Varma M, Srigley JR. Postatrophic hyperplasia of the prostate gland: a detailed analysis of its morphology in needle biopsy specimens. *Am J Surg Pathol* 1999; 23: 925–931.

Anton RC, Kattan MW, Chakraborty S, Wheeler TM. Postatrophic hyperplasia of the prostate: lack of association with prostate cancer. *Am J Surg Pathol* 1999; 23: 932–936.

Baltaci S, Orhan D, Ozer G, Tolunay O, Gogous O. Bcl-2 proto-oncogene expression in low- and high- grade prostatic intraepithelial neoplasia. *BJU Int* 2000; 85: 155–159.

Banach-Petrosky W, Ouyang X, Gao H, Nader K, Ji Y, Suh N, DiPaola RS, Abate-Shen C. Vitamin D inhibits the formation of prostatic intraepithelial neoplasia in Nkx3.1;Pten mutant mice. *Clin Cancer Res* 2006; 12: 5895–5901.

Baretton GB, Vogt T, Blasenbreu S, Lohrs U. Comparison of DNA ploidy in prostatic intraepithelial neoplasia and invasive carcinoma of the prostate: an image cytometric study. *Hum Pathol* 1994; 25: 506–513.

Berney DM, Fisher G, Kattan MW *et al.* Pitfalls in the diagnosis of prostatic cancer: retrospective review of 1791 cases with clinical outcome. *Histopathology* 2007; 51; 452–457.

Bettuzzi S, Brausi M, Rizzi F, Castagnetti G, Peracchia G, Corti A. Chemoprevention of human prostate cancer by oral administration of green tea catechins in volunteers with high-grade prostate intraepithelial neoplasia: a preliminary report from a one-year proof-of-principle study. *Cancer Res* 2006; 66: 1234–1240.

BillisA. Prostatic atrophy:an autopsy study of a histologic mimic of adenocarcinoma.*Mol Pathol* 1998;11:47-54

Boag AH, Young ID. Increased expression of the 72-kd type IV collagenase in prostatic adenocarcinoma. Demonstration by immunohistochemistry and in situ hybridization. *Am J Pathol* 1994; 144: 585–591.

Bonkhoff H. Role of the basal cells in premalignant changes of the human prostate: a stem cell concept for the development of prostate cancer. *Eur Urol* 1996; 30: 201–205.

Bostwick DG, Qian J. Effect of androgen deprivation therapy on prostatic intraepithelial neoplasia. *Urology* 582 (Suppl 1): S91–S93.

Bostwick DG, Brawer MK. Prostatic intra-epithelial neoplasia and early invasion in prostate cancer. *Cancer* 1987; 59: 788–794.

Bostwick DG. Prostatic intraepithelial neoplasia (PIN). *Urology* 1989; 34(Suppl 6): S16–S22.

Bostwick DG, Amin MB, Dundore P, Marsh W, Schultz DS. Architectural patterns of high-grade prostatic intraepithelial neoplasia. *Hum Pathol* 1993; 24: 298–310.

Bostwick DG, Dousa MK, Crawford BG, Wollan PC. Neuroendocrine differentiation in prostatic intraepithelial neoplasia and adenocarcinoma. *Am J Surg Pathol* 1994; 18: 1240–1246.

Bostwick DG, Qian J. Atypical adenomatous hyperplasia of the prostate. Relationship with carcinoma in 217 whole-mount radical prostatectomies. *Am J Surg Pathol* 1995; 19: 506–518.

Bostwick DG, Qian J, Frankel K. The incidence of high grade prostatic intraepithelial neoplasia in needle biopsies. *J Urol* 1995; 154: 1791–1794.

Bostwick DG. Prospective origins of prostate carcinoma. Prostatic intraepithelial neoplasia and atypical adenomatous hyperplasia. *Cancer* 1996; 78: 330–336.

Bostwick DG, Pacelli A, Lopez-Beltran A. Molecular biology of prostatic intraepithelial neoplasia. *Prostate* 1996; 29: 117–134

Bostwick DG, Shan A, Qian J, Darson M, Maihle NJ, Jenkins RB, Cheng L. Independent origin of multiple foci of prostatic intraepithelial neoplasia: comparison with matched foci of prostatic carcinoma. *Cancer* 1998; 83: 1995–2002.

Bostwick DG. Prostatic intraepithelial neoplasia is a risk factor for cancer. *Semin Urol Oncol* 1999; 17: 187–198.

Bostwick DG, Cheng L. Overdiagnosis of prostatic adenocarcinoma. *Semin. Urol. Oncol. 1999; 17; 199–205*

Bostwick DG. Prostatic intraepithelial neoplasia. *Curr Urol Rep* 2000; 1: 65–70.

Bostwick DG, Cheng L. *Urologic Surgical Pathology*. New York: Elsevier/Mosby, *2008*.

Bourdoumis A, Papatsoris AG, Chrisofos M, Efstathiou E, Skolarikos A, Deliveliotis C.The novel prostate cancer antigen 3 (PCA3) biomarker. Int *Braz J Urol* 2010; 36: 665-9.

Brausi M, Castagnetti G, Dotti A, De Luca G, Olmi R, Cesinaro AM. Immediate radical prostatectomy in patients with atypical small acinar proliferation. Over treatment? *J Urol* 2004; 172: 906–908.

Carver BS, Tran J, Gopalan A, Chen Z, Shaikh S, Carracedo A, Alimonti A, Nardella C, Varmeh S, Scardino PT, Cordon-Cardo C, Gerald W, Pandolfi PP. Aberrant ERG expression cooperates with loss of PTEN to promote cancer progression in the prostate *Nat Genet.* 2009 May; 41: 619–624.

Chan TY, Epstein JI. Follow-up of atypical prostate needle biopsies suspicious for cancer. *Urology* 1999; 53: 351–355.

Cheng L, Shan A, Cheville JC, Qian J, Bostwick DG. Atypical adenomatous hyperplasia of the prostate: a premalignant lesion? *Cancer Res* 1998; 58: 389–391.

Cheng L, Cheville JC, Pisansky TM, Sebo TJ, Slezak J, Bergstralh EJ, Neumann RM, Singh R, Pacelli A, Zincke H, Bostwick DG. Prevalence and distribution of prostatic intraepithelial neoplasia in salvage radical prostatectomy specimens after radiation therapy. *Am J Surg Pathol* 1999; 23: 803–808.

Cheng Liang, Bostwick D.G. Atypical sclerosing adenosis of the prostate : a rare mimic of adenocarcinoma. *Histopathology* 2010; 56: 627-631.

Cheville JC, Bostwick DG. Postatrophic hyperplasia of the prostate. A histologic mimic of prostate adenocarcinoma. *Am J Surg Pathol* 1995; 19: 1068–1076.

Cohen RJ, McNeal JE, Baillie T. Patterns of differentiation and proliferation in intraductal carcinoma of the prostate: significance for cancer progression. *Prostate* 2000; 43: 11–19.

Collina G, Botticelli AR, Martinelli AM, Fano RA, Trentini GP. Sclerosing adenosis of the prostate. Report of three cases with electronmicroscopy and immunohistochemical study. *Histopathology* 1992; 20; 505–510.

Coogan C, Bostwick D, Bloom K, Gould V. Glycoprotein A-80 in the human prostate: immunolocalization in prostatic intraepithelial neoplasia, carcinoma, radiation failure, and after neoadjuvant hormonal therapy. *Urology* 2003; 61: 248–252.

Cote RJ, Skinner EC, Salem CE, Mertes SJ, Stanczyk FZ, Henderson BE, Pike MC, Ross RK. The effect of finasteride on the prostate gland in men with elevated serum prostate-specific antigen levels. *Br J Cancer* 1998; 78: 413–418.

Chrisofos M, Papatsoris AG, Lazaris A, Deliveliotis C. Precursor leasions of prostate cancer. *Crit Rev Clin Lab Sci* 2007; 44: 243-270.

Darson MF, Pacelli A, Roche P, Rittenhouse HG, Wolfert RL, Young CYF, Klee GG, Tindall DJ, Bostwick BG. Human glandular kallikrein 2 (hK2) expression in prostatic intraepithelial neoplasia and adenocarcinoma: A novel prostate cancer marker *Urology* 1997; 49: 857-862.

Darson MF, Pacelli A, Roche P, Rittenhouse HG,Wolfert RL, Saeid MS, Young CY, Klee GG, Tindall DJ, Bostwick DG. Human glandular kallikrein 2 expression in prostate adenocarcinoma and lymph node metastases. *Urology* 1999; 53: 939–944.

Davidson D, Bostwick D, Qian J, Wollan PC, Oesterling JE, Rudders RA, Siroky M, Stilmant M. Prostatic intraepithelial neoplasia is a risk factor for adenocarcinoma: predictive accuracy in needle biopsies. *J Urol* 1995; 154: 1295–1299.

DeMarzo AM, Marchi VL, Epstein JI, NelsonWG. Proliferative inflammatory atrophy of the prostate: implications for prostatic carcinogenesis. *Am J Pathol* 1999; 155: 1985–1992.

De Marzo AM, Platz EA, Epstein JI. A working group classification of focal prostate atrophy lesions. *Am J Surg Pathol.* 2006 30: 1281-1291.

Dovey Z, Corbishley CM, Kirby RS. Prostatic intraepithelial neoplasia: a risk factor for prostate cancer. *Can J Urol* 2005; 12(Suppl 1): 49–52.

Drivalos A, Papatsoris AG, Chrisofos M, Efstathiou E, Dimopoulos MA.The role of the cell adhesion molecules (integrins / cadherins) in prostate cancer. MA. *Int Braz J Urol.* 2011; 37: 302-326.

Ellis WJ, Brawer MK. Repeat biopsy: who needs it? *J Urol* 1995; 153: 1496–1498.

Epstein JI, Grignon DJ, Humphrey PA, McNeal JE, Sesterhenn IA, Troncoso P, Wheeler TM. Interobserver reproducibility in the diagnosis of prostatic intraepithelial neoplasia. *Am J Surg Pathol* 1995; 19: 873–886.

Epstein JI. Pathology of prostatic neoplasia. In Walsh PC, Retik AB, Vaughan ED, Wein AJ, Eds. *Campell's Urology, 8th Ed.* Pp 3025–3037. Philadelphia: Saunders, 2002.

Epstein JI. What's new in prostate cancer disease assessment in 2006? *Curr Opin Urol* 2006; 16: 146–151.

Epstein JI, Herawi M. Prostate needle biopsies containing prostatic intraepithelial neoplasia or atypical foci suspicious for carcinoma: implications for patient care. *J Urol* 2006; 175: 820–834.

Fadare O, Wang S, Mariappan MR. Practice patterns of clinicians following isolated diagnoses of atypical small acinar proliferation on prostate biopsy specimens. *Arch Pathol Lab Med* 2004; 128: 557–560.

Franks LM. Atrophy and hyperplasia in the prostate proper. *J Pathol Bacteriol* 1954; 68: 617–621.

Gallo F, Chiono L, Gastaldi E, Venturino E, Giberti C. Prognostic Significance of High-Grade Prostatic Intraepithelial Neoplasia (HGPIN): Risk of Prostatic Cancer on Repeat Biopsies *Urology* September 2008; 72: 628-632.

Gaudin PB, Epstein JI. Adenosis of the prostate. Histologic features in transurethral resection specimens. *Am J Surg Pathol* 1994; 18: 863–870.

Gaudin PB, Epstein JI. Adenosis of the prostate Histological features in needle biopsy specimens. *Am J Surg Pathol* 1995; 19: 737–747.

Gaudin PB, Sesterhenn IA, Wojno KJ, Mostofi FK, Epstein JI. Incidence and clinical significance of high-grade prostatic intraepithelial neoplasia in TURP specimens. *Urology* 1997; 49: 558–563.

Goeman L, Joniau S, Ponette D, Van der Aa F, Roskams T, Oyen R, Van Poppel H. Is low-grade prostatic intraepithelial neoplasia a risk factor for cancer? *Prostate Cancer Prostatic Dis* 2003; 6: 305–310.

Grignon DJ, Ro JY, Srigley JR, Troncoso P, Raymond AK, Ayala AG. Sclerosing adenosis of the prostate gland. A lesion showing myoepithelial differentiation. *Am. J. Surg. Pathol. 1992; 16; 383–391.*

Grignon DJ, Sakr WA. Atypical adenomatous hyperplasia of the prostate: a critical review. *Eur Urol* 1996; 30: 206–211.

Hailemariam S, Vosbeck J, Cathomas G, Zlobec I, Mattarelli G, Eichenberger T, Zellweger T, Bachmann A, Gasser T, Bubendorf L. Can molecular markers stratify the diagnostic value of high-grade prostatic intraepithelial neoplasia? *Human Pathology* 2011; 42: 702-709.

Haggman MJ, Macoska JA, Wojno KJ, Oesterling JE. The relationship between prostatic intraepithelial neoplasia and prostate cancer: critical issues. *J Urol* 1997; 158: 12–22.

Hellpap B, Kollermann J. Atypical acinar proliferation of the prostate. *Pathol Res Pract* 1999; 195: 795–799. Helpap B, Kollermann J, Oehler U. Limiting the diagnosis of atypical small glandular proliferations in needle biopsies of the prostate by the use of immunohistochemistry. *J Pathol* 2001; 193: 350–353.

Iczkowski KA, MacLennan GT, Bostwick DG. Atypical small acinar proliferation suspicious for malignancy in prostate needle biopsies: clinical significance in 33 cases. *Am J Surg Pathol* 1997; 21: 1489–1495.

Iczkowski KA, Bassler TJ, Schwob VS, Bassler IC, Kunnel BS, Orozco RE, Bostwick DG. Diagnosis of "suspicious for malignancy" in prostate biopsies: predictive value for cancer. *Urology* 1998; 51: 749–758. Iczkowski KA, Bostwick DG. Criteria for biopsy diagnosis of minimal volume prostatic adenocarcinoma: analytic comparison with nondiagnostic but suspicious atypical small acinar proliferation. *Arch Pathol Lab Med* 2000; 124: 98–107.

Iczkowski KA, Chen HM, Yang XJ, Beach RA. Prostate cancer diagnosed after initial biopsy with atypical small acinar proliferation suspicious for malignancy is similar to cancer found on initial biopsy. *Urology* 2002; 60: 851–854

Jones EC, Clement PB, Young RH. Sclerosing adenosis of the prostate gland. A clinicopathological and immunohistochemical study of 11 cases. *Am. J. Surg. Pathol. 1991; 15; 1171–1180.*

Joniau S, Goeman L, Pennings J, Van Poppel H. Prostatic intraepithelial neoplasia (PIN): importance and clinical management. *Eur Urol* 2005; 48: 379–385.

Joniau S, Goeman L, Roskams T, Lerut E, Oyen R, Van Poppel H. Effect of Nutritional Supplement Challenge in Patients with Isolated High-Grade Prostatic Intraepithelial Neoplasia *Urology* 2007; 69: 1102-1106.

Kang GH, Lee S, Lee HJ, Hwang KS. Aberrant CpG island hypermethylation of multiple genes in prostate cancer and prostatic intraepithelial neoplasia. *J Pathol* 2004; 202: 233–240.

Keetch DW, Humphrey P, Stahl D, Smith DS, Catalona WJ. Morphometric analysis and clinical follow up of isolated prostatic intraepithelial neoplasia in needle biopsy of the prostate. *J Urol* 1995; 154: 347–351.

Kelloff GJ, Lieberman R, Brawer MK, Crawford ED, Labrie F, Miller GJ, Kelloff GJ. Strategies for chemoprevention of prostate cancer. *Prostate Cancer Prostatic Dis* 1999; 2 (Suppl): S27–S33.

Koivisto PA, Schleutker J, Helin H, Ehren-van Eekelen C, Kallioniemi OP, Trapman J. Androgen receptor gene alterations and chromosomal gains and losses in prostate carcinomas appearing during finasteride treatment for benign prostatic hyperplasia. *Clin Cancer Res* 1999; 5: 3378–3382.

Kopelovich L, Crowell JA, Fay JR. The epigenome as a target for cancer chemoprevention. *J Nat Cancer Inst* 2003; 95: 1747–1757.

Kronz JD, Allan CH, Shaikh AA, Epstein JI. Predicting cancer following a diagnosis of high grade prostatic intraepithelial neoplasia on needle biopsy: data on men with more than one follow-up biopsy. *Am J Surg Pathol* 2001 ; 25: 1079–1085.

Langer JE, Rovner ES, Coleman BG, Yin D, Arger PH, Malkowicz SB, Nisenbaum HL, Rowling SE, Tomaszewski JE, Wein AJ, Jacobs JE. Strategy for repeat biopsy of patients with prostatic intraepithelial neoplasia detected by prostate needle biopsy. *J Urol* 1996; 155: 228–231.

Lefkowitz GK, Taneja SS, Brown J, Melamed J, Lepor H. Follow-up interval prostate biopsy 3 years after diagnosis of high grade prostatic intraepithelial neoplasia is associated with high likelihood of prostate cancer, independent of change in prostate specific antigen levels. *J Urol* 2002; 168: 1415–1418.

Lieberman R, Bermejo C, Akaza H, Greenwald P, Fair W, Thompson I. Progress in prostate cancer chemoprevention: modulators of promotion and progression. *Urology* 2001; 58: 835–842

Marks P, Rifkind RA, Richon VM, Breslow R, Miller T, Kelly WK. Histone deacetylases and cancer: causes and therapies. *Nat Rev Cancer* 2001; 1: 194–202.
McNeal JE. Morphogenesis of prostatic carcinoma. *Cancer* 1965; 18: 1659–1666.
McNeal JE, Bostwick DG. Intraductal dysplasia: a premalignant lesion of the prostate. *Hum Pathol* 1986; 17: 64–71.
McNeal JE, Bostwick DG. Intraductal dysplasia: a pre-malignant lesion of the prostate. *Hum Pathol* 1986; 17: 64–71.
Montironi R, Galluzzi CM, Diamanti L, Taborro R, Scarpelli M, Pisani E. Prostatic intraepithelial neoplasia. Qualitative and quantitative analyses of the blood capillary architecture on thin tissue sections. *Pathol Res Pract* 1993; 189: 542–548.
Montironi R, Magi-Galluzzi C, Muzzonigro G, Prete E, Polito M, Fabris G. Effects of combination endocrine therapy on normal prostate, prostatic intraepithelial neoplasia, and prostatic adenocarcinoma. *J Clin Pathol* 1994; 47: 906–913.
Montironi R, Mazzuccelli R, Marshall JR, Bartels PH. Prostate cancer prevention: review of target populations, pathological biomarkers, and chemopreventive agents. *J Clin Pathol* 1999; 52: 793–803. Montironi R, Santinelli A, Mazzucchelli R. Prostatic intraepithelial neoplasia and prostate cancer. *Panminerva Med* 2002; 44: 213–220.
Moore CK, Karikehalli S, Nazeer T, Fisher HAG, Kaufman RP Jr, Mian BM. Prognostic significance of high grade prostatic intraepithelial neoplasia and atypical small acinar proliferation in the contemporary era. *J Urol* 2005; 173: 70–72.
Myers RB, Grizzle WE. Biomarker expression in prostatic intraepithelial neoplasia. *Eur Urol* 1996; 30: 153–166.
Nelson WG, De Marzo AM, Isaacs WB. Prostate cancer. *N Engl J Med* 2003; 349: 366–381.
Newling DW. PIN I-II: when should we interfere? *Eur Urol* 1999; 35: 504–507.
O'Dowd GJ, Miller MG, Orozco R & Veltri RW. Analysis of repeated biopsy results within 1 year after noncancer diagnosis. *Urology* 2000; 55: 553–559.
Orteil H. Involutionary changes in prostate and female breast cancer in relation to cancer development. *Can Med Assoc J* 1926; 16: 237.
O'Shaughnessy JA, Kelloff GJ, Gordon GB, Dannenberg AJ, Hong WK, Fabian CJ, Sigman CC, Bertagnolli MM, Stratton SP, Lam S, Nelson WG, Meyskens FL, Alberts DS, Follen M, Rustgi AK, Papadimitrakopoulou V, Scardino PT, Gazdar AF, Wattenberg LW, Sporn MB, Sakr WA, Lippman SM, Von Hoff DD. Treatment and prevention of intraepithelial neoplasia: an important target for accelerated new agent development. *Clin Cancer Res* 2002; 8: 314–346.
Pacelli A, Bostwick DG. Clinical significance of high-grade prostatic intraepithelial neoplasia in transurethral resection specimens. *Urology* 1997; 50: 335–359.
Papatsoris AG, Papavassiliou AG. Prostate cancer: horizons in the development of novel anti-cancer strategies. *Curr Med Chem Anticancer Agents* 2001; 1: 47–70.
Papatsoris AG, Karamouzis MV, Papavassiliou AG. Novel insights into the implication of the IGF-1 network in prostate cancer. *Trends Mol Med* 2005; 11: 52-55.
Papatsoris AG, Karamouzis MV, Papavassiliou AG. Novel biological agents for the treatment of hormone-refractory prostate cancer (HRPC). *Curr Med Chem* 2005; 12: 277–296.
Papatsoris AG, Karamouzis MV, Papavassiliou AG. The power and promise of "rewiring" the mitogen-activated protein kinase network in prostate cancer therapeutics. *Mol Cancer Ther* 2007; 6: 811-819.

Papatsoris AG, Liolitsa D, Deliveliotis C. Manipulation of the nerve growth factor network in prostate cancer. *Expert Opin Investig Drugs* 2007; 16: 303-309.

Papatsoris AG, Anagnostopoulos F. Prostate cancer screening behaviour. *Public Health* 2009; 123: 69-71.

Patra SK, Patra A, Dahiya R. Histone deacetylase and DNA methyltransferase in human prostate cancer. *Biochem Biophys Res Commun* 2001; 287: 705–713.

Powell IJ, Bock CH, Ruterbusch JJ. & Sakr W. Evidence Supports a Faster Growth Rate and/or Earlier Transformation to Clinically Significant Prostate Cancer in Black Than in White American Men, and Influences Racial Progression and Mortality Disparity. *J Urol* 2010; 183: 1792-1797.

Qian J, Bostwick DG, Takahashi S, Borell TJ, Herath JF, Lieber MM, Jenkins RB. Chromosomal anomalies in prostatic intraepithelial neoplasia and carcinoma detected by fluorescence in situ hybridization. *Cancer Res* 1995; 55: 5408–5414.

Qian J,Wollan P, Bostwick DG. The extent and multicentricity of high-grade prostatic intraepithelial neoplasia in clinically localized prostatic adenocarcinoma. *Hum Pathol* 1997; 28: 143–148.

Raghow S, Hooshdaran MZ, Katiyar S, Steiner MS. Toremifene prevents prostate cancer in the transgenic adenocarcinoma of mouse prostate model. *Cancer Res* 2002; 62: 1370–1376.

Ravery V. Towards early and more specific diagnosis of prostate cancer? Identifying a Key Target Population for Chemoprevention and Available Strategies *European Urology Supplements* 2010; 8: 103-107.

Ronnett BM, Carmichael MJ, Carter HB, Epstein JI. Does high-grade prostatic intraepithelial neoplasia result in elevated serum prostate specific antigen levels? *J Urol* 1993; 150: 386–389.

Rubin MA, Zhou M, Dhanasekaran SM, Varambally S, Barrette TR, Snada MG, Pienta KJ, Ghosh D, Chinnaiyan AM. Alpha-Methylacyl coenzyme A racemase as a tissue biomarker for prostate cancer. *JAMA* 2002; 287: 1662–1670.

Sakamoto N, Tsuneyoshi M, Enjoji M. Sclerosing adenosis of the prostate. Histopathologic and immunohistochemical analysis. *Am. J. Surg. Pathol.* 1991; 15; 660–667.

Sakr WA, Haas GP, Cassin BJ, Pontes JE, Crissman JD. Frequency of carcinoma and intraepithelial neoplasia of the prostate in young male patients. *J Urol* 1993; 150: 379–385

Sakr WA, Grignon DJ, Haas GP, Schomer KL, Heilbrun LK, Cassin BJ, Powell J, Montie JA, Pontes JE, Crissman JD. Epidemiology of high grade prostatic intraepithelial neoplasia. *Pathol Res Pract* 1995; 191: 838–841.

Sakr WA, Grignon DJ, Haas GP, Heilbrur LK, Pontes JE, Crissman JD. Age and racial distribution of prostatic intraepithelial neoplasia. *Eur Urol* 1996; 30: 138–144.

Sakr WA, Brawer MK, Moul JW, Donohue R, Schulman CG, Sakr D. Pathology and bio markers of prostate cancer. *Prostate Cancer Prostatic Dis* 1999; 2(Suppl): S7–S14.

Sandor V, Bakke S, Robey RW, Kang MH, Blagosklonny MV, Bender J, Brooks R, Piekarz RL, Tucker E, Figg WD, Chan KK, Goldspiel B, Fojo AT, Balcerzak SP, Bates SE. Phase I trial of the histone deacetylase inhibitor, depsipeptide (FR901228, NSC 630176), in patients with refractory neoplasms. *Clin Cancer Res* 2002; 8: 718–728.

Sardana G, Dowell B, Diamandis EP. Emerging Biomarkers for the diagnosis and prognosis of prostate cancer. *Clinical Chemistry* 2008 54 : 1951-1960

Scattoni V, Roscigno M, Freschi M, Deho F, Raber M, Briganti A, Fantini G, Nava L, Montorsi F, Rigatti P. Atypical small acinar proliferation (ASAP) on extended prostatic biopsies: predictive factors of cancer detection on repeat biopsies. *Arch Ital Urol Androl* 2005; 77: 31–36.

Shah RB, Kunju LP, Shen R, LeBlanc M, Zhou M, Rubin MA. Usefulness of basal cell cocktail (34beta E12+p63) in the diagnosis of atypical prostate glandular proliferations. *Am J Clin Pathol* 2004; 122: 517–523.

Shepherd D, Keetch DW, Humphrey PA, Smith DS, Stahl D. Repeat biopsy strategy in men with isolated prostatic intraepithelial neoplasia on prostate needle biopsy. *J Urol* 1996; 156: 460-463.

Shin SS, Gould VE, Gould JE, Warren WH, Gould KA, Yaremko ML, Manderino GL, Rittenhouse HG, Tomita JT, Jansson DS. Expression of a new mucin-type glycoprotein in select epithelial dysplasias and neoplasms detected immunocytochemically with Mab A-80. *APMIS* 1989; 97: 1053–1067.

Signoretti S, Waltregny D, Dilks J, Isaac B, Lin D, Garraway L, Yang A, Montironi R, McKeonand F & Loda M. *Am J Pathol* 2000; 157: 1769–1775.

Singh PB, Nicholson CM, Ragavan N, Blades RA, Martin FL, Matanhelia SS. Risk of prostate cancer after isolated high-grade prostatic intraepithelial neoplasia (HGPIN) detected on extended core needle biopsy : a UK hospital experience. *BMC Urol* 2009; 9: 3.

Sinha AA, Quast BJ, Reddy PK, Lall V, Wilson MJ, Qian J, Bostwick DG. Microvessel density as a molecular marker for identifying high-grade prostatic intraepithelial neoplasia precursors to prostate cancer. *Exp Mol Pathol* 2004; 77: 153–159.

Sporn MB. Prevention of cancer in the next millennium: report of the chemoprevention working group to the American Association for Cancer Research. *Cancer Res* 1999; 59: 4743–4758

Steiner MS. High-grade prostatic intraepithelial neoplasia and prostate cancer risk reduction.*World J Urol* 2003; 21: 15–20.

Swinnen JV, Roskams T, Joniau S, Van Poppel H, Oyen R, Heyns W, Verhoeven G. Overexpression of fatty acid synthase is an early and common event in the development of prostate cancer. *Int J Cancer* 2002; 98: 19–22.

Tomlins SA, Rhodes DR, Perner S, Dhanasekaran SM, Mehra R, Sun XW, Varambally S, Cao X, Tchinda J, Kuefer R, Lee C, Montie JE, Shah RB, Pienta KJ, Rubin MA, Chinnaiyan AM. Recurrent fusion of TMPRSS2 and ETS transcription factor genes in prostate cancer. *Science* 2005; 310: 644–648.

Van der Kwast TH, Labrie F, Tetu B. Prostatic intraepithelial neoplasia and endocrine manipulation. *Eur Urol* 1999; 35: 508–510.

Vis AN, Van Der Kwast TH. Prostatic intraepithelial neoplasia and putative precursor lesions of prostate cancer: a clinical perspective. *BJU Int* 2001; 88: 147–157.

Vis AN, Hoedemaeker RF, Roobol M, Schroder FH, van der Kwast TH. The predictive value for prostate cancer of lesions that raise suspicion of concomitant carcinoma: an evaluation from a randomized population-based study of screening for prostate cancer. *Cancer* 2001; 92: 524–534.

Weinstein MH, Epstein JI. Significance of high-grade prostatic intraepithelial neoplasia on needle biopsy. *Hum Pathol* 1993; 24: 624–629.

Yamanaka M, Watanabe M, Yamada Y, Takagi A, Murata T, Takahashi H, Suzuki H, Ito H, Tsukino H, Katoh T, Sugimura Y, Shiraishi T. Altered methylation of multiple genes in carcinogenesis of the prostate. *Int J Cancer* 2003; 106: 382–387.

Yamauchi A, Kawai K, Tsukamoto S, Ideyama Y, Shirai T, Akaza H. Persistence of prostatic intraepithelial neoplasia after effective chemoprevention of microscopic prostate cancer with antiandrogen in a rat model. *J Urol* 2006; 175: 348–352.

Yang XJ, Lecksell K, Short K, Gottesman J, Peterson L, Bannow J, Schellhammer PF, Fitch WP, Hodge GB, Parra R, Rouse S, Waldstreicher J, Epstein JI. Does long-term finasteride therapy affect the histologic features of benign prostatic tissue and prostate cancer on needle biopsy? PLESS Study Group. Proscar Long-Term Efficacy and Safety Study. *Urology* 1999; 53: 696–700.

Yoshimoto M, Joshua AM, Cunha IW, Coudry RA, Fonseca FP, Ludkovski O, Zielenska M, Soares FA, Squire JA. Absence of TMPRSS2: ERG fusions and PTEN losses in prostate cancer is associated with a favorable outcome. *Mod Pathol* 2008; 21: 1451-1460.

Young RH, Clement PB. Sclerosing adenosis of the prostate. *Arch. Pathol. Lab. Med.* 1987; 111; 363–366.

Young RH, Clement PB. 'Pseudoadenomatoid' tumour of prostate. *Histopathology* 1990; 16: 420.

Zeng L, Kyprianou N. Apoptotic regulators in prostatic intraepithelial neoplasia (PIN): value in prostate cancer detection and prevention. *Prostate Cancer Prostatic Dis* 2005; 8: 7–13.

7

Diagnosis of Prostatic Intraepithelial Neoplasia in Luminal Cells Using Raman Spectroscopy

Suneetha Devpura[1], Jagdish Thakur[1], Seema Sethi[2], Vaman M. Naik[3], Fazlul Sarkar[2], Wael Sakr[2] and Ratna Naik[1]
[1]Wayne State University, Detroit, MI
[2]Pathology, Karmanos Cancer Institute, Detroit, MI
[3]Univeristy of Michigan-Dearborn, Dearborn, MI, USA

1. Introduction

Prostate cancer is the second most common cancer among men in worldwide based on the statistics in 2008 (Jemal, 2011). In 2008, 903,500 (14%) new cases are recorded and about 258,400 (6%) people died. The highest incidence rates are observed in the developed countries in Oceania, Europe, and North America. Since the introduction of Prostate Specific Antigen (PSA) test, which measures the level of PSA in patients' blood, for prostate cancer screening the mortality rate has decreased due to its early detection and treatment (Oesterling, 1991, Shroder, 2009). The other method for detecting the prostate cancer involves a Digital Rectal Examination (DRE) to check for growths in or enlargement of the prostate gland in men. If there is a tumor growth in the prostate, it can often be felt as a hard lump. To further confirm the tumor, a pathological examination is performed on surgically removed tissues from the suspected areas of prostate and grade of the cancer (Humphrey, 2004) is determined. According to the current policy, the age limit to obtain PSA has been lowered to 40 years. In addition, decision to perform biopsies is not followed by PSA and DRE alone, other factors such as patient age, PSA velocity, PSA density, family history, ethnicity, etc are also considered (Caroll, 2009). One of the common tissue extraction methods is needle biopsy. A recent study has shown that a Target Scan biopsy method has better accuracy over conventional practice to locate the malignant tissues (Andriole, 2007). Combined examination of PSA, DRE, and pathological tests provides a better diagnostic ability for prostate cancer (Partin, 1997). Once a patient is diagnosed with cancer, there are a few early therapeutic procedures available for patient depending on a variety of different factors, like the stage of the tumor, health of the patient and his age etc. These procedures are: radical prostatectomy, external beam radiotherapy, brachytherapy, high intensity focused ultrasound, and cryotherapy (Hricak, 2009). After radical prostatectomy, number of biopsies containing tumor and biopsy perineural invasion are found to be independent predictors of the recurrence of the disease, provided that the patients' PSA is more than 10ng/ml (Quinn, 2003). Prostate instraepethelial neoplasia (PIN) is a precursor lesion in prostate cancer which can be of high or low grade category. Usually PIN is referred to as high grade if it is capable of developing into cancer within the next 10 years (Bostwick &

Qian, 2004) or so. A study has suggested that antiactivity of certain dietary flavonoids prevents the progression of high grade PIN to cancer (Kandaswami, 2005). However, this hypothesis could not be established in a randomized double-blind study performed with 303 men in twelve Canadian centers. These men were given soy, vitamin E, and selenium on daily basis for three years. The results were not statistically significant to show their effects on decreasing the progression of cancer or eliminating it (Fleshner, 2011).

Detection and confirmation of prostate cancer is very crucial for its successful treatment and survival rate. Sometimes the standard screening programs can provide misleading results leading to wrong or over-treatments and occasionally to fatal consequences. The interpretations of histological examination of biopsies, considered as the "gold standard" for diagnosis, are often subjective and can vary significantly from one pathologist to another (Allbrook, 2001). Hence, it is imperative to detect the state of the disease with a method which is objective and capable of providing results within a very short period of time (1-2 minutes). Optical spectroscopy techniques are very well suited for these types of goals, and in addition, they are also capable of probing disease at cellular level. Raman spectroscopy is one of the optical techniques which is currently extensively investigated as a diagnostic tool for detection of different types of cancers (Laserna, 1996). This optical method can provide information about the changes in the concentrations of the constituent biomolecules of tissues and detect the progression or state of the disease. In Raman spectroscopy measurements, a laser light is incident on a sample which interacts with its molecules and gets scattered. Majority of the light scatters elastically; however a very small fraction of it scatters inelastically carrying information about the nature of the sample's molecules, their mutual interaction, and their relative concentrations in the sample (Raman, 1928). The chemical nature of molecules can be uniquely determined from a set of their vibrational energy levels and Raman spectroscopy has the capability to measure these vibrational energy levels (Gelder, 2007, Movasaghi, 2007). This powerful capability of the Raman spectroscopy provides a fundamental motivation to develop this optical technique as an objective diagnostic tool for early detection of cancers. The changes in biochemical composition of a cancerous tissue could be detected through the observed changes in Raman band intensities compared to those of normal tissue. As the biochemical compositions of a tissue or cell begin to change from its normal values, it can trigger the onset of a cancer, and Raman spectroscopy has the potential to detect those initial compositional changes. So this technique can be used to diagnose pathological condition of organs and progression of disease. Currently, the potential of this technique are being tested to detect different types of cancers: breast, prostate, bladder, cervix, skin, larynx, head and neck squamous cell carcinoma, etc. and determine their unique spectra features (Stone, 2003, Keller, 2006, Devpura, 2010, 2011). Raman spectroscopy is able to identify prostate cancer from benign with 89% accuracy in snap frozen biopsies *in vitro* (Crow, 2003). Reduction in glycogen and increment in nucleic acid contents of malignant areas are observed through Raman bands. Sensitivity of differentiating cancer grades, Gleason score 7, less than 7, and greater than 7 are more than 81%. In another study, prostate cancer was identified with 94% accuracy compared to benign and prostate intraepithelial neoplasia (Devpura, 2010). In addition, Gleason score 6, 7, and 8 were distinguished with more than 81%. However, this needs to be validated with additional studies on more tissue specimens. Bladder and prostate cancers were also investigated using a fiber optic near-infrared Raman spectrometer and an overall accuracy of 84% and 86%, respectively, was observed (Crow, 2005). An attempt to construct an integrated Raman and angular-scattering microscope was made to collect both Stokes-shifted light and elastic light (Smith & Berger, 2009) to improve the detection performance and accuracy. This will allow characterizing simultaneously the size of cell and its chemical information. Recently, Raman spectroscopy was successfully used to determine the variation of chemical composition of a cell in response to a drug treatment. A threshold concentration of a toxic amount of *Nerium Oleander* was determined (Saha, 2009). This demonstrates that this technique can be used in drug designing application.

Due to advancement in diagnostic technologies and treatment modalities, most of the cancers can be cured if detected in their early stages. Cancer is basically a disease in which abnormal cells divide without any control and these cancerous cells are able to invade other tissues, and by this process the disease spreads to other organs. Hence, it certainly will be of great advantage to detect biomolecular compositional changes at cellular level, particularly in these proliferating cells. In this study, we have focused our study on luminal cells of PIN and compare their spectral features of benign epithelia (BE) and cancerous cells of the prostate tissues. To the best of our knowledge, this is the first report of such an investigation. It is important to compare luminal cells of each pathological category since basal cells are absent in the epithelium of microacinar structures of the prostate cancer. In addition, we have investigated the stroma surrounding BE, PIN, and cancerous micro acinar clusters.

The interaction between prostatic stroma and the epithelial cells is somewhat different from the stromal cells in prostate tumors (Bowsher & Carter, 2006). The prostatic stroma, which consists of fibromuscular matrix enclosing the prostatic ducts, limits the proliferation of the epithelia unlike the stroma in the prostatic tumors which contain fibroblasts or myofibroblasts. The stroma bordering prostatic tumors is called "reactive stroma" or "carcinoma associated fibroblasts" (Bowsher & Carter, 2006). It is imperative to explore the spectral features of the stromal cells in BE, PIN, and tumor stages and understand its linkage with cancer and its progression. It appears that the reactive stroma in prostate initiates the carcinogenesis and helps its progression (Olumi, 1999, Hayward, 2001, Niu & Zia, 2009).

2. Materials and methods

In this study, we used a Renishaw RM1000 Raman microscope-spectrometer with a 785 nm laser excitation source. RM1000 is equipped with a CCD (charged-coupled device) detector, an automated *xyz* stage (ProScan II) with WIRE 2.0 software to control the recording of the Raman spectra. 50x objective was used to collect data from the tissue specimens with laser power of about 20 mW focused to a spot size of ~ 2 μm diameter on the tissue specimens. Each Raman spectrum was averaged over three scans with 20 s integration time to obtain a good signal-to-noise ratio. The scattered light was collected in a back scattering geometry and dispersed using a 1200 lines/mm grating.

2.1 Preparation of tissues for Raman spectroscopy

Tissue specimens which are embedded in paraffin wax were obtained from Karmanos Cancer Center and Harper University Hospital in Detroit, MI, USA, and were processed at the University Pathology Services at Karmanos Cancer Center. In this study, we specifically selected the tissue specimens which were purely BE, PIN or cancerous. For each specimen, two parallel adjacent sections were cut. One 5 µm thick section was stained with Haematoxylin and Eosin (H&E) and was used for pathological examination, and the second 10 µm thick layer was used for Raman spectroscopic measurements. The H&E stained slides were reviewed by three experienced pathologists and none of the cases studied here found to be in dispute. The paraffin wax was removed from the 10 µm thick tissue sections using xylene and ethanol baths following the procedures described in Devpura, 2010 and 2011. It is noted that the incomplete removal wax residues gives rise to strong and sharp Raman bands that interfere with the Raman bands of the tissue samples at 1063, 1130, 1296, 1436, and 1465 cm^{-1} (Ó Faoláin, 2005). In our spectra, we did not observe any of the sharp bands associated with wax. Assuming that the morphological features do not change across a few micrometer thick layers, the H&E stained layer was used as a guide to collect the Raman spectra from the specific sites of the adjacent unstained deparaffinized tissue section.

2.2 Raman spectroscopic measurements

A total of 34 tissue specimens obtained from 33 patients were used in this study. Out of these, 12 specimens were benign, 11 were PIN, and 11 were cancerous with a grade of 3. The Raman spectra were recorded from the unstained tissue section. The appropriate regions on the unstained tissue section were identified with the help of the adjacent stained section with regions marked by pathologist as BE, PIN, cancer, and stroma. The identification of these regions was done with an optical microscope to make sure the data were collected only from the marked regions. When collecting Raman spectra, the laser beam was focused only on the luminal cells (Figure 1). The regions marked with elliptical symbols in the Figure 1 show the regions from where the Raman spectra were collected. In addition, it was made sure that each Raman spectrum was taken from a different region of luminal cells. The Raman spectra were collected in the 500-1900 cm^{-1} region. The 600-1800 cm^{-1} region is commonly known as the "biological window" where most of the biomolecules show intense Raman excitations. An extra 100 cm^{-1} extended region were recorded at both ends of the Raman spectra to avoid any artifacts which may occur while removing the fluorescence background

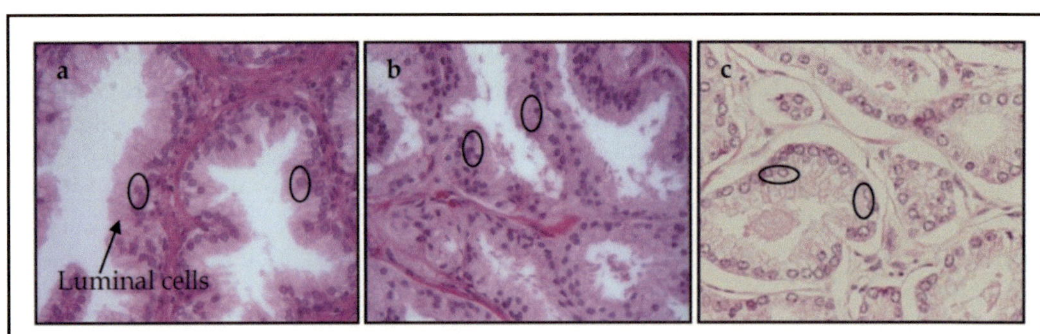

Fig. 1. Pathology pictures of (a) BE tissue, (b) PIN, and (c) Cancer (images are taken with 40x magnification). Elliptical symbols represent locations of the Raman measurements from the corresponding unstained tissue.

from each spectrum. A total of 1220 Raman spectra were collected from the tissue samples in which 207, 202, and 208 are from the luminal cells of BE, PIN, and cancer (grade 3), respectively, and the remaining (201 spectra each) from the corresponding stromal regions. The Raman measurements of stromal cells in cancer tissues were obtained from the bordering regions of the grade 3 micro acinar clusters.

2.3 Raman data processing and chemometric analysis

The collected Raman spectra were examined for non-standard noise and those with such noise were discarded from the database used for analysis. The spectra used in the analyses were cleaned from any spurious bands due to cosmic rays and noise by using wavelets method (Cao, 2007). The fluorescence background from each spectrum was removed with minmax adaptive algorithm that requires no apriori knowledge of the spectra. Finally, each spectrum was normalized with respect to the highest intensity band in the spectrum. Multivariate/chemometric statistical method, like principal component analysis, PCA, (Jolliffe, 2002) which determines correlation in the variance, was used to detect trends in the data set. The data was further analyzed using discriminant function analysis, DFA (Klecka, 1980) to classify the data. First, the data was analyzed using PCA which reduces the dimensionality of the original data set from 601 variables to 19 new variables, called the eigenvectors. These new variables captured 97% of the variance of the data. Examination of the first two eigenvectors show distinct trends in the data representing BE, PIN, and cancer. These new fewer variables carrying most of the variance of the data are useful for determining the groups in the data. To find classes in the data, we have performed DFA using 19 eigenvectors as the input variables. The classification of each pathological state is done using the leave-one-out method, where each data set is considered a new case and compared with the rest of the data pool.

3. Results and discussion

The average Raman spectral features of BE, PIN, and cancer are shown in Figure 2. We see changes in the peak intensities of most of the Raman bands (Raman band assignments are listed in the table 1) in the spectra of PIN compared to the spectra of BE and cancer tissues. These changes are fundamentally related to the changes in the concentrations of the biochemicals of BE luminal cells. Significant changes are in the region from 600 cm^{-1} to 1145 cm^{-1} which are shown in the lower panel of the Figure 2. Some of the changes are noteworthy: the band at 726 cm^{-1} (assigned to ring breathing mode of DNA/RNA bases) becomes quite intense in PIN, and in addition the Raman bands at 853 cm^{-1}, 931 cm^{-1} ($\nu_{C\text{-}C}$ stretching mode of protein), 960 cm^{-1}, and 1090 cm^{-1} (symmetric phosphate stretching vibrations) also show an increase in their intensities when pathological state of cell changes from BE to PIN. While the bands at 1605 cm^{-1} and 1667 cm^{-1} (amide I) showed decrease in their intensities. When comparing the average spectral changes of PIN with cancer, we see that the peak intensities at 780 cm^{-1}, 1240 cm^{-1} (proline, tyrosine), 1330 cm^{-1} and 1605 cm^{-1} are enhanced when pathological state of luminal cells changes from PIN to cancer, while the bands at 726, 853, 931, 960, and 1090 cm^{-1} show decrease in their intensities which show similar trend like the bands of BE. The Raman bands at 780 cm^{-1} and 878 cm^{-1} showed progressive increase in their intensities when cells changes from BE to PIN and then to cancer. These Raman bands should be further investigated for their possible association with progression of prostate cancer and perhaps their use as diagnostic variables.

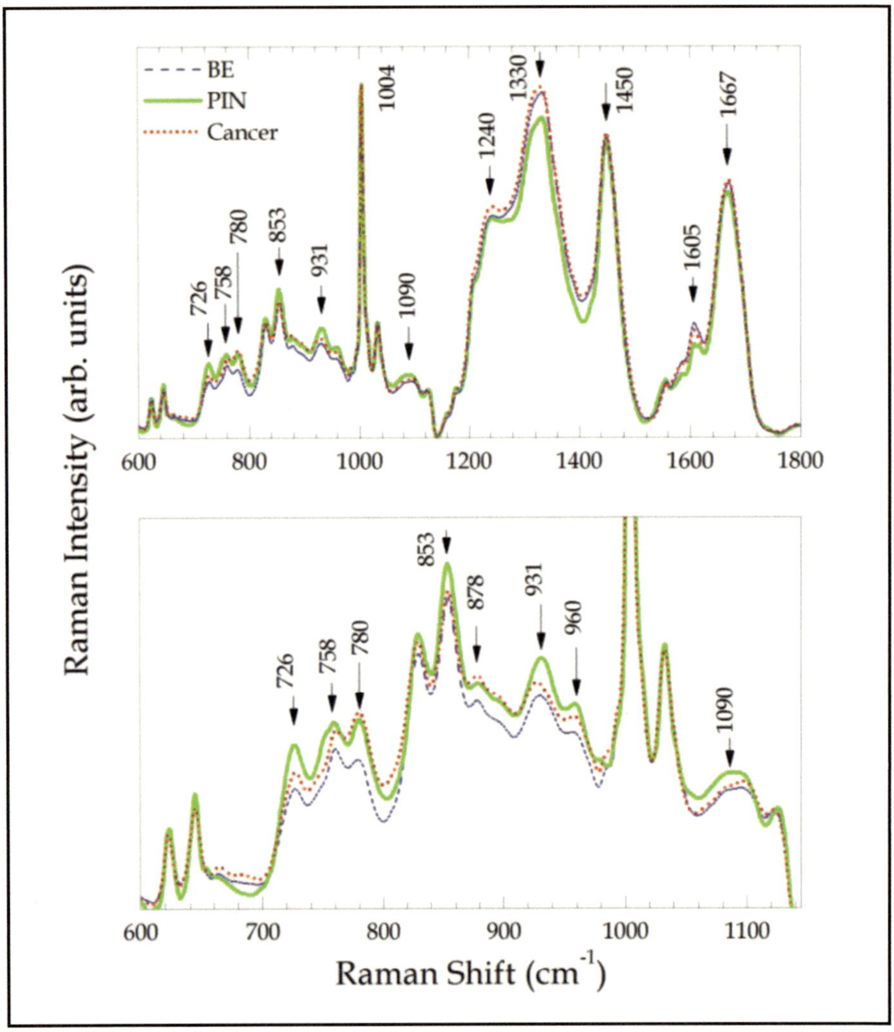

Fig. 2. Average Raman spectra of BE (blue dash line), PIN (green), and Cancer (red dotted line). The lower panel shows the Raman spectral range of 600-1145 cm^{-1}.

Raman Shift (cm^{-1})	Peak Assignment
726	A ring breathing mode of DNA/RNA bases
758	Symmetric breathing of tryptophan
780	DNA/uracil ring breathing mode
829	Tyrosine, phosphodiester, O-P-O stretching DNA/RNA
853	Ring breathing mode of tyrosine, C-C stretch of proline ring, glycogen
878	Tryptophan, hydroxyproline, C-O-C ring
931	C-C stretch, α-helix, protein band
960	Cholesterol, phosphate of HA
1004	Phenylalanine
1032	Phenylalanine, proline
1081	Typical phospholipids, phosphodiester groups in nucleic acids/collagen
1090	Symmetric phosphate stretching vibrations
1240	RNA, Amide III, collagen
1313	Lipid/protein
1330	Collagen, nucleic acids & phospholipids
1450	CH_2 bending mode of proteins & lipids, methylene deformation
1557	Tryptophan, tyrosine
1605	Cytocine, phenylalanine, tyrosine, C=C stretch
1667	Protein, C=C stretch, amide I

Table 1. Raman peak assignment (Gelder, 2007, Movasaghi, 2007).

3.1 Statistical analysis of the PIN, BE, and cancer data

The first three eigenvectors or the principal components (PCs) are plotted against each other in Figure 3. The left panel is the plot of PC2 vs. PC1 and the right panel represents PC3 vs. PC1. These three PCs contain 76% of the variance in the data showing different trends for each pathological state. Although some of the data seem to be overlapping with each other, the different trends are still very clear in the data. The largest variance in the data is captured by the PC1 which is shown by the spread of the BE, PIN and cancer along the PC1 axis. PC3 shows distinct trend present in the spectral data of PIN.

The average spectra of BE, PIN, and cancer showed distinct variations in the intensities of certain peaks while the spectral features of individual spectrum of each category are expected to spread about its average value and must also be different from other categories. As tissue changes from BE to PIN and then to cancer, the spectral variances in the data must exhibit some distinct classes if each of these categories is pathologically different. The classification results are shown in Figure 4 where we clearly see three distinct classes with their centroids (marked with black squares) far away from each other. It is interesting to note that PIN class is very distinct class from other classes and does not have much overlap with others. There are only three pathological states (Klecka, 1980), which means there are two discriminant functions (DFs). So the DF1 shows the maximum variance in the Raman data, and the DF2 contains the rest of the variances.

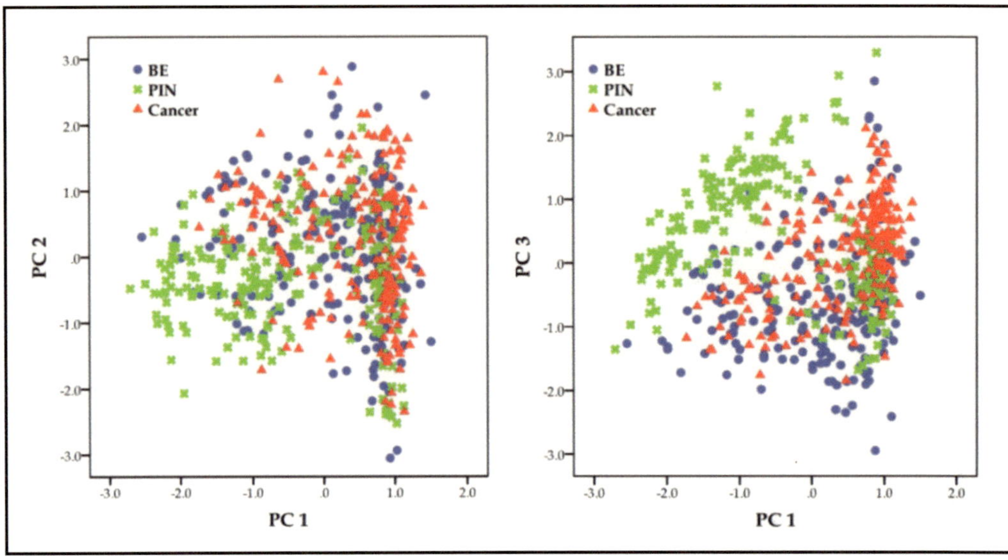

Fig. 3. PCA results of BE, PIN, and cancer. PC2 vs PC1 is on the left panel and the PC3 vs. PC1 is on to the right.

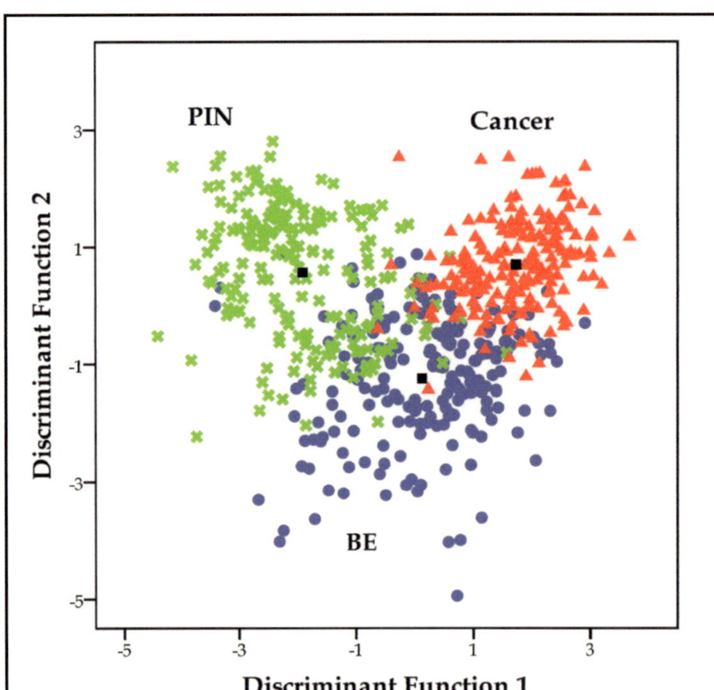

Fig. 4. DF plot of BE, PIN, and cancer.

			Predicted Group Membership			
		Group	BE	PIN	Cancer	Total
Cross-validated	Count	BE	158	20	29	207
		PIN	33	165	4	202
		Cancer	16	2	190	208
	%	BE	**76.3**	9.7	14.0	100.0
		PIN	16.3	**81.7**	2.0	100.0
		Cancer	7.7	1.0	**91.3**	100.0

Table 2. Classification results of BE, PIN, and cancer. Centre the values of "BE", "PIN" and "Cancer"

The group prediction of the Raman spectroscopy data using DFA is compared with that of pathological diagnosis: the "gold standard" for diagnosing cancer. To test the validity of our predicted classifications, we have performed leave-one-out cross-validation where the group classification for each spectrum with one of the known pathological states is determined while using the remaining data as a training set. The results of cross-validation classification results are shown in Table 2. We see that the PIN is predicted with 82% accuracy while the prediction accuracies for BE and cancer are 76% and 91 %, respectively.

3.2 Comparison of Raman spectra of stroma in BE, PIN, and cancer

It is interesting to study the stroma surrounding each of the pathological states as it could provide useful information about the onset of cancer. The nature of stroma observed was found to depend on its environment (Bowsher & Carter, 2006). Figure 5 shows the average Raman spectra of stroma surrounding BE, PIN, and cancer. The stroma surrounding cancer shows a significant enhancement in the intensity of Raman bands at 726, 758, 931, 1240, 1313, and 1330 cm^{-1} compared to stroma surrounding PIN and BE whereas bands at 1081, 1450 and 1667 cm^{-1} show a slight reduction in intensity. The Raman spectra of stromal regions in cancer and BE seem to show similarity in their biochemicals compared to that of the stroma of PIN. When comparing spectral features of the luminal cells of PIN with surrounding stroma, the Raman bands associated with DNA/RNA (726, 780, 829, and 1330 cm^{-1}) are suppressed and the bands arising from amino acids/protein/collagen (853, 931, 960, and 1240 cm^{-1}) are significantly enhanced. This can also be observed in the stroma of BE, and cancer.

The chemometric analysis was also performed on the stromal data. The PC plots of stromal investigation are shown in Figure 6. Here, the analysis generated 15 principal scores containing 98% of the variance in the Raman data. The plot is based on the first three PCs which consist of 86% of the Raman spectral information. Here, we see clear trends for stroma associated with each epithelial category: BE, PIN, and cancer.

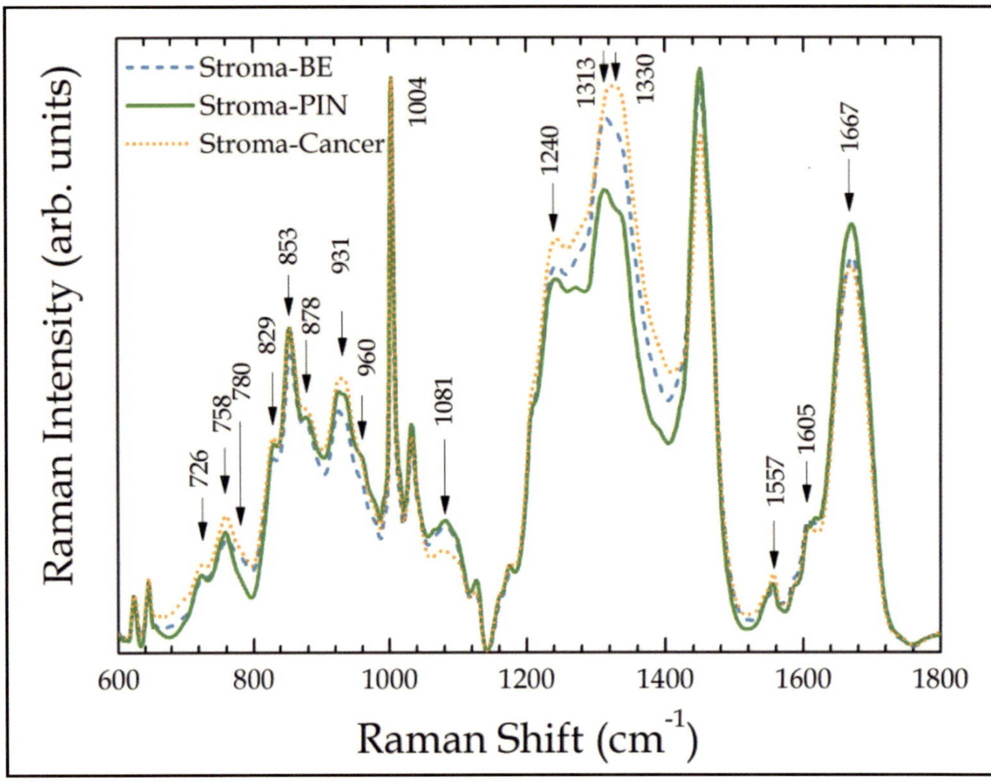

Fig. 5. Average Raman spectra of stroma surrounding BE, PIN, and cancer.

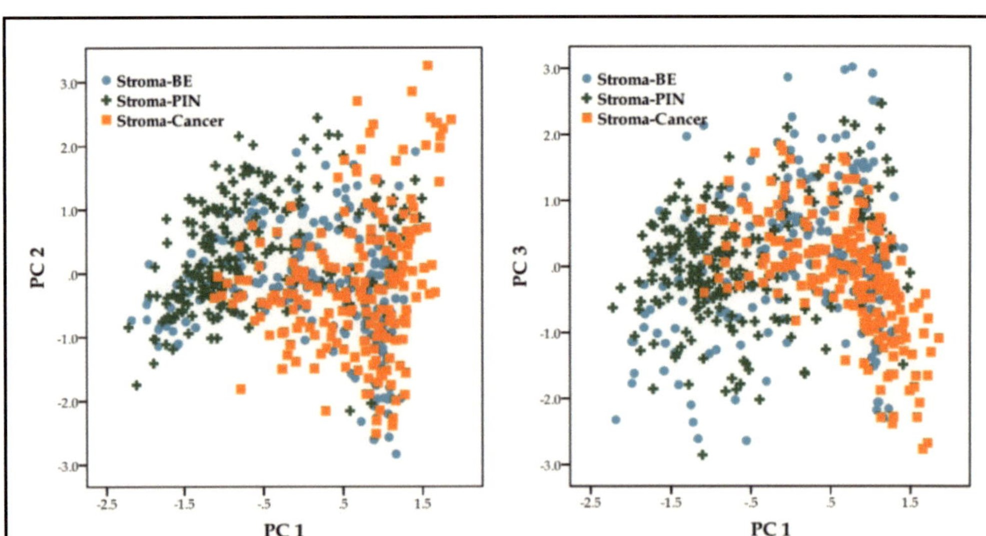

Fig. 6. PCA analysis of the Raman data of stroma.

Apparently, the stroma surrounding BE, PIN, and cancer are quite distinct as shown in the DF plot together with the overlapping average Raman spectra of stroma in BE, stroma in PIN, and stroma in cancer (see Figures 6 and 7). Here, the DFA is performed with 15 eigenvectors which contained 98% of the variance in the stromal data. Table 3 shows predicted group membership using leave-one out classification method for stromal investigation, we find that the stroma surrounding PIN is 83.6% correctly identified. The stroma in BE and cancer is classified with 81.6% and 87.1% accuracy, respectively.

It seen that when comparing stroma surrounding PIN with that of cancer, the intensities of Raman bands at 853, 931, 1240, and 1330 cm^{-1} have increased whereas the Raman bands at 1081 cm^{-1} and 1450 cm^{-1} have decreased. Thus, Raman spectroscopy can be used to distinguish easily the stroma associated with BE, PIN, and cancer accuracy. It is interesting to note when spectral data of all the pathologies are combined and analyzed statistically to find their distinct classes, we see a clear separation of stroma from BE, PIN and cancer. In addition stroma of BE, PIN, and cancer are also well separated (see Figure 8).

It should be noted that DFA constructs one less number of discriminant functions for the user-defined categories. Thus, this analysis created 5 discriminat functions due to 6 categories, and figure 8 shows only the first two discriminant functions which carry 89% of the variance in the Raman spectra. Thus, the overlapping of data in this 2-D plot may not be the same for the other dimensions. This study shows that the Raman spectroscopy can be used to distinguish the luminal cells in their normal, BE and PIN states. Further, the stroma surrounding these regions can also be distinguishes as they exhibit distinct characteristic spectral features of their own.

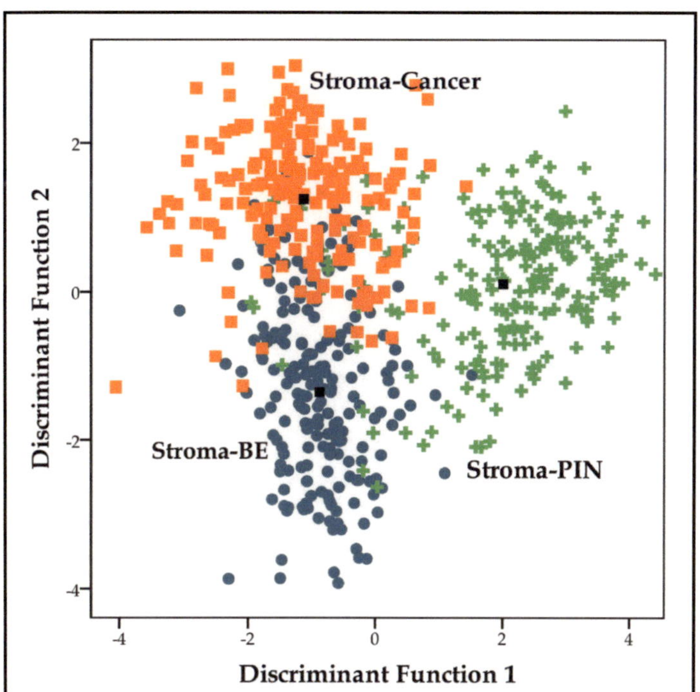

Fig. 7. DF plot of stroma surrounding BE, PIN, and cancer.

		Group	Predicted Group Membership			Total
			Stroma-BE	Stroma-PIN	Stroma-Cancer	
Cross-validated	Count	Stroma-BE	164	3	34	201
		Stroma-PIN	14	168	19	201
		Stroma-Cancer	18	8	175	201
	%	Stroma-BE	**81.6**	1.5	16.9	100.0
		Stroma-PIN	7.0	**83.6**	9.5	100.0
		Stroma-Cancer	9.0	4.0	**87.1**	100.0

Table 3. Classification results of stroma in BE, PIN, and cancer.

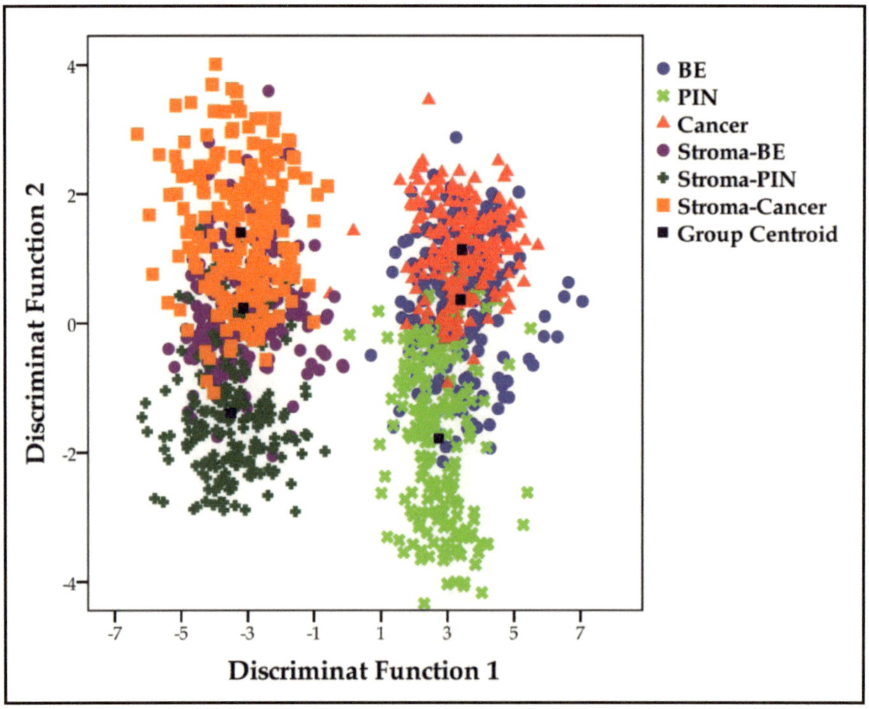

Fig. 8. DF plot of all the categories: BE, PIN, and cancer, and their surrounding stroma.

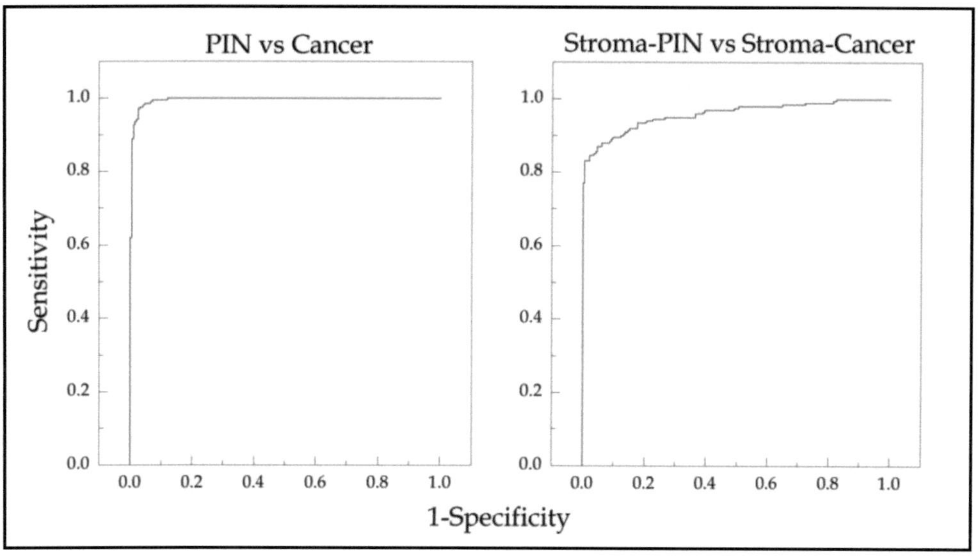

Fig. 9. ROC curves for PIN vs cancer and stromal PIN vs stromal cancer.

We also constructed Receiver Operating Characteristic (ROC) curves (Mason & Graham, 2002) for both the analyses, PIN compared to cancer and comparison between stroma around PIN and stroma associated with cancer. In an ROC graph, the sensitivity and 1-specificity are plotted against each other. Sensitivity is the ratio of true positives (cancer measurements which are correctly identified as cancer) over the total PIN data and the specificity is the ratio of true negatives (PIN measurements which are correctly identified as PIN) over the total PIN data. The sensitivity and specificity for luminal cell investigation of PIN and cancer are 98% and 99%. For the stromal investigation, the sensitivity and specificity are about 90% and 94%, respectively. The area under the curves (AUC) infers the validity of the test. An AUC = 1, indicates a perfect test whereas AUC = 0.5 implies a null result. As shown in Figure 9, both the AUC's are more than 0.96 indicating a very good test for PIN and stroma investigations.

4. Conclusions and future work

In this study, we have investigated using Raman spectroscopy, luminal cells from the tissues which are purely either BE, PIN or cancerous. We particularly focused on PIN and compared its spectral features with BE and cancer. Significant and noticeable changes in the Raman spectra of BE, PIN, and cancerous tissues are observed. As luminal cells become cancerous, the intensities of the most Raman bands in the 700-1000 cm^{-1} increase and the intensity changes can be interpreted in terms of changes in the biochemical composition of the tissues. In particular, the intensity of the 780 cm^{-1} (possibly arising from nucleic acids) Raman band increases considerably in the spectrum of cancerous tissue compared to the BE. Additionally, we also studied stromal cells surrounding each pathological state of the tissues, namely, BE, PIN and cancer and, we observed enhancement in protein contents and reduction in DNA contents when compared to the luminal cells. Chemometric analysis of the data shows that the spectral variations in the data are quite pronounced and can easily be classified with very high accuracies into distinct pathological groups. The sensitivity and specificity of luminal cells of PIN and cancer are about 98% for each and for the stroma associated with these pathologies, both the sensitivity and specificity are more than 90%. Current study suggests further investigation of different pathology grades (low and high grade) of PIN, including basal cells, are needed and to expand the Raman spectral database for better prediction capability. Since some of the PIN structures may not lead to carcinoma, by spectroscopic investigation one can explore the Raman signatures of a PIN structure which can lead to cancer.

5. Acknowledgement

We thank Dr. D. Shi, Detroit Medical Center, Detroit, for her help with prostate samples and Dr. M. D. Klein, Children's Hospital of Michigan, Detroit, for providing access to the Raman Spectroscopy facility. We express our sincere thanks to Richard A. Barber Foundation for the financial support of this work.

6. References

Allsbrook, W. C. , Mangold, K. A., Johnson, M. H., Lane, R. B., Lane, C. G. & Epstein, J. I. (2001). Interobserver reproducibility of Gleason grading of prostatic carcinoma: General Pathologists. *Human Pathology*, Vol. 32, No. 1, (January 2001), pp. (81-88)

Andriole, G. L., Bullock, T. L., Belani, J. S., Traxel, E., Yan, Y., Bostwick, D. G. & Humphrey, P. A. (2007). Is there a better way to biopsy the prostate? Prospects for a novel Transrectal systematic biopsy approach. *Urology*, Vol. 70, No. 6, Supp 6A, (December 2007), pp. (22-26).

Bostwick, D. G. & Qian, J. (2004). High-grade prostatic intraepithelial neoplasia. *Modern Pathology*, Vol. 17, (January 2004), pp. (360–379).

Bowsher, W & Carter, A. (2006). *Challenges in prostate cancer* (Second edition), Blackwell Publishing, ISBN 978-4051-0752-5, Massachusetts, USA.

Cao, A., Pandya, A. K., Serhatkulu, G. K., Weber, R. E., Dai, H., Thakur, J. S., Naik, V. M., Naik, R., Auner, G. W. & Rabah, R. J. (2007). A robust method for automated background subtraction of tissue fluorescence. *J Raman Spectrosc.*, Vol. 38, (May 2007), pp. (1199–1205)

Carroll, P., Alnerstein , P. C., Greene, K., Babalan, R. J. , Carter, H. B., Gann, P. H., Han, M., Kuban, D. A., Sartor, A. O., Stanford, J. L. & Zletman, A. (2009). In: *Prostate-Specific Antigen Best Practice Statement*, http://www.auanet.org/content/guidelines-and-quality-care/clinical-guidelines/main-reports/psa09.pdf.

Crow, P., Molckovsky, A., Stone, N., Uff, J., Wilson, B. & Wongkeesong, L.-M. (2005). Assesment of fiberoptic near-infrared Raman spectroscopy for diagnosis of bladder and prostate cancer. *Urology*, Vol. 65, (June 2005), pp. (1126-1130)

Crow, P., Stone, N., Kendall, C. A., Uff, J. S., Farmer, J. A. M., Barr, H. & Wright, M. P. J. (2003). The use of Raman spectroscopy to identify and grade prostatic adenocarcinoma in vitro. British J of Cancer, Vol. 89, pp. (106-108)

Devpura, S., Thakur, J. S., Sarkar, F. H., Sakr, W. A., Naik, V. M. & Naik, R. (2010). Detection of benign epithelia, prostatic neoplasia, and cancer regions in radical prostatectomy tissues using Raman spectroscopy. *Vibrational Spectrosc.*, Vol. 53, (July 2010), pp. (227-232)

Devpura, S., Thakur, J. S., Sethi, S, Naik, V. M. & Naik, R. (2011). Diagnosis of head and neck squamous cell carcinoma using Raman spectroscopy: tongue tissues. *J Raman Spectrosc.* (DOI: 10.1002/jrs.3070)

Fleshner, N. E., Kapusta, L., Donnelly, B., Tanguay, S., Chin, J., Hersey, K., Farley, A., Jansz, K., Siemens, R., Trpkov, K., Lacombe, L., Gleave, M., Tu D. & Parulekar, W. R. (2011). Progression From High-Grade Prostatic Intraepithelial Neoplasia to Cancer: A Randomized Trial of Combination. *J Clin. Oncol.*, Vol. 29, (June 2011), pp. (2386-2390)

Gelder, J. D., Gussem, K. D., Vandenabeele, P & Moens, L. (2007). Reference database of Raman spectra of biological molecules. *J Raman Spectrosc.* Vol. 38, (September 2007), pp. (1133-1147).

Hayward, S. W., Wang, Y., Cao, M., Hom, Y. K. & Zhang, B. (2001). Malignant transformation in a nontumorigenic human prostatic epithelial cell line. *Cancer Res.*, Vol. 61, (November 2001), pp. (8135–8142).

Hricak, H., Scardino, P. T. & Reznek, R. H. (2009). *Prostate Cancer*, Cambridge University Press, ISBN 978-0-521-88704-5, New York, USA.

Humphrey, P. A. (2004). Gleason grading and prognostic factors in carcinoma of the prostate. *Modern Pathology*, Vol. 17, (March 2004), pp. (292–306), doi:10.1038/modpathol.3800054.

Jemal, A., Siegel, R., Bray, F., Center, M. M., Ferlay, J., Ward, E. & Forman, D. (2011). Global Cancer Statistics. *Cancer J Clin.* Vol. 5961, (March/April 2011), pp. (225-249), doi:0.3322/caac.20107 doi: 10.3322/caac.20006.

Jolliffe, I. T. (2002). *Principal Components Analysis* (Second edition), Springer-Verlag, New York, USA.

Kandaswami, C., Lee, L. T., Lee, P. P, Hwang, J. J., Ke, F. C., Huang, Y. T. & Lee, M. T. (2005). The antitumor activities of flavonoids. *In Vivo*, Vol. 19, (September-October 2005), pp. (895-909).

Keller, M. D., Kanter, E. M. & Mahadevan-Jansen A. (2006). Raman spectroscopy for cancer diagnosis. Spectroscopy, Vol. 21, No. 11, (November 2006), pp. (33-41)

Klecka, W. R. (1980). *Discriminant Analysis, Series: Quantitative applications in the social sciences*, Sage Publications Inc., Newbury Park.

Laserna, J. J. (1996). *Modern Techniques in Raman spectroscopy*, John Wiley& Sons, New York, USA.

Mason, S. J.& Graham, N. E. (2002). Areas beneath the relative operating characteristics (ROC) and relative operating levels (ROL) curves: Statistical significance and interpretation. *Q. J. R. Meteor. Soc.* Vol. 128, pp. (2145-2166).

Movasaghi, Z., Rehman, S. & Rehman, I. U. (2007). Raman spectroscopy of biological tissues. *Applied. Spectroscopy Reviews*, Vol. 42, (September 2007), pp. (493-541), doi: 10.1080/05704920701551530.

Niu, Y. -N. & Zia, S. -J. (2009). Stroma–epithelium crosstalk in prostate cancer. *Asian Journal of Andrology*, Vol. 11, (December 2008), pp. (28–35).

Oesterling, J. E. (1991). Prostate specific antigen: a critical assessment of the most useful tumor marker for adenocarcinoma of the prostate. *J Urol*, Vol. 145, No. 5, (May 1991), pp. (907-923).

Ó Faoláin, E., Hunter, M. B., Byrne, J. M., Kelehan, P., Lambkin, H. A., Byrne, H. J. & Lyng, F.M. (2005). Raman Spectroscopic Evaluation of Efficacy of Current Paraffin Wax

Section Dewaxing Agents *J Histochem Cytochem* Vol. 53(1), (March 2005), pp. (121-129).

Olumi, A. F., Grossfeld, G. D., Hayward, S. W., Carroll, P. R., Tlsty, T. D. & Cunha, G. R. (1999). Carcinoma-associated fibroblasts direct tumor progression of initiated human prostatic epithelium. *Cancer Res*, Vol. 59, (October 1999) pp. (5002–5011).

Partin A. W., Kattan, M. W., Subong, E. N., Walsh, P. C., Wojno, K. J., Oesterling, L. E., Scardino, P. T., & Pearson, J. D. (1997). Combination of prostate-specific antigen, clinical stage, and Gleason score to predict pathological state of localized prostate cancer. A multi-institutional update. *J. Am. Med. Assoc.*, Vol. 277, (May 1997), pp. (1445–1451).

Quinn, D. I., Henshall, S. M., Brenner, P. C., Kooner, R., Golovsky, D., O'Neill, G. F., Turner, J. J., Delprado, W., Grygiel, J. J., Sutherland, R. L. & Stricker, P. D. (2003). Prognostic significance of preoperative factors in localized prostate carcinoma treated with radical prostectomy. *Cancer*, Vol. 97, No. 8, (April 2003), p.p. (1884-1893).

Raman, C. V. (1928). A new type of secondary radiation. *Nature*, Vol. 121, No. 3048, (March 1928), pp. (501-502).

Saha, A. & Yakovlev, V. V. (2009). Towards a rational drug design: Raman micro-spectroscopy analysis of prostate cancer cells treated with an aqueous extract of Nerium Oleander. *J. Raman Spectrosc.*, Vol. 40, (December 2008), pp. (1459–1460).

Shroder, F. H., Hugosson, J. & Roobol, M. J. (2009). Screening and prostate-cancer mortality in a randomized European study. *New Eng J Med*, Vol. 360, (March 2009), pp. (1320-1328).

Smith, Z. J. & Berger, A. J. (2009). Construction of an integrated Raman- and angular-scattering microscope. *Review of Scientific Instruments*, Vol. 80, No. 044302, (April 2009), pp. (1-8).

Stone, N., Kendall, C., Smith, J., Crow, P. & Barr, H. (2003). Raman spectroscopy for identification of epithelial cancers. *Faraday Discuss*, Vol. 126, (September 2003), pp. (141–157).

Chemopreventive Target for Prostate Cancer: Prostatic Intraepithelial Neoplasia

J. Arunakaran[1], S. Banudevi[1] and A. Arunkumar[2]
[1]*Department of Endocrinology, Dr. ALM Post Graduate Institute of Basic Medical Sciences, University of Madras, Sekkizhar Campus, Taramani, Chennai Tamilnadu,*
[2]*Center of Excellence in Cancer Research, Department of Biomedical Sciences, Texas Tech University Health Sciences Center, Texas*
[1]*India*
[2]*USA*

1. Introduction

Prostate cancer is one of the most frequently diagnosed malignancies among the male population and the second common cancer-related death worldwide after lung cancer (Jemal *et al.*, 2010). It is estimated that 30% of male older than 50 years are harboring microscopic transformation of adenocarcinoma within the prostate gland. Because of the dramatic rise in the incidence of prostate cancer with the rate increasing approximately 6% per year worldwide (Eschenbach, 1996), the study of precursor lesions of prostate cancer is emerging concept in the field of prostate cancer prevention.

2. Prostatic intraepithelial neoplasia

John McNeal introduced the term *intraductal dysplasia of the prostate* in the early 1960s, postulating that carcinoma of the prostate arose from active ductal/acinar epithelium and not from atrophic acini (McNeal, 1965, 1988; Amin *et al.*, 1993). Later various terms have been rasied such as *large acinar atypical hyperplasia with malignant change* (Allam *et al.*, 1996) and *ductacinar dysplasia* (McNeal, 1988). None of these have gained popularity. The term Prostatic intraepithelial neoplasia (PIN) was first proposed by Bostwick and Brawer in 1987, and this term was accepted at the 1989 Workshop on Prostatic Dysplasia (Bethesda, Md; March 1989) as the preferred nomenclature for this preneoplastic change (Bethesda, Md; March 1989; Drago *et al.*, 1989). PIN refers to the putative precancerous end of the continuum of cellular proliferations within the lining of prostatic ducts, ductules and acini (Bostwick and Amin, 1996; Bostwick and Qian, 2004).

PIN is the most likely precursor of prostate cancer and has been described as a premalignant or pre-invasive form of prostate cancer (Sakr *et al.*, 1993; Bostwick, 1996). Although two histopathologic lesions in the prostate were proposed as being premalignant (PIN and atypical adenomatous hyperplasia, AAH), there is less evidence of a premalignant role for AAH than there is for PIN (De La Torre *et al.*, 1993; Jones and Young, 1994; Epstein, 1994; Bostwick, 1996). Within these lesions, studies have identified impaired and abnormal differentiation, increased proliferation, and abnormal DNA content and elevated *ras* protooncogene mRNA expression (Jones and Young, 1994). There are two grades of PIN (low-grade and high-grade), although the term PIN is usually used to indicate high-grade PIN (HGPIN). The high level of interobserver variability with low-grade PIN (LGPIN) limits its clinical utility, and many pathologists do not report this finding except in research studies. Low grade PIN (LGPIN) is only a very early precursor, and might even not be considered as a precancerous lesion. Moreover, the distinction between LGPIN and normal epithelium might be observer related (Lipski *et al.*, 1996; Zlotta and Schulman, 1999; Vis and Van der Kwast, 2001).

PIN lesions can only be diagnosed by histopathological examination of prostatic tissue. It is impossible to detect PIN clinically by digital rectal examination (DRE), prostate specific antigen (PSA) or ultrasound. Cytologically, LGPIN and HGPIN have clear and reproducible features (Table 1). Histologically, however, different architectural variations exist for HGPIN (Fig. 1). At least four distinct patterns can be distinguished: flat, tufting, micropapillary and cribriform (Bostwick, 1989). Less frequent are signet cell pattern, small cell neuroendocrine pattern, mucinous pattern and microvacuolar pattern. In the big majority of PIN-lesions, a tufting pattern can be found. Frequently, multiple patterns can be found at the same time.

Structural pattern	Low grade PIN (LGPIN)	High grade PIN (HGPIN)
Architecture	Crowding, stratification, irregular spacing	More changes, 4 patterns (T, MP, cribriform, flat)*
Nuclei Chromatin Nucleoli	Slight enlargement, size variation Normal Rarely prominent	Definite enlargement, less size variation Increased density and clumping Frequently prominent
Basal cell layer	Intact	May show some disruption
Basement membrane	Intact	Intact

* T indicates tufting; MP- micropapillary.

Table 1. Prostatic intraepithelial neoplasia (PIN): diagnostic criteria modified from Bostwick and Brawer (1987)

HGPIN is the most significant risk factor for prostate cancer in needle biopsy specimens. Its role as the preinvasive stage of cancer was recently confirmed conclusively in two separate mouse models (Kasper *et al.*, 1998; Garabedian *et al.*, 1998). PIN coexists with cancer in more than 85% of cases (McNeal and Bostwick, 1986; Qian *et al.*, 1997) but retains an intact or fragmented basal cell layer, unlike cancer, which lacks a basal cell layer (Bostwick and Brawer, 1987). PIN is strongly predictive of adenocarcinoma, and its identification in biopsy specimens of the prostate warrants further search for concurrent cancer. PIN alone has no apparent influence on serum PSA concentration, and it is not apparently visible by current imaging techniques.

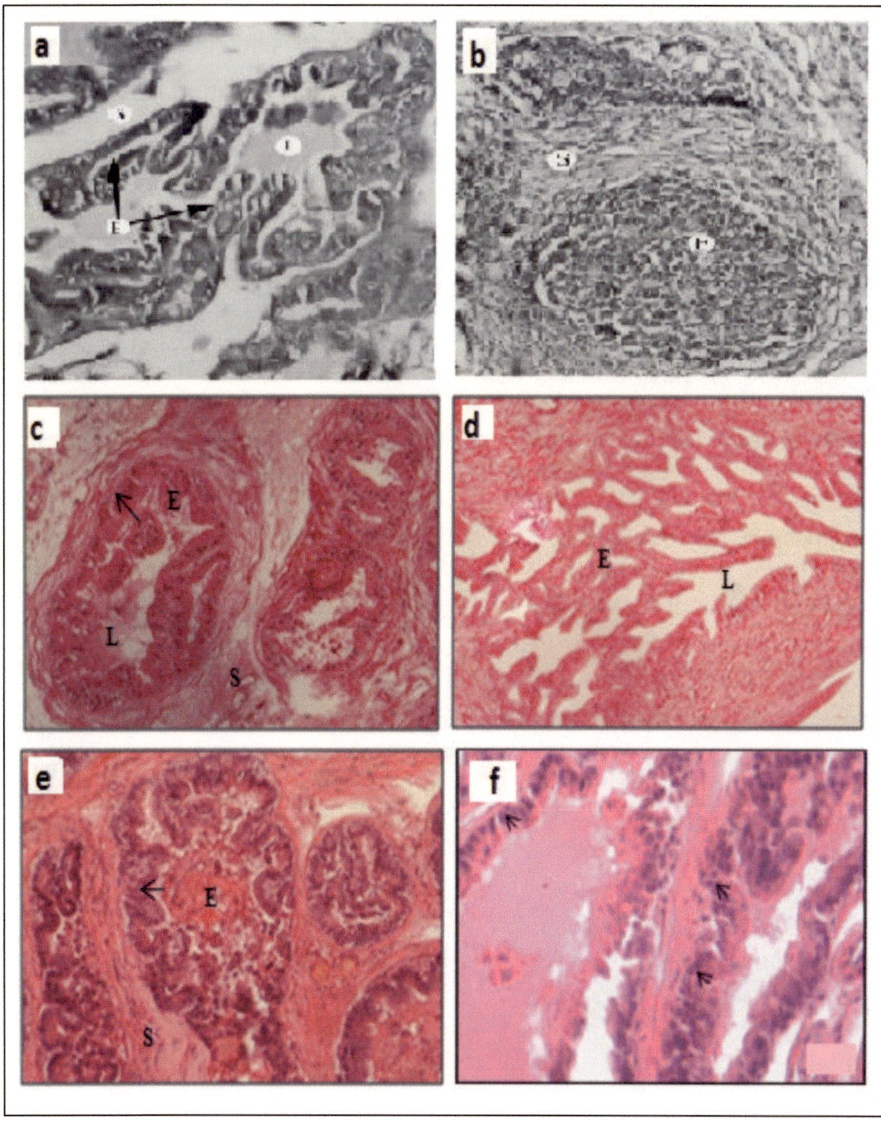

Fig. 1. **Prostatic intraepithelial neoplasia Histology**. **(a)**. Multiple dysplastic and hyperplastic sites were seen within the same glandular epithelium (×200 magnifications; H&E) **(b)**. Fully developed PIN with loss of basal epithelial cells (×200 magnifications; H&E) (Arunkumar *et al.*, 2006). Architectural pattern of high grade prostatic intraepithelial neoplasia (PIN) such as tufting **(c)**, cribriform **(d)**, and micropapillary **(e)** structures were observed (×200 magnifications; H&E) **(f)**. The cell number in PIN was markedly increased, and cell density with sparse cytoplasm (arrow headed) (×400 magnifications; H&E) (Banudevi *et al.*, 2011a & b). E- Epithelium; L- Lumen; S-Stroma

3. Identification of PIN: Histological criteria

The classification of PIN into low grade and high grade is based mainly on the cytological characteristics of the cells. The nuclei of cells composing LGPIN are enlarged, vary in size, have normal or slightly increased chromatin content, and possess small or inconspicuous nucleoli (Figs. 2 and 3). HGPIN is characterised by cells with large nuclei of relatively uniform size, an increased chromatin content, which might be irregularly distributed, and prominent nucleoli that are similar to those of carcinoma cells (Fig. 4). The basal cell layer is intact or rarely interrupted in LGPIN, but may have frequent disruptions in high grade lesions. Although the cytological features of LGPIN and HGPIN are fairly constant, the architecture shows a spectrum, varying from a flattened epithelium to a florid cribriform proliferation. Four basic patterns that often coexist have been described by Bostwick and colleagues (Bostwick *et al.*, 1993): flat, tufting, micropapillary, and cribriform. Familiarity with this diverse architectural spectrum may facilitate the histological recognition of PIN, even though these various architectural patterns have no apparent clinicopathological relevance (Bostwic *et al.*, 1993).

Neuroendocrine differentiation occurs in PIN, where it is intermediate in degree between normal prostate (which has the most cells with neuroendocrine differentiation) and carcinoma (Bostwick *et al.*, 1994a; Di Sante Agnese, 1996). Paneth cell like change of the prostatic epithelium (neuroendocrine cells with large eosinophilic granules) is considered to be a distinct form of neuroendocrine differentiation characterised by isolated cells or small groups of cells with prominent eosinophilic cytoplasmic granules.

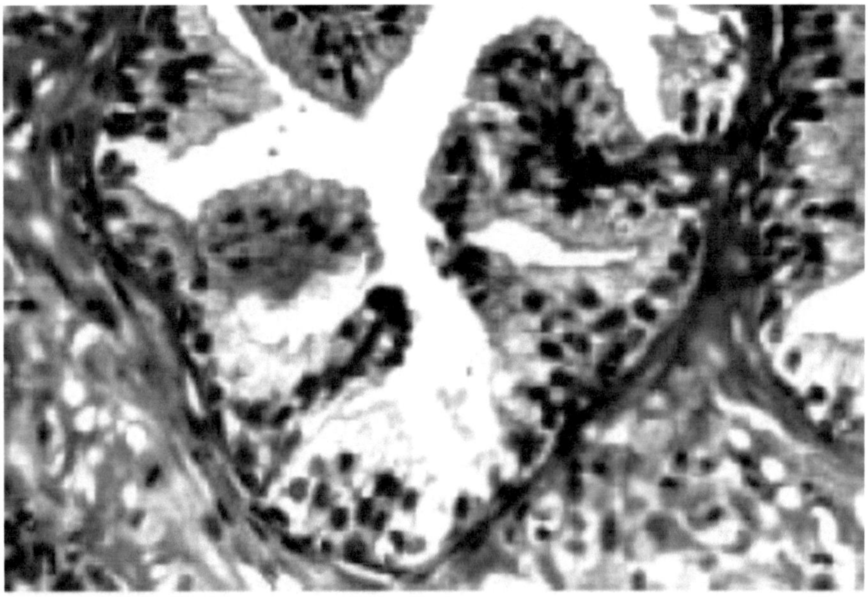

Fig. 2. **Normal prostate**. The duct is lined by a two cell layer– for example, the basal cell and the secretory or luminal cell layers.

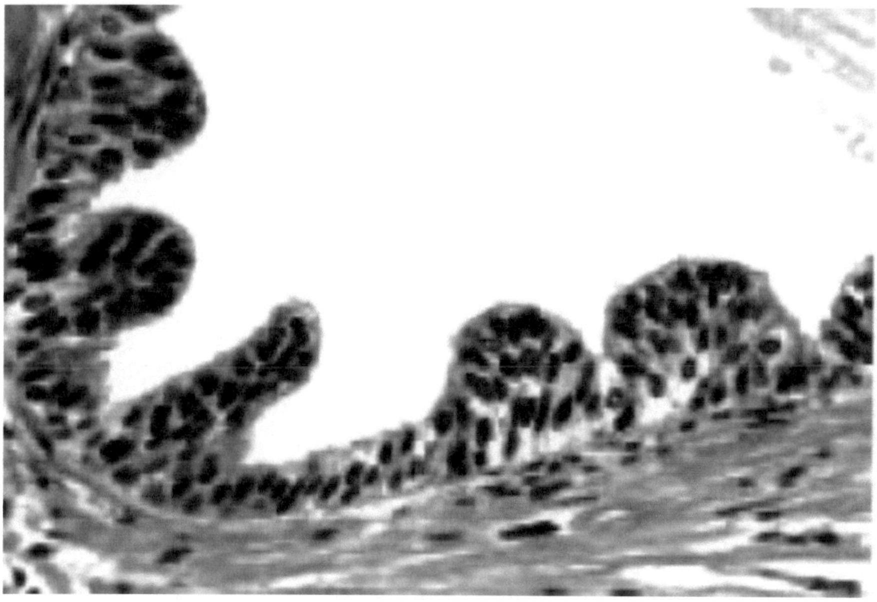

Fig. 3. Low grade prostatic intraepithelial neoplasia. The nuclei of the secretory cells are enlarged, vary in size, have normal or slightly increased chromatin content, and possess small or inconspicuous nucleoli. The basal cell layer is almost intact.

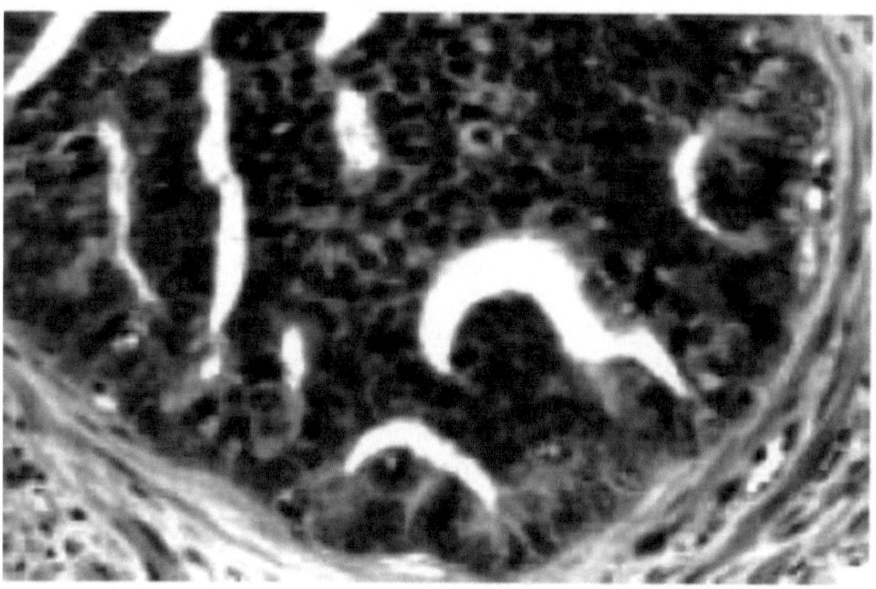

Fig. 4. **High grade prostatic intraepithelial neoplasia** with cribriform patterns. The perimeter cells show features of clearly dysplastic cells, whereas, going from the periphery towards the centre, the nuclei become smaller and the nucleoi become less apparent ("maturation phenomenon"). The basal cell layer is disrupted.

4. PIN incidence

The incidence of PIN varies according to the male population. The lowest likelihood is in men participating in PSA screening and early detection studies, with an incidence of PIN in biopsies ranging from 0.7% to 20% (Bostwick *et al.*, 1996; Langer *et al.*, 1996; Wills *et al.*, 1997; Skjorten *et al.*, 1997). Men seen by urologists in practice have PIN in 4.4% to 25% of contemporary 18-gauge needle biopsies obtained by urologists. Those undergoing transurethral resections have the highest likelihood of PIN, varying from 2.8% to 33% (Pacelli *et al.*, 1997). In such cases, all tissues should be examined, but serial sections of suspicious foci are probably not usually necessary. Select anti-keratin antibodies such as 34β-E12 (high molecular weight keratin) may be used to stain tissue sections for the presence of basal cells, recognizing that PIN retains intact or fragmented basal cell layer, whereas cancer does not (Bostwick and Brawer, 1987). By immunohistochemical analysis, Prostate tumor overexpressed-1 (PTOV1) was considered as good marker for PIN which shows strong immunoreactivity in areas of carcinoma and HGPIN (Morote *et al.*, 2008)

5. PIN distribution

Prostatic intraepithelial neoplasia is found predominantly in the peripheral zone of the prostate (75%-80%), rarely in the transition zone (10%-15%), and extremely rarely in the central zone (< 5%). This distribution parallels the frequency of the zonal predilection for prostatic carcinoma (Bostwick *et al.*, 1995; Gaudin *et al.*, 1997,; Pacelli *et al.*, 1997). The frequency of HGPIN in needle biopsy series ranges from 5% to 16% and in transurethral resection of the prostate specimens between 2.3% and 4.2% (Bostwick *et al.*, 1995; Gaudin *et al.*, 1997; Melissari *et al.*, 2006) McNeal in 1969 mentioned the multifocality of this process (McNeal, 1969; 1988); this observation has since been corroborated by others.

6. Immunohistochemistry in PIN

Numerous studies to highlight the basal cells and the secretory cells have been done (Brawer *et al.*, 1985; McNeal *et al.*, 1988a, 1988b; Perlman and Epstein, 1990; Abhrams *et al., 2002;* Zhou *et al.*, 2003; Wu *et al.*, 2004). The basal cells and luminal cells of the prostatic glands display different keratin immunoreactivity. The high-molecular-weight cytokeratin monoclonal antibody (clone 34βE12, also referred to as CK903) recognizes keratin proteins of 49, 51, 57, and 66 kD and labels the basal cells but not the luminal/secretory cells of the prostatic glands that stain with prostate-specific antigen and prostatic acid phosphatase. α-Methylacyl CoA-racemase (AMACR) stains the cells of adenocarcinoma but usually does not stain benign prostate glands (Brawer *et al.*, 1985; McNeal *et al.*, 1988a, 1988b; Perlman and Epstein, 1990; Abhrams *et al.*, 2002; Zhou *et al.*, 2003; Wu *et al.*, 2004).

Other antibodies that also mark basal cells include p63 (McNeal, 1969) and CK5/6 (Abhrams *et al.*, 2002). p63 is a nuclear stain, whereas CK5/6 stains the cytoplasm (Abhrams *et al.*, 2002; Zhou *et al.*, 2003). The basal cell layer is present in benign epithelial proliferations, may be disrupted in HGPIN, and is absent in invasive carcinoma (Bostwick and Brawer , 1987). Bostwick and Brawer in 1987 have shown that the frequency and extent of basal cell disruption in PIN is related to the PIN grade and is greatest in HGPIN.

A numerous of Immuno histochemical studies (McNeal *et al.*, 1988a; Perlman and Epstein, 1990; Deschenes and Weidner, 1990; Nagle *et al.*, 1991; Sesterhenn *et al.*, 1991) have been done to correlate the relationship between HGPIN and invasive carcinoma, Including evaluation of monoclonal antikeratin antibody, KA4, *Ulex europaeus* lectin (UEA-l), lectin binding pattern, and vimentin. Wu *et al.* demonstrated that a significantly higher P504S (AMACR) positive rate (56.0%) was found in isolated HGPIN glands adjacent to cancer (distance less than 5 mm) compared with those away from cancer (distance more than 5 mm; 14%, $P < 0.001$) (Wu *et al.*, 2004). High-grade PIN glands adjacent to cancer also showed a higher ($P <0 .001$) P504S intensity than did those away from cancer.

Other studies including argyrophilic nucleolar organizer regions and static DNA flow cytometry suggest that HGPIN and carcinoma have similar proliferative activity and DNA content, and hence HGPIN is the most likely precursor of cancer (Sesterhenn *et al.*, 1991; Weinberg and Weidner, 1993; Amin *et al.*, 1994). Cytogenetic abnormalities (involving 7q, 8q, 10q, 16q) and numerical chromosomal changes are noted in HGPIN and carcinoma (Emmert-Buck *et al.*, 1995; Macoska *et al.*, 1995; Qian *et al.*, 1999; Al-Maghrabi *et al.*, 2002). High-grade PIN and prostate cancer share genetic and molecular markers as well, with PIN representing an intermediate stage between benign epithelium and invasive carcinoma (Brawer, 2005).

PIN offers promise as an intermediate endpoint in studies of chemoprevention of prostatic carcinoma (Bostwick *et al.*, 1994b; Aquilina *et al.*, 1997). Recognizing the slow growth rate of prostate cancer and the considerable amount of time needed in animal and human studies for adequate follow-up, the non-invasive precursor lesion PIN is a suitable intermediate histologic marker to indicate subsequent likelihood of cancer (Aquilina *et al.*, 1997).

7. Chemoprevention strategies

Chemoprevention is the administration of agents to prevent induction of cancer, or to inhibit or delay its progression. In prostatic neoplasia, the time from tumour initiation and progression to invasive carcinoma often begins in men in the fourth and fifth decades of life and extends across decades. This phenomenon represents a unique opportunity to arrest or reverse the process of carcinogenesis with the use of chemopreventive agents. Animal models in defining efficacy of chemoprevention agents against prostate cancer. Detection of inhibitory effects on de novo prostate cancer development requires a high cancer incidence and similarity of induced tumors to human prostate carcinomas. The following animal models have produced high incidences of multifocal prostate adenocarcinoma: transgenic mice with oncogenes expressed in a prostate specific fashion; Noble rats that have been treated chronically with combination of 17β-estradiol and testosterone; and Wistar or F344 rats treated sequentially with a single injection of *N*-methyl-*N*-nitrosourea (MNU) and chronic administration of testosterone.

PIN most often occurs in the first two models, and metastases are frequent in some transgenic models and the MNU-testosterone model (Shirai *et al.*, 1991; Pollard *et al.*, 1992; Kadomatsu *et al.*, 1993; Slayter *et al.*, 1994; Ingles *et al.*, 1997). The chemopreventive efficacy of a series of agents using a model in which hormone dependent prostate cancer is induced in the Wistar-Unilever rat (McCormick, 1998). This is achieved by sequential treatment with an antiandrogen (cyproterone acetate), and androgen (testosterone propionate) and a direct acting chemical carcinogen (N-methyl-N-nitrosourea), followed by chronic androgen stimulation (testosterone). This regimen reproducibly induces a high incidence (< 75%) of prostate cancer, with no gross toxicity and a low incidence of neoplasia in the seminal vesicles and other non-target tissue.

Dehydroepiandrosterone (DHEA) and 9-cis-retinoic acid (9-cis-RA) are the most active chemopreventive agents identified to date. DHEA inhibits the induction of prostate cancer when administration is started before carcinogen exposure, and when it is delayed until incipient neoplastic lesions are present. Chronic administration of 9-cis-RA starting before carcinogen exposure is highly effective in the chemoprevention of prostate cancer. Liarozole fumarate confers modest protection against induction of prostate cancer, whereas N-(4-hydroxyphenyl) retinamide (4-HPR), a-difluoromethylornithine, DL-α-tocopherol acetate (vitamin E), oltipraz, and L-selenomethionine are inactive. The differential activity of 9-cis-RA and 4-HPR suggests the ligand specificity may be a determinant of retinoid action in prostate cancer chemoprevention. Chemoprevention of MNU +T induced prostate carcinogenesis at low dose level (0.5 μg/kg body weight) of calcitriol has significant potency to inhibit prostatic hyperplasia, dysplasia and PIN, and also decreased serum PAcP activity. Calcitriol may be an effective therapy for the treatment of early prostate cancer (Senthil kumar *et al.*, 2006).

Christov *et al.* (2002) studied that PIN can be used for assessing the efficacy of chemopreventive agents on prostate carcinogenesis. Dially disulfide, an organosulfur compound of garlic, has significant potency as an inhibitor of cancer induction in Sprague Dawley rat prostate by inhibiting PIN, hyperplastic and dysplastic foci (Arunkumar *et al.*, 2006). Zinc also acts as a chemopreventive agent against prostate cancer by inducing regression in PIN (Banudevi *et al.*, 2011a). Zinc inhibits PIN an early stage of prostate cancer. This study proves the ability of zinc to restore the PIN changes particularly in the rat ventral prostate induced by carcinogen and testosterone thereby indicating its anticarcinogenic potential (Banudevi *et al.*, 2011a). As the dorsolateral prostate is most likely homologue to the human prostate (Bosland *et al.*, 1990), in our recent study we proved that zinc was found to inhibit the growth and decrease dorsolateral prostatic acid phosphatase, zinc, citrate levels, phase I drug metabolizing enzyme activities, lipid peroxide, H_2O levels, proliferating cell nuclear antigen (PCNA), Bcl2, Bcl-X_L expressions with concomitant increase in phase II enzyme activities, GSH levels, p53, Bax, caspase-3 expressions in MNU testosterone induced model of prostate carcinogenesis (Banudevi *et al.*, 2011b). Signs of dysplasia, a characteristic of prostatic intraepithelial neoplasia, were evident in the dorsolateral prostatic histoarchitecture. Thus, zinc may act as an essential trace element against MNU and testosterone induced prostatic preneoplastic progression in Sprague Dawley rats.

The most efficient strategy for developing a chemoprevention programme is to perform two clinical trials concurrently, each based on the modulation of high grade PIN but in different target populations (Nelson *et al.*, 1996; Bostwick, 1997). In patients with high grade PIN associated with prostate cancer, a prospective, double blind, placebo controlled chemoactive pilot study designed to measure the response of a potential chemopreventive agent in the period (three to six weeks) before radical prostatectomy could easily be performed.

Androgen deprivation treatment is commonly used in this population to downsize the prostate before radical prostatectomy. This study may provide information regarding the effectiveness of proposed agents on surrogate endpoint biomarkers, premalignant lesions, and cancer. In particular, such an investigation would determine the response of PIN to the agent in whole mounted radical prostatectomy specimens. In some preliminary investigations it has been shown that there is a marked decrease in the prevalence and extent of PIN in prostates after androgen deprivation treatment, as compared with untreated prostates (Ferguson *et al.*, 1994). This is accompanied by regressive changes in the secretory epithelium. Apoptotic bodies are more often seen in the treated normal prostate, PIN, and prostate cancer than in untreated cases. This suggests that androgen ablation induces epithelial regression by enhancing apoptosis. The low proliferating cell nuclear antigen (PCNA) and Ki67 related values and the absence of mitoses in PIN as well as in normal prostate and prostate cancer in the treated cases indicates suppressed proliferation activity as a consequence of androgen deprivation treatment (Armas *et al.*, 1993; Montironi *et al.*, 1994). It has been reported that angiogenesis is inhibited in prostate lesions when total androgen ablation induces cell regression and activation of the apoptosis (Montironi *et al.*, 1996). Consequently, the epithelial cells are blocked from expressing, producing, or exporting angiogenic molecules. All these findings indicate that the dysplastic prostatic epithelium is hormone dependent.

A short term prospective, double blind, placed controlled phase II chemopreventive trial with cancer as an endpoint could be done in patients with high grade PIN without cancer. Chemoprevention trials designed to reverse high grade PIN may be confounded by the presence of underlying but undetected addressed by requiring a second biopsy with negative findings for cancer before entry into the study (preferably sextant biopsies with special attention to areas of abnormality on ultrasonogram or digital rectal examination), and by including enough subjects in the study and control groups to equalise the risk of coexistent cancer between the two groups.

PIN is routinely monitored by repeat biopsy in contemporary urological practice. Periodic re-evaluation would be necessary, including physical examination, rebiopsy, and evaluation of surrogate intermediate endpoint biomarkers. If subsequent biopsy reveals prostate cancer, these patients need definitive treatment. Those with PIN or no malignancy need continued observation (Bostwick, 1997).

8. Clinical chemoprevention studies

Table 2 reports agents, the treatment periods, and the primary endpoints used in clinical chemoprevention studies sponsored or funded by the National Cancer Institute (Kellof, 1997).

Green tea catechins

Epidemiological and case-control studies have garnered support for the chemopreventive properties of green tea (Jian *et al.*, 2004). A recent study was conducted on 60 volunteers with high-grade prostate intraepithelial neoplasia, a putative precursor of prostate adenocarcinoma (Bettuzzi *et al.*, 2006). Patients received green tea compounds in capsule form 200 mg three times per day. Following 1 year of treatment, only 3% of patients that received the green tea polyphenols were diagnosed with cancer compared with 30% in the placebo group. Furthermore, patients that received the green tea capsules exhibited a longer latency to tumor detection and exhibited an improved quality of life. Another phase II study, in which 6 g/day of tea was administered to 42 patients with asymptomatic, androgen- independent prostate cancer, has demonstrated that a single patient achieved a PSA response of >50% that lasted for approximately 1 month. These patients suffered with side effects that include diarrhea, nausea and fatigue (Jatoi *et al.*, 2003). Another clinical study used 250 mg dose of green tea polyphenols twice daily. In this study, 6 out of 19 patients had disease control for 3 to 5 months and there was only 1 patient whose PSA rise was affected by green tea supplementation. The dose used in this study did not discernibly alter the course of hormone-refractory prostate cancer (Choan *et al.*, 2005). These results suggest that green tea possesses cancer chemopreventive properties and minimal anti-neoplastic activity against advance stage prostate cancer.

Agent	*Cohort (treatment period)*	*Primary endpoints*
Phase II		
DFMO	Scheduled for prostate cancer surgery (4–8 weeks)	Histopathology (PIN grade, nuclear polymorphism, nucleolar polymorphism, ploidy), proliferation biomarkers (PCNA, Ki-67)
	Scheduled for prostatectomy (stage A or B prostatic carcinoma or bladder cancer without prostatic carcinoma and scheduled for cystoprostatectomy) (14 days)	Drug effect measurements: ODC activity (skin and prostate), polyamine levels (prostate). Histopathology (TRUS guided biopsies). Biochemical biomarkers: PSA, PAP, testosterone
	Serum PSA 3–10 ng/ml (includes patients with prostatic carcinoma and PIN) (14 days–l year)	Drug effect measurements: ODC activity (skin and prostate) Polyamine levels (prostate). Histopathology (TRUS-guided biopsies) Biochemical biomarkers: PSA, PAP, testosterone
DHEA	Scheduled for prostate cancer surgery (28 days)	Histopathology (PIN grade, nuclear polymorphism, nucleolar polymorphism, ploidy). Proliferation biomarkers (PCNA, Ki-67). Genetic/regulatory biomarkers (p53, *bc1-2*, pc-l, chromosome 8p loss)
Flutamide	Patients with high grade PIN (12 months)	PIN grade and incidence, cancer incidence, nuclear polymorphism, nucleolar size, ploidy. Other endpoints: PCNA, angiogenesis, apoptosis, LOH chromosome 8; growth factors, PSA
4-HPR	Biopsy proven non-metastatic prostate adenocarcinoma, scheduled for radical prostatectomy (4 weeks)	Genetic/regulatory biomarkers: TGFβ, c-myc, p53, plasminogen activators (tPA, uPA), apoptosis
	Scheduled for prostate cancer surgery (4–8 weeks)	Histopathology: PIN grade, nuclear polymorphism, nucleolar polymorphism, ploidy. Proliferation biomarkers: PCNA, Ki-67. Differentiation biomarkers: Lewis^{Y} antigen. Genetic/regulatory biomarkers: p53, EGFR, TGFα
Phase III		
Finasteride	Men ≥ 55 years of age with normal DRE and PSA < 3.0 ng/ml (7 years)	Prostate cancer incidence (grade and stage), BPH incidence and severity, overall and prostate-specific mortality, TURP, PSA levels
Selenised yeast	Skin cancer (melanoma, non-melanoma) patients, low Se areas in USA (~1 year)	PSA levels

BPH, benign prostatic hypertrophy; DFMO, difluoromethyllornithine; DHEA, dehydroepiandrosterone; DRE, digital rectal examination; EGFR, epidermal growth factor receptor; PAP, prostatic acid phosphatase; PCNA, proliferating cell nuclear antigen; PIN, prostatic intraepithelial neoplasia; PSA, prostate specific antigen; Se, selenium; TGF, transforming growth factor; TRUS, transrectal ultrasound; TURP, transurethral resection of the prostate; 4-HPR, *N*-(4-hydroxyphenyl)retinamide.

(Kellof, 1997).

Table 2. National Cancer Institute Chemoprevention Branch: sponsored od funded phase II/III clinical chemoprevention trials: prostate cancer

Selective estrogen receptor modulators (SERMs)

Interest in SERMs as preventive agents has been stimulated by an apparent role of estrogens in the pathogenesis of prostate cancer, through promotion of cell growth. SERMs are generally considered to be 'weak estrogens' because they possess both agonist and antagonist activities depending on the specific tissue type and on the relative ER subtype interactions. Consequently this class of agents has been called selective estrogen receptor modulators or SERMs. As with phytoestrogens, SERMs appear to possess the ability to suppress prostate carcinogenesis. Toremifene has been evaluated in a phase IIa exploratory trial in men with high-grade PIN (Steiner and Pound, 2003). After 4 months of treatment with a daily oral dose of toremifene, 18 men with high-grade PIN underwent a repeat prostate biopsy. The prostate biopsy specimens showed significantly less high-grade PIN than historical controls. This trial provided the proof-of-concept support behind a currently open 485 patient placebo controlled, randomized dose finding phase IIb/III clinical trial

(Price *et al.*, 2006). This trial is investigating the efficacy of toremifene in reducing prostate cancer incidence in men with high-grade PIN. Men with high-grade PIN are treated for 12 months with placebo or toremifene and will undergo a repeat prostate biopsy at 6 and 12 months (the trial details are available at http://www.gtxinc.com/tech/clinical.htm). In addition, the National Cancer Institute is evaluating the effects of toremifene versus placebo in men with prostate cancer prior to radical prostatectomy. The objective of this phase II clinical trial is to evaluate the effects of a toremifene on biomarkers of prostate cancer. The trial details are available at http://www.cancer.gov/search/ViewClinicalTrials.

Difluoromethyl ornithine (DFMO)

DFMO is an irreversible inhibitor of ornithine decarcoxylase involved in the synthesis of polyamines; it possesses cytostatic and cytotoxic effects (Messing *et al.*, 1999). At the clinical level, interest in exploring DFMO as a chemoprevention agent for prostate cancer has recently increased as the administration of DFMO at 0.5 g/m2 daily for 4 weeks to men scheduled for surgical interventions to treat either prostatic hyperplasia or neoplasia resulted in reduction of polyamine pools, including spermine (Simoneau *et al.*, 2001). These results confirm that DFMO reaches the target tissue and hence may warrant further study as a possible chemopreventive agent for prostate cancer.

Selective COX-2 inhibitors

Inhibition of COX-2 expression blocks its pro-inflammatory effects, reduces expression of androgen receptors and androgen inducible genes and promotes apoptosis in prostate cancer cells. Selective COX-2 expression has been observed in high-grade PIN, a putative precursor of prostate cancer, suggesting a role early in carcinogenesis (Hussain *et al.*, 2003). These results support the hypothesis that inhibition of COX-2 may be an effective preventive strategy for prostate cancers; however, an industry-sponsored large-scale trial of rofecoxib was closed after the drug was withdrawn from the market because of concerns over its cardiovascular safety.

Selenium

Many of the cellular processes and molecular markers shown to be modified by selenium play key roles in prostate cancer progression. Two clinical trials are examining the role of selenium in other groups of high-risk individuals: men who have had negative prostate biopsies and men with HGPIN. The Negative Biopsy study, which includes men who have had at least one negative sextant prostate biopsy, will be using selenium supplementation in the form of selenium yeast, SeY (200 or 400 μg) (Marshall, 2001). The high-grade PIN study will determine the incidence of prostate cancer in men with biopsy-proven high grade intraepithelial neoplasia supplemented daily with 200 μg selenomethionine (Marshall, 2001). The results of these studies will be critical in defining a role for intervention with selenium in high-risk individuals, for whom there is no current treatment.

Bicalutamide

Intermittent (weekly), low-dose bicalutamide on prostate morphology revealed a tendency to a favorable modulation of high-risk proliferative lesions such as HGPIN. Namely, HGPIN status improved in 26% of treated subjects as compared with 4% of subjects in the no-treatment arm. These findings must be interpreted with extreme caution due to the inherent limitations of prostate sampling with needle biopsy. However, our analysis including all changes in HGPIN status (i.e., both HGPIN resolution and HGPIN development after 6 months of treatment) may account, at least in part, for sampling errors, supporting the worth of our findings although they derive from a post hoc analysis. The 28% incidence of HGPIN found in our study was unusually high compared with that reported in the general population, which ranges from 0.7% to 25% in noncancerous prostate biopsies (Bubendorf *et al.*, 1998). HGPIN incidence increases with age and is higher in men seen in clinical practice compared with men participating in screening programs (Bostwick and Qian, 2004). As most subjects in our study were in their seventies and as all were urological practice outpatients, this could partly explain our findings. Moreover, whereas HGPIN by itself does not seem to increase PSA (Bostwick and Qian, 2004), the incidence of HGPIN in homogeneous cohorts of men with elevated PSA is largely unknown. Once-a-week administration of bicalutamide in men at risk for prostate cancer is feasible and reasonably safe. This finding, coupled with the encouraging signal of activity emerging from the analysis of HG-PIN changes, supports further studies of this schedule at the lowest dose for prostate cancer prevention in men at high risk despite the negative primary end-point findings on Ki-67 (Zandari *et al.*, 2009).

Nutraceuticals and Micronutrients

Nutraceutical compounds most commonly show antioxidant properties combined with other anti-neoplastic actions (Syed *et al.*, 2008). Table 3 presents the most notable nutraceutical compounds examined in prostate cancer prevention, including vitamin D, vitamin E, selenium, lycopene, soy, and green tea (Trottier *et al.*, 2010a & b).

Compound	*Origin*	*Proposed mechanism*	*Strength of evidence*	*Outcomes*	*Selected references*
Vitamin D (calcitriol)	Sunlight, meats, fish	Vitamin D receptor activation: cancer homeostasis, cell proliferation and differentiation	Case–control and cohort studies	Conflicting when levels are normal; modest evidence when levels are low	Trottier *et al.*, 2010 Schwartz *et al.*, 2006
Vitamin E (tocopherols and tocotrienols)	Nuts, vegetable oils, palm oil, oats, rye, wheat, rice bran	Antioxidant, proapoptotic	Cohort studies, 2 RCTS[a]	No difference from placebo in RCTS	Gaziano *et al.*, 2009 Lippman *et al.*, 2009
Lycopene	Tomatoes	Carotenoid antioxidant	Case–control and cohort studies, meta-analysis	Positive meta-analysis, but negative results from the PLCO screening trial	Etminan *et al.*, 2004 Kirsh *et al.*, 2006 Peters *et al.*, 2007
Soy and isoflavanoids	Soybeans	Phytoestrogens and tyrosine kinase inhibition causing apoptosis, limited cell growth, reduced inflammation	Case–control and cohort studies, meta-analysis	Positive effect noted with non-fermented soy and mainly in non-Western men	Yan and Spitznagel, 2009
Green tea	*Camellia sinensis* plant	EGCG is the likely active ingredient: antioxidant polyphenol and 5ARI activity	Case–control and cohort studies, 1 RCT	Conflicting for overall PCa diagnosis; possible positive effect on advanced PCa diagnosis	Kurahashi *et al.*, 2008 Brausi *et al.*, 2008

[a] SELECT (Selenium and Vitamin E Cancer Prevention Trial) and Physician's Health Study II.
RCT = randomized control trial; PLCO = Prostate, Lung, Colorectal, and Ovarian Cancer; EGCG = epigallocatechin-3-gallate; 5ARI = 5α-reductase inhibitor; PCa = prostate cancer.

Table 3. Primary prostate cancer prevention with selected nutraceutical (Trottier *et al.*, 2010)

9. Signal anomalies of human prostate cancer

Prostatic intraepithelial neoplasia (PIN) lesions could be described as low grade (LG) or high grade (HG) and it is widely perceived that HGPIN is a precursor of prostatic adenocarcinoma (Isaacs *et al.*, 2002). Since the initial growth of prostate tumor or cancer is dependent on androgens, hormone therapy in the form of medical or surgical castration constitutes a common approach for systemic treatment. However over a period of time, most cancer will develop androgen-independence, thereby making the continued androgen deprivation therapy ineffective (Taplin and Balk, 2004). While the mechanisms that drive the genesis of subclinical, microscopic PIN lesions, their progression to invasive cancer and androgen independence remain largely unknown and evidence collected in recent years point to certain molecular aberrations that pave the path of disease progression.

For example, anomalies in specific signaling molecules, including extracellular growth factors, protein tyrosine kinase cell surface receptors, intracellular transcription factors, nuclear factors and their ligands, growth suppressors, cell cycle regulators and others have indicated in some prostate carcinomas (Abate Shen and Shen, 2000; Gao and Isaacs, 2000; Roy-Burman *et al.*, 2004)

There is currently a strong focus on the genetic alterations or aberrations in gene expression that are frequently encountered in human prostate cancer in the design of mouse models. Although both men and mice harbour functionally equivalent prostate glands, there are similarities as well as differences in the anatomy and histology of the prostate in the two species. Similar epithelial cell types namely secretory, basal and neuroendocrine are found in both mouse and human prostate, although their proportions vary. While human prostate has a robust fibromuscular stroma, the mouse contains a modest stromal component. Anatomically the human prostate gland is a single, alobular structure with central, peripheral and transitional zones. In contrast, the mouse prostate is composed of four paired lobes namely anterior (AP), dorsal (DP), lateral (LP) and ventral (VP) prostate. Since DP and LP share a ductal system they are often dissected together and referred to as the dorsolateral prostate (DLP). The mouse DLP is perceived to be the most similar to the human peripheral zone in which the majority of clinically diagnosed prostate cancers are found. The mouse VP does not appear to have a human homologue and the human transitional zone does not have a murine homologue. The transitional zone constitutes a site where human nodular hyperplasia (BPH) is commonly seen. The mouse AP is analogous to the human central zone, which only infrequently represents a site of neoplasia in humans (Roy-Burman *et al.*, 2004).

10. Cell surface signaling molecules

Signaling interactions between various extracellular growth factors and the corresponding cell surface receptors converge to determine the fate of the cell with respect to proliferation, survival or death. In this context, dysregulation of several growth factors or their receptors has been implicated in prostate tumorigenesis. A number of transgenic mouse lines have been produced in which genes that are known to be overexpressed in human prostate cancer are targets. The survival factor, insulin like growth factor-I (IGF-I) which is generally overexpressed in human prostate and which may potentially be a good tumor marker in prostate cancer was a target in a transgenic line (Woodson et al., 2003). Its expression in the mouse tissues was designed by using the bovine keratin 5 promoter (Di Giovanni et al., 2000). These mice develop squamous papillomas some of which progress to carcinomas of the skin. The increased IGF I levels also lead to pathologic changes in the prostate and in other male accessory glands of these animals (Di Giovanni et al., 2000a).The severity of the lesions in the prostate ranges from PIN to carcinoma in Situ as well as tumors with neuroendocrine differentiation.

11. Fibroblast Growth Factors (FGFs)

The FGF family of heparin binding proteins is intercellular signaling molecules of which atleast 23 different members (FGF-1 - FGF-23) have been identified to date. FGF proteins are generally secreted and their effects are mediated by a complex system of FGF receptor (FGFR) tyrosine kinases, either through autocrine or paracrine mechanisms, or both (Wilkie et al., 1995; McKeehan et al., 1998). While dysregulation of several FGFs has been described in prostate development and tumorigenesis, two members, FGF 7 and FGF 8 have been further pursued through mouse modeling experiments (Djakiew, 2000; Thomson, 2001).

FGF 8b has been demonstrated to possess the most transforming and tumorigenic potential (Daphna-Iken et al., 1998). While expression of FGF 8b appears to represent the primary species in prostatic epithelium, its expression is practically undetected in the stromal component of prostate cancer (Valve et al., 2001). Increased expression of FGF 8b in prostatic lesions beginning from PIN to adenocarcinoma and its persistence in androgen independent disease has been described. The overexpression of FGF8b in prostate cancer cells has been shown to increase proliferative and invasive properties of the affected cells directly and proliferation of prostatic stromal cells indirectly (Song et al., 2000). Consistent with these results antisense down regulation of FGF8b mRNA reduces the growth rate, inhibits cologenic activity and decreases in vivo tumorigenicity of prostate tumor cells (Rudra-Ganguly et al., 1998). FGF 8 expressions in prostate cancer is regulated by the androgen receptor at the transcriptional level and that FGF 8 is angiogenic further enhance the biological relevance of the factor in prostate cancer.

Prostatic hyperplasia appears in the LP and VP in some FGF 8b transgenic animals as early as 2 to 3 months and in DP and AP between 6 to 16 months. LGPIN lesions manifest from 5 to 7 months. 100% of the mice display multifocal prostatic epithelial hyperplasia during the first 14 months with 35% also having areas of LGPIN. In subsequent months (15 to 24 months) the profile changes to a higher incidence of LGPIN (66%) along with HGPIN (51%). Ocassionally HGPIN lesions resemble the histopathology of human prostatic carcinoma *in situ*.

12. P27kip, regulator of cyclin-cdk activity

Activation of AKT through deregulated phosphatidylinositol 3- kinase (PI3K) signaling resulting from genetic inactivation of phosphatase and tensin homolog (PTEN), mutational activation of PI3K, or the activation of upstream oncogenic tyrosine kinases is a frequent molecular event in human cancer (Brugge *et al.*, 2007; Lee *et al.*, 2007). Transgenic expression of activated AKT1 in the murine prostate induces prostatic intraepithelial neoplasia (PIN) that does not progress to invasive prostate cancer. In human epithelial cancers, reduced levels of $p27^{Kip1}$ expression are frequently observed (Slingerland and Pagano, 2000) and are correlated with tumor progression and poor survival (Loda *et al.*, 1997; Porter *et al.*, 1997; Yang *et al.*, 1998). $p27^{Kip1}$ functions primarily as a negative regulator of cyclin-CDK activity and thus likely participates in tumor suppression by inhibiting cell-cycle progression (Chu *et al.*, 2008). Targeted disruption of $p27^{Kip1}$ (Cdkn1b$_{-/-}$) in mice leads to prostatic hyperplasia (Cordon-Cardo *et al.*, 1998) and development of pituitary adenomas (Fero *et al.*, 1996, 1998) as the mice age. However, Cdkn1b$_{-/-}$ mice do not typically develop other spontaneous tumors (Fero *et al.*, 1996; Kiyokawa *et al.*, 1996; Nakayama *et al.*, 1996).

In many human cancer cells, oncogene-induced senescence (OIS) is associated with known tumor suppressor pathways such as p53, VHL, and Rb (Serrano et al., 1997; Young *et al.*, 2008). It has been reported that OIS occurs in many human and mouse precursors of cancer and that this phenomenon can be reversed by the inactivation of tumor suppressor pathways (Braig *et al.*, 2005; Chen *et al.*, 2005; Collado *et al.*, 2005; Michaloglou *et al.*, 2005). Majumder *et al.* investigated the role of $p27^{Kip1}$ in tumor suppression in prostate cancer using both genetically engineered mice and human prostate samples (Majumder *et al.*, 2008). They have identified a relationship among senescence induction, $p27^{Kip1}$ expression, and PIN that supports the notion that $p27^{Kip1}$ induction in the context of early neoplastic lesions may represent a preinvasive checkpoint linked to cellular senescence.

Importantly, is study is highly relevant to human prostate cancer (Majumder *et al.*, 2008). Indeed, we show that $p27^{Kip1}$ is overexpressed in human PIN not associated with invasive cancer, presumably representing the earliest phase of neoplastic transformation. In contrast, PIN adjacent to invasive cancer, where checkpoint loss may have already occurred, is associated with low levels of $p27^{Kip1}$. The role of $p27^{Kip1}$ in this process is further supported by a body of data showing that loss of $p27^{Kip1}$ is commonly found in human cancers (Chu *et al.*, 2008) and that invasive tumor cells specifically degrade $p27^{Kip1}$. This in turn results in increased CDK2 activity (Loda *et al.*, 1997).

As many as 30% of men with a diagnosis of PIN on biopsy are subsequently found to harbor an invasive prostatic adenocarcinoma on repeat biopsy (Gokden *et al.*, 2005). Thus the CDK inhibitors might have utility in preventing cancer progression from *in situ* dysplasia to invasion.

13. Conclusions

High-grade PIN is the most likely precursor of prostatic adenocarcinoma, according to virtually all available evidence. PIN is associated with progressive abnormalities of phenotype and genotype that are intermediate between normal prostatic epithelium and cancer, indicating impairment of cell differentiation and regulatory control with advancing stages of prostatic carcinogenesis. There is progressive loss of some markers of secretory differentiation, whereas other markers show progressive increase. The clinical importance of recognizing PIN is based on its strong association with prostatic carcinoma. PIN has a high predictive value as a marker for adenocarcinoma, and its identification in biopsy specimens of the prostate warrants further search for concurrent invasive carcinoma. Studies to date have not determined whether PIN remains stable, regresses, or progresses, although the implication is that it can progress. Chemoprevention of early stage of prostate cancer, PIN may be useful strategy in the prostate cancer prevention.

14. Acknowledgements

The financial assistance provided by University of Madras as UWPFEP Fellowship to one of the authors Mr. A. Arunkumar and Council of Scientific and Industrial Research (CSIR), India, in the form of CSIR-SRF to Ms. S. Banudevi are gratefully acknowledged.

15. References

Abate Shen C, Shen MM. Molecular genetics of prostate cancer. *Genes Dev.* 2000; 14:2410-2434.

Abrahams NA, Ormsby AH, Brainard J. Validation of cytokeratin 5/6 as an effective substitute for keratin 903 in the differentiation of benign from malignant glands in prostate needle biopsies. *Histopathology* 2002; 41:35–41.

Allam CK, Bostwick DG, Hayes JA, *et al.* Interobserver variability in the diagnosis of high grade prostatic intraepithelial neoplasia and adenocarcinoma. *Mod Pathol.* 1996; 9:742–751.

Al-Maghrabi J, Vorobyova L, Toi A, *et al.* Identification of numerical chromosomal changes detected by interphase fluorescence in situ hybridization in high-grade prostate intraepithelial neoplasia as a predictor of carcinoma. *Arch Pathol Lab Med.* 2002; 126:165–169.

Amin MB, Ro JY, Ayala AG. Ideas in pathology: putative precursor lesions of prostatic adenocarcinoma: fact or fiction? *Mod Pathol.* 1993; 6:476–483.

Amin MB, Schultz DS, Zarbo RJ. Computerized static DNA ploidy analysis of prostatic intraepithelial neoplasia. *Arch Pathol Lab Med.* 1994; 118:260–264.

Aquilina JW, Lipsky JJ, Bostwick DG: Androgen deprivation as a strategy for prostate cancer chemoprevention. *J Natl Cancer Inst.* 1997; 89:689–696.

Armas OA, Melamed A, Aprikian A, *et al.* Effect of preoperative androgen deprivation therapy in prostatic carcinoma [abstract]. *Lab Invest.* 1993; 68:55A.

Arunkumar A, Vijayababu MR, Venkataraman P, Senthilkumar K, Arunakaran J. Chemoprevention of rat prostate carcinogenesis by diallyl disulfide, an organosulfur compound of garlic. *Biol Pharm Bull.* 2006; 29:375−379.

Banudevi S, Elumalai P, Arunkumar R, Senthilkumar K, Gunadharini DN, Sharmila G, Arunakaran J. Chemopreventive effects of zinc on N-methyl-N-nitrosourea and testosterone induced prostatic intraepithelial neoplasia in the dorsolateral prostate of male Sprague-Dawley rats. *J Cancer Res Clin Oncol.* 2011a; 137:677-686.

Banudevi S, Elumalai P, Sharmila G, Arunkumar R, Senthilkumar K, Arunakaran J. Protective effects of zinc on prostate carcinogenesis induced by N-methyl-N-nitrosourea and testosterone in adult male Sprague-Dawley rats. *Exp Biol Med.* 2011b; *in press.*

Bethesda Md. Prostatic intraepithelial neoplasia: significance and correlation with prostate-specific antigen and transrectal ultrasound. Proceedings of a workshop of the

National Prostate Cancer Detection Project; March 13, 1989; Bethesda, Md. *Urol.* 1989; 34:2–69.

Bettuzzi S, Brausi M, Rizzi F, Castagnetti G, Peracchia G, Corti A. Chemoprevention of human prostate cancer by oral administration of greentea catechins in volunteers with high-grade prostate intraepithelial neoplasia: a preliminary report from a one-year proof-of-principle study. *Cancer Res.* 2006; 6:1234–1240.

Bosland MC, Prinsen MK. Induction of dorsolateral prostate adenoma carcinomas and other accessory sex gland lesions in male Wistar rats by N-methyl-N-nitrosourea, 7,12-dimethylbenz(a) anthracene, and 3,2′-dimethyl-4-aminobiphenyl after sequential treatment with cyproterone acetate and testosterone propionate. *Cancer Res.* 1990; 50:691–699.

Bostwick DG, Amin MB, Dundore P, *et al.*: Architectural patterns of high-grade prostatic intraepithelial neoplasia. *Hum Pathol.* 1993; 24:298–310.

Bostwick DG, Amin MB. Prostate and seminal vesicles. In: Damjanov I, Linder J (eds.), Anderson's pathology, 10th edn, Vol. II, Chapter.67. St. Louis: Mosby, 1996, 2166-230.

Bostwick DG, Brawer MK. Prostatic intra-epithelial neoplasia and early invasion in prostate cancer. *Cancer* 1987; 59:788–794.

Bostwick DG, Burke HB, Wheeler TM, *et al.*: The most promising surrogate endpoint biomarkers for screening candidate chemopreventive compounds for prostatic adenocarcinoma in short-term phase II clinical trials. *J Cell Biochem.* 1994b; 19 (suppl):283–289.

Bostwick DG, Dousa M, Crawford, *et al.* Neuroendocrine differentiation in prostatic intraepithelial neoplasia and adenocarcinoma. *Am J Surg Pathol.* 1994a; 18:1240-1246.

Bostwick DG, Qian J, Frankel K. The incidence of high-grade prostatic intraepithelial neoplasia in needle biopsies. *J Urol.* 1995; 154:1791–1794.

Bostwick DG, Qian J. High-grade prostatic intraepithelial neoplasia. *Mod Pathol.* 2004; 17(3):360–379.

Bostwick DG. Phase II efficacy trials for chemoprevention in patients with PIN: strategies with androgen deprivation therapy. In: Crawford ED (ed.), Proceedings of 7th International Prostate Cancer Update. Beaver Creek, Colorado, 22-26 January 1997.Pp 485-490.

Bostwick DG. Prospective origins of prostate carcinoma. Prostatic intraepithelial neoplasia and atypical adenomatus hyperplasia. *Cancer* 1996; 78:330.

Bostwick DG. Prostatic intraepithelial Neoplasia (PIN). *Urol.* 1989; 34:16-22.

Bostwick DG. Target populations and strategies for chemoprevention trials of prostate cancer. *J Cell Biochem.* 1994; 19(suppl): 191-196.

Braig M, Lee S, Loddenkemper C, Rudolph C, Peters AH, SchlegelbergerB, Stein H, Dorken B, Jenuwein T, Schmitt CA. Oncogene- induced senescence as an initial barrier in lymphoma development. *Nature* 2005; 436:660–665

Brawer MK, Peehl DM, Stamey TA, Bostwick DG. Keratin immunoreactivity in the benign and neoplastic human prostate. *Cancer Res.* 1985; 45:3663– 3667.

Brawer MK. Prostatic intraepithelial neoplasia: an overview. *Rev Urol.* 2005; 7(suppl 3):S11–S18.

Brugge J, Hung MC, Mills GB. A new mutational AKT activation in the PI3K pathway. *Cancer Cell* 2007; 12:104–107.

Bubendorf L, Tapia C, Gasser TC, *et al.* Ki67 labeling index in core needle biopsies independently predicts tumor-specific survival in prostate cancer. *Hum Pathol.*1998; 29:949–54.

Chen Z, Trotman LC, Shaffer D, Lin HK, Dotan ZA, Niki M, Koutcher JA, Scher HI, Ludwig T, Gerald W, *et al.* Crucial role of p53-dependent cellular senescence in suppression of Pten-deficient tumorigenesis. *Nature* 2005; 436:725–730.

Choan E, Segal R, Jonker D, Malone S, Reaume N, Eapen L, Gallant V.2005. A prospective clinical trial of green tea for hormone refractory prostatecancer: an evaluation of the complementary/alternative therapy approach.*Urol Oncol.* 2005; 23:108–113.

Christov KT, Moon RC, Lantvit DD, Boone CW, Steele VE, Lubet RA, Kelloff GJ, Pezzuto JM. *Cancer Res.* 2002; 62:5178-5182.

Chu IM, Hengst L, Slingerland JM. The Cdk inhibitor p27 in human cancer: prognostic potential and relevance to anticancer therapy. *Nat Rev Cancer* 2008; 8:253–267.

Collado M, Gil J, Efeyan A, Guerra C, Schuhmacher AJ, Barradas M, Benguria A, Zaballos A, Flores JM, Barbacid, M, *et al.* Tumour biology: senescence in premalignant tumours. *Nature* 2005: 436: 642.

Cordon-Cardo C, Koff A, Drobnjak M, Capodieci P, Osman I, Millard SS, Gaudin PB, Fazzari M, Zhang ZF, Massague J, Scher HI. Distinct altered patterns of p27KIP1 gene expression in benign prostatic hyperplasia and prostatic carcinoma. *J Natl Cancer Inst.* 1998; 90:1284–1291.

Daphna-Iken D, Shankar DB, Lawshe A, Ornitz DM, Shackleford GM, MacArthur CA. FGF-8 isoforms differ in NIH3T3 cell transforming potential. *Cell Growth Differ.* 1998; 6:817-825.

De La Torre M, Haggman M, Brandstedt S, Busch C. Prostatic intraepithelial neoplasia and invasive carcinoma in total prostatectomy speciemens: distribution, volumes and DNA ploidy. *Br J Urol.* 1993; 72:207.

Deschenes J, Weidner N. Nucleolar organizer regions (NOR) in hyperplastic and neoplastic prostate disease. *Am J Surg Pathol.* 1990; 14:1148–1155.

Di Giovanni J, Boe DK, Wilker E *et al.* Constitutive expression of insulin like growth factor 1 in epidermal basal cells of transgenic mice leads to spontaneous tumor promotion. *Cancer Res.* 2000a; 63:3991-3994.

Di Giovanni J, Kiguchi K, Frijhoft A *et al.* Deregulated expression of IGF I in prostate epithelium leads to neoplasia in transgenic mice. *Cancer Res.* 2000b; 60:1561-1570.

Di Sant' Agnese PA. Neuroendocrine differentiation in the precursor of prostate cancer. *Eur Urol.* 1996; 30: 185-190.

Djakiew D. Dysregulated expression of growth factors and their receptors in the development of prostate cancer. *Prostate* 2000; 42: 150-160.

Drago JR, Mostofi FK, Lee F. Introductory remarks and workshop summary. *Urol.* 1989; 34:2–3.

Emmert-Buck MR,Vocke CD, Pozzatt RO, et al. Allelic loss of chromosome 8p12-21 in microdissected prostatic intraepithelial neoplasia. *Cancer Res.* 1995; 55:2959–2962.

Epstein JI. Adenosis (atypical adenomatous hyperplasia): histopathology and relationship to carcinoma. *Path Res Pathol.* 1994; 191:888.

Eschenbach AC. The biologic dilemma of early carcinoma of the prostate. *Cancer* 1996; 78: 326.

Ferguson J, Zincke H, Ellison E, *et al.* Decrease of prostatic intraepithelial neoplasia (PIN) following androgen deprivation therapy in patients with stage T3 carcinoma treated by radical prostatectomy. *Urol.* 1994; 44:91-95.

Fero ML, Randel E, Gurley KE, Roberts JM, Kemp CJ. The murine gene p27Kip1 is haplo-insufficient for tumour suppression. *Nature* 1998; 396:177–180.

Fero ML, Rivkin M, Tasch M, Porter P, Carow CE, Firpo E, Polyak K, Tsai LH, Broudy V, Perlmutter RM, *et al.* A syndrome of multiorgan hyperplasia with features of gigantism, tumorigenesis, and female sterility in p27(Kip1)-deficient mice. Cell 1996; 85: 733–744.

Gao A, Isaccs JT. The molecular basis of prostate carcinogenesis. In: Coleman WB, Tsongalis GJ (eds.), Molecular basis of human cancer, The Humana Press. Inc., Totowa NJ, 2000. Pp 365-379.

Garabedian EM, Humphrey PA, Gordon JI. A transgenic mouse model of metastatic prostate cancer originating from neuroendocrine cells. *Proc Natl Acad Sci USA* 1998; 95:15382–15387.

Gaudin PB, Sesterhenn IA, Wojno K, Mostofi FK, Epstein JI. Incidence and clinical significance of high grade prostatic intraepithelial neoplasia in TURP specimens. *Urol.* 1997; 49:558–563.

Gokden N, Roehl KA, Catalona WJ, Humphrey PA. Highgrade prostatic intraepithelial neoplasia in needle biopsy as risk factor for detection of adenocarcinoma: current level of risk in screening population. *Urol.* 2005; 65:538–542.

Hussain T, Gupta S, Mukhtar H. Cyclooxygenase-2 and prostate carcinogenesis. *Cancer Lett.* 2003; 191:125–135.

Ingles SA, Ross RK, Yu MC, *et al.* Association of prostate cancer risk with genetic polymorphisms in vitamin D receptor and androgen receptor. *J Natl Cancer Inst.* 1997; 89:166-170.

Isaacs W, De Marzo A, Nelson WG. Focus on prostate cancer. *Cancer Cell* 2002; 2:113-116.

Jatoi A, Ellison N, Burch PA, Sloan JA, Dakhil SR, Novotny P, TanW, Fitch TR, Rowland KM, Young CY, Flynn PJ. A phase IItrial of green tea in the treatment of patients with androgen independent metastatic prostate carcinoma. *Cancer* 2003; 97:1442–1446.

Jemal A, Siegel R, Ward E, Murray T, Xu J, Thun, MJ. Cancer statistics, 2010. CA. *Cancer J Clin.* 2010; 57:43-66.

Jian L, Xie LP, Lee AH, Binns CW. Protective effect of green tea against prostate cancer: a case-control study in southeast China. *Int J Cancer* 2004; 108:130–135.

Jones EC, Young RH. The differential diagnosis of prostatic carcinoma. Its distinction from premalignant and pseudocarcinomatous lesions of the prostate gland. *Am J Clin Pathol.* 1994; 101:148.

Kadomatsu K, Anzano MA, Slayter MV, *et al.* Expression of sulfated glycoprotein 2 is associated with carcinogenesis induced by N-nitroso-M-methylurea in rat prostate and seminal vesicle. *Cancer Res.* 1993; 53:1480-1483.

Kasper S, Sheppard PC, Yan Y, *et al.*: Development, preogression, and androgen-dependence of prostate tumors in probasin-large T antigen transgenic mice: A model for prostate cancer. *Lab Invest.* 1998; 78:319–333.

Kellof GJ. Chemoprevention strategies for prostate cancer. In: Crawford ED, (ed.), Proceedings of 7th International Prostate Cancer Update. Beaver Creek, Colorado, 22-26 January 1997.Pp 134-135.

Kelloff GJ, Hawk ET, Crowell JA, *et al.* Strategies for identification and clinical evaluation of promising chemoprevention agents. *Oncology* 1996; 10:1471-1481.

Kiyokawa H, Kineman RD, Manova-Todorova KO, Soares VC, Hoffman ES, Ono M, Khanam D, Hayday AC, Frohman LA, Koff A. Enhanced growth of mice lacking the cyclin-dependent kinase inhibitor function of p27(Kip1). *Cell* 1996; 85:721–732.

Langer JE, Rovner ES, Coleman BG, *et al.*: Strategy for repeat biopsy of patients with prostatic intraepithelial neoplasia detected by prostate needle biopsy. *J Urol.* 1996; 155:228–231.

Lee JY, Engelman JA, Cantley LC.Biochemistry. PI3K charges ahead. *Science* 2007; 317:206–207.

Lipski B, Garcia R, Brawer M. Prostatic intraepithelial neoplasia: significance and management. *Semin Urol Oncol.* 1996; 14:149–155.

Loda M, Cukor B, Tam SW, Lavin P, Fiorentino M, Draetta GF, Jessup JM, Pagano M. Increased proteasome-dependent degradation of the cyclin-dependent kinase inhibitor p27 in aggressive colorectal carcinomas. *Nat Med.*1997; 3:231–234.

Macoska JA, Trybus TM, Benson PD, et al. Evidence for three tumor suppressor gene loci on chromosome 8p in human prostate cancer. *Cancer Res.* 1995; 55:5390–5395.

Majumder PK, Grisanzio C, O'Connell F, Barry M, Brito JM, Xu Q, Guney I, *et al.* A Prostatic Intraepithelial Neoplasia-Dependent p27Kip1 Checkpoint Induces Senescence and Inhibits Cell Proliferation and Cancer Progression. *Cancer Cell 2008;* 14:146–155.

Mashall JR. Larry Clark's Legacy: Randomized, controlled, selenium-based, prostate cancer chemopreventiontrials. *Nutr Cancer* 2001; 40:74–77.

Mc Keehan WL, Wang F, Kan M. The heparin sulfate- fibroblast growth factor family: diversity of structure. *Prog Nucleic Acid Res Mol Biol.* 1998; 59 135-176.

McCormick DL. Chemoprevention of hormone-dependent prostate cancer in the Wistar-Unilever rat. In: Schulman C, Kelloff G (eds.), Proceedings of the International Symposium "Strategies for the chemoprevention of prostate cancer". Brussels, 30-31 October 1998. Pp 38.

McNeal JE, Alroy J, Leav I, Redwine EA, Freiha FS, Stamey TA. Immunohistochemical evidence for impaired cell differentiation in the premalignant phase of prostate carcinogenesis. *Am J Clin Pathol.* 1988b;90:23–32.

McNeal JE, Bostwick DG. Intraductal dysplasia: a premalignant lesion of the prostate. *Hum Pathol.* 1986; 17:64–71.

McNeal JE, Leav I, Alroy J. Differential lectin staining of central and peripheral zones of the prostate and alterations in dysplasia. *Am J Clin Pathol.* 1988a; 89:41–48.

McNeal JE. Morphogenesis of prostate carcinoma. *Cancer* 1965; 18:1659–66.

McNeal JE. Origin and development of carcinoma in the prostate. *Cancer.* 1969; 23:24–34.

McNeal JE. Significance of duct-acinar dysplasia in prostatic carcinogenesis. *Prostate* 1988; 13:91–102.

Melissari M, Lopez-Beltran A, Mazzucchelli R, Froio E, Bostwick DG, Montironi R. High grade prostatic intraepithelial neoplasia with squamous differentiation. *J Clin Pathol.* 2006; 59:437–439.

Messing EM, Love RR, Tutsch KD, Verma AK, Douglas J, Pomplun M, Simsiman R, Wilding G. Low-dose difluoromethylornithine and polyamine levels in human prostate tissue. *J Natl Cancer Inst.* 1999; 91:1416–1417.

Michaloglou C, Vredeveld LC, Soengas MS, Denoyelle C, Kuilman T,van der Horst CM, Majoor DM, Shay JW, Mooi WJ, Peeper DS. BRAFE600-associated senescence-like cell cycle arrest of human naevi. *Nature* 2005; 436:720–724.

Montironi R, Diamanti L, Thompson D, *et al.* Analysis of the capillary architecture in the precursors of prostate cancer: recent findings and new concepts. *Eur Urol.* 1996; 30:191-200.

Montironi R, Galluzzi CM, Scarpelli M, *et al.* Quantitative characterization of the frequency and location of cell proliferation and death in prostate pathology. *J Cell Biochem.* 1994; 19(suppl):238-45.

Morote J, Fernandez S, Alan L, Iglesias C, Planas J, Reventos J, Cajal SR, Paciucci R, and de Torres IM. PTOV1 Expression Predicts Prostate Cancer in Men with Isolated High-Grade Prostatic Intraepithelial Neoplasia in Needle Biopsy. *Clin Cancer Res.* 2008; 14: 2617-2622.

Nagle RB, Brawer MK, Kittelson J. Phenotypic relationships of prostatic intraepithelial neoplasia to invasive prostatic carcinoma. *Am J Pathol.* 1991; 138: 119–128.

Nakayama K, Ishida N, Shirane M, Inomata A, Inoue T, Shishido N, Horii I, Loh DY. Mice lacking p27(Kip1) display increased body size, multiple organ hyperplasia, retinal dysplasia, and pituitary tumors. *Cell* 1996; 85:707–720.

Nelson PS, Gleason TP, Brawer MK. Chemoprevention for prostatic intraepithelial neoplasia. *Eur Urol.* 1996; 30:269- 278.

Pacelli A, Bostwick DG. Clinical significance of high-grade prostatic intraepithelial neoplasia in transurethral resection specimens. *Urol.* 1997; 50:355–359.

Perlman EJ, Epstein JI. Blood group antigen expression in dysplasia and adenocarcinoma of the prostate. *Am J Surg Pathol.* 1990; 14:810–818.

Pollard M. The Lobund-Wistar rat model of prostate cancer. *J Cell Biochem.* 1992; 16(suppl):84-88.

Porter PL, Malone KE, Heagerty PJ, Alexander GM, Gatti LA, Firpo EJ, Daling JR, Roberts JM.. Expression of cell-cycle regulators p27Kip1 and cyclin E, alone and in combination, correlate with survival in young breast cancer patients. *Nat Med.* 1997; 3:222–225.

Price D, Stein B, Sieber P, Tutrone R, Bailen J, Goluboff E, Burzon D,Bostwick D, Steiner M. Toremifene for the prevention of prostate cancer in men with high grade prostatic intraepithelial neoplasia: results of a double-blind, placebo controlled, phase IIB clinical trial. *J Urol.* 2006; 176:965–970.

Qian J, Jenkins RB, Bostwick DG. Genetic and chromosomal alterations in prostatic intraepithelial neoplasia and carcinoma detected by fluorescence in situ hybridization. *Eur Urol.* 1999; 35:479–483.

Qian J, Wollan P, Bostwick DG. The extent and multicentricity of high grade prostatic intraepithelial neoplasia in clinically localized prostatic adenocarcinoma. *Hum Pathol.* 1997; 28:143–148.

Roy-Burman P, Wu H, Powell WC, Hagenkord J, Cohen MB. Genetically7 defined mouse models that mimic natural aspects of human prostate cancer development. *Endocrine Relat Cancer* 2004; 11:225-254.

Rudra-Garsguly N, Zheng J, Hoang AT, Roy-Burman P. Down regulation of human FGF 8 activity by antisense constructs in murine fibroblastic and human prostatic carcinoma cell systems. *Oncogene* 1998; 16:1487-1492.

Sakr WA, Haas GP, Cassin BF, Pontes JE, Crissman JD. The frequency of carcinoma and intraepithelial neoplasia of the prostate in young male patients. *Br J Urol.* 1993; 150:379.

Senthilkumar K, Arunkumar A, Sridevi N, Vijayababu MR, Kanagaraj P, Venkataraman P, Aruldhas MM, Srinivasan N, Arunakaran J. Chemoprevention of MNU and testosterone induced prostate carcinogenesis by calcitriol (vitamin D_3) in adult male albino wistar rats. *Ann Cancer Res Therap.* 2006; 14:12–18

Serrano M, Lin AW, McCurrach ME, Beach D, Lowe SW. Oncogenic ras provokes premature cell senescence associated with accumulation of p53 and p16INK4a. *Cell* 1997; 88:593–602.

Sesterhenn IA, Becker RL, Avallone FA. Image analysis of nucleoli and nucleolar organizer regions in prostatic hyperplasia, intraepithelial neoplasia, and prostatic carcinoma. *J Urogenital Pathol.* 1991; 1:61–74.

Shirai T, Yamamoto A, Iwasaki S, *et al.* Induction of invasive carcinomas of the seminal vesicles and coagulating glands of F344 rats by administration of N-methylnitrosourea or N-nitroso-bis (2-oxypropyl) amine and followed by testosterone propionate with or without high-fat diet. *Carcinogenesis* 1991;12:2169-2173.

Simoneau AR, Gerner EW, Phung M, McLaren CE, Meyskens Jr. FL. Alpha difluoromethylornithine and polyamine levels in the human prostate: results of a phase IIa trial. *J Natl Cancer Inst.* 2001; 93:57–59.

Skjorten FJ, Berner A, Harvei S, *et al.*: Prostatic intraepithelial neoplasia in surgical resections. Relationship to coexistent adenocarcinoma and atypical adenomatous hyperplasia of the prostate. *Cancer* 1997; 79:1172–1179.

Slayter MV, Anzano MA, Kadomatzu K, *et al.* Histogenesis of induced prostate and seminal vesicle carcinoma in Lobund-Wistar rats: a system for histological scoring and grading. *Cancer Res.* 1994; 54:1440-1445.

Slingerland J, Pagano M. Regulation of the cdk inhibitor p27 and its deregulation in cancer. *J Cell Physiol.* 2000; 183:10–17.

Song Z, Powell WC, Kasahara N, van Bokhoven A, Miller GJ, Roy-Burman P. The effect of fibroblast growth factor 8, isoform b, on the biology of prostate carcinoma cells and their interaction with stromal cells. ***Cancer*** *Res.* 200; 60: 6730-6736.

Steiner MS, Pound CR. Phase IIA clinical trial to test the efficacy and safety of toremifene in men with high-grade prostatic intraepithelial neoplasia. *Clin Prostate Cancer* 2003; 2:24–31.

Syed DN, Suh Y, Afaq F, Mukhtar H. Dietary agents for chemoprevention of prostate cancer. Cancer Lett 2008; 265:167–76.

Taplin ME, Balk SP. Androgen receptor: a key molecule in the progression of prostate cancer to hormone independence. *J Cell Biochem.* 2004; 91:483-490.

Thomson AA. Role of androgens and fibroblast growth factors in prostatic development. *Reproduction* 2001; 121:187-195.

Trottier G, Bostrom PJ, Lawrentschuk N, Fleshner NE. Nutraceuticals and prostate cancer prevention: a current review. *Nat Rev Urol.* 2010; 7:21–30.

Trottier G, Lawrentschuk N, Fleshner NE. Prevention strategies in prostate cancer. *Current Oncol.* 2010; 17 (Suppl 2):S4-10.

Valve EM, Nevalainenen MT, Nurmi MJ, Laato MK, MArtikainen PM, Harkonen PL. Increased expression of FGF-8 isoforms and FGF receptors in human premalignant prostatic intraepithelial neoplasia lesions and prostate cancer. *Lab Invest.* 2001; 81:815-826.

Vis AN, Van der Kwast TH. Prostatic intraepithelial neoplasia and putative precursor lesions of prostate cancer: a clinical perspective. *BJU Int.* 2001; 88:147–157.

Weinberg DS, Weidner N. Concordance of DNA content between prostatic intraepithelial neoplasia and concomitant invasive carcinoma: evidence that prostatic intraepithelial neoplasia is a precursor of invasive prostatic carcinoma. *Arch Pathol Lab Med.* 1993; 117:1132–1137.

Wilke AO, Morriss-Kay GM, Jones EY, Health JK. Functions of fibroblast growth factors and their receptors. *Curr Biol.* 1995; 5: 5000-5007.

Wills ML, Hamper UM, Partin AW, *et al.*: Incidence of highgrade prostatic intraepithelial neoplasia in sextant needle biopsy specimens. *Urol.* 1997; 49:367–373.

Woodson K, Tangrea JA, Pollak M *et al.* Models of metastatic prostate cancer: a transgenic perspective. *Prostate Cancer Prostatic Dis.* 2003; 6:204-211.

Wu CL, Yang XJ, Tretiakova M, et al. Analysis of alpha-methylacyl-CoA racemase (P504S) expression in high-grade prostatic intraepithelial neoplasia. *Hum Pathol.* 2004; 35:1008–1101.

Yang RM, Naitoh J, Murphy M, Wang HJ, Phillipson J, deKernion JB, Loda M, Reiter RE. Low p27 expression predicts poor diseasefree survival in patients with prostate cancer. *J Urol.* 1998; 159:941–945.

Young AP, Schlisio S, Minamishima YA, Zhang Q, Li L, Grisanzio C, Signoretti S, Kaelin WG. VHL loss actuates a HIF-independent senescence programme mediated by Rb and p400. *Nat Cell Biol.* 2008; 10:361–369.

Zanardi S, Puntoni M, Maffezzini M, Bandelloni R, Mori M, Argusti A, Campodonico F, Turbino L, Branchi D, Montironi R Decensi A. Phase I-II Trial of Weekly

Bicalutamide in Men with Elevated Prostate-Specific Antigen and Negative Prostate Biopsies. *Cancer Prev Res.* 2009; 2:377.

Zhou M, Shah R, Shen R, Rubin MA. Basal cell cocktail (34betaE12 _ p63) improves the detection of prostate basal cells. *Am J Surg Pathol.* 2003; 27: 365–371.

Zlotta A, Schulman C. Clinical evolution of prostatic intraepithelial neoplasia. *Eur Urol.* 1999; 35:498–503.

Part 5

Intraepithelial Neoplasia of Uterus

9

Endometrial Intraepithelial Neoplasia

Nisreen Abushahin[1,4], Shuje Pang[1,2], Jie Li[1,3],
Oluwole Fadare[5] and Wenxin Zheng[1,6,7]
[1]*Department of Pathology, University of Arizona College of Medicine, Tucson, AZ,*
[2]*Department of Pathology, Tianjin Central Hospital of Obstetrics and Gynecology, Tianjin,*
[3]*Department of Obstetrics and Gynecology, Qilu Hospital,*
Shandong University, Jinan, Shandong,
[4]*Department of Pathology, Jordan University Hospital- University of Jordan, Amman,*
[5]*Department of Pathology, Vanderbilt University School of Medicine, Nashville, TN*
[6]*Department of Obstetrics and Gynecology, University of Arizona, Tucson, AZ*
[7]*Arizona Cancer Center, University of Arizona, Tucson, AZ,*
[1,5,6,7]*USA*
[2,3]*China*
[4]*Jordan*

1. Introduction

Endometrial cancers are the most common malignancies of the female genital tract in the United States, with 42,160 new cases diagnosed and 7780 cancer-associated deaths in 2009 (Jemal, Siegel et al. 2009). The histopathological classifications of endometrial cancers are numerous, but in 1983, two broad clinico-pathologic categories of endometrial carcinomas were delineated (Bokhman 1983). This conceptual classification has largely been based on light microscopic appearance, clinical behavior and epidemiology, and had been subsequently supported by molecular-cytogenetic data, which has facilitated the acceptance of the so-called *dualistic model* of endometrial carcinogenesis(Deligdisch and Holinka 1987; Lax and Kurman 1997; Sherman 2000; Matias-Guiu, Catasus et al. 2001; Lax 2004; Liu 2007), a modified and more comprehensive comparison of both types is illustrated in Table 1.

According to that model, the first and the most common type of endometrial carcinoma is called *Type I endometrial cancer*. These Type I cancers, of which the pathologic prototype is endometrioid carcinoma, represent at least 80% of newly diagnosed cases of endometrial cancer. The much less common mucinous carcinomas are also generally classified as a Type I cancer. Overall, they occur in comparatively younger age group (40-50 years)(Deligdisch and Holinka 1987; Lax and Kurman 1997; Sherman 2000; Matias-Guiu, Catasus et al. 2001; Lax 2004; Liu 2007). The tumor cells frequently express estrogen and progesterone receptors (Demopoulos, Mesia et al. 1999; Lax 2004), and their evolution appears to be driven by unopposed estrogen stimulation from either endogenous (e.g. ovarian estrogen-producing tumors) and/or exogenous sources (e.g. hormonal therapy)(Ettinger, Golditch et al. 1988; Potischman, Hoover et al. 1996; Demopoulos, Mesia et al. 1999). These tumors, therefore, mostly arise in a background of endometrial glandular hyperplasia(Lax 2004; Liu 2007). *Type*

I endometrial cancers have a relatively favorable prognostic profile compared to *type II endometrial cancer* (Creasman, Odicino et al. 2003). Several kinds of genetic alterations had been detected in *Type 1 endometrial cancers*, including PTEN inactivation(Tashiro, Blazes et al. 1997; Mutter, Ince et al. 2001), beta-catenin (CTNNB1) mutations (Konopka, Janiec-Jankowska et al. 2007), and to a lesser degree, microsatellite instability (related to inactivation of the MLH1 gene) (Esteller, Levine et al. 1998), and activational mutations of the K-ras gene (Velasco, Bussaglia et al. 2006).

Parameters	**Type I**	**Type II**
Incidence	80%	15%
Peak Age	50-60	60-70
Obesity	Common	Uncommon
Estrogen stimuli	Common	Uncommon
Precancer	EIN (classic)	EmGD (serous type & clear cell type)
Latent Precancer	PTEN null glands	P53 signature glands
Progression	Slow	Rapid
Histology	Endometrioid, mucinous	Serous, Clear cell, and Carcinosarcoma
Genetic changes	PTEN, MSI	p53, BRCA, 1pDel
Familial	HNPCC	Unknown
Prognosis	Good	Poor

Table 1. Dualistic model of endometrial cancer as modified by Zheng et al (Zheng, Xiang et al. 2011).

Type II endometrial cancer in the dualistic model are significantly less common than their Type I counterparts, and represent only10- 15% of cases. The pathologic prototype of this category is the endometrial serous carcinoma (ESC) [previously termed uterine papillary serous carcinoma (UPSC)]. *Type II endometrial cancer* typically occurs in an older age group (60-70 years) (Lax and Kurman 1997; Sherman 2000; Matias-Guiu, Catasus et al. 2001). They frequently arise in a background of inactive or resting endometrium(Lax and Kurman 1997; Sherman 2000; Matias-Guiu, Catasus et al. 2001), display a low frequency of expression of hormonal receptors, are not associated with the estrogen-associated clinical factors (such as obesity)and generally are not thought to be directly influenced by hormones (Sasano, Comerford et al. 1990; Lax, Pizer et al. 1998; Demopoulos, Mesia et al. 1999; Lax 2004; Shang 2006). Definitive risk factors for *type II endometrial cancer* are still unclear, however. In one recent study, we found that women 55 years of age or under with a personal history of breast cancer, had an increased risk of ESC as compared with controls (Liang, Pearl et al. 2010), and an earlier study by Chan et al came to comparable conclusions 2006 (Chan, Manuel et al. 2006). These Type II cancers, most notably ESC, also exhibit frequent mutation and overexpression of the p53 (Sherman, Bur et al. 1995; Nordstrom, Strang et al. 1996) and HER2/neu (Rolitsky, Theil et al. 1999) genes and proteins, respectively. They also show alterations of intercellular adhesion molecules like E-cadherin (Holcomb, Delatorre et al.

2002; Mell, Meyer et al. 2004) and claudin(Santin, Bellone et al. 2007; Konecny, Agarwal et al. 2008), and display over-expression of p16 (Chiesa-Vottero, Malpica et al. 2007; Yemelyanova, Ji et al. 2009) and IMP-3(Reid-Nicholson, Iyengar et al. 2006; Zheng, Yi et al. 2008). Overall, *type II endometrial cancer* have a relatively poor prognosis independent of other factors, and a higher mortality rate in comparison to type I cancers(Lauchlan 1981; Eifel, Ross et al. 1983; Sherman, Bitterman et al. 1992). This dualistic model has provided a valuable academic framework for the subsequent studies of myriad aspects of endometrial carcinogenesis and progression and a conceptual basis for the differential deployment of histotype-specific treatment modalities.

1.1 Endometrial Intraepithelial neoplastic lesions: The nomenclature dilemma

Endometrial cancers, especially *type II endometrial cancer*, are a significant cause of morbidity and mortality in women (Jemal, Siegel et al. 2009). This has prompted the long-standing search for optimal approaches for their prevention; one aspect of prevention is the early recognition of occult *precursor lesions* or *precancers* (Berman, Albores-Saavedra et al. 2006), along with the administration of therapeutic interventions prior to the development of overt malignancy. To establish any lesion as a precursor lesion or a precancer to one neoplasm, the putative lesion should meet some basic criteria that defines a precancer, as recognized by participants at a consensus conference on the subject sponsored by the National Cancer Institute in 2006 (Berman, Albores-Saavedra et al. 2006). This definition modifies and generalizes a definition initially proposed for endometrial intraepithelial neoplasia (Mutter 2000; Mutter, Baak et al. 2000; Mutter, Ince et al. 2001; Mutter 2002; Hecht and Mutter 2006; Mutter, Zaino et al. 2007) . The following five defining criteria must all be met: "(1) Evidence exists that the precancer is associated with an increased risk of cancer. (2) When a precancer progresses to cancer, the resulting cancer arises from cells within the precancer. (3) A precancer is different from the normal tissue from which it arises. (4) A precancer is different from the cancer into which it develops, although it has some, but not all, of the molecular and phenotypic properties that characterize the cancer. (5) There is a method by which the precancer can be diagnosed". In the last two decades, there have been significant advances made in the study of the precursors of *Type I endometrial cancer*, and this precancerous lesion is currently considered as endometrial atypical hyperplasia in the WHO classification system (that is still the most frequently used by pathologists) and the "endometrial intraepithelial neoplasia (EIN)" system that was originally proposed by Mutter et al (Mutter 2000; Mutter, Baak et al. 2000; Mutter, Ince et al. 2001; Mutter 2002; Hecht and Mutter 2006; Mutter, Zaino et al. 2007). On the other hand, studies of *Type II endometrial cancer* precursors have been relatively limited. The prototype of *Type II endometrial cancer, which is* ESC, usually arises in a background of atrophic or resting endometrium. This is in contrast to *Type I endometrial cancer*, which generally have a hyperplastic (or at least non-atrophic) background and show a strong relation to high estrogen levels. For this and a variety of other reasons, the precancers of *type I endometrial cancer* are highly unlikely to constitute the precancer lesions for *Type II endometrial cancer*. Numerous lines of evidence developed during the last decade point toward a newly recognized lesion called "endometrial glandular dysplasia (EmGD)" as the actual precursor of Type II cancers, including serous and clear cell types (Zheng, Liang et al. 2004). These lines of evidence include pathologic, genetic as well as clinical factors. Accordingly, the precancer of *type I endometrial cancer* and *type II endometrial cancer* are two distinct entities at the morphologic and molecular levels and are not related to each other. In this chapter, we explore the current state of knowledge on all types of precancerous lesions of the endometrium, based on our interpretation and modification of the dualistic model of endometrial carcinogenesis. Clinical and pathological experience in endometrial carcinogenesis had shown a significant impact of histologic subtype (endometrioid, serous, clear cell etc) on overall prognosis and survival. Considering the multiple conflicting nomenclatures that existed in studies of endometrial carcinogenesis, which lead to the inappropriate inclusion of some entities as 'precancers' (as discussed in following sections),we plan to propose a unified terminology and classification scheme for the precancerous lesions in the endometrium, which will be biology-based and clinically oriented for better patient care. Accordingly, the discussion of intraepithelial neoplastic lesions of the endometrium would embrace the precancer of *type I endometrial cancer*, which we will refer to as endometrioid EIN; as well as the precancers of *type II endometrial cancer*, that is, serous EmGD and clear cell EmGD, which will be referred to as serous EIN and clear cell EIN respectively. As summarized in Figure 1.

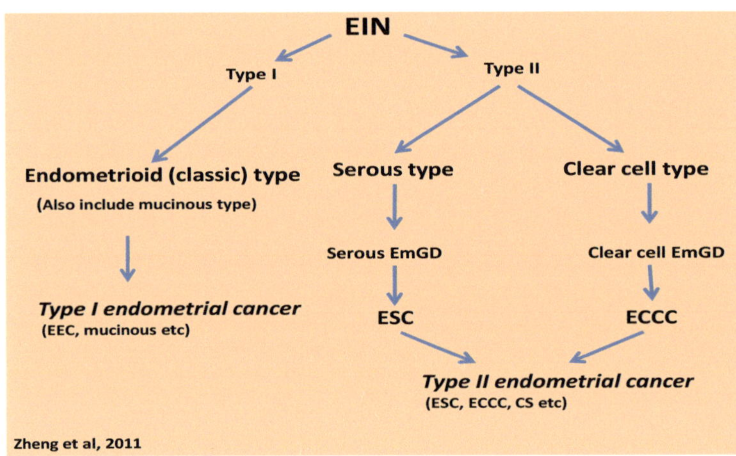

Fig. 1. A proposed unified model of endometrial carcinogenesis. Endometrial intraepithelial neoplasia (EIN) encompass a broad spectrum of morphologically and biologically distinct entities, categorized as type I, referring to the classic EIN lesion described by Mutter, and type II that include serous EmGD and clear cell EmGD as precancers of type II endometrial cancer.

2. Precancers of type I endometrial cancers

2.1 Historical backgrounds

In the past, *Type I endometrial cancer* was thought to be preceded by pan-endometrial hormonally induced changes referred to as endometrial hyperplasia. The term endometrial hyperplasia encompasses a broad spectrum of polyclonal proliferations that result from a physiological response of the endometrium to an abnormal estrogenic stimulus. The magnitude of such proliferations, reflects the quantity and duration of unopposed estrogen exposure (Trial 1996; Mutter, Zaino et al. 2007), resulting in architecturally variable glands covering a surface area that is equal or exceeds that of the stroma (i.e. gland-stroma ratio more than 1:1). The most widely observed histological features include irregular architectural remodeling of endometrial glands in functionalis layer, vascular thrombi, and stromal breakdown. A critical feature of benign hyperplasia is that no significant cytological changes are seen between the hyperplastic glands and the surrounding glands (Mutter, Zaino et al. 2007). Benign endometrial hyperplasia is most frequent around the time of the menopause, due to alterations of the normal cycle of sequentially regulated estrogen and progesterone. It may also occur following anovulatory cycles for the same reason. The most common symptoms of hyperplasia are prolonged or excessive bleeding at intervals that are initially longer than normal. Microinfarcts and estrogen withdrawal are responsible for symptomatic bleeding (Song, Rutherford et al. 2002; Ferenczy 2003). Other patients may complain of intermittent spotting, commonly attributed to patchy stromal breakdown secondary to estrogen-induced microthrombi. A rapid decline in the prolonged estrogen stimulation causes massive apoptosis of the endometrial glands and stroma resulting in heavy shedding. Occasionally, the decrease in estrogen levels is sufficiently gradual that generalized apoptosis and shedding fail to take place as regular menstruation.

The World Health Organization (WHO) 1994 classification system subdivided endometrial hyperplasia according to architectural complexity and cytological atypia into 4 subgroups: simple, simple hyperplasia without atypia, complex, and atypical complex hyperplasia (Scully RE 1994), as illustrated in Figure 2. The WHO 1994 endometrial hyperplasia schema confines most precancers of *type I endometrial cancer* in the atypical hyperplasia subgroup, but in the opinion of many pathologists and investigators, there are several problems associated with this classification. First, this classification system is poorly reproducible among pathologists (Hunter, Tritz et al. 1994; Skov, Broholm et al. 1997; Zaino 2000). Second, this system is missing diagnostic elements that have only become clear in recent years. Of these elements, the localizing topographic distribution of a clonally expanding precancer and the need to establish size thresholds for diagnosis. Third, it is a purely morphology-based system without any supporting molecular and morphometric studies that precisely quantifies diagnostic architectural changes. The search for an alternative classification system for endometrial carcinomas had lead to the introduction of the Endometrial Intraepithelial Neoplasia (EIN) entity.

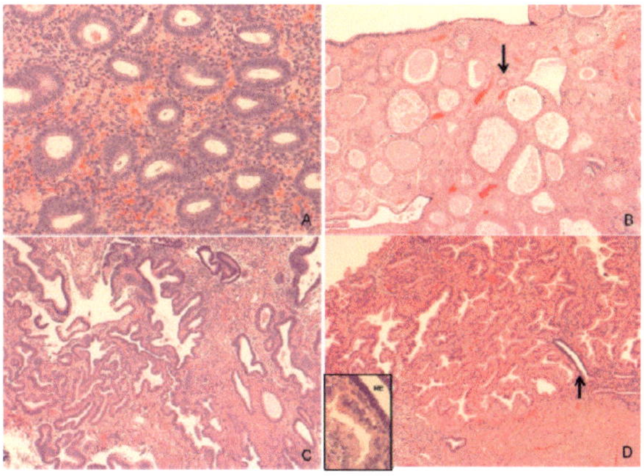

Fig. 2. A: simple hyperplasia, B: simple hyperplasia without atypia, C: complex hyperplasia, D: atypical complex hyperplasia. Arrows indicate residual uninvolved glands. Inset: magnified area with arrow, a hyperplastic gland shows atypical distinct morphology compared to adjacent resting endometrial gland (RE).

2.2 EIN: Mutter's model for *type I endometrial cancer*

The concept of EIN and the diagnostic schema was introduced by Mutter and the Endometrial Collaborative Group in 2000 (Mutter 2000); and later launched at Brigham and Women's Hospital in 2002 (Mutter 2002; Hecht, Ince et al. 2005), to replace the older hyperplasia-based nomenclature, the currently used terminology by WHO 1994 classification system(Scully RE 1994), which implies endometrial hyperplasia as the precancerous lesion of type I cancers. This concept was the result of cautious correlation of genetically ascertained pre-malignant lesions with histopathologic feature and clinical outcomes. A better vision of the carcinogenesis of *type I endometrial cancer* was achievable with the advent of polymerase chain reaction–based clonal assays and relevant biomarkers that facilitated a molecular, rather than purely morphologic approach to precancer diagnosis. The molecular entity of EIN is thought to be a clinically pertinent lesion that can be reproducibly diagnosed by pathologists and targeted for therapeutic intervention. According to this model, the premalignant lesions are referred to as EIN to distinguish them from the diffuse estrogen associated changes of benign endometrial hyperplasia. EIN is a" histologically recognizable localized lesion composed of a clonal proliferation of glands and that usually carry one or several of the genetic abnormalities associated with endometrioid carcinoma" (Mutter, Boynton et al. 1996; Mutter, Baak et al. 2000) . This model had been supported by molecular and morphometric studies. First, the monoclonality of EIN lesions was proven utilizing nonrandom X-chromosome inactivation (HUMARA assay) and clonal propagation of altered microsatellites (Mutter, Chaponot et al. 1995; Jovanovic, Boynton et al. 1996). Second, the identification of lineage continuity with subsequent carcinomas that occur in the same patient, fulfilling a vital standard for molecular definition of precancers(Mutter, Baak et al. 2000). Third, the application of computer based morphometry has been successful at further improving diagnostic reproducibility of precursor diagnosis, and have a better correlation between morphologic features and patient actual clinical outcome(Baak, Nauta et al. 1988; Baak, Wisse-Brekelmans et al. 1992). The applied morphometric measures were combined into a threshold D-score (detailed below). In 2005, a meta-analysis study of the cumulative outcome prediction experience of the D-score (Baak, Mutter et al. 2005), showed that patients with a D-score less than 1 have an overall 89-fold increased cancer risk than those with D-score more than 1. Even if one excludes concurrent cancers, those diagnosed within 12 months of EIN, cancer risk over the next two decades is 45-fold that of controls. Comparison of the WHO 94 and the EIN systems, with correlation of the clinical outcome reveals a degree of overlapping. Mutter et al (Hecht, Ince et al. 2005) had found that, for the simple non-atypical hyperplasia, only a minimal risk for endometrial cancer is believed to be present (only 5% are re-diagnosed as EIN upon review). Complex atypical hyperplasia has the highest risk of cancer and 80% of cases are rediagnosed as EIN (the greatest overlap). Therefore, majority of EIN lesions are actually equivalent to most of the WHO atypical complex hyperplasia category. Detailed relationship is illustrated in Figure 3.

2.2.1 Diagnostic features of EIN

As defined by Mutter et al, EIN is 'the premalignant clone of an endometrial lesion that is characteristically offset from the background endometrium by its altered cytology and crowded architecture'. This definition implies the use of an internal control for cytologic atypia, which is the benign resting endometrium, combined with the distinctive topography of a clonal process. The average age of women with EIN is 52 years (Baak, Mutter et al.

2005), almost a decade younger than the average age for cases of endometrioid endometrial carcinoma in patients with concurrent endometrioid carcinoma (Baak, Mutter et al. 2005; Hecht and Mutter 2006), and when those patients are excluded, the average time following EIN detection to carcinoma diagnosis is 4 years(Baak, Mutter et al. 2005). The clinical significance of EIN lesions is that they represent a long-term cancer risk that is 45-fold greater than that of their benign endometrial hyperplasia counterparts (Hecht and Mutter 2006; Mutter, Zaino et al. 2007). This distinctive clinical profile, is further supported by morphometric measures, summed up under the term D-score, which includes the volume percent stroma (a measure of gland crowding); standard deviation of the shortest nuclear axis (a measure of nuclear pleomorphism); and gland outer surface density (a measure of branching and folding). The morphometric techniques were effective at discriminating those endometrial lesions which progress to adenocarcinoma from those that do not (Baak, Nauta et al. 1988). However, we would like to point out that the morphometric techniques are so far mainly limited to research applications rather than in general practice.

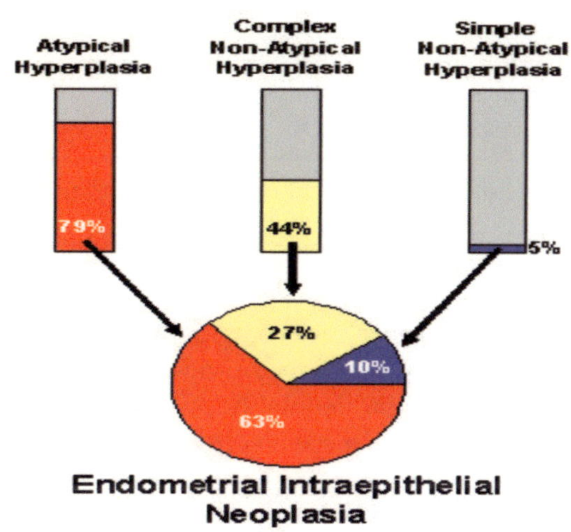

Fig. 3. Mutter's diagram (Hecht, Ince et al. 2005) for overlaps between WHO and EIN classification systems.

Based on the model of EIN, 5 strict morphologic features are applied, and all 5 criteria must be met in each case to maintain a high level of diagnostic specificity and predictive value. The diagnostic criteria are summarized in Table 2.

Architecture

A feature that makes EIN lesions readily visible under low magnification. Area of glands exceeds that of stroma, thus, the surface area of glands (combined epithelium and lumen) is greater than that of the stroma that contains them, and the tissue proportion occupied by stroma is less than 50%. However, this ratio is also used as a diagnostic feature for benign endometrial hyperplasias. To overcome the potential source of diagnostic confusion, strict search for the other 4 criteria is critical to confirm the lesion in question is EIN and not a focus of endometrial hyperplasia. Another important point to mention is the condition of the endometrial stroma within the area of question.

EIN feature	Definitions
Architecture	Area of glands exceeds that of stroma (glands/stroma > 1). Lesion composed of individual glands, which may branch slightly and vary in shape.
Cytology	Nuclear and/or cytoplasmic features of epithelial cells differ between glands with abnormal architecture and those with normal background. May include change in nuclear polarity, nuclear pleomorphism, or altered cytoplasmic differentiation state. Highly abnormal cytology if no normal comparison glands are present
Size	Maximum linear dimension exceeds 1 mm
Exclude benign mimics	Benign conditions with overlapping criteria :disordered proliferative, basalis, secretory, polyps, repair, etc.
Exclude cancer	Carcinoma if mazelike glands, solid areas, or significant cribriform growth.

Table 2. Essential diagnostic criteria of EIN as outlined by Mutter et al (Mutter, Zaino et al. 2007).

Cytologic Changes

This must be judged individually in each case using the native background endometrium as the internal control (Figure 4 A). No unified diagnostic cytologic features are settled for EIN, this is due to several factors. First, the variability of the cytological characteristics of the endometrial glandular epithelium among specimens, according to fixation, processing, and staining. Second, this inconsistency also depends largely on the fluctuating hormonal environment. Third, not all EIN lesions maintain endometrioid differentiation (Mutter, Zaino et al. 2007), and commonly acquire metaplastic changes, including mucinous,

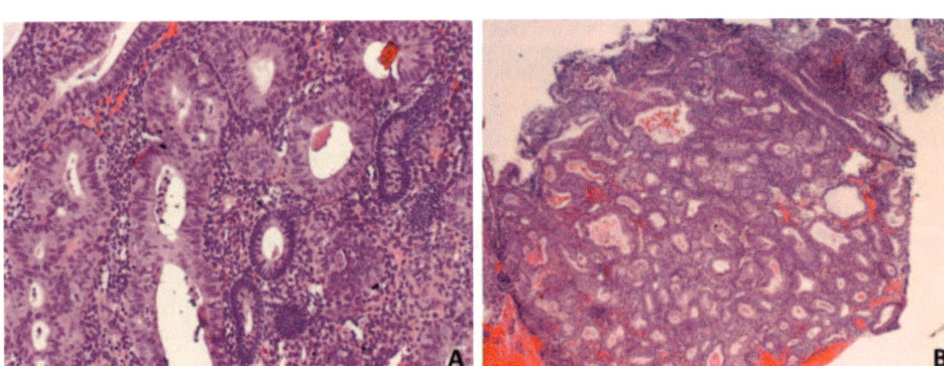

Fig. 4. Diagnostic features to look for in EIN lesions. EIN glands are cytologically distinct from the surrounding normal endometrial glands (A, 200x). The lesion should be at least 1mm in dimension (B, 40x).

squamous morular, tubal, eosinophilic, or micropapillary changes. The practicing pathologist should be careful, however, not to confuse the relatively mild cytologic atypia of EIN lesions with the striking atypia with possibly hobnailed nuclei seen in the precancer of *type II endometrial cancer* (serous EmGD and clear cell EmGD).

Size

The lesion must be at least 1 mm in dimension in a single tissue fragment (Figure 4B). This "golden" number needs to be present in only one dimension of the lesion. Separate foci cannot be added to achieve this minimum size, it must be met in a single focus(Mutter, Zaino et al. 2007). The reason why a size parameter is needed in such a lesion, is probably to confer reproducibility and predictive value in pathological and the clinical sides, respectively. It may also significantly reduce the risk of EIN overdiagnosis in minute randomly detected foci of glandular crowding. One problem of the size limit is that about 20% of EIN lesions are diffuse and non-localized by the time they are detected(Mutter, Zaino et al. 2007), such a diagnostic difficulty might be overcome by largely depending on the other diagnostic criteria. Lesions that have most of the diagnostic criteria for EIN but are <1mm in dimension are still of unknown clinical significance, but are thought to be a good indication for subsequent follow-up endometrial sampling. However, in a recent study by Huang et al(Huang, Mutter et al. 2010), 71 579 consecutive gynecological pathology reports were retrieved, of which, 206 (0.3%) cases with 'gland crowding' were identified, in which 69% (143/206) had follow-up sampling. Of these, 33 (23%) had an outcome diagnosis of EIN (27 cases; 19%) or carcinoma (6 cases; 4%). Included were 18 cases (55%) diagnosed within the first year and presumed concurrent, and an additional 15 (45%) discovered after 1 year and interpreted as a later phase of disease or new events (Huang, Mutter et al. 2010). The authors suggested that such "gland crowding" is significant and deserves mention in pathologic reports.

Exclusion of benign mimics

Many innocent conditions are frequently encountered during routine examination of endometrial specimens, and these may be the source of diagnosticdifficulty in the exclusion of a potential EIN lesion. These may include (but are not limited to) artifactually pushed together or telescoped endometrial glands; or crowding related to the late secretory endometrium, in which the gland density may be very high in the deep functionalis where predecidual change is minimal (Figure 5A). Some portions of specialized but otherwise normal endometrium such as lower uterine segment or uterine basalis may also cause confusion, these are usually identified by their fibrous stromal context and quiescent epithelium. Another more serious misinterpretation comes when dealing with endometria under the influence of estrogen withdrawal, either during the normal menstruation or as a result of hormonal imbalances, the resulting microscopic picture is collapsed glands and stromal condensation. This frequently results in irregular glands lacking much stromal separation, giving an EIN-like picture (Figure 5B). Overall, the most commonly overdiagnosed lesions as EIN are probably endometrial polyps (as well as with endometrial hyperplasia), yet, their characteristic altered stroma and thick vessels, are readily distinct from the stromal features of EIN.

Exclusion of cancer

EIN lesions are composed of clusters of individually recognizable glands, whereas endometroid carcinoma show more complex growth patterns not seen in EIN, such as solid, cribriform, or complex interlacing mazelike growth (Figure 6A &B). The presence of myoinvasion is also diagnostic of carcinoma (Figure 6C), but this is better applied to hysterectomy specimens where intact myometrial wall is present. Overly malignant cytologic features beyond that seen in EIN are also present (Figure 4D).

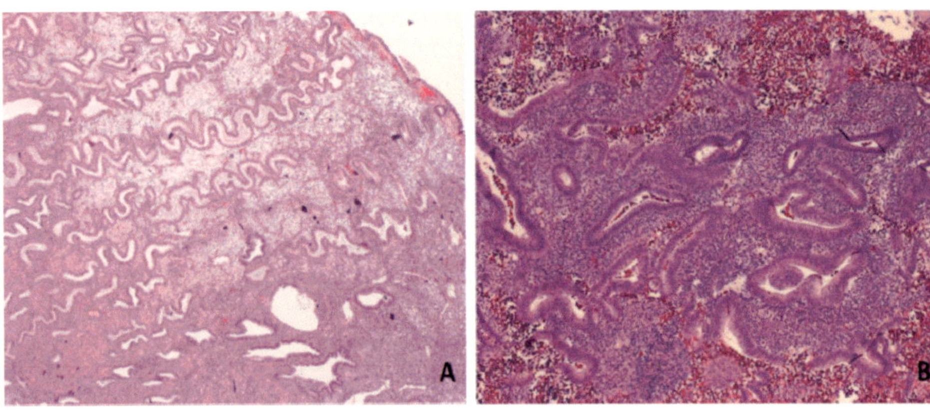

Fig. 5. Benign mimics of EIN. Late secretory endometrium displays prominent tortuous glands and crowding (A, 40x). Breakdown changes with artificially crowded irregular glands due to stromal collapse (B, 100x).

In our current proposal for a unified and simplified nomenclature for the precancers of endometrial cancers, we prefer to refer to this classic EIN entity described above as 'endometrioid EIN'.

2.2.2 Differential diagnosis

Many of the important mimics of EIN lesions have been discussed in the preceding sections (exclusion of benign mimics and exclusion of cancer). Another differential diagnostic consideration that is worth mention is the precancer of *type II endometrial cancer* (in our opinion, serous EmGD and clear cell EmGD). Unlike *type II endometrial precancers*, endometrioid EIN cells lack high-grade cytologic features, including hobnail nuclei. Also endometrioid EIN usually has a high-level estrogen stimulation, yet this is not the usual scenario in serous or clear cell EIN. Immunohistochemical studies with p53 and IMP3 are useful as these markers are positive in serous EmGD but not in endometrioid EIN.

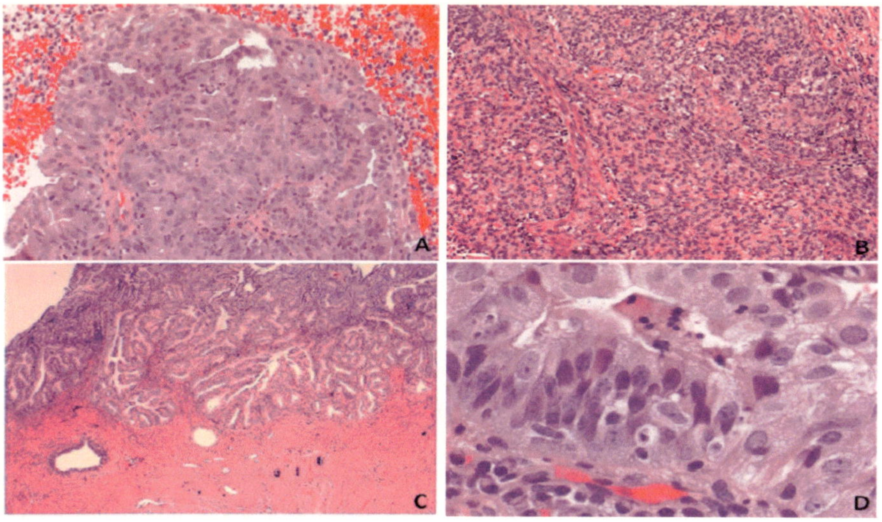

Fig. 6. Features of endometrioid carcinoma, and not EIN. Cribriform glands (A,100x), solid growth pattern (B, 40x), presence of muscular invasion (C, 20x), or frankly malignant cytologic features (D, 200x).

2.3 Molecular insights

2.3.1 *Type I endometrial cancer* and sex hormones

The normal endometrial epithelial cells are highly responsive to sex hormones, namely, estrogens and progesterone; and the morphology of the endometrium at any point is the sum of these responses and interactions. Consequently, the risk for *type I endometrial cancer* is significantly affected by the reciprocal and "opposing"actions of estrogens and progesterones, and is a dynamic process that depends on temporal changes in tissue responsiveness. The same is true for the resultant cancer in which the neoplastic cells retain this feature of hormone-responsiveness. Studies of the expression profiling of *type 1 endometrial cancer* cells had shown resemblance to the expression profile seen in estrogen-driven proliferative endometrium, it also lacks expression of some genes induced by progestins (Hecht and Mutter 2006).

On one hand, estrogens are promoters of cell proliferation and inhibitors of apoptosis, the effect of which is a manifestation of a complex downstream sequence of transcription changes that may involve modulation of tumor suppressor genes. These changes may include alterations in PTEN, PAX2, and HOXB13 among others. PTEN expression in normal endometrial glands is greatly elevated by estrogens and reduced by progestins during hormonal fluctuations of the normal menstrual cycle(Mutter, Lin et al. 2000). As promoters of proliferative activity, estrogens may also increase probability of arbitrary mutations(Cairns 1998), as well as increase the rate of mutagenesis through free radical formation (Burcham 1999), although the magnitude of this effect is minimal. Overall, large-scale population studies had shown that women exposed to "unopposed" estrogens have 2 to 10 folds increased risk for *type I endometrial cancer*, and this wide range is influenced by the dose and duration of exposure (Parazzini, La Vecchia et al. 1991; Potischman, Hoover et al. 1996; Trial 1996; Zeleniuch-Jacquotte, Akhmedkhanov et al. 2001). Moreover, EIN lesions are thought to attain high levels of nuclear estrogen receptors (Mutter, Ince et al. 2001), thus, estrogens may also act as growth positive selectors of the previously mutated cells, allowing their clonal expansion.

On the other hand, progestins have the ability to "oppose" the biologic effects of coexisting estrogens through down-regulation of the estrogen receptor itself in the endometrial epithelial cells. This is actually the basis of combined estrogen/progesterone therapies, in which the net effect is dominated by the progestin component. It is also known to be the reason behind the protective influence of combined oral contraceptives, women who uses these drugs are said to have 0.5 to 0.7 fold risk of *type I endometrial cancer* compared to controls (Grimes and Economy 1995; Weiderpass, Adami et al. 1999). Other protective effects of circulating progestins are due to downregulation of proliferative promoters like PTEN, thus it was found that PTEN mutant clones have a tendency to involute under the influence of progestins (Zheng, Baker et al. 2004). The anti-cancer role of progestins is further mediated by induction of apoptosis through the increased expression of Bcl-2 and BAX (Vereide, Kaino et al. 2005).

2.3.2 Molecular alterations in *type I endometrial cancer* and endometrioid EIN

Type I endometrial cancer demonstrate large numbers of genetic changes in which the sequential order of mutation, and the final combination of defects differ considerably between individual examples (Hecht and Mutter 2006). Common genetic changes in endometrioid carcinoma include, but are not limited to, microsatellite instability (MSI) (Risinger, Berchuck et al. 1993; Duggan, Felix et al. 1994; Kobayashi, Matsushima et al. 1996; Mutter, Boynton et al. 1996; Catasus, Bussaglia et al. 2004), or specific mutation of *PTEN* (Risinger, Hayes et al. 1997; Tashiro, Blazes et al. 1997; Levine, Cargile et al. 1998; Maxwell, Risinger et al. 1998; Gurin, Federici et al. 1999; Mutter, Lin et al. 2000), *K-ras* (Enomoto, Inoue et al. 1991; Fujimoto, Shimizu et al. 1993; Duggan, Felix et al. 1994; Sakamoto, Murase et al. 1998; Mutter, Wada et al. 1999; Swisher, Peiffer-Schneider et al. 1999; Lax, Kendall et al. 2000; Lagarda, Catasus et al. 2001), and β-catenin genes (Kobayashi, Matsushima et al. 1996; Fukuchi, Sakamoto et al. 1998; Mirabelli-Primdahl, Gryfe et al. 1999; Schlosshauer, Pirog et al. 2000). As previously described, it is the clonal origin of EIN that supports its definition as a precancer. Moreover, studies by Mutter et al gave considerable evidence that comparison of the type and magnitude of genomic damage between endometrioid EIN and *type I endometrial cancer* (Mutter, Boynton et al. 1996; Esteller, Catasus et al. 1999; Mutter, Baak et al. 2000; Mutter, Lin et al. 2000), indicates a greater cumulative mutational burden in the later , a feature considered one milestone in the definition of precancer (Berman, Albores-Saavedra et al. 2006). Below is a discussion of the most commonly encountered molecular alterations.

PTEN

Inactivation of the *PTEN* tumor-suppressor gene (formerly known as *MMAC1*) is the most common genetic defect in endometrioid carcinoma and is seen in up to 83% of tumors that are preceded by a histologically discrete premalignant phase (Mutter, Lin et al. 2000). It acts as tumor suppressor genes because their proteins may counteract the effect of the proteins encoded by the protein kinase group of protooncogenes (Matias-Guiu, Catasus et al. 2001).

The most frequently encountered alterations of PTEN in endometrial cancers are LOH at chromosome 10q23 (40% of EC) (Jones, Koi et al. 1994; Peiffer, Herzog et al. 1995); and somatic mutation, which are almost exclusively found in *type I endometrial cancer* (37 to 61%) (Kong, Suzuki et al. 1997; Tashiro, Blazes et al. 1997; Maxwell, Risinger et al. 1998; Bussaglia, del Rio et al. 2000). A number of investigators have found a concordance between microsatellite instability status and PTEN mutations; the mutations occur in 60% to 86% of MSI (+) endometrioid carcinoma, but in only 24% to 35% of the MSI (-) tumors (Matias-Guiu, Catasus et al. 2001). Such results have led to the assumption that PTEN could be a likely target for mutations in MSI (+) EC. PTEN inactivation was detected frequently in EIN lesions (63% of cases) (Mutter, Ince et al. 2001). However, the routine application of PTEN as an informative marker of premalignant lesions is still questionable due to several facts. First, PTEN mutations have been detected in endometrial hyperplasia with and without atypia (19% and 21% respectively) (Levine, Cargile et al. 1998; Maxwell, Risinger et al. 1998; Bussaglia, del Rio et al. 2000). Second, the lack of PTEN inactivation in about one third of studied EIN lesions(Mutter, Zaino et al. 2007). And finally, the finding of somatic inactivation of PTEN in scattered benign endometrial gland in 43% of cases.(Mutter, Ince et al. 2001)

B-catenin (CTNNB1)

Gain of function mutations in exon 3 of *CTNNB1* gene at 3p21 are seen in 25% to 38% of *type I endometrial cancer*s (Fukuchi, Sakamoto et al. 1998; Schlosshauer, Pirog et al. 2000). B-catenin is a component of the E-cadherin-catenin unit essential for cell differentiation and maintenance of normal tissue architecture, and plays an important role in signal transduction (Hecht and Mutter 2006). B-catenin mutation may represent a pathway to endometrial carcinogenesis characterized by squamous differentiation and independent of PTEN (Su, Vogelstein et al. 1993). B-catenin expression change is usually a diffuse process seen in all tumor cells, and is present in some premalignant lesions (Hecht and Mutter 2006). This suggests that B-catenin mutation is an early step of endometrial tumorigenesis that is clonally represented in all tumor cells (Matias-Guiu, Catasus et al. 2001; Saegusa, Hashimura et al. 2001; Hecht and Mutter 2006). Furthermore, B-catenin might regulate the expression of the matrix metalloprotease-7, which would have a role in the establishment of the microenvironment necessary for the initiation and maintenance of growth of the primary tumors and their metastasis. (Brabletz, Jung et al. 1999). Further studies are needed to explore the role of B-catenin in *type I endometrial cancer* carcinogenesis.

K-RAS

K-RAS mutations have been identified in 10% to 30% of *type I endometrial cancer* (Sasaki, Nishii et al. 1993; Swisher, Peiffer-Schneider et al. 1999; Lax, Kendall et al. 2000). There is a higher frequency of *K-ras* mutations in cancers with microsatellite instability (MSI), and many of these are characterized by methylation related GC3AT transitions(Lagarda, Catasus et al. 2001). Several investigators had previously found associations between k-RAS mutations and the presence of coexistent endometrial hyperplasia, (Tsuda, Jiko et al. 1995) lymph node metastases, and clinical outcome in postmenopausal patients over 60 years of age (Ito, Watanabe et al. 1996). In addition, some investigators have reported an almost complete absence of k-RAS mutations in serous and clear cell carcinomas of the endometrium (Caduff, Johnston et al. 1995). In the study by Mutter et al (Lagarda, Catasus et al. 2001), the authors reported k-RAS mutations in 18.9% of 58 endometrial cancers, all of them were of endometrioid type. They also described a higher frequency of k-RAS mutations in MSI (+) carcinomas (6 of 14, 42.8%) than in MSI (-) tumors (5 of 44, 11.3%), which lead to the assumption that k-RAS mutations are common in endometrial cancer with the microsatellite mutator phenotype. In the same series, k-RAS mutations were detected in only one of 22 endometrial hyperplasia cases. In this case, atypical hyperplasia coexisted with carcinoma; interestingly, both lesions exhibited MLH-1 promoter hypermethylation, MSI, and identical PTEN mutations, but they had different k-RAS mutations; of the remaining 21 endometrial hyperplasias, 6 had shown MLH-1 promoter hypermethylation and one had both MLH 1 methylation and MSI. Accordingly, the authors hypothesized that "both k-RAS and MSI are closely related phenomena that may occur simultaneously before and during clonal expansion".

Microsatelite instability (MSI)

Among sporadic *type I endometrial cancer* of all grades, approximately 20% demonstrate a molecular phenotype referred to as Microsatelite instability (MSI) (Risinger, Berchuck et al. 1993; Burks, Kessis et al. 1994; Duggan, Felix et al. 1994; Mutter, Boynton et al. 1996). MSI is rare (< 5%) in *type II endometrial cancer* (Faquin, Fitzgerald et al. 2000; Goodfellow, Buttin et al. 2003). Microsatellites are short segments of repetitive DNA bases that are scattered throughout the genome; they are found predominantly in noncoding DNA. Due to DNA repair errors made during replication, the tendency to develop changes in the number of repeat elements as compared with normal tissue is termed MSI. MLH1 inactivation, a component of the mismatch repair system, is the most common mechanism in endometrial carcinoma and is accomplished by hypermethylation of CpG islands in the gene promoter, a process known as epigenetic silencing.(Esteller, Levine et al. 1998) Inherited or somatically acquired mutations of *MSH6*, another mismatch repair element, are also common in patients with MSI endometrial cancers.(Goodfellow, Buttin et al. 2003) MSI in general, and abnormal methylation of MLH1 in particular, is an early event in endometrial carcinogenesis that has been described in precancerous lesions (Mutter, Boynton et al. 1996; Levine, Cargile et al. 1998; Esteller, Catasus et al. 1999). The significance of MSI may also be a result of its ability to specifically inactivate other genes which contain susceptible repeat elements, such as transforming growth factor receptor type II, (TGF-âRII), BAX, insulin-like growth factor II receptor (IGFIIR), and hMSH3, resulting in secondary tumor sub-clones with an increased capacity to invade and metastasize (Ouyang, Shiwaku et al. 1997; Catasus, Matias-Guiu et al. 2000).

p53

p53 is a nuclear phosphoprotein that provoke cell cycle arrest or apoptosis through induction of P21Waf1/Cip1 and hMdm2 in response to cellular stress (Hecht and Mutter 2006). Mutations involving p53 are among the most commonly encountered molecular abnormalities in *type II endometrial cancer* (detailed in subsequent sections), and are usually due to p53 truncation mutations (Alkushi, Lim et al. 2004). On the other hand, only 5% of *type I endometrial cancers* show aberrant accumulation of inactivated p53 protein (Lax, Kendall et al. 2000), may be secondary to changes in its upstream regulatory proteins (Soslow, Shen et al. 1998) rather than truncation mutations. Examples of such upstream regulatory molecules include *MDM2* and *p14 ARF*, that regulate p53 levels and their dysregulation had been shown to cause detectable levels of p53 in the absence of p53 mutation, and may be associated with adverse clinical outcomes(Soslow, Shen et al. 1998; Schmitz, Hendricks et al. 2000; Pijnenborg, van de Broek et al. 2006). p53 overexpression and high protein levels are thought to be associated with high grade and stage, but is also an independent prognostic factor (Alkushi, Lim et al. 2004). Other possible causes for p53 accumulation in *type I endometrial cancers* may be nonspecific DNA damage such as that induced by irradiation which is known to induce accumulation of wild-type *p53* (MacCallum and Hupp 1999).

3. Precancers of type II endometrial cancer

3.1 Precursor of endometrial serous carcinoma

3.1.1 Historical backgrounds

Endometrial carcinoma with papillary features and psammoma bodies had been described in the literature as early as 1960s (Karpas and Bridge 1963; Hameed and Morgan 1972; Factor 1974). Nevertheless, the concept of "serous" differentiation and the distinguished aggressive behavior of such cancers were recognized 2 decades later by Lauchlan in 1981 (Lauchlan 1981), and shortly followed by Kempson and Hendrickson (Hendrickson, Ross et al. 1982). These concepts were further established by subsequent studies and case series focusing on morphologic features and patient survival relative to *type I endometrial cancer* (Lauchlan 1981; Eifel, Ross et al. 1983; Sherman, Bitterman et al. 1992). In 1992, Sherman et al illustrated 32 cases of endometrial cancer with a serous component (13 pure and 19 mixed histotypes), the author noted the presence of "cytologically malignant cells closely resembling the invasive serous carcinoma in the surface endometrium adjacent to the tumor" in 28 out of the 32 studied cases, and were entitled "intraepithelial carcinoma" (Sherman, Bitterman et al. 1992). Spiegel et al described a similar lesion in 1995,and designated it as "endometrial carcinoma in-situ" (Spiegel 1995).Within the same year, Ambros et al introduced the designationof endometrial intraepithelial carcinoma (EIC), as a lesion that was repeatedly and distinctively associated with endometrial carcinoma with a serous differentiation (Ambros, Sherman et al. 1995). Main histologic patterns illustrated in Figure 7.

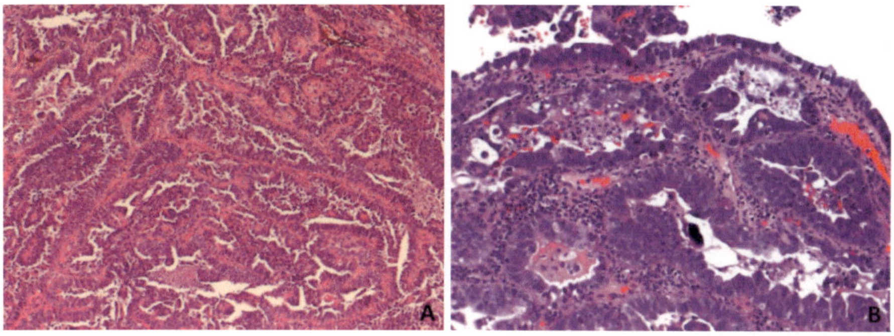

Fig. 7. Morphology of endometrial serous carcinoma. Papillary pattern (A) and glandular pattern (B).

However, in 1998, Zheng et al used the designation "uterine surface carcinoma" instead to describe that lesion, with emphasis on the multicentricity and relatively worse behavior in comparison to carcinoma in-situ per se, questioning the appropriateness of such a lesion as a precancer (Zheng, Khurana et al. 1998). A similar approach had been published in 2000 by Wheeler et al, who proposed the term "minimal uterine serous carcinoma", adding the size parameter (<1cm) to the definition of that lesion (Wheeler, Bell et al. 2000).

3.1.2 Zheng's model for precursors of type II endometrial cancer

Serous EIC is still used in the most recent (2003)WHO classification as the precancerous lesion for serous endometrial carcinoma (Tavassoli FA 2003). However, in our opinion, the fact that stage 1A non-myoinvasive serous carcinomas are known to display extrauterine disease in 17-67% of studied cases (Carcangiu, Tan et al. 1997; Gehrig, Groben et al. 2001; Zheng and Schwartz 2005), strongly argues against the designation of serous EIC as a true "precancer". Many years of gynecological surgical experience and studies of patient outcome have show that many patients diagnosed with serous EIC and treated with simple hysterectomy without surgical staging, had recurrences or intra-abdominal carcinomatosis (Carcangiu, Tan et al. 1997; Gehrig, Groben et al. 2001; Chan, Loizzi et al. 2003; Zheng and Schwartz 2005). Consequently, serous EIC is better recognized as an endometrial serous carcinoma with an early, non-myoinvasive growth pattern (Zheng and Schwartz 2005).

Careful examination of the definition of a precancer established in the National Cancer Institute Consensus in 2006, resulted in the conclusion that EmGD fulfills most of the defined criteria as a precancer of *Type II endometrial cancer*. The diagnostic criteria of serous EmGD were established by Zheng et al in 2004 (Zheng, Liang et al. 2004). Using morphological as well as immunohistochemical features, the EmGD lesions display changes that bridge the gap between benign endometrium and frankly malignant epithelium of serous EIC (Figure 8); the dysplastic epithelium of EmGD has cytologic features that are more atypical than resting endometrium but fall short of serous EIC (Figure 9), as discussed in Table 3.

Macroscopic features

Grossly, no visible lesions could be identified in the corresponding areas of EmGD (Zheng, Liang et al. 2004).

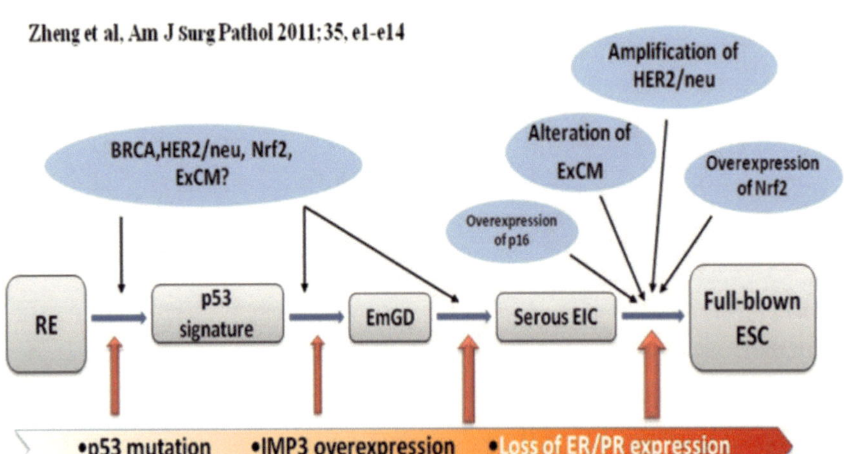

Fig. 8. Proposed model for endometrial serous carcinogenesis by Zheng et al (Zheng, Xiang et al. 2011).

3.1.3 Diagnostic criteria of serous EmGD

Serous EmGD Criterion	Comments
Patient age	Postmenopausal women, classically elder than 55 years old
Architecture & Cytology	Atypical endometrial glandular epithelium. The degree of atypia falls short of serous EIC. Many in endometrial polyp
Size limit and background	No size limit. Background is often atrophic or weakly proliferative, could be proliferative and rarely hyperplastic.
Exclude mimics	Benign conditions with overlapping features: bleeding or curettage associated atypia, repair, polyp with metaplastic changes
Exclude cancer	Serous EIC has frankly malignant cells same as in ESC/UPSC

Table 3. Serous EIN (serous EmGD) fact sheet

Microscopic features

The EmGD lesions are frequently multifocal (86% of cases) (Fadare and Zheng 2008). Classically, EmGD is characterized by glands and/or surface endometrial epithelium with atypical cytologic features. The cells of EmGD shows oval or round nuclei with a 2-3 folds nuclear enlargement compared with the benign resting endometrium. The nuclei are either hyperchromatic or with open chromatin patterns. When hyperchromasia is present, the degree of hyperchromasia is less than that of frankly malignant cells seen in serous EIC. Nucleoli are usually conspicuous instead of prominent. Partial loss of cell polarity is seen when nuclear stratification is present. A few stratifications may be seen. Mitotic figures and apoptotic bodies are appreciable, but not easily identified. Small papillary structures can be identified in EmGD glands, the thin fibrovascular cores of the EmGD papillae are also lined by dysplastic cells instead of malignant cells as in serous EIC or ESC. Occasional mitotic figures are present, but no abnormal mitoses are seen in EmGD lesions. Apoptotic bodies are scarce and in one of our series ranged from 0 to 5 per gland with an average of 1.5/gland (Zheng, Liang et al. 2004). The most common microscopic patterns include glandular involvement, either as a single or a group of EmGD glands within the endometrium or within an endometrial polyp. Another pattern is surface epithelial involvment of the endometrium or lining a polyp. EmGD foci are usually smaller than 1 mm in size. This may be related to the fact that they often presented as a single or a group of a few glands. However, occasionally, potential serous EmGD glands form clusters. When in endometrial polyps, the overall size of serous EmGD lesions may reach several millimeters. The stroma around the serous EmGD glands is usually fibrotic, but desmoplastic reactions are not seen. Background endometrium is often atrophic or weakly proliferative endometrium, but it could also be proliferative or rarely hyperplastic. This is actually a significant point to keep in mind, since nowadays; a considerable number of post-menopausal women are using hormonal replacement therapy compared to those who did 2 or 3 decades ago. In clinical practice, this is translated to the fact that about 40% of women with serous EIC or ESC have a non-atrophic endometrium as a background (Zheng, Liang et al. 2004) (34% proliferative,

6% hyperplastic endometrium). The significance of these findings is, in one hand, it provides further evidence that hormones are not risk factors for *type II endometrial cancer*; and on the other hand, pathologists should keep endometrial serous carcinoma as a differential diagnosis even in the existence of endometrial hyperplasia, in order to avoid the misdiagnosis of *type I endometrial cancer*, and the substantial consequences on patient management and outcome.

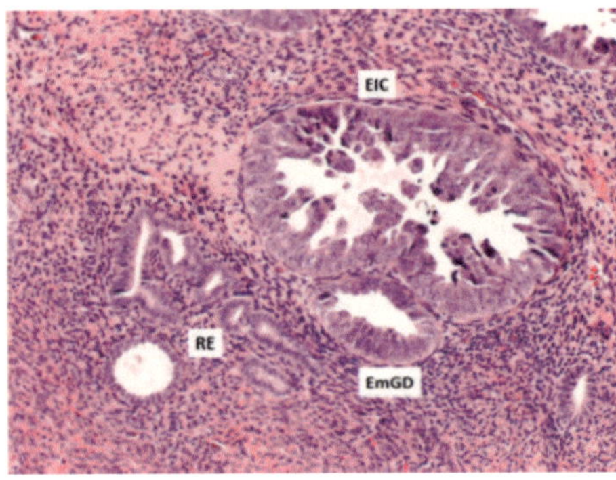

Fig. 9. Endometrial glandular dysplasia (EmGD) morphology. EmGD bridges the morphologic gap between benign resting endometrium (RE) and endometrial intraepithelial carcinoma (EIC).

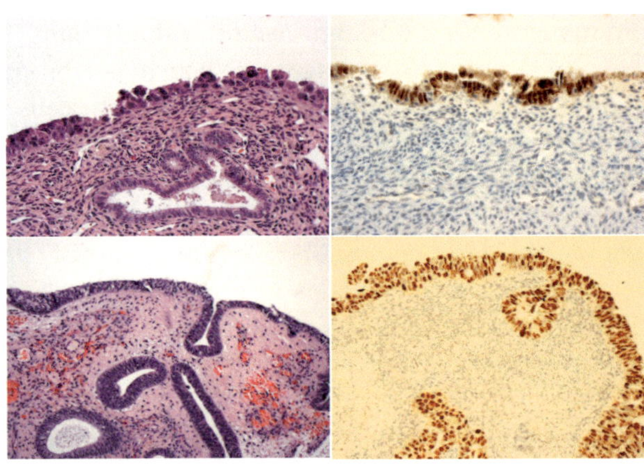

Fig. 10. p53 immunohistochemical stain in EmGD lesions. EmGD may involve the surface epithelium (upper left) or endometrial glands (lower left). The right panel shows diffuse nuclear positivity for p53 stain in areas corresponding to those in the left panel.

3.1.4 Molecular alterations of serous EIN

p53 Mutations. The p53 tumor suppressor gene, located on chromosome 17p 13.1, is probably the most commonly altered gene in human cancers (Harris 1993; Pietsch, Sykes et al. 2008), with the mutations commonly resulting in p53 protein over-expression (Darvishian, Hummer et al. 2004; Liang, Chambers et al. 2004; Jia, Liu et al. 2008). An extremely high rate of p53 alteration and over-expression (90% of our studied cases) had been detected in endometrial serous carcinoma, as evaluated by immunohistochemical staining (Figure 10) (Zheng, Cao et al. 1996; Zheng, Khurana et al. 1998). In 2008, our group studied the frequency of TP53 gene mutations in exons 5 and 8 from laser-captured microdissected endometrial samples (Jia, Liu et al. 2008). In that specific context, the TP53 gene mutations had shown a successive increment from p53 signature glands (42%) to EmGD (43%), to serous EIC (63 to 72%), and to ESC (96%) (Jia, Liu et al. 2008). The benign endometria from the control group, in contrast, showed no mutation in non-signature glands. Analogous findings were found in a later study by Zhang et al in 2009 (Zhang, Liang et al. 2009). It is concluded that p53 gene mutation is a critical and early step in endometrial serous carcinogenesis, and that p53 is an important diagnostic immunohistochemical tool in this situation (Liang, Chambers et al. 2004; Jia, Liu et al. 2008; Zheng, Xiang et al. 2011).

BRCA Mutations

A subset of relatively younger women with hereditary breast cancers are also at increased risk for the development of subsequent ovarian/tubal serous malignancies as a manifestation of hereditary breast-ovarian syndrome (Hall, Jamison et al. 2001; Arai, Utsunomiya et al. 2004), and in patients with BRCA mutations (Lavie, Hornreich et al. 2004). An earlier paper by Curtis et al in 1973, had described other malignancies that may follow breast cancer, including endometrial cancer (Inskip and Curtis 2007). The exact nature of this link between breast and endometrial cancer is still unclear; however, a few foundational studies had shed some light on evidences for such a relationship. In 1999, Hornreich et al reported a case of "uterine serous papillary carcinoma" in 2 siblings with both endometrial and ovarian serous carcinomas who were carrying identical mutation in BRCA1 gene (Hornreich, Beller et al. 1999). Genetic analysis showed loss of the wild-type allele, suggesting a link between germline BRCA1 mutation and serous cancer. A following study of Ashkenazi Jewish patients with endometrial serous carcinoma confirmed a high incidence of BRCA1 mutation and LOH (75% of tumor samples) (Lavie, Hornreich et al. 2004). A contradictory result was found in a study by the same group on a population of germline-BRCA mutation carriers, showing no relationship to increased risk of endometrial cancer. Another disagreement was reported by Liu et al, who found no significant increase in BRCA1 mutation in sporadic endometrial cancers (Liu, Ho et al. 1997).

Based on epidemiologic data, Chan et al had reported an association between breast cancer and endometrial cancers with aggressive histological types (Chan, Manuel et al. 2006). In 2007, a Swedish study found that 7.28% of patients undergoing genetic counseling for an increased risk of breast cancer, had family histories of both endometrial and breast cancers (von Wachenfeldt, Lindblom et al. 2007). We recently published a large cohort study that had found a history of a prior breast cancer in 20% of women with ESC, with the incidence being significantly higher in patients who were 55 years old or younger (41.5%) in comparison to those older than 55 years (16%) (Liang, Pearl et al. 2010).

In the light of the current controversy, further studies are absolutely needed to clarify the possible role of BRCA mutations in ESC. Contemporary data regarding BRCA mutations in serous EIC and EmGD lesions are still lacking.

Alteration of extracellular adhesion molecules

Studies of the role of extracellular adhesion molecules in the development of ESC are limited relative to studies of tumor supressor genes and oncogens. As aforementioned, ESC has the unusual capacity to metastasize outside the uterus even in the absence of myometrial invasion. This might be linked to alterations of the extracellular adhesion molecules of the neoplastic serous epithelium. Such alterations likely assist the transtubal spread of ESC into the peritoneum, and consequently result in the advanced stage of disease at time of diagnosis, even with limited uterine disease. The phenomenon of transtubal spread of serous carcinoma cells had been emphasized by our study of serous EIC lesions in 2005 (Zheng and Schwartz 2005). In that study, 67% (6 out of 9) serous EIC cases had peritoneal carcinomatosis, and among these cases, 50% showed free-floating serous malignant cells and cell clusters in the tubal lumena (Zheng and Schwartz 2005). Our suggestion was further supported by the former findings of identical clones of cells in serous EIC and serous carcinomas at extrauterine sites (Kupryjanczyk, Thor et al. 1996; Baergen, Warren et al. 2001).

Of these extracellular molecules, *E-cadherin* and *claudins* had been described as potential contributors to the biological aggressiveness of ESC. E-cadherin downregulation had been previously reported to be associated with the progression of endometrial cancers (Sakuragi, Nishiya et al. 1994; Holcomb, Delatorre et al. 2002; Mell, Meyer et al. 2004). Holocomb et al described a reduction of E-cadherin expression in 62% and 87% of their studied serous carcinoma and clear cell carcinoma, respectively (Holcomb, Delatorre et al. 2002). A recent study showed that loss of E-cadherin may be attributed to L1CAM upregulation in the aggressive subtype of endometrial cancer (Huszar, Pfeifer et al.). Claudins are a family of extracellular tight junction proteins that are said to be up regulated in ovarian cancers (Rangel, Agarwal et al. 2003), and possibly related to cancer progression (Santin, Bellone et al. 2007). Expression of claudins, especially claudin-3 and claudin-4, is also higher in *type II endometrial cancers* relative to *type I endometrial cancers* (Konecny, Agarwal et al. 2008). *CD44* is a protein involved in cell adhesion and leukocyte homing, CD44v6 is one of its isoforms that may be related to lymphovascular space invasion and metastasis. A significant loss of CD44 and that particular isoform CD44v6 had been detected in ESC compared to EEC (Soslow, Shen et al. 1998). *β-catenin* is a transcriptional activator downstream of the Wnt signaling pathway. Many types of human cancers harbor mutations of β-catenin, including endometrial cancers. Fukuchi et al (Fukuchi, Sakamoto et al. 1998)detected B-catenin mutations in 13% (10 out of 76) of their ESC cases. Whether or not serous EmGD show such alterations of extracellular adhesion molecules is still unclear and is the subject of future studies.

Amplification of HER2/neu

HER2/neu, also known as c-erb B2, is a protoncogen that encodes the human epidermal growth factor receptor (Gehrig, Groben et al. 2001). Amplification of HER2/neu and the overexpression of its protein had been shown in many human malignancies, including ESC (Santin, Bellone et al. 2002; Casalini, Iorio et al. 2004), some studies even described that in association with advanced stage and poor prognosis in ESC (Santin, Bellone et al. 2002; Villella, Cohen et al. 2006). Although similar overexpression of HER2/neu by immunohistochemistry had been shown by the authors in serous EmGD and serous EIC in the studied cases, no data regarding the gene amplification is available so far.

Overexpression of IMP-3

Insulin-like growth factor m-RNA binding protein 3, or IMP-3 is a protoncogen expressed predominantly in embryonic tissues and rarely in adult tissues except for the placenta and gonads (Nielsen, Christiansen et al. 1999; Yaniv and Yisraeli 2002). Some studies have revealed that IMP-3 is associated with cell migration and tumor invasion (Yaniv and Yisraeli 2002; Vikesaa, Hansen et al. 2006), and it could predict metastasis and prognosis in renal cell carcinoma(Jiang, Chu et al. 2006). In 2008, our group studied the expression of this oncofetal protein in serous endometrial carcinoma and its proposed precursor lesions using immunohistochemical staining (Zheng, Yi et al. 2008), we found that IMP-3 was overexpressed in 14% (3 of 21) EmGD lesions, 89% (16 of 18) serous EIC, and 94% (48 of 51) ESC cases. This was significantly higher than the expression detected in only 5 out of 70 (7%) EEC cases, and was not identified in its precancer lesion (EIN) (0 of 35 cases). These findings imply that IMP-3 overexpression may contribute in the early steps of ESC development and aggressive behavior (Zheng, Yi et al. 2008).

Overexpression of Nrf2

NF-E2-related factor 2, or for simplicity, Nrf2, is a newly described transcription factor that is thought to boost the chemo-resistance of cancer cells (Wang, Sun et al. 2008). Nrf2 has been the subject of multiple studies by our group. In one of these studies in 2010 (Jiang, Chen et al.), Nrf2 showed high expression in 89% (41 of 46) of ESC cases, compared to marginal expression of Nrf2 in 28% (14 of 51) of EEC cases, while none of the studied benign endometria showed such an expression (0 of 20). Transient silencing of endogenous Nrf2 enhanced the sensitivity to chemotherputic agents in SPEC-2 cells derived from ESC (Zheng, Xiang et al. 2011). In addition, Overexpression of Keap1, a negative regulatory gene of Nrf2, significantly sensitized those ESC-derived SPEC-2 cells and its xenografts to chemotherapeutic drugs. More recently, we have also examined Nrf2 expression in precursor lesions of ESC, and found that Nrf2 was expressed in 40% of EmGD lesions, and 44% of serous EIC lesions in the studied cases (Chen, Yi et al.); it also showed a lesser degree of expression in clear cell carcinoma (13%) and its proposed precursor lesions, clear cell EmGD and EIC (10% and 25%), respectively. In the same study, only 6% of EEC (3 out of 50) and none of the atypical endometrial hyperplasia/EIN showed overexpression of Nrf2 (Chen, Yi et al.). The relationship between Nrf2 and early steps of ESC carcinogenesis and p53 mutations is currently under exploration in our laboratory.

Overexpression of p16

p16, also known as CDKN2A, is a tumor supressor gene that had been extensively studied in the context of HPV-related cancers and their precursors (Keating, Cviko et al. 2001; Keating, Ince et al. 2001; Negri, Egarter-Vigl et al. 2003). In cervical HPV-related cancers, the mechanism of p16 overexpression may be mediated by HPV E7 viral protein. More recently, p16 has been also shown to be overexpressed in the cells of ESC in multiple studies (Reid-Nicholson, Iyengar et al. 2006; Chiesa-Vottero, Malpica et al. 2007; Yemelyanova, Ji et al. 2009). The mechanism of this overexpression, however, is probably different from that described in viral- related malignancies, since HPV DNA in situ hybridization has been negative in all studied cases (Chiesa-Vottero, Malpica et al. 2007). ESC, it is rather linked to the inactivation of RB gene through dysregulation of the p16INK4a/cyclin D-CDK/pRb-E2F pathway (Reid-Nicholson, Iyengar et al. 2006). Reid- Nicholson et al, (Reid-Nicholson, Iyengar et al. 2006) reported that p16 overexpression was detected in 92% (22 of 24) of ESC cases, compared with 7% (3 of 42) FIGO grade 1and 2 EEC, and 25% (10 of 40) of FIGO grade 3 EEC cases. Unpublished data from our laboratory also show p16 overexpression in lesions of EmGD and serous EIC (Zheng w et al, unpublished), however, it was also diffusely present in benign endometrial samples, raising the question of the practical relevance of this biomarker in serous carcinogenesis.

3.1.5 Differential diagnosis

The diagnosis of serous EIN can be difficult because it does not present as a mass. It may be a focal finding in an otherwise unremarkable endometrial polyp. This is particularly true when a biopsy sample is encountered. The overall clinico-pathologic picture is significant to avoid misdiagnosis (Table 3). The recognition of serous EmGD in an endometrial biopsy or a curettage specimen may aid the pathologist to diagnose serous EIC or to raise concerns for the presence of concurrent ESC before a hysterectomy is undertaken. Attention should be paid in the interpretation of endometrial specimens not to confuse EmGD with any of the following pathologic entities:

Reparative epithelial changes in benign endometrium

These benign changes are frequently encountered post –endometrial curettage or biopsy and rarely show the architectural patterns seen in EmGD. The cytologic atypia is minimal. Numerous mitotic figures are lacking as well. In difficult cases, the use of immunohistochemical stains for p53, IMP-3 and ki-67 can be very useful (Figure 11 A &11B).

Serous EIC

The most useful criterion here is nuclear atypia, which is marked in serous EIC, even identical to that of invasive ESC. Mitotic figures are also more frequent in EIC.

Benign endometrial metaplasias

These may include hobnail metaplasia, papillary metaplasia and also some cases of Arias-Stella reaction. The cytologic atypia in these various types of metaplasia are minimal and they are usually associated with bleeding or breakdown changes in adjacent endometrium. Mitotic activity is rarely seen. Other characteristic cytologic features, such as hobnail nuclei

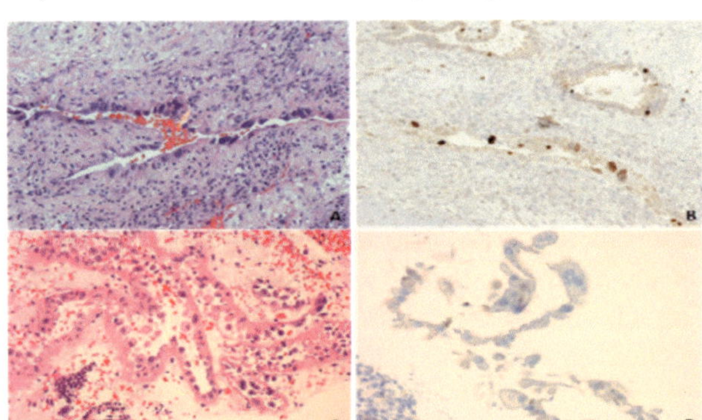

Fig. 11. Reactive endometrial changes. Post-abortive decidulized endometrium may show atypical glandular cells (A), but immunostaining with p53 is weak and focal (B). Hobnail metaplasia in endometrial curretings (C), lack of mitoses and negative p53 stain (D) helps to rule out malignancy.

or cytoplasmic clearing or eosinophilia can further help in the distinction. Pathologic examination should always keep pace with the clinical data and presentation, as a history of a preceeding conception or dilation and curettage will help minimize the misdiagnosis of such benign changes with serous EmGD. An example is illustrated in Figure 11C & 11D.

Endometrial hyperplasia

As previously mentioned, it is of clinical significance to accurately differentiate between the precursors of type I and *type II endometrial cancer*, due to the influence on management and patient outcome. In most of the cases, this should be straightforward, bearing in mind that *type I endometrial cancer* precursors usually lack the highly atypical nuclear features seen in type II precancers, including hobnail appearance, round large nuclei and prominent nucleoli. However, in case of doubt, correlation with positive immunohistochemical stains for p53, IMP-3 would help diagnose *type II endometrial cancer* precancers.

3.1.6 Clinical significance and future management

At present, there are no standard management guidelines for patients with EmGD. The approach at our institute is based on our consideration of these patients to be at a significantly higher risk for the development of endometrial malignancy than their counterparts without EmGD, and that this risk is accentuated by factors such as a personal history of breast cancer or BRCA mutations(Chan, Manuel et al. 2006; Liang, Pearl et al. 2010). For patients without breast cancer history and/or BRCA mutations, if the diagnosis of EmGD is confirmed in a biopsy, we recommend complete dilation and curettage (D&C) for larger sampling. If the diagnosis was made on an endometrial curettage, we recommend periodic follow-up (no more than every 6 months) with transvaginal ultrasound and pelvic examinations. The presence of any abnormalities during this period that may be a harbinger for neoplasia, such as persistent abnormal uterine bleeding, abnormal glandular cells on Papanicolaou tests, palpable pelvic masses, or ultrasound abnormalities, should warrant a complete D and C. For those patients with BRCA mutations or a personal history of breast cancer, our gynecologic oncologists typically offer the option for a hysterectomy. Whether or not complete staging is performed would then be dependent on the intraoperative frozen section findings. If a serous cancer is identified, irrespective of its size in representative sections of the uterus, a complete staging, including omentectomy is performed. If no such focus is identified, the procedure is limited to the hysterectomy with or without the salpingoophorectomies. It should be emphasized, however, that additional studies are required to more clearly define the clinical significance of the lesion in everyday practice. This would entail a larger systematic study of endometrial biopsies to establish the time frame between the development of EmGD and ESC, the proportion of EmGD cases that evolve to ESC, and follow-up of prospectively diagnosed cases to confirm that they are never associated with extrauterine disease in a short term.

3.2 Clear cell EmGD

3.2.1 Historical background

Endometrial clear cell carcinoma (ECCC) is a rare variant of endometrial type II cancer, accounting for 1% to 6% of all endometrial carcinomas cases (Webb and Lagios 1987; Abeler and Kjorstad 1991). It is now established that precursor lesions exist for the more common and more thoroughly studied types of endometrial cancers, including the spectrum of atypical hyperplasia and classic (endometrioid) EIN for *type I endometrial cancer* (Kurman, Kaminski et al. 1985; Mutter 2000; Mutter 2002; Mutter, Zaino et al. 2007; Scully RE 1994); and serous endometrial glandular dysplasia (EmGD) for ESC (Zheng, Liang et al. 2004; Zheng, Liang et al. 2007; Fadare and Zheng 2009; Zheng, Xiang et al. 2011). However, the other rarer and accordingly less studied variants of endometrial carcinoma, including ECCC, has not been the focus of similar searches. A few pioneer studies are mentioned in the following sections.

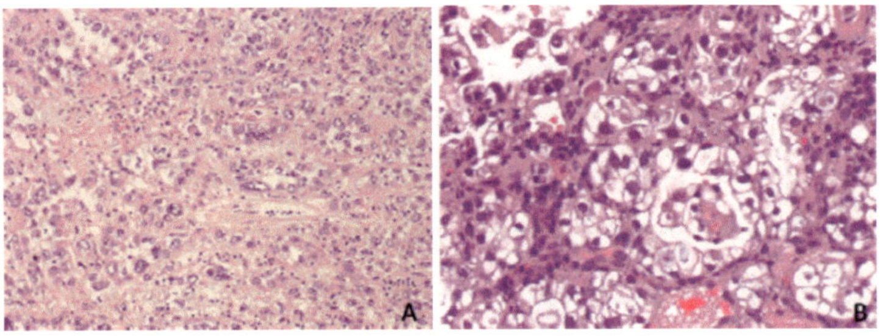

Fig. 12. Clear cell carcinoma of the endometrium.

3.2.2 Putative precursor for endometrial clear cell carcinoma: Clear cell EmGD

In 2004, Moid and Berezowski (Moid and Berezowski 2004) described a distinctive lesion in a hysterectomy specimen from a 70-year-old woman which they designated endometrial intraepithelial carcinoma, clear cell type (EIC, clear cell type). The lesion comprised surface epithelium and glands that were lined by cells with "clear cytoplasm, marked nuclear pleomorphism, coarse chromatin, irregular nuclear membranes, and prominent eosinophilic nucleoli" and an occasional hobnail appearance. No mitotic figures were recognized. There was no evidence of stromal or myometrial invasion. The lesions showed "focal" staining for p53, a "moderate to high proliferative index," and no evidence of extrauterine extension. In 2006, our group studied the characteristic clinicopathologic features of these putative precursor lesions (Fadare, Liang et al. 2006). 14 cases of pure ECCC and 16 endometrial carcinomas with a greater than 10% clear cell component were evaluated, the adjacent benign endometria were searched for lesions that were morphologically distinct from the background benign endometrium and which were not clearly classifiable as a non-neoplastic process. A total of 38 benign uteri and 30 uteri with EEC served as the control groups. In 90% of cases, we identified a spectrum of atypical endometrial glandular and surface changes that were distinct from both the background benign endometrium and the adjacent ECCC. These changes were not identified in any of the control group cases. Transition from resting endometrium to clear cell EmGD, or from clear cell EmGD to clear cell EIC, was detected in 11 (41%) of 27 cases(Fadare, Liang et al. 2006). These morphological changes were also maintained by immunohistochemical stains, which showed that the clear cell EmGD lesions had p53 staining scores and MIB1 proliferative indices that were intermediate between the resting endometrium in which they were identified and the adjacent ECCC. The lesions also showed markedly reduced frequency of ER and PR expression compared with the background endometrium. According to our findings, we hypothesized that these lesions represent precancerous lesions of ECCC. There has been an inadequate number of cases described to know if clear cell EIC in isolation, like serous EIC, has any capacity or propensity for extrauterine extension. Additional studies, as have previously been carried out on serous EmGD(Zheng, Liang et al. 2007; Zheng, Xiang et al. 2011), are required to conclusively establish the precancerous nature of these per National Cancer Institute criteria(Berman, Albores-Saavedra et al. 2006).

3.2.3 Morphologic features of clear cell EmGD

The features of clear cell EmGD are a spectrum of morphological changes involving a single gland, a few glandular clusters or surface epithelium lined by cells with cytoplasmic clarity or eosinophilia, or hobnail nuclei, and varying degrees of nuclear atypia. These changes were graded on a scale of 1 to 3 (Fadare, Liang et al. 2006), primarily depending on the level of cytologic atypia of the constituent cells. A lesion is grade 1 if there is nuclear enlargement (2- to 3-fold compared with resting endometrium) (Figure 13). Grade 3 nuclei show marked pleomorphism and prominent nucleoli comparable to frank ECCC (Figure 12). Grade 2 changes display intermediate features. Mitotic figures were rare in grade 1 and 2 lesions but were easily seen in grade 3 lesions. Morphologically and conceptually, grade 3 lesions were classifiable as clear cell EIC, whereas grade 1 and 2 lesions were designated clear cell endometrial glandular dysplasia (clear cell EmGD).

3.2.4 Molecular alterations of clear cell EmGD

The genetic aspects of ECCC are not fully understood, and further studies are required to establish the exact pathogenesis of this unusual tumor. The information assembled from previous efforts suggests that the molecular pathogenesis of ECCC is different from that of EEC and ESC, and that the molecular alterations frequently detected in EEC and ESC, including PTEN, K-ras, and TP53 mutations, are not commonly seen in ECCC. Lax et al (Lax, Pizer et al. 1998); noted that a division of ECCC cases display morphologic features suggestive of ESC (ECCC with serous features) and that the latter showed a higher Ki-67 proliferative index than did typical ECCC. Furthermore, ECCC with serous features were associated with serous endometrial intraepithelial carcinoma (EIC) in 50% of cases. In 2004, An et al (An, Logani et al. 2004), studied 16 ECCCs (including 11 pure and 5 mixed cases) for mutations in the PTEN and p53 genes, and for microsatellite instability. These alterations were detected in only a minority of the pure cases, but they were present in the mixed tumors. In addition, in the 2 cases of mixed ECCC/ESC, identical p53 mutations were identified in the 2 histologically distinct parts of the tumor. In one case of a mixed ECCC/EEC, identical p53 and PTEN mutations, as well as microsatellite instability, were identified in the 2 components. The authors concluded that ECCC "represent a heterogeneous group of tumors that arise via different pathogenetic pathways."

As previously noted, molecular alterations that are characteristic of ESC, such as p53 mutations or down-regulation of E-cadherin, may also be seen in ECCC but at a significantly lower frequency (Lax, Pizer et al. 1998; Holcomb, Delatorre et al. 2002; Yalta, Atay et al. 2009). On the other hand, expression of ER and PR is seen at a considerably lower rate in ECCC than is typical of EEC. Other alterations that have been reported in ECCC include decreased expression of the metastasis suppressor CD82 (Kangai-1) and frequent hypermethylation of the stem cell-related transcription factor (SOX2), and up-regulation of the oncogenesis-related protein HNF-1A. The first 2 of these alterations are considered to be linked to type II cancers in general, rather than ECCC in particular(Wong, Huo et al.). The precise molecular alterations in clear cell EmGD and clear cell EIC are still uncertain and further molecular and genetic studies are necessary to elucidate them.

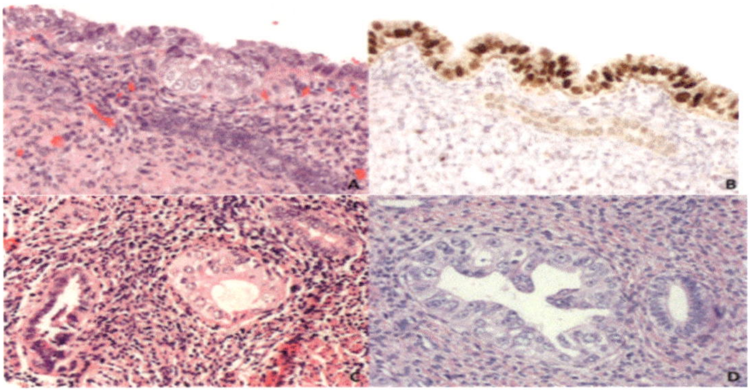

Fig. 13. Clear cell endometrial glandular dysplasia (clear cell EmGD). It can be seen in the surface epithelium (A), or single glands (C&D). Imunohistochemical stain for p53 is positive (B).

3.2.5 Clinical significance and future management

Due to limited number of clear cell EmGD cases that have been studied,the practical clinical impact of this diagnosis, especially if it is found in isolation in an endometrial biopsy sample, is simply unclear. Guidelines on how to manage such cases will not be available until more retrospective and prospective studies are done. Clear cell carcinoma is a rare type of endometrial type II carcinoma. Studies of precursor lesions are so far scarse. We previously proposed clear cell EmGD as a putative precursor due to similarities in morphologic and immunophenotypic features of clear cell carcinoma. However, follow-up and molecular studies are required to establish an ancestry connection between the clear cell EmGD, clear cell EIC, and ECCC and to illuminate the genetic pathways involved in the development and progression of these putative precursor lesions.

4. Conclusion

Endometrial carcinomas encompass a wide spectrum of morphologically and biologically distinct entities. These can be categorized into 2 major pathways (*type I* and *type II endometrial cancer*) according to the dualistic model of endometrial carcinogenesis. Both types have histologic subtypes, and are distinct in their risk factors, molecular background, precancerous lesions and overall patient outcome. The histologic subtype of endometrial cancer has been demonstrated as a significant prognostic factor. The previously used contradicting nomenclature systems for endometrial precancers had been a basis for confusion and low reproducibility among pathologists. They also resulted in the inappropriate inclusion of certain lesions as precancer lesions that did not qualify as such (e.g. simple hyperplasia without atypia for *type I endometrial cancer*, and serous EIC for *type II endometrial cancer*); which in our opinion makes it essential to search for a more simple and unified nomenclature system in this context. Based on the previously detailed dualistic model of endometrial carcinogenesis, and with emphasis on the strict criteria of a precancer as defined by the 2006 National Cancer Institute consensus; we believe that endometrioid EIN (as defined by Mutter et al) is the precancer lesion for *type I endometrial cancer*. For *type II endometrial cancer,* on the other hand, our recent studies confirmed that serous EIN (serous EmGD as previously defined) is the precancerous lesion for serous carcinoma. Similarly, clear cell EIN (previously defined as clear cell EmGD) as a putative precancer for clear cell carcinoma. The precancers of type I and type II endometrial cancer are morphologically and biologically distinct entities, and to the best of our knowledge do not overlap or function as precancer of their cancer counterparts. Much is still to be explored regarding the nature, clinical significance, and appropriate management of those precancer lesions. The newly proposed unified endometrial intraepithelial neoplasia classification system, hopefully, will reduce the confusion in clinic and ultimately benefit patients.

5. References

Abeler, V. M. and K. E. Kjorstad (1991). "Clear cell carcinoma of the endometrium: a histopathological and clinical study of 97 cases." *Gynecol Oncol* 40(3): 207-17.

Alkushi, A., P. Lim, et al. (2004). "Interpretation of p53 immunoreactivity in endometrial carcinoma: establishing a clinically relevant cut-off level." *Int J Gynecol Pathol* 23(2): 129-37.

Ambros, R. A., M. E. Sherman, et al. (1995). "Endometrial intraepithelial carcinoma: a distinctive lesion specifically associated with tumors displaying serous differentiation." *Hum Pathol* 26(11): 1260-7.

An, H. J., S. Logani, et al. (2004). "Molecular characterization of uterine clear cell carcinoma." *Mod Pathol* 17(5): 530-7.

Arai, M., J. Utsunomiya, et al. (2004). "Familial breast and ovarian cancers." *Int J Clin Oncol* 9(4): 270-82.

Baak, J. P., G. L. Mutter, et al. (2005). "The molecular genetics and morphometry-based endometrial intraepithelial neoplasia classification system predicts disease progression in endometrial hyperplasia more accurately than the 1994 World Health Organization classification system." *Cancer* 103(11): 2304-12.

Baak, J. P., J. J. Nauta, et al. (1988). "Architectural and nuclear morphometrical features together are more important prognosticators in endometrial hyperplasias than nuclear morphometrical features alone." *J Pathol* 154(4): 335-41.

Baak, J. P., E. C. Wisse-Brekelmans, et al. (1992). "Assessment of the risk on endometrial cancer in hyperplasia, by means of morphological and morphometrical features." *Pathol Res Pract* 188(7): 856-9.

Baergen, R. N., C. D. Warren, et al. (2001). "Early uterine serous carcinoma: clonal origin of extrauterine disease." *Int J Gynecol Pathol* 20(3): 214-9.

Berman, J. J., J. Albores-Saavedra, et al. (2006). "Precancer: a conceptual working definition -- results of a Consensus Conference." *Cancer Detect Prev* 30(5): 387-94.

Bokhman, J. V. (1983). "Two pathogenetic types of endometrial carcinoma." *Gynecol Oncol* 15(1): 10-7.

Brabletz, T., A. Jung, et al. (1999). "beta-catenin regulates the expression of the matrix metalloproteinase-7 in human colorectal cancer." *Am J Pathol* 155(4): 1033-8.

Burcham, P. C. (1999). "Internal hazards: baseline DNA damage by endogenous products of normal metabolism." *Mutat Res* 443(1-2): 11-36.

Burks, R. T., T. D. Kessis, et al. (1994). "Microsatellite instability in endometrial carcinoma." *Oncogene* 9(4): 1163-6.

Bussaglia, E., E. del Rio, et al. (2000). "PTEN mutations in endometrial carcinomas: a molecular and clinicopathologic analysis of 38 cases." *Hum Pathol* 31(3): 312-7.

Caduff, R. F., C. M. Johnston, et al. (1995). "Mutations of the Ki-ras oncogene in carcinoma of the endometrium." *Am J Pathol* 146(1): 182-8.

Cairns, J. (1998). "Mutation and cancer: the antecedents to our studies of adaptive mutation." *Genetics* 148(4): 1433-40.

Carcangiu, M. L., L. K. Tan, et al. (1997). "Stage IA Uterine Serous Carcinoma: A Study of 13 Cases." *The American Journal of Surgical Pathology* 21(12): 1507-1514.

Casalini, P., M. V. Iorio, et al. (2004). "Role of HER receptors family in development and differentiation." *J Cell Physiol* 200(3): 343-50.

Catasus, L., E. Bussaglia, et al. (2004). "Molecular genetic alterations in endometrioid carcinomas of the ovary: similar frequency of beta-catenin abnormalities but lower rate of microsatellite instability and PTEN alterations than in uterine endometrioid carcinomas." *Hum Pathol* 35(11): 1360-8.

Catasus, L., X. Matias-Guiu, et al. (2000). "Frameshift mutations at coding mononucleotide repeat microsatellites in endometrial carcinoma with microsatellite instability." *Cancer* 88(10): 2290-7.

Chan, J. K., V. Loizzi, et al. (2003). "Significance of comprehensive surgical staging in noninvasive papillary serous carcinoma of the endometrium." *Gynecol Oncol* 90(1): 181-5.

Chan, J. K., M. R. Manuel, et al. (2006). "Breast cancer followed by corpus cancer: is there a higher risk for aggressive histologic subtypes?" *Gynecol Oncol* 102(3): 508-12.

Chen, N., X. Yi, et al. "Nrf2 expression in endometrial serous carcinomas and its precancers." *Int J Clin Exp Pathol* 4(1): 85-96.

Chiesa-Vottero, A. G., A. Malpica, et al. (2007). "Immunohistochemical overexpression of p16 and p53 in uterine serous carcinoma and ovarian high-grade serous carcinoma." *Int J Gynecol Pathol* 26(3): 328-33.

Creasman, W. T., F. Odicino, et al. (2003). "Carcinoma of the corpus uteri." *Int J Gynaecol Obstet* 83 Suppl 1: 79-118.

Darvishian, F., A. J. Hummer, et al. (2004). "Serous endometrial cancers that mimic endometrioid adenocarcinomas: a clinicopathologic and immunohistochemical study of a group of problematic cases." *Am J Surg Pathol* 28(12): 1568-78.

Deligdisch, L. and C. F. Holinka (1987). "Endometrial carcinoma: two diseases?" *Cancer Detect Prev* 10(3-4): 237-46.

Demopoulos, R. I., A. F. Mesia, et al. (1999). "Immunohistochemical comparison of uterine papillary serous and papillary endometrioid carcinoma: clues to pathogenesis." *Int J Gynecol Pathol* 18(3): 233-7.

Duggan, B. D., J. C. Felix, et al. (1994). "Microsatellite instability in sporadic endometrial carcinoma." *J Natl Cancer Inst* 86(16): 1216-21.

Eifel, P. J., J. Ross, et al. (1983). "Adenocarcinoma of the endometrium. Analysis of 256 cases with disease limited to the uterine corpus: treatment comparisons." *Cancer* 52(6): 1026-31.

Enomoto, T., M. Inoue, et al. (1991). "K-ras activation in premalignant and malignant epithelial lesions of the human uterus." *Cancer Res* 51(19): 5308-14.

Esteller, M., L. Catasus, et al. (1999). "hMLH1 promoter hypermethylation is an early event in human endometrial tumorigenesis." *Am J Pathol* 155(5): 1767-72.

Esteller, M., R. Levine, et al. (1998). "MLH1 promoter hypermethylation is associated with the microsatellite instability phenotype in sporadic endometrial carcinomas." *Oncogene* 17(18): 2413-7.

Ettinger, B., I. M. Golditch, et al. (1988). "Gynecologic consequences of long-term, unopposed estrogen replacement therapy." *Maturitas* 10(4): 271-82.

Factor, S. M. (1974). "Papillary adenocarcinoma of the endometrium with psammoma bodies." *Arch Pathol* 98(3): 201-5.

Fadare, O., S. X. Liang, et al. (2006). "Precursors of endometrial clear cell carcinoma." *Am J Surg Pathol* 30(12): 1519-30.

Fadare, O. and W. Zheng (2008). "Endometrial Glandular Dysplasia (EmGD): morphologically and biologically distinctive putative precursor lesions of Type II endometrial cancers." *Diagn Pathol* 3: 6.

Fadare, O. and W. Zheng (2009). "Insights into endometrial serous carcinogenesis and progression." *Int J Clin Exp Pathol* 2(5): 411-32.

Faquin, W. C., J. T. Fitzgerald, et al. (2000). "Sporadic microsatellite instability is specific to neoplastic and preneoplastic endometrial tissues." *Am J Clin Pathol* 113(4): 576-82.

Ferenczy, A. (2003). "Pathophysiology of endometrial bleeding." *Maturitas* 45(1): 1-14.

Fujimoto, I., Y. Shimizu, et al. (1993). "Studies on ras oncogene activation in endometrial carcinoma." *Gynecol Oncol* 48(2): 196-202.

Fukuchi, T., M. Sakamoto, et al. (1998). "Beta-catenin mutation in carcinoma of the uterine endometrium." *Cancer Res* 58(16): 3526-8.

Gehrig, P. A., P. A. Groben, et al. (2001). "Noninvasive papillary serous carcinoma of the endometrium." *Obstet Gynecol* 97(1): 153-7.

Goodfellow, P. J., B. M. Buttin, et al. (2003). "Prevalence of defective DNA mismatch repair and MSH6 mutation in an unselected series of endometrial cancers." *Proc Natl Acad Sci U S A* 100(10): 5908-13.

Grimes, D. A. and K. E. Economy (1995). "Primary prevention of gynecologic cancers." *Am J Obstet Gynecol* 172(1 Pt 1): 227-35.

Gurin, C. C., M. G. Federici, et al. (1999). "Causes and consequences of microsatellite instability in endometrial carcinoma." *Cancer Res* 59(2): 462-6.

Hall, H. I., P. Jamison, et al. (2001). "Second primary ovarian cancer among women diagnosed previously with cancer." *Cancer Epidemiol Biomarkers Prev* 10(9): 995-9.

Hameed, K. and D. A. Morgan (1972). "Papillary adenocarcinoma of endometrium with psammoma bodies. Histology and fine structure." *Cancer* 29(5): 1326-35.

Harris, C. C. (1993). "p53: at the crossroads of molecular carcinogenesis and risk assessment." *Science* 262(5142): 1980-1.

Hecht, J. L., T. A. Ince, et al. (2005). "Prediction of endometrial carcinoma by subjective endometrial intraepithelial neoplasia diagnosis." *Mod Pathol* 18(3): 324-30.

Hecht, J. L. and G. L. Mutter (2006). "Molecular and pathologic aspects of endometrial carcinogenesis." *J Clin Oncol* 24(29): 4783-91.

Hendrickson, M., J. Ross, et al. (1982). "Uterine papillary serous carcinoma: a highly malignant form of endometrial adenocarcinoma." *Am J Surg Pathol* 6(2): 93-108.

Holcomb, K., R. Delatorre, et al. (2002). "E-cadherin expression in endometrioid, papillary serous, and clear cell carcinoma of the endometrium." *Obstet Gynecol* 100(6): 1290-5.

Hornreich, G., U. Beller, et al. (1999). "Is Uterine Serous Papillary Carcinoma a BRCA1-Related Disease? Case Report and Review of the Literature." *Gynecologic Oncology* 75(2): 300-304.

Huang, E. C., G. L. Mutter, et al. (2010). "Clinical outcome in diagnostically ambiguous foci of /`gland crowding/' in the endometrium." *Mod Pathol* 23(11): 1486-1491.

Hunter, J. E., D. E. Tritz, et al. (1994). "The prognostic and therapeutic implications of cytologic atypia in patients with endometrial hyperplasia." *Gynecol Oncol* 55(1): 66-71.

Huszar, M., M. Pfeifer, et al. "Up-regulation of L1CAM is linked to loss of hormone receptors and E-cadherin in aggressive subtypes of endometrial carcinomas." *J Pathol* 220(5): 551-61.

Inskip, P. D. and R. E. Curtis (2007). "New malignancies following childhood cancer in the United States, 1973-2002." *Int J Cancer* 121(10): 2233-40.

Ito, K., K. Watanabe, et al. (1996). "K-ras point mutations in endometrial carcinoma: effect on outcome is dependent on age of patient." *Gynecol Oncol* 63(2): 238-46.

Jemal, A., R. Siegel, et al. (2009). "Cancer statistics, 2009." *CA Cancer J Clin* 59(4): 225-49.

Jia, L., Y. Liu, et al. (2008). "Endometrial glandular dysplasia with frequent p53 gene mutation: a genetic evidence supporting its precancer nature for endometrial serous carcinoma." *Clin Cancer Res* 14(8): 2263-9.

Jiang, T., N. Chen, et al. "High levels of Nrf2 determine chemoresistance in type II endometrial cancer." *Cancer Res* 70(13): 5486-96.

Jiang, Z., P. G. Chu, et al. (2006). "Analysis of RNA-binding protein IMP3 to predict metastasis and prognosis of renal-cell carcinoma: a retrospective study." *Lancet Oncol* 7(7): 556-64.

Jones, M. H., S. Koi, et al. (1994). "Allelotype of uterine cancer by analysis of RFLP and microsatellite polymorphisms: frequent loss of heterozygosity on chromosome arms 3p, 9q, 10q, and 17p." *Genes Chromosomes Cancer* 9(2): 119-23.

Jovanovic, A. S., K. A. Boynton, et al. (1996). "Uteri of women with endometrial carcinoma contain a histopathological spectrum of monoclonal putative precancers, some with microsatellite instability." *Cancer Res* 56(8): 1917-21.

Karpas, C. M. and M. F. Bridge (1963). "Endometrial Adenocarcinoma with Psammomatous Bodies." *Am J Obstet Gynecol* 87: 935-41.

Keating, J. T., A. Cviko, et al. (2001). "Ki-67, cyclin E, and p16INK4 are complimentary surrogate biomarkers for human papilloma virus-related cervical neoplasia." *Am J Surg Pathol* 25(7): 884-91.

Keating, J. T., T. Ince, et al. (2001). "Surrogate biomarkers of HPV infection in cervical neoplasia screening and diagnosis." *Adv Anat Pathol* 8(2): 83-92.

Kobayashi, K., M. Matsushima, et al. (1996). "Mutational analysis of mismatch repair genes, hMLH1 and hMSH2, in sporadic endometrial carcinomas with microsatellite instability." *Jpn J Cancer Res* 87(2): 141-5.

Konecny, G. E., R. Agarwal, et al. (2008). "Claudin-3 and claudin-4 expression in serous papillary, clear-cell, and endometrioid endometrial cancer." *Gynecol Oncol* 109(2): 263-9.

Kong, D., A. Suzuki, et al. (1997). "PTEN1 is frequently mutated in primary endometrial carcinomas." *Nat Genet* 17(2): 143-4.

Konopka, B., A. Janiec-Jankowska, et al. (2007). "Molecular genetic defects in endometrial carcinomas: microsatellite instability, PTEN and beta-catenin (CTNNB1) genes mutations." *J Cancer Res Clin Oncol* 133(6): 361-71.

Kupryjanczyk, J., A. D. Thor, et al. (1996). "Ovarian, peritoneal, and endometrial serous carcinoma: clonal origin of multifocal disease." *Mod Pathol* 9(3): 166-73.

Kurman, R. J., P. F. Kaminski, et al. (1985). "The behavior of endometrial hyperplasia. A long-term study of "untreated" hyperplasia in 170 patients." *Cancer* 56(2): 403-12.

Lagarda, H., L. Catasus, et al. (2001). "K-ras mutations in endometrial carcinomas with microsatellite instability." *J Pathol* 193(2): 193-9.

Lauchlan, S. C. (1981). "Tubal (serous) carcinoma of the endometrium." *Arch Pathol Lab Med* 105(11): 615-8.

Lavie, O., G. Hornreich, et al. (2004). "BRCA germline mutations in Jewish women with uterine serous papillary carcinoma." *Gynecol Oncol* 92(2): 521-4.

Lax, S. F. (2004). "Molecular genetic pathways in various types of endometrial carcinoma: from a phenotypical to a molecular-based classification." *Virchows Arch* 444(3): 213-23.

Lax, S. F., B. Kendall, et al. (2000). "The frequency of p53, K-ras mutations, and microsatellite instability differs in uterine endometrioid and serous carcinoma: evidence of distinct molecular genetic pathways." *Cancer* 88(4): 814-24.

Lax, S. F. and R. J. Kurman (1997). "A dualistic model for endometrial carcinogenesis based on immunohistochemical and molecular genetic analyses." *Verh Dtsch Ges Pathol* 81: 228-32.

Lax, S. F., E. S. Pizer, et al. (1998). "Clear cell carcinoma of the endometrium is characterized by a distinctive profile of p53, Ki-67, estrogen, and progesterone receptor expression." *Hum Pathol* 29(6): 551-8.

Levine, R. L., C. B. Cargile, et al. (1998). "PTEN mutations and microsatellite instability in complex atypical hyperplasia, a precursor lesion to uterine endometrioid carcinoma." *Cancer Res* 58(15): 3254-8.

Liang, S. X., S. K. Chambers, et al. (2004). "Endometrial glandular dysplasia: a putative precursor lesion of uterine papillary serous carcinoma. Part II: molecular features." *Int J Surg Pathol* 12(4): 319-31.

Liang, S. X., M. Pearl, et al. (2010). "Personal history of breast cancer as a significant risk factor for endometrial serous carcinoma in women aged 55 years old or younger." *Int J Cancer* 128(4): 763-70.

Liu, F. S. (2007). "Molecular carcinogenesis of endometrial cancer." *Taiwan J Obstet Gynecol* 46(1): 26-32.

Liu, F. S., E. S. Ho, et al. (1997). "Mutational analysis of the BRCA1 tumor suppressor gene in endometrial carcinoma." *Gynecol Oncol* 66(3): 449-53.

MacCallum, D. E. and T. R. Hupp (1999). "Induction of p53 protein as a marker for ionizing radiation exposure in vivo." *Methods Mol Biol* 113: 583-9.

Matias-Guiu, X., L. Catasus, et al. (2001). "Molecular pathology of endometrial hyperplasia and carcinoma." *Hum Pathol* 32(6): 569-77.

Maxwell, G. L., J. I. Risinger, et al. (1998). "Mutation of the PTEN tumor suppressor gene in endometrial hyperplasias." *Cancer Res* 58(12): 2500-3.

Mell, L. K., J. J. Meyer, et al. (2004). "Prognostic significance of E-cadherin protein expression in pathological stage I-III endometrial cancer." *Clin Cancer Res* 10(16): 5546-53.
Mirabelli-Primdahl, L., R. Gryfe, et al. (1999). "Beta-catenin mutations are specific for colorectal carcinomas with microsatellite instability but occur in endometrial carcinomas irrespective of mutator pathway." *Cancer Res* 59(14): 3346-51.
Moid, F. and K. Berezowski (2004). "Pathologic quiz case: a 70-year-old woman with postmenopausal bleeding. Endometrial intraepithelial carcinoma, clear cell type." *Arch Pathol Lab Med* 128(11): e157-8.
Mutter, G. L. (2000). "Endometrial intraepithelial neoplasia (EIN): will it bring order to chaos? The Endometrial Collaborative Group." *Gynecol Oncol* 76(3): 287-90.
Mutter, G. L. (2002). "Diagnosis of premalignant endometrial disease." *J Clin Pathol* 55(5): 326-31.
Mutter, G. L., J. P. Baak, et al. (2000). "Endometrial precancer diagnosis by histopathology, clonal analysis, and computerized morphometry." *J Pathol* 190(4): 462-9.
Mutter, G. L., K. A. Boynton, et al. (1996). "Allelotype mapping of unstable microsatellites establishes direct lineage continuity between endometrial precancers and cancer." *Cancer Res* 56(19): 4483-6.
Mutter, G. L., M. L. Chaponot, et al. (1995). "A polymerase chain reaction assay for non-random X chromosome inactivation identifies monoclonal endometrial cancers and precancers." *Am J Pathol* 146(2): 501-8.
Mutter, G. L., T. A. Ince, et al. (2001). "Molecular identification of latent precancers in histologically normal endometrium." *Cancer Res* 61(11): 4311-4.
Mutter, G. L., M. C. Lin, et al. (2000). "Altered PTEN expression as a diagnostic marker for the earliest endometrial precancers." *J Natl Cancer Inst* 92(11): 924-30.
Mutter, G. L., M. C. Lin, et al. (2000). "Changes in endometrial PTEN expression throughout the human menstrual cycle." *J Clin Endocrinol Metab* 85(6): 2334-8.
Mutter, G. L., H. Wada, et al. (1999). "K-ras mutations appear in the premalignant phase of both microsatellite stable and unstable endometrial carcinogenesis." *Mol Pathol* 52(5): 257-62.
Mutter, G. L., R. J. Zaino, et al. (2007). "Benign endometrial hyperplasia sequence and endometrial intraepithelial neoplasia." *Int J Gynecol Pathol* 26(2): 103-14.
Negri, G., E. Egarter-Vigl, et al. (2003). "p16INK4a is a useful marker for the diagnosis of adenocarcinoma of the cervix uteri and its precursors: an immunohistochemical study with immunocytochemical correlations." *Am J Surg Pathol* 27(2): 187-93.
Nielsen, J., J. Christiansen, et al. (1999). "A family of insulin-like growth factor II mRNA-binding proteins represses translation in late development." *Mol Cell Biol* 19(2): 1262-70.
Nordstrom, B., P. Strang, et al. (1996). "Endometrial carcinoma: the prognostic impact of papillary serous carcinoma (UPSC) in relation to nuclear grade, DNA ploidy and p53 expression." *Anticancer Res* 16(2): 899-904.
Ouyang, H., H. O. Shiwaku, et al. (1997). "The insulin-like growth factor II receptor gene is mutated in genetically unstable cancers of the endometrium, stomach, and colorectum." *Cancer Res* 57(10): 1851-4.
Parazzini, F., C. La Vecchia, et al. (1991). "The epidemiology of endometrial cancer." *Gynecol Oncol* 41(1): 1-16.

Peiffer, S. L., T. J. Herzog, et al. (1995). "Allelic loss of sequences from the long arm of chromosome 10 and replication errors in endometrial cancers." *Cancer Res* 55(9): 1922-6.

Pietsch, E. C., S. M. Sykes, et al. (2008). "The p53 family and programmed cell death." *Oncogene* 27(50): 6507-21.

Pijnenborg, J. M., L. van de Broek, et al. (2006). "TP53 overexpression in recurrent endometrial carcinoma." *Gynecol Oncol* 100(2): 397-404.

Potischman, N., R. N. Hoover, et al. (1996). "Case-control study of endogenous steroid hormones and endometrial cancer." *J Natl Cancer Inst* 88(16): 1127-35.

Rangel, L. B., R. Agarwal, et al. (2003). "Tight junction proteins claudin-3 and claudin-4 are frequently overexpressed in ovarian cancer but not in ovarian cystadenomas." *Clin Cancer Res* 9(7): 2567-75.

Reid-Nicholson, M., P. Iyengar, et al. (2006). "Immunophenotypic diversity of endometrial adenocarcinomas: implications for differential diagnosis." *Mod Pathol* 19(8): 1091-100.

Risinger, J. I., A. Berchuck, et al. (1993). "Genetic instability of microsatellites in endometrial carcinoma." *Cancer Res* 53(21): 5100-3.

Risinger, J. I., A. K. Hayes, et al. (1997). "PTEN/MMAC1 mutations in endometrial cancers." *Cancer Res* 57(21): 4736-8.

Rolitsky, C. D., K. S. Theil, et al. (1999). "HER-2/neu amplification and overexpression in endometrial carcinoma." *Int J Gynecol Pathol* 18(2): 138-43.

Saegusa, M., M. Hashimura, et al. (2001). "beta- Catenin mutations and aberrant nuclear expression during endometrial tumorigenesis." *Br J Cancer* 84(2): 209-17.

Sakamoto, T., T. Murase, et al. (1998). "Microsatellite instability and somatic mutations in endometrial carcinomas." *Gynecol Oncol* 71(1): 53-8.

Sakuragi, N., M. Nishiya, et al. (1994). "Decreased E-cadherin expression in endometrial carcinoma is associated with tumor dedifferentiation and deep myometrial invasion." *Gynecol Oncol* 53(2): 183-9.

Santin, A. D., S. Bellone, et al. (2002). "Overexpression of HER-2/neu in uterine serous papillary cancer." *Clin Cancer Res* 8(5): 1271-9.

Santin, A. D., S. Bellone, et al. (2007). "Overexpression of claudin-3 and claudin-4 receptors in uterine serous papillary carcinoma: novel targets for a type-specific therapy using Clostridium perfringens enterotoxin (CPE)." *Cancer* 109(7): 1312-22.

Sasaki, H., H. Nishii, et al. (1993). "Mutation of the Ki-ras protooncogene in human endometrial hyperplasia and carcinoma." *Cancer Res* 53(8): 1906-10.

Sasano, H., J. Comerford, et al. (1990). "Serous papillary adenocarcinoma of the endometrium. Analysis of proto-oncogene amplification, flow cytometry, estrogen and progesterone receptors, and immunohistochemistry." *Cancer* 65(7): 1545-51.

Schlosshauer, P. W., E. C. Pirog, et al. (2000). "Mutational analysis of the CTNNB1 and APC genes in uterine endometrioid carcinoma." *Mod Pathol* 13(10): 1066-71.

Schmitz, M. J., D. T. Hendricks, et al. (2000). "p27 and cyclin D1 abnormalities in uterine papillary serous carcinoma." *Gynecol Oncol* 77(3): 439-45.

Scully RE, B. T., et al., Ed. (1994). *Histological Typing of Female Genital Tract Tumors* Uterine corpus. New York, NY, Springer Verlag.

Shang, Y. (2006). "Molecular mechanisms of oestrogen and SERMs in endometrial carcinogenesis." *Nat Rev Cancer* 6(5): 360-8.

Sherman, M. E. (2000). "Theories of endometrial carcinogenesis: a multidisciplinary approach." *Mod Pathol* 13(3): 295-308.

Sherman, M. E., P. Bitterman, et al. (1992). "Uterine serous carcinoma. A morphologically diverse neoplasm with unifying clinicopathologic features." *Am J Surg Pathol* 16(6): 600-10.

Sherman, M. E., M. E. Bur, et al. (1995). "p53 in endometrial cancer and its putative precursors: evidence for diverse pathways of tumorigenesis." *Hum Pathol* 26(11): 1268-74.

Skov, B. G., H. Broholm, et al. (1997). "Comparison of the reproducibility of the WHO classifications of 1975 and 1994 of endometrial hyperplasia." *Int J Gynecol Pathol* 16(1): 33-7.

Song, J., T. Rutherford, et al. (2002). "Hormonal regulation of apoptosis and the Fas and Fas ligand system in human endometrial cells." *Mol Hum Reprod* 8(5): 447-55.

Soslow, R. A., P. U. Shen, et al. (1998). "Distinctive p53 and mdm2 immunohistochemical expression profiles suggest different pathogenetic pathways in poorly differentiated endometrial carcinoma." *Int J Gynecol Pathol* 17(2): 129-34.

Soslow, R. A., P. U. Shen, et al. (1998). "The CD44v6-negative phenotype in high-grade uterine carcinomas correlates with serous histologic subtype." *Mod Pathol* 11(2): 194-9.

Spiegel, G. W. (1995). "Endometrial carcinoma in situ in postmenopausal women." *Am J Surg Pathol* 19(4): 417-32.

Su, L. K., B. Vogelstein, et al. (1993). "Association of the APC tumor suppressor protein with catenins." *Science* 262(5140): 1734-7.

Swisher, E. M., S. Peiffer-Schneider, et al. (1999). "Differences in patterns of TP53 and KRAS2 mutations in a large series of endometrial carcinomas with or without microsatellite instability." *Cancer* 85(1): 119-26.

Tashiro, H., M. S. Blazes, et al. (1997). "Mutations in PTEN are frequent in endometrial carcinoma but rare in other common gynecological malignancies." *Cancer Res* 57(18): 3935-40.

Tavassoli FA, D. P., (Eds), Ed. (2003). *World Health Organization Classification of Tumors.* Pathology and Genetics of Tumors of the Breast and Female genital Organs. Lyon, IARC Press.

Trial, T. W. G. f. t. P. (1996). "Effects of hormone replacement therapy on endometrial histology in postmenopausal women. The Postmenopausal Estrogen/Progestin Interventions (PEPI) Trial. The Writing Group for the PEPI Trial." *JAMA* 275(5): 370-5.

Tsuda, H., K. Jiko, et al. (1995). "Frequent occurrence of c-Ki-ras gene mutations in well differentiated endometrial adenocarcinoma showing infiltrative local growth with fibrosing stromal response." *Int J Gynecol Pathol* 14(3): 255-9.

Velasco, A., E. Bussaglia, et al. (2006). "PIK3CA gene mutations in endometrial carcinoma: correlation with PTEN and K-RAS alterations." *Hum Pathol* 37(11): 1465-72.

Vereide, A. B., T. Kaino, et al. (2005). "Bcl-2, BAX, and apoptosis in endometrial hyperplasia after high dose gestagen therapy: a comparison of responses in patients treated with intrauterine levonorgestrel and systemic medroxyprogesterone." *Gynecol Oncol* 97(3): 740-50.

Vikesaa, J., T. V. Hansen, et al. (2006). "RNA-binding IMPs promote cell adhesion and invadopodia formation." *EMBO J* 25(7): 1456-68.

Villella, J. A., S. Cohen, et al. (2006). "HER-2/neu overexpression in uterine papillary serous cancers and its possible therapeutic implications." *Int J Gynecol Cancer* 16(5): 1897-902.

von Wachenfeldt, A., A. Lindblom, et al. (2007). "A hypothesis-generating search for new genetic breast cancer syndromes--a national study in 803 Swedish families." *Hered Cancer Clin Pract* 5(1): 17-24.

Wang, X. J., Z. Sun, et al. (2008). "Nrf2 enhances resistance of cancer cells to chemotherapeutic drugs, the dark side of Nrf2." *Carcinogenesis* 29(6): 1235-43.

Webb, G. A. and M. D. Lagios (1987). "Clear cell carcinoma of the endometrium." *Am J Obstet Gynecol* 156(6): 1486-91.

Weiderpass, E., H. O. Adami, et al. (1999). "Use of oral contraceptives and endometrial cancer risk (Sweden)." *Cancer Causes Control* 10(4): 277-84.

Wheeler, D. T., K. A. Bell, et al. (2000). "Minimal uterine serous carcinoma: diagnosis and clinicopathologic correlation." *Am J Surg Pathol* 24(6): 797-806.

Wong, O. G., Z. Huo, et al. "Hypermethylation of SOX2 Promoter in Endometrial Carcinogenesis." *Obstet Gynecol Int* 2010.

Yalta, T., L. Atay, et al. (2009). "E-cadherin expression in endometrial malignancies: comparison between endometrioid and non-endometrioid carcinomas." *J Int Med Res* 37(1): 163-8.

Yaniv, K. and J. K. Yisraeli (2002). "The involvement of a conserved family of RNA binding proteins in embryonic development and carcinogenesis." *Gene* 287(1-2): 49-54.

Yemelyanova, A., H. Ji, et al. (2009). "Utility of p16 expression for distinction of uterine serous carcinomas from endometrial endometrioid and endocervical adenocarcinomas: immunohistochemical analysis of 201 cases." *Am J Surg Pathol* 33(10): 1504-14.

Zaino, R. J. (2000). "Endometrial hyperplasia: is it time for a quantum leap to a new classification?" *Int J Gynecol Pathol* 19(4): 314-21.

Zeleniuch-Jacquotte, A., A. Akhmedkhanov, et al. (2001). "Postmenopausal endogenous oestrogens and risk of endometrial cancer: results of a prospective study." *Br J Cancer* 84(7): 975-81.

Zhang, X., S. X. Liang, et al. (2009). "Molecular identification of "latent precancers" for endometrial serous carcinoma in benign-appearing endometrium." *Am J Pathol* 174(6): 2000-6.

Zheng, W., H. E. Baker, et al. (2004). "Involution of PTEN-null endometrial glands with progestin therapy." *Gynecol Oncol* 92(3): 1008-13.

Zheng, W., P. Cao, et al. (1996). "p53 overexpression and bcl-2 persistence in endometrial carcinoma: comparison of papillary serous and endometrioid subtypes." *Gynecol Oncol* 61(2): 167-74.

Zheng, W., R. Khurana, et al. (1998). "p53 immunostaining as a significant adjunct diagnostic method for uterine surface carcinoma: precursor of uterine papillary serous carcinoma." *Am J Surg Pathol* 22(12): 1463-73.

Zheng, W., S. X. Liang, et al. (2007). "Occurrence of endometrial glandular dysplasia precedes uterine papillary serous carcinoma." *Int J Gynecol Pathol* 26(1): 38-52.

Zheng, W., S. X. Liang, et al. (2004). "Endometrial glandular dysplasia: a newly defined precursor lesion of uterine papillary serous carcinoma. Part I: morphologic features." *Int J Surg Pathol* 12(3): 207-23.

Zheng, W. and P. E. Schwartz (2005). "Serous EIC as an early form of uterine papillary serous carcinoma: recent progress in understanding its pathogenesis and current opinions regarding pathologic and clinical management." *Gynecol Oncol* 96(3): 579-82.

Zheng, W., L. Xiang, et al. (2011). "A proposed model for endometrial serous carcinogenesis." *Am J Surg Pathol* 35(1): e1-e14.

Zheng, W., X. Yi, et al. (2008). "The oncofetal protein IMP3: a novel biomarker for endometrial serous carcinoma." *Am J Surg Pathol* 32(2): 304-15.

Part 6

Intraepithelial Neoplasia of Cervix

10

Cervical Intraepithelial Neoplasia – Clinical and Etiological Aspects

Raghad Samir[1] and Dan Hellberg[2]
[1]*Department of Obstetrics and Gynecology*
Falun Hospital, Falun,
[2]*Center for Clinical Research, Falun and*
Department of Women´s and Children´s Health
Uppsala University, Uppsala,
Sweden

1. Introduction

Cervical cancer is one of the most common cancers among women worldwide. According to the most recent data, an estimated 466,000 new cases of cervical cancer occur among women worldwide each year, the vast majority of them in developing countries[1]. Overall global mortality rate is 60%, with large differences between industrialized countries and low-income countries. Of the 231,000 women who are deceased from cervical cancer annually, approximately 80 percent are from developing countries, where cervical cancer is the most common cause of cancer morbidity among women [2].

Organized screening programmes for cervical cancer using cervical cytology, papsmears, have been shown to be effective in decreasing mortality and incidence, and gynecological mass-screening has reduced the present incidence by more than half since the 1960s and 1970s in many high income countries [3-5].

Organized cervical cancer screening was implemented in Sweden in the mid 60s and since then a significant decrease in cervical cancer has been observed. Annually around 700,000 papsmears are taken in Sweden, with a total population of 9,000,000. Approximately 600,000 are taken within the mass-screening screening program, while the remaining is taken as part other gynaecological examinations. The overall incidence of cervical cancer declined by 67% over a 40-year period, from 20 Cases per 100 000 women (world standard rate) in 1965 to 6.6 per 100 000 women in 2005 [6]. During the last decade, however, the incidence has stabilized [7, 8]. Cancer of the ovaries, on the other hand, is decreasing by 1% to 2% annually based on data for the last 20 years. The increase of HPV infections are one cause that explain the present stability in the incidence of cervical cancer.

2. Background

Hippocrates in 450 b.c. was the first to describe cervical cancer as cancer of the uterus and added that it was a disease so destructive that it should better be left uncured than treated.

Aretaeus of Cappodocia 130-200 a.c. and in particular Aetius of Amida in 600 a.c. described uterine cancer as superficial and deep ulcers that would eventually infiltrate the uterus. He also described another type of cancer, which did not present with ulcers, but rather as a tumor in the uterus. In 1793, Mathew Baillie observed that cervical cancer did not cause enlargement of the uterus, but rather continuous ulceration of the uterus until the whole organ is destroyed [9].

In the early 19th, Rigoni-Stern, an Italian physician, examined the death records of the city of Verona between the years of 1760 and 1839. He noted that cancer of the cervix was common among married ladies and widows, but less among Jewish women, rare in unmarried ladies, and absent in nuns. This was the first report that incriminated reproductive and sexual events in the genesis of cervical neoplasms. Later, Rigoni-Stern found that the disease was very common among prostitutes, and cervical cancer thus became the poor and socially deprived women's disease [10]. von Scazoni, a German physician, reported in 1861 that female sexual activity outside marriage and sex not directed towards reproduction was the cause of cervical cancer development. Accordingly, woman who developed cervical cancer aroused suspicions of having engaged in 'too much sex' or having committed 'self-pollution'.

During the late 19th century, deaths due to cervical cancer in South Carolina, US, were observed to be much higher in black women, and socio-economic status was regarded as one of the risk factors. In 1895, John Clark examined 20 cases of cervical cancer treated by hysterectomy, Clark found that the disease in 15 hysterectomy specimens had extended past the margins of resection and he described the cervical tumor as 'peculiar cauliflower excrescence'.

Virchow stated in 1855 that 'every cell is derived from a cell' (*cellula a cellula*) and that human disease processes were essentially a disease of the cells. Virchow is considered the protagonist of the concept of *Zellular pathologie*, or pathology based on the study of cells. Virchows work can be considered a fore-runner to cervical cytological screening.

Background to cervical cytology screening

The papsmear (vaginal cytology) was developed by George Papanicolaou in the 1920s. Later, G. Papanicolou and the gynecologist Herbert Traut, in 1941 published the first major article on the use of vaginal smears for the diagnosis of cancer of the uterus. Soon thereafter, the papsmear (named after Papanicolou), was born and it is still one of the most sensitive, simple and effective cancer screening tests.

Simultaneously, Hans Hinselman and Leitz technicians devised the first working binocular colposcope. In 1925, he published the first paper on colposcopy, and later on in 1933 the book 'Einfurthrung in die Kolposcopi' was published. Colposcopy was developed furthermore in 1925 by Hinselman and Eduardwirth, but routine colposcopic examinations were confined to Germany until the 1960s. In the United States, as early as 1929, Levy described the importance to study the genital tract with some degree of magnification and subsequently Emmert published an article introducing the colposcope to North American physicians. By 1932 the colposcopic technique was used in a few centers. The present form of colposcopy started in 1953 when Bolten introduced the modern colposcope in United States. Initially, it served as a tool to identify women with asymptomatic early invasive disease. Subsequently, it has also helped physicians identify preinvasive squamous neoplasia of the cervix [11]. At a meeting of the American College of Obstetricians and Gynecologists in Miami in 1964, a group of enthusiastic colposcopists identified the need for a colposcopy society. Thereafter, through the dedicated efforts of many members of the society, various colposcopy courses were initiated. In 1981, Hamou introduced the microhystreoscope for the examination of the cervix and endocervical canal. This provided a panoramic and contact microscopical observation of stained cells in vivo at high magnification.

Treatment: Historical background

The first radical hysterectomy was described by John G. Clark at the Johns Hopkins Hospital, US in 1895. At a pathological examination of 20 cases treated by hysterectomy, Clark found that the disease had extended past the margins of resection in 15 cases. Influenced by the surgical doctrines of William Halsted, he developed an operative technique that is today recognized as the first true radical hysterectomy [12]. The operation was modified and popularized by Ernst Wertheim, whose experience was impressive in magnitude, follow-up, and descriptions of complications associated with the procedure. In 1898, Wertheim introduced abdominal radical hysterectomy with the removal of the adjacent medial portion of parametria and the upper part of the vagina. In 1945, pelvic lymphadenectomy was added to radical abdominal hysterectomy and its gained the name modified Wertheim. [13].

Screening program in Sweden

Cervical cancer screening has been linked to population- and pathological registers in specific counties since the beginning of the 1960s, and all Swedish counties had computerized screening programs in 1993. The screening is free of charge. All women aged 23-50 are invited every third year for gynecological screening. Women between 51-60 years of age are invited at 5 years intervals. The papsmear is taken by midwives and all results are reported to the patient. If the smear shows abnormal findings or CIN, the patient will be referred to a gynecologist for colposcopical examination. HPV DNA-testing is used with triage of ASCUS and CIN1 and in the follow up of CIN2 and CIN3 (see below).

Histopathology

The most common type of the cervical cancer is squamous cell carcinomas and these represent 80% of all cervical cancer, while 15-20% are adenocarcinomas.

Dysplasia is the premalignant squamous cell abnormalities that range from mild, moderate and severe dysplasia, and eventually carcinoma in situ, but this classification has been replaced by cervical intraepithelial neoplasia (CIN). CIN is also used for histological abnormalities that are histopathologically diagnosed in cervical biopsies.

CIN1 (mild dysplasia) is a low grade lesion with atypical cells in the basal, lower third, of the epithelium. Viral cytopathic effects by HPV (koilocytotic atypia) are often present. Another name is low-grade SIL (squamous epithelial lesion).

CIN 2 (moderate dysplasia) is also called high grade lesion HSIL. It refers to moderately atypical cellular changes confined to the basal two-thirds of the epithelium, with preservation of epithelial maturation in the superficial parts of the epithelium.

CIN 3 (severe dysplasia and cancer in situ), also HSIL, refers to severely atypical cellular abnormalities encompassing more than two-thirds or the complete epithelium.

Prognosis

Most dysplasias remain stationary or regress, but some dysplasias progress to carcinoma in situ and subsequently to invasive cancer. The progress of HPV infection/CIN1 to CIN3 is estimated to 10 years, but progression in 1-3 years is not uncommon. Similar estimates are considered for the progress of carcinoma in situ to invasive cancer. The progression rate of CIN 3 to invasive squamous cell cancer has been reported to be 12-30% in different investigations, and might depend on the size of lesion, the age of patient, immunological factors and the characteristics of the study population.

Management of the abnormal papsmear

Management differs between countries, hospital and economical resources. Liquid cytology is increasingly used instead of papsmear, as cells could be spared for HPV diagnosis. A colposcopically directed cervical biopsy undergoes histopathological examination. When the microscopical examination is normal, repeated papsmear shall be performed within 12 months, and when negative, no further controls are required. When the papsmear continuous to be abnormal, a new colopscopical examination is required. When the initial HPV-DNA test was positive, if evaluated, but with no cytological CIN is found, a directed colposcopical biopsy shall be performed and further management depends on the results.

An alternative strategy has been suggested, i.e. that all women above 35 years of age with cytological ASCUS (atypical cells of undermined significance) or CIN1 shall be examined for detection of HPV-DNA, as this test has a high sensitivity for CIN 2 and CIN3 compared to repeated papsmears.

When biopsy has been taken with directed colposcopy without HPV testing, the approach according to this alternative management will include colposcopy and a new cytological test (PAP) within 6 months in women with ASCUS or CIN1.

See-and-treat

See-and-treat is based on colposcopical findings without previous histopathological grading. This includes an electrosurgical loop excision of the cervical transformation zone (ELECTZ), a superficial cone biopsy, that facilitates the subsequent histological diagnosis and might be the sole treatment of CIN if microscopically radical, thus eliminating the need for a preliminary cervical biopsy and additional patient visits. Requirements for the procedure are an abnormal cervical papsmear and a colposcopical suspicion of CIN. This procedure is not recommended in case of ASCUS and CIN1, as in general there is spontaneous regression of mild lesions. See-and-treat could also be used when the colposcopy findings after an abnormal papsmear are not conclusive.

In CIN2 and CIN3 colposcopically directed examinations including the vagina are essential. When indicated, a biopsy should be taken. If no lesion can be detected, papsmear shall be taken and if it positive, a diagnostic conisation is preferred. When the biopsy shows CIN2 or CIN3 a therapeutic conisation should be performed.

Management of glandular cell atypia or AIS (adenocarcinoma in situ) is similar to that of squamous cell high grade lesions, but should include endometrial biopsy in women above 40 years of age. The conisation should be extended higher in the cervical canal than in squamous cell lesions.

Treatment methods

All methods of treatment of cervical intraepithelial neoplasia are surgical, and might differ with histological findings, extension of lesion, adverse reactions and cost effectiveness [14]the age of the patient, the possibility of pregnancy, as extensive treatment methods can decrease fertility and pregnancy outcome. Treatment methods are ablative or excisions.

Ablative methods

Cryotherapy: By using liquid nitrogen at -270 C° in a closed cylinder with cervical application for 5-10 minutes the abnormal tissue are frozen to temperatures as low as -29, and the tissue will be removed.

Laser ablation: A laser beam is used to evaporate the abnormal tissue with the aid of application of acetic acid and colposcopy in order to visualize the affected area in the cervix.

Excisional

Cold knife, using a scalpel, or laser conization: The affected area and the complete transformation zone are removed with a cone biopsy, where the size depends on the lesion, by traditional surgery.

Loop electrosurgical excision [LEEP, LLETZ]): This is a surgical procedure that uses an electrified wire to remove tissue from the cervix. It is done under local anaesthesia and colposcopy examination.

There were no differences in the effectiveness and outcome between ablative or excisional surgery according to a systematic review of randomized controlled trials in women who underwent treatment of low- and high-grade CIN with cryotherapy, laser ablation, or LEEP 15. Cold knife or laser conization is by many investigators considered as the most effective treatments.

Topical treatment with Acyclovir (nucleotide analogue), cyclooxygenase inhibitors and other pharmaceutical treatments have been suggested and tried. The success rates have been poor.

Vaccination

Prevention by vaccination will probably decrease the incidence of HPV infections, CIN and cervical cancer in the future. The identification of the HPV oncogenes E6 and E7 led to the development of effective vaccines with immunological activation of HPV antibodies, but is at present only directed against HPV 16 and HPV 18. Some cross reactions with other high risk HPV types have, however, been observed against other high risk HPV types [16]. As 13-18 HPV types are considered high-risk, conclusive results will not be available in 10-20 years.

Clinical studies have demonstrated that HPV 16 L1 VLP vaccines are well tolerated and generate high level of antibodies against HPV 16. The prophylactic polyvalent vaccine against oncogenic HPVs in young girls prior to the onset of sexual activity is the key for prevention and avoidance of the disease. An early double-blind, randomized study showed that the vaccine was well tolerated and with high immunological response [17]. In another study 2392 young women 16-23 years of age with negative HPV-16 DNA were included. They were randomly assigned to receive the HPV-16LVLP vaccine or placebo at day 0, and at 2, and 6 months. Forty-one women (3.8 per 100 woman years) in the placebo group acquired HPV-16 infections, including 9 cases of CIN, during follow-up, while no woman who received the HPV-16 vaccine, developed infection or CIN. In one study, HPV types 16, 18, 42, 31, 33, 52 and 35 were in descending order of frequency the most common types in cervical cancer.[18]

3. Risk factors for cervical neoplasia

Among risk factors for CIN, human papillomavirus infection, smoking and sex steroid hormones, in general hormonal contraceptives are the most studied and important. In countries and areas associated with many childbirths, like in developing countries or where the use of contraceptives because of religion, parity is still a major risk factor

Human papillomavirus infections

HPV infections are the most common genital infection worldwide. It is sexually transmitted and mostly clinically silent and self-limiting. Some women remain persistent carriers of the viral infection and become at high risk of progression to CIN and invasive cervical cancer [19].

The lifetime risk of genital HPV infection is approximately 80%. For many HPV infected women (80%), the immune defence will eliminate the infection in general after approximately 12 months. In the remaining cases, progression to cytological abnormalities and CIN is observed in 5% to 10% of persistent HPV infections. After an interval of 7-15 years less than 1% of these infections lead to carcinoma.

Human papillomavirus belongs to the family Papillomaviridae, which includes viruses infecting many different vertebrates. They are strictly species- and organ-specific. HPV are small DNA viruses. The relatively small viral genome of 8000 base pairs are organized in three different regions: the long control region, also called the non-coding region, and the two coding regions, the late (L) and the early (E) regions. The early coding region in human HPV types is divided into E1, E2, E4, E5, E6 and E7. and encodes for the proteins with different regulatory functions [20].

Different HPV types exhibit a type-specific tropism either for squamous epithelium or mucosal sites. Viremia or systemic infections are absent. Despite low or undetectable antibody levels following infection, It is unknown if the HPV type-specific immunity is [21] is lifelong.

The HPV life cycle in the cervix is confined to the epithelium. The border between squamous cell epithelium covering the vagina and glandular epithelium covering the uterus, the transformation zone is the target for HPV invasion. Most HPV-related lesions resolve spontaneously, and progression to cervical neoplasia is a relatively rare event. A key factor in allowing disease to progress is the ability of HPV to evade the immune system and establish a persistent infection. Approximately 50% of infected individuals fail to demonstrate or produce a detectable antibody response to HPV. In those who respond there is no full protection from future HPV infections.

High risk HPV infections

Among more than approximately 150 HPV types, 13 HPV types are considered high-risk and 5 HPV types as moderate-risk for cervical neoplasia. Globally, HPV 16 and HPV 18 are the predominant oncogenic types, accounting for more than 70% of all cervical infections [18, 22]. Low-risk types are rarely found in cervical neoplasias, but some types, in particular HPV 6 and 11 are associated to benign genital condylomas.

High-risk HPV DNA is according to our own studies, detected in 37% in low-grade lesions (CIN1 and borderline lesions), 89% in high-grade lesions (CIN2 and CIN3), and in 40% of cytological CIN in papsmears, but with no information of histological CIN grade [23]. In invasive cancer HPV DNA are detected in close to 100%. This indicates that while HPV is a necessary factor for cervical cancer, other factors could be responsible for development of CIN.

There are several steps in the pathway from HPV infection to CIN and cervical cancer. The initial viral entry is the target cells of the basal epithelium. HPV DNA integrates into the host genome and the HPV oncogenes E6 and E7 are expressed in some cases of CIN2 and in most cases of CIN3 (carcinoma in situ). The results of integration are cytogenetic instability and uncontrolled cell growth (immortalization). For malignant transformation, CIN3 or invasive cancer, HPV DNA integration is necessary. HPV itself may transform cervical cells from normal into CIN3, but is not sufficient in developing CIN3 into invasive cancer. Co-factors are needed and will be discussed below.

Integration of the HPV genome into the host genome frequently leads to disruption of the E2 gene that regulates the expression of the two major oncogenes, E6 and E7. Protein products of these oncogenes are responsible for transforming and immortalizing cells, which may lead to CIN3 or invasive cervical cancer. The viral oncoproteins E6 and E7 degrade two key tumor suppressors, p53 and retinoblastoma protein, respectively [24]. p53 and retinoblastoma proteins cause cell cycle arrest, allowing for repair of mutant DNA or inducing apoptosis, programmed cell death. Inactivation leads to unscheduled progression through the cell cycle and proliferation, which is required for development and maintenance of malignant cells.

4. Smoking

Epidemiological studies

During the 1980s, studies started to appear, where the correlation between smoking and cervical neoplasia, independent of sexual risk factors was evaluated. As far back as 1966 it was reported that smoking was twice as common among women with CIN as those without, but it was regarded as a confounder for sexual risk behaviour [25].

A number of studies from 1980 and onwards confirmed that smoking was an risk factor, independent of sexual risk behaviour, for CIN [26]. The first report on smoking and CIN that adjusted for sexual risk behaviour on CIN estimated relative risks for smokers to be above 2.0 in multivariate analyses, and slightly, but not substantially, higher in crude analyses. Thus, the association between smoking and sexual risk behaviour was not very strong [27].

In 1983 followed three studies on CIN, one by us and another two independent studies (Hellberg, Valentin et al. 1983; Lyon, Gardner et al. 1983; Trevathan, Layde et al. 1983). They all confirmed the results of the initial study. We suggested, and later performed, studies on cervical mucus in smokers. There was a slight decrease in odds ratios between crude and multivariate analyses in these studies. Independent odds ratios in all three studies were between 2.0 and 3.0. In addition, our results indicated that passive smoking could play a role. Many confirmatory studies where proper adjustments were made have followed these four initial studies smoking habits might ever be more important in CIN than in invasive cancer. Thus, there are reports of a higher relative risk with CIN compared to invasive cancer, and smoking. It suggests that smoking is particularly involved in early carcinogenesis and might be a biological co-factor to a progressive HPV infection[28]. In some studies, women above 40 years of age show lower odds ratios for smoking and CIN compared to younger women [29, 30]. The role of the hormonal environment in premenopausal women will be discussed below.

One study [30] also found a strong trend with increased risk by pack-years of smoking and age of starting smoking. A number of early, unadjusted studies were also able to show a dose-response relationship, a prerequisite in most epidemiological studies where exposure is analysed. A number of later studies have confirmed the dose-response relationship for smoking [31]. Some studies on previous smokers have reported substantially decreased risk to acquire CIN after some years of smoking cessation [31-33].

Decreasing odds ratios in multivariate analyses compared to crude analyses are of some concern. There is always a possibility of residual confounding, i.e. variables that was not controlled for. Age at first intercourse and number of lifetime sexual partners may not entirely reflect sexual risk behaviour. Factors such as sex at first date, sex with casual and unknown partners, sex tourism and anal sex all increase the risk for acquiring a sexually transmitted infection. Moreover, the male's sexual risk behaviour is rarely, if ever, controlled for. As in most epidemiological studies they must be confirmed by similar studies *and* additional biological and experimental evidence is necessary to support the results, to be considered conclusive.

An interesting finding in one study was that smoking attributed little to the risk in women with many sexual partners, but was an important risk factor in women who had only had 0-1 sexual partners and also with increasing risks by years of smoking. The relative risk was impressingly 3.7 in women who had smoked for more than 20 years. The results adds to the findings that smoking also has a role independent of HPV, as these women could not be supposed to practising a sexual risk behaviour [34].

In a calculation of attributable risk (PAR) for CIN for a large number of risk factors, smoking (29%) was second to number of sexual partners (57%), while attributable risk for long-term oral contraceptive use was only 8%. [35].

Finally, a number of meta-analyses on the role of smoking in CIN and cervical cancer have been performed [36-39]. All meta-analyses concluded that smoking epidemiologically seemed to be an independent risk factor for cervical cancer. There were some indications that the risk was higher in HPV-infected compared to non-infected women. Calculated pooled odds ratios ranged from 1.95 to 2.17.

Smoking and human papillomavirus infections

It has been suggested to evaluate the importance of smoking only in women with negative HPV status. HPV detection in both CIN III and invasive cervical cancer is approaching 100% why such studies would be hard to conduct. The presence of HPV is lower in low-grade CIN, and searching for a correlation to smoking might give new information. An epidemiological association between HPV infection and smoking has been searched for in numerous studies. In most studies there are significant corrrelations between smoking habits and HPV infection. It has been speculated that smoking-induced impaired immune defence is behind the correlation. Declining odds ratios after adjustments raise suspicions of residual confounding, i.e. risk behaviours or factors that were not adjusted for. [26].

HPV, smoking and cervical neoplasias

More important, also clinically, than a possible association between a cervical HPV infection with normal epithelium and smoking, would be if smoking in addition to HPV is also involved in the transformation from normal to cervical neoplasia. One approach is to study if smoking is more prevalent in HPV infected women with high-grade CIN compared to HPV infected women with low-grade CIN. Indeed, some studies that found that there was a higher (4.4) correlation between smoking and CIN II-III than to CIN I. [40]. Smoking frequency was reported to be increased from 16% in women having no CIN or CIN I, to 41% in those who had CIN III [41]. There are also studies with discrepant results.

Of interest in this review are some studies that investigated the association between CIN and smoking after adjustment for current HPV infection and this was claimed to insignificantly decrease the correlation between CIN II-III and smoking habits. With presence of HPV infection odds ratios (3.0) were unchanged after adjustments which is somewhat surprising. In studies where HPV negative and positive women were analysed separately, odds ratio for HPV negative women was still significantly increased in smokers [42]. Similar results have been reported in other studies. If these results are true carcinoma in situ (CIN III) can develop in smokers, maybe in combinations with other potential carcinogens, even without a current HPV infection.

Experimental studies

As stated above, experimental results must be added to epidemiological findings. The first biological explanation in humans was our finding of nicotine levels that were 40 times higher in cervical mucus, directly collected from the cervical canal with a syringe, compared to serum levels in healthy smokers. In addition, the stable nicotine metabolite cotinine were found in almost four times higher concentrations in mucus than in serum [43]. In a larger study on smoking women with current CIN we could confirm the results. While nicotine and cotinine could not be measured in serum of non-smokers and passive smokers both substances were found in small amounts in cervical mucus. There was a dose-response relationship by smoking intensity and nicotine/cotinine levels in the cervix [44]. In addition, we measured these tobacco constituents in another female genital gland, the follicle fluid of the ovaries. Nicotine and cotinine levels were found to be equal to those in serum [45]. Subsequent studies confirmed the results of the finding of tobacco constituents in the cervix [46, 47]. A problem was that these studies used a cervical flush technique and direct nicotine levels in mucus could not be estimated.

It is unclear whether nicotine and cotinine in itself exert carcinogenic effects. In cell lines derived from human normal, HPV transfected cells nicotine was added to tissue culture plates at concentrations we found in cervical mucus and in higher concentrations. Nicotine enhanced cell proliferation in all three lines [48].

We tried to analyse carcinogenic tobacco products, during the mid-eighties there was not enough sensitive methods to detect tobacco carcinogens, in particular tobacco-specific nitrosamines and polynuclear aromatic hydrocarbons (PAH), i.e. benzpyrenes. During the late 1990s, the presence of the highly carcinogenic, tobacco-specific nitrosamine NNK and benzo(a)pyrene in smoker's cervical mucus were finally found by our previous collaborating laboratory (Prokopczyk, Cox et al. 1997; Melikian, Sun et al. 1999).

During the 1950s and the 1960s a number of animal studies aimed at transforming normal cervical epithelium to malignant. Coal-tar PAHs, like benzpyrenes was reported to induce invasive squamous cell carcinoma [49], but studies of human cervical cell lines have been difficult to interpret [50, 51].

Smoke condensate - in vitro studies

Smoke condensate has been administered to HPV immortalized cell lines. When two human HPV 16 containing cell lines underwent condensate treatment for each passage up to 26 months, they progressed to malignant tumours with few exceptions. Treatment with smoke condensate, but not without, formed invasive cervical cancer when injected in nude mice [52]. The same research group reported that in a HPV 18 immortalized cell line from the transformation zone, that addition of smoke condensate, but not without, was followed by malignant transformation [53].

Tumor markers - in vivo studies

There are still few cervical tissue studies specifically investigating smoking and the levels of proteins considered to be tumor markers in invasive cancer, and in particular in CIN. We studied 17 tumor markers in CIN and normal epithelium, correlated to smoking habits. Some of the tumor markers showed no or entire expression, but most were possible to evaluate. In normal epithelium there were no correlations to expression of tumor markers. In CIN, the tumor suppressors p53 and FHIT, and the immunologic marker IL-10 were underexpressed, while the proliferation marker Ki-67, and Cox-2, involved in many carcinogenic processed, were overexpressed. Thus, this provides in vivo biological evidence for a direct promoter role of smoking in CIN [54].

In another study of women with normal histology, or CIN I to CIN III, smoking was significantly associated to CIN, while they could not confirm our results of smoking and Ki-67 expression. Odds ratios were, however, 2.0-4.2 depending on smoking intensity which indicates that the study did not have enough power. Trend for number of cigarettes per day was of borderline significance [55].

We also studied expression of 14 tumor markers and correlation to smoking in invasive cervical cancer tissue. Many of these markers were also included in the study of CIN. Interestingly, only decreased p53 and increased Cox-2 expression were significantly correlated to smoking both in CIN and cancer. In cancer, also decreased expression of the tumor suppressor LRIG1, and increased expressions of the angiogenesis protein VEGF correlated to smoking, in contrast to CIN [54, 56, 57]. This indicates that the biological roles of smoking might not be entirely similar in CIN and invasive cancer.

Sex steroids - hormonal contraceptives

Multiparity is a classic risk factor for CIN and cancer, but might be a confounder for high-risk sexual behavior, in particular before the introduction of commonly used modern contraceptives, but that is still not the situation in many parts of the world. It still gave an indication that reproductive factors were involved in the etiology of CIN. Most of the major studies restricting the analysis to HPV-positive women, also report an increased risk for cervical neoplasia with increasing parity. It has been suggested that the increased exposure of the cervical transformation zone, where cervical neoplasia is initiated, after pregnancy might facilitate HPV infection [58]. In that case, the hormonal influence would only be secondary.

Oral contraceptive (OC) use early emerged as an epidemiological risk factor for cervical neoplasia, but only in the early 1980s, studies with adjustment for other risk factors, i.e. sexual risk behavior and smoking, appeared [27, 59]. It might be expected that women with oral contraceptive use are more sexually active than women without. Sexual abstinence, marriages or other characteristics will decrease the necessity of contraceptive use. Parity could be lower among oral contraceptive users and could introduce a negative bias. Smoking habits might correlate to sexual risk behavior, and detection bias due to frequent papsmear evaluations, must be taken into account. Thus, there are numerous pitfalls in epidemiological studies.

Oral contraceptives increase serum levels of sex steroid hormones. In epidemiological studies it is not possible, to confirm the theory of sex steroid hormones as causal co-factors to HPV in the transition of normal epithelium to CIN and invasive cancer. When the first epidemiological studies with adjustment for sexual risk behavior were published, that also included smoking habits [59], it became clear that OC use, but only long-term use, i.e. more than 4-5 years, was independently correlated to cervical neoplasia, irrespective of sexual risk behavior and smoking [27, 59]. Odds ratios were in general moderate, 1.5-2.0, but significant. Discrepant results were found in some subsequent studies, but in those cases commonly a tendency of a correlation was observed.

OC use must be investigated for a possible correlation to HPV infection, to exclude that OCs are merely bystanders to HPV. If OC use is a risk factor independent of HPV infection, it strengthens the evidence that OCs are true biological co-factors. Several studies have investigated an eventual correlation to HPV infection and adjusted the results for sexual risk behavior [23, 60-62]. These studies found independent correlations between OC use and cervical neoplasia. Interestingly, we found that use of high dose OCs, but not low dose OCs, was significantly associated with HPV infection [60]. Available studies does not indicate that any hormonal contraceptive influence prognosis in CIN or invasive cancer.

Immunity

Sex steroid hormones exert effects on immune responses. Overall, progesterone is associated with tumor suppression, allowing for immunological escape for HPV infected cells. Estradiol seems to be associated with an increased immune defense. During pregnancy, the natural killer cell activity is suppressed, indicating a decreased immunological response. The clinical role of such findings is unclear.

In an early study, progesterone and glucocorticoid response elements were identified in the long region of several types of the HPV genome, and administration of progestins increased expression of the oncogenes E6 and E7, considered crucial in cell transformation [63] . In another study on HPV positive cell lines, progesterone treatment enhanced the colony formation, while no effect was observed on HPV negative cell lines [64]. These studies on human cell lines support the notion that progesterone is the major sex steroid co-factor in cervical cancer. It was, however, also reported that estrogen treatment stimulated HPV 16 transcripts in another cell line, while progesterone did not [65]. Finally, p53 expression was increased in HPV cervical cancer cell lines after treatment with high doses of estradiol, a favorable effect, but not with low or medium doses, a possible favorable effect in tumor suppression [66].

Serum levels of progesterone and estradiol

The idea of studying cervical neoplasms by correlating clinical variables to serum hormone levels is attracting as it reflects physiologic conditions. We performed two studies on premenopausal women with cancer. Outcome in the first experimental study was S-phase fraction in tissue, a marker of proliferation. High serum progesterone, but not estradiol, levels directly correlated to a high S-phase fraction and after adjustment for eight variables, only serum progesterone and smoking emerged significantly correlated to proliferation [67].

In a clinical study, mortality was studied and adjustment was made for a number of variables, e.g. clinical cancer stage, the most important variable for prognosis. Premenopausal women, who eventually died from cervical cancer, with high serum estradiol showed increased survival-months, compared to those with low serum estradiol, while women with high progesterone levels showed decreased survival-months than those with low levels. A estradiol-progesterone ratio was constructed and the combination of high estradiol and low progesterone correlated significantly to a longer survival, and vice verse [68].

We performed two studies, one clinical and one laboratory, where the above criteria were taken care of. In both studies, all women were analysed together, and pre- and postmenopausal women were also analysed separately. Analyses in the former group showed no differences regarding the variables included, and results were presented only for the premenopausal group. Outcome was S-phase fraction, i.e. the percentage of dividing cells in the cancer tissue that is a marker of proliferation and cancer growth. Close to all tumors where serum progesterone was high, had a high S-phase fraction. There were no correlations to serum estradiol levels and after adjustment for eight variables, only serum progesterone and smoking emerged significantly correlated to proliferation. This supports the theory that progestins are promoters of cancer growth and correlated to poor prognosis [67].

In a clinical study, women with high serum estradiol, but who eventually died from the disease, however, showed increased survival-months, compared to those with low serum estradiol, but this was nonsignificant. Women with high progesterone levels, on the other hand, showed decreased survival-months than those with low levels. A estradiol-progesterone ratio was constructed and the combination of high estradiol and low progesterone increased the prognosis prediction [68].

To find evidence that estradiol or progesterone correlates to CIN grade a study where both cases and controls were HPV positive was conducted. None of the hormones measured did correlate to lesions more or equal to CIN2 compared to low-grade CIN. Serum levels of sex steroids thus have not proved to be useful in distinguishing low- and high-grade lesions [69].

We evaluated tumor marker expression and serum progesterone levels in CIN, and found a significantly higher expression of Cox-2, low retinoblastoma protein (tumor suppressor) and low p16 (tumor suppressor) expression with high progesterone levels, the former were independent of CIN grade. No correlations between serum estradiol and tumor marker expressions were found. It could be concluded that progesterone levels CIN are associated with a negative tumor marker pattern, as was the case in oral contraceptive users [70]. In summary, available results indicate that oral contraceptives and high serum progesterone levels exert unfavorable effects in CIN, both epidemiologically and in laboratory studies, while the role of estrogens are unclear [70].

5. References

[1] Gustafsson L, Ponten J, Bergstrom R, Adami HO. International incidence rates of invasive cervical cancer before cytological screening. Int J Cancer 1997;71:159-65.

[2] Sankaranarayanan R, Ferlay J. Worldwide burden of gynaecological cancer: the size of the problem. Best Pract Res Clin Obstet Gynaecol 2006;20:207-25.

[3] Laara E, Day NE, Hakama M. Trends in mortality from cervical cancer in the Nordic countries: association with organised screening programmes. Lancet 1987;1:1247-9.

[4] Hakama M, Rasanen-Virtanen U. Effect of a mass screening program on the risk of cervical cancer. Am J Epidemiol 1976;103:512-7.

[5] Fidler HK, Boyes DA, Worth AJ. Cervical cancer detection in British Columbia. A progress report. J Obstet Gynaecol Br Commonw 1968;75:392-404.

[6] Andrae B, Kemetli L, Sparen P, et al. Screening-preventable cervical cancer risks: evidence from a nationwide audit in Sweden. J Natl Cancer Inst 2008;100:622-9.

[7] National Board of Health and Welfare. Cancer incidence in Sweden. Official statistic of Sweden 2008.

[8] Cancer incidence in Sweden. National Board of Health and Welfare. Official statistic of sweden 2008.

[9] Gasparini R, Panatto D. Cervical cancer: from Hippocrates through Rigoni-Stern to zur Hausen. Vaccine 2009;27 Suppl 1:A4-5.

[10] De Palo G. Cervical precancer and cancer, past, present and future. Eur J Gynaecol Oncol 2004;25:269-78.

[11] Nyberg R, Tornberg B, Westin B. Colposcopy and Schiller's iodine test as an aid in the diagnosis of malignant and premalignant lesions of the squamous epithelium of the cervix uteri. Acta Obstet Gynecol Scand 1960;39:540-56.

[12] Grigsby PW, Herzog TJ. Current management of patients with invasive cervical carcinoma. Clin Obstet Gynecol 2001;44:531-7.

[13] Gaffney DK, Erickson-Wittmann BA, Jhingran A, et al. ACR Appropriateness Criteria(R) on Advanced Cervical Cancer Expert Panel on Radiation Oncology-Gynecology. Int J Radiat Oncol Biol Phys 2011.

[14] Salani R, Backes FJ, Fung Kee Fung M, et al. Posttreatment surveillance and diagnosis of recurrence in women with gynecologic malignancies: Society of Gynecologic Oncologists recommendations. Am J Obstet Gynecol 2011;204:466-78.

[15] Nuovo J, Melnikow J, Willan AR, Chan BK. Treatment outcomes for squamous intraepithelial lesions. Int J Gynaecol Obstet 2000;68:25-33.

[16] Borysiewicz LK, Fiander A, Nimako M, et al. A recombinant vaccinia virus encoding human papillomavirus types 16 and 18, E6 and E7 proteins as immunotherapy for cervical cancer. Lancet 1996;347:1523-7.

[17] Koutsky LA, Ault KA, Wheeler CM, et al. A controlled trial of a human papillomavirus type 16 vaccine. N Engl J Med 2002;347:1645-51.

[18] Munoz N, Bosch FX, de Sanjose S, et al. Epidemiologic classification of human papillomavirus types associated with cervical cancer. N Engl J Med 2003;348:518-27.

[19] Trottier H, Franco EL. Human papillomavirus and cervical cancer: burden of illness and basis for prevention. Am J Manag Care 2006;12:S462-72.

[20] Syrjanen SM, Syrjanen KJ. New concepts on the role of human papillomavirus in cell cycle regulation. Ann Med 1999;31:175-87.

[21] Viscidi RP, Snyder B, Cu-Uvin S, et al. Human papillomavirus capsid antibody response to natural infection and risk of subsequent HPV infection in HIV-positive and HIV-negative women. Cancer Epidemiol Biomarkers Prev 2005;14:283-8.
[22] Smith JS, Lindsay L, Hoots B, et al. Human papillomavirus type distribution in invasive cervical cancer and high-grade cervical lesions: a meta-analysis update. Int J Cancer 2007;121:621-32.
[23] Samir R, Asplund A, Tot T, Pekar G, Hellberg D. High-Risk HPV Infection and CIN Grade Correlates to the Expression of c-myc, CD4+, FHIT, E-cadherin, Ki-67, and p16INK4a. J Low Genit Tract Dis 2011.
[24] Munger K, Baldwin A, Edwards KM, et al. Mechanisms of human papillomavirus-induced oncogenesis. J Virol 2004;78:11451-60.
[25] Naguib SM, Lundin FE, Jr., Davis HJ. Relation of various epidemiologic factors to cervical cancer as determined by a screening program. Obstet Gynecol 1966;28:451-9.
[26] Hellberg D. Smoking and cervical cancer. in Research focus on smoking and women´s health, eds Tolson, KP and Veksler EB 2008:19-60.
[27] Harris RW, Brinton LA, Cowdell RH, et al. Characteristics of women with dysplasia or carcinoma in situ of the cervix uteri. Br J Cancer 1980;42:359-69.
[28] La Vecchia C, Franceschi S, Decarli A, Fasoli M, Gentile A, Tognoni G. Cigarette smoking and the risk of cervical neoplasia. Am J Epidemiol 1986;123:22-9.
[29] Lyon JL, Gardner JW, West DW, Stanish WM, Hebertson RM. Smoking and carcinoma in situ of the uterine cervix. Am J Public Health 1983;73:558-62.
[30] Trevathan E, Layde P, Webster LA, Adams JB, Benigno BB, Ory H. Cigarette smoking and dysplasia and carcinoma in situ of the uterine cervix. JAMA 1983;250:499-502.
[31] Ylitalo N, Sorensen P, Josefsson A, et al. Smoking and oral contraceptives as risk factors for cervical carcinoma in situ. Int J Cancer 1999;81:357-65.
[32] Brinton LA, Schairer C, Haenszel W, et al. Cigarette smoking and invasive cervical cancer. JAMA 1986;255:3265-9.
[33] Kjaer SK, Engholm G, Dahl C, Bock JE. Case-control study of risk factors for cervical squamous cell neoplasia in Denmark. IV: role of smoking habits. Eur J Cancer Prev 1996;5:359-65.
[34] Nischan P, Ebeling K, Schindler C. Smoking and invasive cervical cancer risk. Results from a case-control study. Am J Epidemiol 1988;128:74-7.
[35] de Vet HC, Sturmans F. Risk factors for cervical dysplasia: implications for prevention. Public Health 1994;108:241-9.
[36] Appleby P, Beral V, Berrington de Gonzalez A, et al. Carcinoma of the cervix and tobacco smoking: collaborative reanalysis of individual data on 13,541 women with carcinoma of the cervix and 23,017 women without carcinoma of the cervix from 23 epidemiological studies. Int J Cancer 2006;118:1481-95.
[37] Franceschi S. The IARC commitment to cancer prevention: the example of papillomavirus and cervical cancer. Recent Results Cancer Res 2005;166:277-97.
[38] Baldwin RL, Green JW, Shaw JL, et al. Physician risk attitudes and hospitalization of infants with bronchiolitis. Acad Emerg Med 2005;12:142-6.
[39] Plummer M, Herrero R, Franceschi S, et al. Smoking and cervical cancer: pooled analysis of the IARC multi-centric case--control study. Cancer Causes Control 2003;14:805-14.

[40] Roteli-Martins CM, Panetta K, Alves VA, Siqueira SA, Syrjanen KJ, Derchain SF. Cigarette smoking and high-risk HPV DNA as predisposing factors for high-grade cervical intraepithelial neoplasia (CIN) in young Brazilian women. Acta Obstet Gynecol Scand 1998;77:678-82.

[41] Rajeevan MS, Swan DC, Nisenbaum R, et al. Epidemiologic and viral factors associated with cervical neoplasia in HPV-16-positive women. Int J Cancer 2005;115:114-20.

[42] Kjellberg L, Hallmans G, Ahren AM, et al. Smoking, diet, pregnancy and oral contraceptive use as risk factors for cervical intra-epithelial neoplasia in relation to human papillomavirus infection. Br J Cancer 2000;82:1332-8.

[43] Sasson IM, Haley NJ, Hoffmann D, Wynder EL, Hellberg D, Nilsson S. Cigarette smoking and neoplasia of the uterine cervix: smoke constituents in cervical mucus. N Engl J Med 1985;312:315-6.

[44] Hellberg D, Nilsson S, Haley NJ, Hoffman D, Wynder E. Smoking and cervical intraepithelial neoplasia: nicotine and cotinine in serum and cervical mucus in smokers and nonsmokers. Am J Obstet Gynecol 1988;158:910-3.

[45] Hellberg D, Nilsson S. Smoking and cancer of the ovary. N Engl J Med 1988;318:782-3.

[46] Holly EA, Petrakis NL, Friend NF, Sarles DL, Lee RE, Flander LB. Mutagenic mucus in the cervix of smokers. J Natl Cancer Inst 1986;76:983-6.

[47] Prokopczyk B, Cox JE, Hoffmann D, Waggoner SE. Identification of tobacco-specific carcinogen in the cervical mucus of smokers and nonsmokers. J Natl Cancer Inst 1997;89:868-73.

[48] Waggoner SE, Wang X. Effect of nicotine on proliferation of normal, malignant, and human papillomavirus-transformed human cervical cells. Gynecol Oncol 1994;55:91-5.

[49] Wentz WB, Reagan JW, Fu YS, Heggie AD, Anthony DD. Experimental studies of carcinogenesis of the uterine cervix in mice. Gynecol Oncol 1981;12:S90-7.

[50] Sizemore N, Mukhtar H, Couch LH, Howard PC, Rorke EA. Differential response of normal and HPV immortalized ectocervical epithelial cells to B[a]P. Carcinogenesis 1995;16:2413-8.

[51] Melikian AA, Wang X, Waggoner S, Hoffmann D, El-Bayoumy K. Comparative response of normal and of human papillomavirus-16 immortalized human epithelial cervical cells to benzo[a]pyrene. Oncol Rep 1999;6:1371-6.

[52] Yang X, Jin G, Nakao Y, Rahimtula M, Pater MM, Pater A. Malignant transformation of HPV 16-immortalized human endocervical cells by cigarette smoke condensate and characterization of multistage carcinogenesis. Int J Cancer 1996;65:338-44.

[53] Nakao Y, Yang X, Yokoyama M, Pater MM, Pater A. Malignant transformation of human ectocervical cells immortalized by HPV 18: in vitro model of carcinogenesis by cigarette smoke. Carcinogenesis 1996;17:577-83.

[54] Samir R, Asplund A, Tot T, Pekar G, Hellberg D. Tissue tumor marker expression in smokers, including serum cotinine concentrations, in women with cervical intraepithelial neoplasia or normal squamous cervical epithelium. Am J Obstet Gynecol 2010;202:579 e1-7.

[55] Harris TG, Kulasingam SL, Kiviat NB, et al. Cigarette smoking, oncogenic human papillomavirus, Ki-67 antigen, and cervical intraepithelial neoplasia. Am J Epidemiol 2004;159:834-42.

[56] Lindstrom AK, Ekman K, Stendahl U, et al. LRIG1 and squamous epithelial uterine cervical cancer: correlation to prognosis, other tumor markers, sex steroid hormones, and smoking. Int J Gynecol Cancer 2008;18:312-7.
[57] Lindstrom AK, Stendahl U, Tot T, Hellberg D. Associations between ten biological tumor markers in squamous cell cervical cancer and serum estradiol, serum progesterone and smoking. Anticancer Res 2007;27:1401-6.
[58] Castellsague X, Munoz N. Chapter 3: Cofactors in human papillomavirus carcinogenesis--role of parity, oral contraceptives, and tobacco smoking. J Natl Cancer Inst Monogr 2003:20-8.
[59] Hellberg D, Valentin J, Nilsson S. Long-term use of oral contraceptives and cervical neoplasia: an association confounded by other risk factors? Contraception 1985;32:337-46.
[60] Sikstrom B, Hellberg D, Nilsson S, Brihmer C, Mardh PA. Contraceptive use and reproductive history in women with cervical human papillomavirus infection. Adv Contracept 1995;11:273-84.
[61] Silins I, Kallings I, Dillner J. Correlates of the spread of human papillomavirus infection. Cancer Epidemiol Biomarkers Prev 2000;9:953-9.
[62] Veress G, Csiky-Meszaros T, Czegledy J, Gergely L. Oral contraceptive use and human papillomavirus infection in women without abnormal cytological results. Med Microbiol Immunol 1992;181:181-9.
[63] Chan WK, Klock G, Bernard HU. Progesterone and glucocorticoid response elements occur in the long control regions of several human papillomaviruses involved in anogenital neoplasia. J Virol 1989;63:3261-9.
[64] Yuan F, Auborn K, James C. Altered growth and viral gene expression in human papillomavirus type 16-containing cancer cell lines treated with progesterone. Cancer Invest 1999;17:19-29.
[65] Mitrani-Rosenbaum S, Tsvieli R, Tur-Kaspa R. Oestrogen stimulates differential transcription of human papillomavirus type 16 in SiHa cervical carcinoma cells. J Gen Virol 1989;70 (Pt 8):2227-32.
[66] Correa I, Cerbon MA, Salazar AM, Solano JD, Garcia-Carranca A, Quintero A. Differential p53 protein expression level in human cancer-derived cell lines after estradiol treatment. Arch Med Res 2002;33:455-9.
[67] Lindstrom A, Backstrom T, Hellberg D, Tribukait B, Strang P, Stendahl U. Correlations between serum progesterone and smoking, and the growth fraction of cervical squamous cell carcinoma. Anticancer Res 2000;20:3637-40.
[68] Hellberg D, Lindstrom AK, Stendahl U. Correlation between serum estradiol/progesterone ratio and survival length in invasive squamous cell cervical cancer. Anticancer Res 2005;25:611-6.
[69] Shields TS, Falk RT, Herrero R, et al. A case-control study of endogenous hormones and cervical cancer. Br J Cancer 2004;90:146-52.
Samir R, Tot T, Asplund A, Pekar G, Hellberg D. Increased serum progesterone and estradiol correlate to increased COX-2 tissue expression in cervical intraepithelial neoplasia. Anticancer Res 2010;30:1217-22.
[70] Samir R, Tot T, Asplund A, Pekar G, Hellberg D. Increased serum progesterone and estradiol correlate to increased COX-2 tissue expression in cervical intraepithelial neoplasia. Anticancer Res 2010;30:1217-22.

11

P16INK4A and MIB-1 Expression in Preneoplasia and Neoplasia of Cervix

Supriya Srivastava
Cancer Science Institute, National University Singapore, Singapore

1. Introduction

Cervical cancer is the third most common cancer and fourth most common cause of cancer related deaths in female population, accounting to approximately 453,300 cases per year and 275,100 deaths in the year 2008. According to the latest WHO global cancer statistics, the cumulative risk (%) (Age 0-74) of cervical carcinoma is 0.9 with age adjusted ratio of 9.0 (Jemal et al., 2011). In India, cervical cancer is the leading cancer among females between 15 and 44 years of age. Current estimates indicate that every year 132,082 women are diagnosed with cervical cancer and that 74,118 die from this disease in India alone (http://www.who.int/hpv). Having said this, however, no form of cancer better documents the remarkable effects of prevention, early diagnosis, and curative therapy on the mortality rate than the cancer of cervix. However, the still very high rate of cervical carcinoma in developing countries like India is because of lack of proper screening methods and lack of health infrastructure which allows for periodical and routine screening. Potential threat of cancer has reduced significantly in developed countries, due to Papanicolaou smear screening programs. Papanicolaou smears or commonly referred as Pap smears is a cost effective and reproducible screening technique for diagnosing precursor lesions of cervical carcinoma. However, Pap test gives significant false positive (30%) (Sherman et al., 1994) and false negative (15-50%) results due to subjective test criteria (Arbyn et al., 2008). Apart from the Pap smear screening test, histopathological diagnosis of cervical intraepithelial neoplasias (CINs) and cervical carcinoma is considered as the age old "gold standard" method of diagnosis of cervical neoplasms. However this can also be biased by interobserver variability as reported before (Stoler & Schiffman, 2001). These factors limit, present screening programs and histopathological examination and emphasizes the need for the identification of specific biomarkers for dysplastic epithelial cells to aid in primary screening and lesion diagnosis.

2. Cervical Intraepithelial Neoplasia (CIN)

Invasive squamous cell carcinoma of cervix is preceded by precancerous changes in the cervical epithelium which can be identified histologically. These precancerous lesions are usually described as Cervical Intraepithelial Neoplasia (Buckley et al., 1982). Papanicolaou classification, using the terms '**atypical cells with abnormal features**' has been adhered to, until recently by some cytologists and gynaecologists. In 1953 Reagan *et al.* proposed the term "**dysplasia**" to replace atypical metaplasia and atypical hyperplasia. Ritton and Christopherson defined the normal and abnormal cells of cervical and vaginal smears in the WHO International classification (1973). The conventional histological terminology of mild, moderate and severe dysplasia and carcinoma in situ was used as well as atypical metaplasia. The British Society for clinical cytology's first Working party on terminology recommended the term "**dyskaryosis**", originally coined by Papanicolaou and translated from the Greek meaning "abnormal nucleus", to describe cells from preinvasive and invasive cancer (Spriggs et al., 1978). In 1986, in a further review, dyskaryosis remained the recommended term, but it was classified as *mild, moderate* and *severe*.

The 1988 Bethesda System for reporting Cervical/Vaginal Cytologic Diagnoses was published by a Workshop of North American Experts convened by the Division of Cancer Prevention and Control of the National Cancer Institute to review existing terminology and to recommend effective methods of reporting. It agreed that the Papanicolaou classification was no longer appropriate and proposed the **Bethesda System,** which recommends three essential components of a cervical or vaginal smear report. It includes a new term, **Squamous intraepithelial neoplasia** (SIL) which is divided into two grades, **low grade SIL** (cells from HPV and CIN-I) and **high grade SIL** (cells from CIN II and CIN III) (Broder et al., 1991). A Bethesda workshop was held in 2001 with further modifications. The descriptions of cytological appearances of the cells of precancerous conditions of the cervix are best understood in relation to the well defined three histological grades of CIN (Solomon et al., 2002).

2.1 Low grade Squamous Intraepithelial Lesion (LSIL)

In LSIL the cells are mature squamous cells, they retain their polygonal shape and for the most part retain their normal size with a peripheral rim of dense cytoplasm. The nuclei are enlarged at least 3-4 times that of the normal intermediate cell nucleus, however, when HPV changes are evident, the cells may be smaller (almost parakeratotic) and the nuclei may also be smaller and somewhat pyknotic appearing with binucleation and/or multinucleation. These pyknotic nuclei also exhibit abnormal features such as hyperchromasia, increased size from that of the normal superficial squamous cell and a slight variation in shape and size. The chromatin appears finely to coarsely granular and is evenly distributed. It is important to stress that an interpretation of LSIL/HPV requires both clear-cut cytoplasmic cavitations accompanied by the abnormal nuclear morphology described above.

Differential diagnoses

Reactive

The cells appear single or in sheets, like LSIL, however unlike LSIL, where only mature squamous cells are affected, in reactive types, all the cells may be affected. The nuclei, may be enlarged from 1.5 to 2 times; bi or multinucleation may be present and the nuclear membrane appear smooth. The chromatin is finely granular, evenly distributed and hyperchromasia may not be evident. The nucleoli are uniform and may be multiple in numbers. Peri-nuclear halo is often present, small and multiple vacuoles may be evident due to degeneration

Reparative changes

The cells appear in flat sheets or groups. Predominantly, endocervical or metaplastic cells are affected. The nuclear size may be variable, ranging from slight to marked enlargement. The nuclei may be bi or multinucleated, and the nuclear membranes appear smooth. The chromatin is finely granular and evenly distributed and hyperchromasia may not be evident. The nucleoli are small to conspicuous and often multiple. The cytoplasm appears vacuolated.

2.2 High grade Intraepithelial Lesion (HSIL)

The criteria for HSIL on the ThinPrep® Pap Test are as follows: The single, most important criterion for HSIL is the presence of asymmetrical 3-D nuclear structural abnormalities. This is a concept that must be clearly understood in order to master the interpretation of HSIL. There will be an abnormality in the structure of the dysplastic nucleus that can be thoroughly appreciated only by focusing up and down on the individual cell. A normal nucleus has a relatively round or ovoid shape and its surface is smooth. A dysplastic cell will have humps, bumps, corrugations, crevices, and strange protuberances. These very distinctive abnormalities are the essence of dysplasia, particularly HSIL. This is the very detail that is most often lost in conventional cytology due to the various artefacts of fixation and staining that limit the ability to interpret these conventional smears. These 3-D nuclear structural abnormalities are to be distinguished from simple, "irregular nuclear outlines" which will often be present as a two-dimensional phenomenon in benign cells on the ThinPrep® Pap Tests.

These 3-D structural abnormalities may not be present in every dysplastic cell on the slide, but they will be obvious in at least some cells somewhere on the slides. Obviously, the ability to see "into" the nucleus of a cell is going to be directly related to the quality of staining. Also, these 3-D structural defects should be asymmetrical, as opposed to nuclear grooves or simple creases that involve the full breadth of the nucleus occasionally creating a difficult "look-alike". The presence of these exaggerated nuclear 3-D abnormalities establishes the diagnosis of HSIL.

Apart from above the N/C ratio is the most reliable indicator of degree (moderate, severe, CIS). With an increasing degree of dysplasia, there is a predictable increasing N/C ratio. This abnormal N/C ratio can be considered a major criterion for the diagnosis of HSIL. However, there are rare exceptions, and ultimately the diagnosis must be made on nuclear changes alone.

Gland neck involvement in HSIL has a distinct appearance on the ThinPrep Pap Test and can be differentiated from lesions of glandular origin. SIL in glands presents predominantly in sheets with increased depth of focus. The cytoplasm is finely vacuolated which initially may give the impression of a glandular process, but on closer inspection these sheets exhibit no glandular differentiation such as basal nuclei, crowded columnar formations, pseudostratification, nor feathered edges or rosettes. These sheets of cells can be deceptively flat, but the nuclei retain the same qualities of SIL that are described above. Because these cells are in sheets and usually are small with no other "clues" of HSIL - only subtle 3-D deformities, they can be the most difficult to identify and evaluate. An important factor in determining whether or not these cells are squamous or glandular in origin is the company they keep. Most of the time these cells will be accompanied by definitely dysplastic squamous epithelial cells.

2.3 Atypical Squamous Cells of Undetermined Significance (ASCUS)

ASCUS in the reproductive woman is defined by a number of criteria. The principal one is nuclear size using either an intermediate squamous cell nucleus or a mature metaplastic squamous cell nucleus as the reference standard. An ASCUS nucleus is 2.5 to 3 times the size of an intermediate cell nucleus or 1.5 times the size of a mature metaplastic cell nucleus. Hyperchromasia is commonly present, nucleoli are not prominent. These nuclear features are most important in diagnosing ASCUS.

3. Etiology of CIN and cervical carcinoma

There are various etiological factors leading to CIN and eventually to cervical carcinoma. Active and passive smoking (Brinton et al., 1986), dietary deficiencies (Butterworth et al., 1992), immunosupression (Zur-Hausen, 1993) and sexually associated factors are a few to name. Among these, sexually associated factors (SAF) are the most important in pathogenesis of cervical carcinoma and CIN. Multiple sexual partners, early marriage (Munoz & Bosch, 1989), male sexual behaviour (Brinton et al., 1989), concurrent penile cancer in males (Li et al., 1982) and sexually transmitted diseases are strongly associated with the development of carcinoma. Viral infections with Herpes simplex virus- 2 (HSV-2) (Fenoglio et al., 1982) and Human Papilloma Virus (HPV) has been implicated and studied extensively in the etiopathogenesis of cervical carcinoma and CIN (Meisels et al., 1981)

3.1 Role of HPV in etiology of cervical neoplasia

Innumerable experimental studies have provided strong evidence that HPV is the long sought venereal cause of cervical neoplasia. These viruses are double stranded DNA viruses (Baltimore Class I) and have been included traditionally in the Papovaviridae (Tomita et al., 1987). HPV is a double stranded Papilloma virus; 70 different types of which are known. Many different HPV types associated with cervical neoplasia have been discovered and around twenty types of HPV are commonly known to infect the human genital tract. These are HPV 6, 11, 16, 18, 30, 31, 33, 34, 35, 39, 40, 42, 51-58 (Crum et al., 1991). However they have been divided into high- and low-risk categories based on their association with invasive cervical carcinoma (Lorincz et al., 1992). Of this HPV 16, 18 and 31 are more commonly implicated in cervical carcinoma (Zur- Hausen, 1991). Experimental data indicate that viral E6 and E7 genes of high-risk HPV E7 protein specifically bind to and inactivate pRB (retinoblastoma gene product).

3.1.1 Structure of HPV

HPV-DNA consists of three different regions: early region (ER), late region (LR) and upstream regulatory regions (URR). The ER is composed of seven genes, E1-E8, that encodes proteins which play a significant role in viral replication and have oncogenic properties. The LR is composed of two genes L1 and L2, which encodes proteins required for assembly of infectious viral particles. The URR is the regulatory region. In preneoplastic lesion like CINs the HPV DNA is not integrated in host DNA, rather it is found in circular or episomal form. Briefly, the episomal HPV produces mostly the E2 protein. The E2 protein encodes for a DNA-binding protein that binds to a specific nucleotide motif found in E6 and E7 region (Ham et al., 1991) (Ward et al., 1989). There therefore the E2 regulates the expression of E6 and E7, so that only low level of these proteins is produced. The episomal form integrates into the host's chromosome at E1/E2 region, typically causing "break" in this region, giving rise to uncontrolled production and expression of E6 and E7 proteins and their high levels are produced. Scheffner et al have shown previously that E6 protein forms a complex with p53 tumor-suppressor gene product, leading to the degradation of p53. Crook et al studied the expression of p53 in several HPV-positive or HPV-negative cell lines, and found that the HPV-negative cell lines had a mutation in a single nucleotide (a point mutation) in the p53 mRNA. These findings suggest that the loss of the wild type p53 protein activity is important in the development of a malignant lesion, and this could be mediated either by point mutation or by the binding of HPV E6 protein to p53. The HPV E7 protein binds to retinoblastoma tumor-suppressor gene product and inactivates the p Rb (Scheffner et al., 1992). The degradation of p53 and functional inactivation of p Rb leads to cell cycle disruption and increased proliferation, ultimately giving rise to carcinoma.

3.1.2 HPV detection techniques

Detection of HPV DNA in CIN and cervical carcinoma is the most popular and well investigated biomarker in management of cervical neoplasia. Various techniques are used to detect DNA. These are:

1. Immunocytochemistry
2. Dot Blot assays
3. Southern Blot
4. In situ Hybridization
5. Hybrid Capture™ 2 (HC2) assay
6. Polymerase chain reaction (PCR) techniques
7. HPV genotyping
8. Immunocytochemical detection of L1 capsid protein.

Among the above mentioned In situ hybridization. HC2 assays and PCR are most commonly used methods to detect HPV. Currently according to the updated guidelines published by American Society for Colposcopy and Cervical Pathology (ASCCP), the "HPV testing" refers only to Hybrid Capture 2 test for high-risk types (HPV16 and 18) (Wright et al., 2007). The HC2 test is the only test presently approved by U. S. Food and Drug Administration.

4. Biomarkers in cervical neoplasia

Cytomorphological interpretation of Pap stained cervical smears is the mainstay of cytological evaluation of the human cervix. A wide array of potential biomarkers is being evaluated for the diagnostic usefulness of cervical cancer and its precursors. One of the needs to identify biomarkers in cervical neoplasia is to distinguish CIN from other non neoplastic cervical lesions, so as to prevent under treatment (Al Nafussi et al., 1990) or overtreatment (Creagh et al., 1995). Second purpose is, that since CIN is a dynamic process (not a static process), that can progress or regress, the conventional haematoxylin and eosin (H&E), gives a false impression of a static process. These points emphasize the need to identify and discover new markers that can aid in distinguishing CIN from other benign conditions and establish it as a dynamic process. Since HPV, disrupts the normal cell cycle, leading to cell death, a number of genes/ proteins are deregulated, thereby such genes/proteins can be used as surrogate diagnostic markers. In the past few years number of genes/proteins has been implicated as suitable biomarkers for cervical neoplasia. Two markers that have shown a potential in this direction are p16 INK4A and MIB1. p16 is a tumor suppressor protein, that is expressed in dysplastic cervical epithelial cells only, while MIB-1 is a marker of active dividing cells (basal and parabasal cells), normally not shed in cervical smears. Therefore presence of p16 and MIB-1 positivity in cervical Pap smear is marker of cervical dyskaryosis. Due to these reasons, p16 and MIB-1 have emerged as the most robust, stable and markers with strong predictive value.

4.1 P16INK4A

P16INK4A (inhibitor of kinase 4A), is a tumor suppressor protein and inhibitor of cyclin-dependant kinase 4 and 6 (CDK 4 and 6). The phosphorylation of pRB (retinoblastoma protein) is a molecular "ON–OFF" switch for the cell cycle. In the hypophosphorylated form, pRB binds to transcription factors (p 16) responsible for cell cycle progression. P16 inhibits the cyclin-dependant kinases and thereby prevents the phosphorylation of RB, keeping it in the hypophosphorylated form, i.e. its active form. However, in HPV infection, the viral gene E7 binds to RB protein and functionally inactivates it. This results in accumulation of p16 protein because, normally, RB inhibits the transcription of p16 (Keating, 2001; Klaes, 2001; Sano, 1998). Because this protein is not expressed in the normal cervical epithelium, p16 overexpression allows to specifically identify dysplastic lesions and will reduce interobserver disagreement of conventional histological or cytological tests.

4.1.1 P16INK4A as a diagnostic biomarker in cervical neoplasia

p16 INK4a is a tumor suppressor protein (cyclin dependant kinase inhibitor) which is known to play a critical role as a negative regulator of cell cycle progression and differentiation by controlling the activity of tumor suppressor protein pRb. We performed a study on the role of p16 and MIB-1 in cervical intraepithelial neoplasia. Our hypothesis was that normal cervical epithelium does not express p16 INK 4a and MIB-1 and there is upregulation of these biomarkers in CINs and cervical carcinomas. We evaluated p16 and MIB-1 in 63 cervical biopsies and corresponding Pap smears. p16INK 4A immunostaining was done using Mouse monoclonal antibody RTU-p16-432 (Novocastra, Lab. Ltd., Newcastle, Tyne, NE 128EW, UK, in all study groups. Immunopositive was considered when there was Either diffuse, strong nuclear and cytoplasmic staining, or focal moderate to weak nuclear staining of tumor cells. p16 INK4A immunohistochemistry revealed that there was a significant over expression and upregulation in different groups and as we move from normal cervical epithelia to dysplasia of varying severity to carcinoma, the p16 positivity was increased. p16 INK4A over expression was seen in all CIN I lesions (15/15), all CIN II lesions (15/15), all CIN III lesions (3/3) and all cases of carcinoma cervix (15/15) of tissue biopsies. In Pap smears p16 positivity was seen in CIN I/LSIL (8/10), CIN II/HSIL (5/5), CIN III/HSIL (3/3) and Ca cervix (15/15). No detectable p16 expression was observed in normal cervical epithelium in both pap smears and tissue biopsies. This was found to be statistically significant finding on making a comparison between control versus different groups ($p<0.05$). However, on making an inter group comparison this was found to be statistically insignificant ($p>0.05$). p16 basically is a nuclear protein hence immunohistochemistry should show nuclear staining. However in dysplasia both nuclear and cytoplasmic staining with p16 is observed possibly because of post transcriptional modification or overproduction of p16 protein forcing its transfer into the cytoplasm (Murphy *et al.*, 2002). In our study it was seen that p16 over-expression was restricted to CIN I, II, III and carcinoma cervix and increased in the same order. Therefore, p16 immunostaining allowed precise identification of even small CIN or cervical cancer lesions in biopsy sections and Pap smears and helped to reduce interobserver variation and also reduce false positive and false negative interpretation and thereby significantly improve cervical cancer and precancer detection (Srivastava, 2010). In our study p16 positivity was 15 of 15 (100%) in invasive carcinoma cervix and it was seen that with increasing severity of CINs, p16 positivity increased. Similar results were seen in a study by Murphy *et al.* who observed 100% p16 positivity in invasive SCC and significant linear relation ($p<0.0001$) between p16 staining and increasing grades of squamous dysplasia (Murphy *et al.*, 2002, 2005). We also observed that two Pap smears with LSIL showed negative p16 staining whereas it was positive in corresponding CIN lesion of their tissue section. p16 may be rarely negative in cervical dyskaryosis that may have important implications for the use of p16 staining as a standalone test and support the use of combination of markers of cervical dyskaryosis (Murphy *et al.* 2005). However in our study we did not find any dysplasia negative for p16 in tissues biopsies. p16 staining in LSIL was found to be negative in 20% of Pap smears, which could possibly be due to the technical error as their corresponding sections showed consistent positivity.

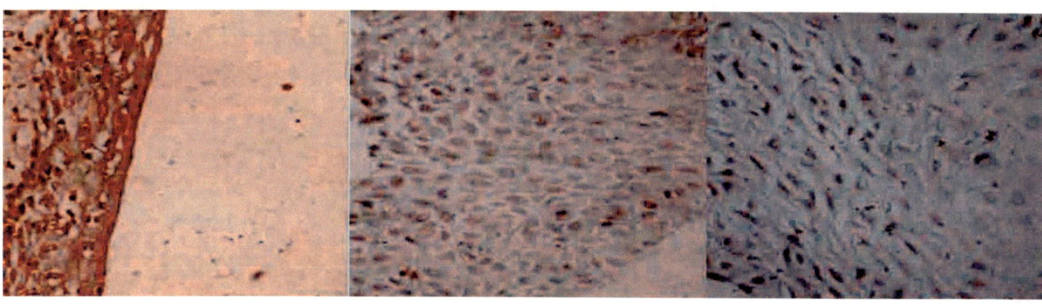

Fig. 1. Images of p16 immunostaining in Cervix tissue biopsy in CINI, CINIII, and Carcinoma cervix (40X)

A study conducted by Trigler *et al.*, in 2004, confirmed that the proportion of pRb positive cells was relatively decreased in premalignant and malignant lesions of the squamous and endocervical mucosa and showed a generally inverse correlation with the expression of p16 at the tissue level. This feedback loop is bypassed via viral E7 interaction and inactivation with pRb, causing p16 to be up regulated which can be detected immunohistochemically. p16 could therefore have a clinical utility as a biomarker because it is a measure of HPV gene expression and activity, rather than solely a detector of viral presence (Stanley 2002). Negri *et al.* in 2003 conducted a study to determine whether immunostaining of p16 is useful in detecting adenocarcinomas of cervix and its precursors in histologic & cytologic routine specimens. A total of 45 patients with glandular lesions including 18 cases of adenocarcinoma in situ (AIS), adenocarcinoma (n=8), endocervical glandular atypia (n=4) and reactive (n=15) lesions were identified. Furthermore, immunocytochemical analysis was performed on 10 Thin Prep Smears with abnormal glandular cells. P16 was detected immunohistochemically on all 26 cases of AIS and adenocarcinoma (100%). Also the immunocytochemical detection on thin prep specimens evidenced a strong expression of p16 in neoplastic endocervical cells. Prior to this study Mc Cluggage *et al.* (2003) investigated the value of p16 immunoreactivity in the distinction between endometrial and endocervical adenocarcinomas. Cases included in this study were endometrial adenocarcinomas of endometrioid type (n=29), and cervical adenocarcinomas of endocervical type (n=23). Twenty-two of 23 endocervical adenocarcinomas showed 100% positive tumor cells. The maximum number of endometrial adenocarcinomas, 9 of 29 showed 21-50% positive tumor cells. They concluded that diffuse strong positivity with p16 suggested an endocervical rather than an endometrial origin of an adenocarcinoma. Endometrial adenocarcinomas are usually positive, but positivity is generally focal and involves less than 50% of cells. Therefore, when there is a morphological doubt then this antibody may be of value as part of a panel for ascertaining the origin of an adenocarcinoma.

Determining the origin of uterine adenocarcinomas can be difficult in biopsy and curettage specimens because the morphologic spectrum of endocervical (ECA) and endometrial adenocarcinomas (EMA) overlap. Ansari Lari *et al.* in 2004 evaluated the utility of immunohistochemistry for P16 in the distinction of ECAs and EMAs. p16 expression was assessed in 24 unequivocal EMA's and 19 unequivocal ECA's and correlated with HPV DNA detected by ISH and PCR. p16 expression was moderate - strong and diffuse in 18 and weak and diffuse in 1 ECA. Fourteen of these were positive for HPV DNA. EMA's displayed weaker staining with patchy distribution and none contained HPV DNA by ISH. Compared with HPV DNA detected by *in situ* hybridization, p16 immunohistochemistry appears to be more sensitive and easier to perform, method for distinguishing ECAs from EMAs. It can be used to assist in the classification of lower uterine segment/endocervical adenocarcinomas of equivocal origin and should be evaluated for its utility in the prospective classification of uterine adenocarcinoma in curettage specimens prior to hysterectomy. Giovanni Negri *et al.* in 2004 evaluated the immunohistochemical expression of p16 as a marker of progression risk in low-grade dysplastic lesions of the cervix uteri. IHC was performed on 32 CIN-I with proven spontaneous regression of lesion in follow up (group A), 31 with progression to CIN-3 (group B) and 33 that were randomly chosen irrespective of the natural history of lesion (Group C). A diffuse staining was detected in 43.8% of CIN-I of group A, 74.2% of group B and 56.3% of group C. Overall 71.4% and 37.8% of p16 negative and diffusely positive CIN-I had regressed, at follow up, where as 26.6% and 62.2% negative and diffusely CIN-I were progressed to CIN-III ($p<0.05$). Although p16 may be expressed in low grade squamous lesion that undergoes spontaneous regression, in this study CIN-I cases with diffuse p16 staining had a significantly higher tendency to progress to a high grade lesion than p16 negative cases. Therefore, p16 may have the potential to support the interpretation of low grade dysplastic lesions of the cervix uteri. Sahebali *et al.* in 2004 examined the potential of p16 INK4a as a potential biomarker for cervical lesions in a study of liquid based cervical cytology. HPV DNA testing by MY09/MY11 consensus PCR and type specific PCRs and p16INK4a immunocytochemistry on a series of 291 patients selected from routine screening was done. Comparison of the number of p16 immunoreactive cells / 1000 cells exhibited a significantly higher mean count (8.80 ± 1.13) than other cytological groups. The mean count of LSIL (1.09 ± 0.18) was significantly higher than other negative groups. Atypical squamous cells, cannot exclude high grade squamous intraepithelial lesion (ASC-H) and HSIL combined showed a significantly higher mean count (6.46 ± 1.17) than negative

ASC, ASCUS and LSIL. Thus p16 immunocytochemistry can be used as an adjunct to LBC in cervical screening, because it has a good diagnostic accuracy to discriminate HSIL and ASC-H (atypical squamous cells - cannot exclude HSIL) from other lesions. It could be used as a surrogate marker of high risk infections.

Kalof *et al.* in 2005 studied the correlation between p16 immunoexpression, grades of CIN and HPV type in 44 cervical biopsies classified as CIN-I and CIN-II/III. In 22 of 25 CIN-I lesions, p16 immuno expression was confined to lower half of the epithelium with sporadic to focal staining in 11 of 25 cases. In CIN-II/III, 15 of 17 showed diffuse 2/3 to full thickness staining of the epithelial. hr HPV were found in 20 CIN-I lesions and 17 CIN-II/III lesions. Punctate signals were detected in 3 of hr HPV positive CIN-I lesions and 17 of 17 CIN-II/III lesions. They found that p16 immunoexpression and the presence of punctate signal on HPV in situ hybridization correlated with degree of cervical neoplasia ($p<0.001$). Thus both increased p16 immunoexpression and punctate signal correlates with CIN-II/III grade, supporting the use of either, or both tests to confirm CIN-II/III.

P16 can be used as a diagnostic marker along with other well known markers implicated in cervical neoplasia. N Murphy *et al.* in 2005 analysed and compared expression patterns of three potential biomarkers p16, CDC6 and MCM5 and evaluated their use as predictive biomarkers in squamous and glandular pre invasive neoplasia. 20 normal cervical biopsies, in addition to 38 CIN-I, 33 CIN-II, 46 CIN-III, 10 SCC, 19 CGIN and 10 adenocarcinoma were included in the study.. In all normal cases cervical epithelia were not stained. Dysplastic epithelial cells showed p16 staining in 100% of CIN-I, CIN-II, CIN-III, SCC and, adenocarcinoma. Simple linear regression analysis revealed a highly significant linear relation between p16 and increasing grades of squamous dysplasia. Among 3 markers p16 was the most reliable marker of cervical dysplasia. It marked all grades of squamous and glandular lesions of the cervix, and its expression was closely associated with high risk HPV infection. However, the failure of p16 to mark an isolated CIN-III case and staining of glandular mimics as tubo endometrioid metaplasia, may limit its use as a standalone test of cervical dysplasia. Thus a combination of dysplastic markers is suggested in difficult cases.

4.2 MIB-1 as a proliferation marker in cervical neoplasia

MIB-1 (Molecular Immunology Borstel) is an important diagnostic marker for CIN. Gerdes *et al.* in 1990 demonstrated that MIB-1 antibody detects Ki-67 antigen (in paraffin embedded biopsies) in G_1, S, G2 and M phase but is absent in G_0 phase. Baak et al formulated a "Stratification Index" (SI, which indicates, how high Ki-67 positive nuclei are located in the epithelium; the higher the SI, the higher the CIN grade) and the number of Ki-67 nuclei per 100 μm basal membrane (the more Ki-67 nuclei, the higher the grade) to distinguish the three CIN grades at the same time.

Ki-67 is an antigen expressed in proliferating cells (Brown, 2002) that can be detected in formalin fixed tissues using the MIB-1 antibody (Cattoretti et al., 1992). MIB-1 is an important immunocytochemical marker to assess the proliferation and has been suggested as a sensitive biological indicator of progression in CIN lesions by Van Hoven et al., 1997. We performed MIB-1 Immunohistochemistry along with p16 in 63 biopsies of cervical neoplasia and their corresponding Pap smears. MIB-I immunohistochemistry revealed that there was a significant over expression of MIB-1 in different groups and as we move from normal cervical epithelia to varying severity of CINs to carcinoma, the MIB-1 positivity increased. This was found to be statistically significant finding on making a comparison between control versus different groups ($p<0.05$). However, on making an intergroup comparison this was found to be statistically insignificant ($p>0.05$). MIB-1 antibody detects Ki-67 Antigen in G1, S, G2 and M phase but is absent in G0 phase. Therefore, this antibody may be a useful marker of proliferative activity of premalignant and malignant lesions of cervix. In our study we found that as we move from normal to carcinoma group via the varying degrees of CIN, labeling index of positively stained nuclei increased with the severity of CIN to carcinoma group. Review of published literature showed that Goel *et al.* (2005) have also observed similar results. Proliferative index was significantly increased in the carcinoma group in comparison with dysplasia. They showed the following trend for both MIB-1 and PCNA.

Normal $<$ LSIL $<$ HSIL $<$ Carcinoma

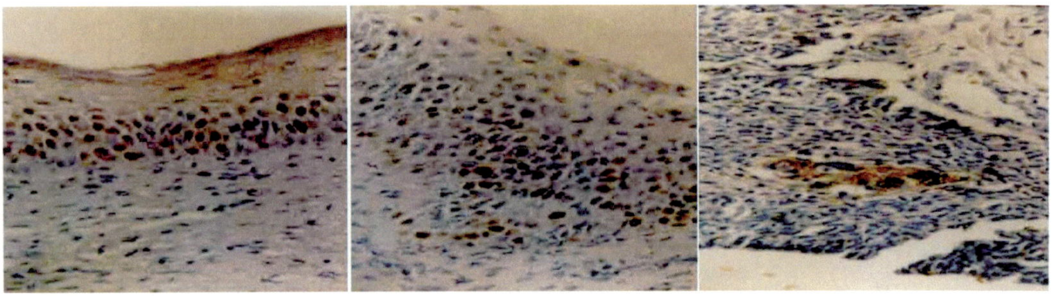

Fig. 2. Images of MIB-1 immunostaining in Cervix tissue biopsz in CINI, CINII, and Carcinoma cervix (40X)

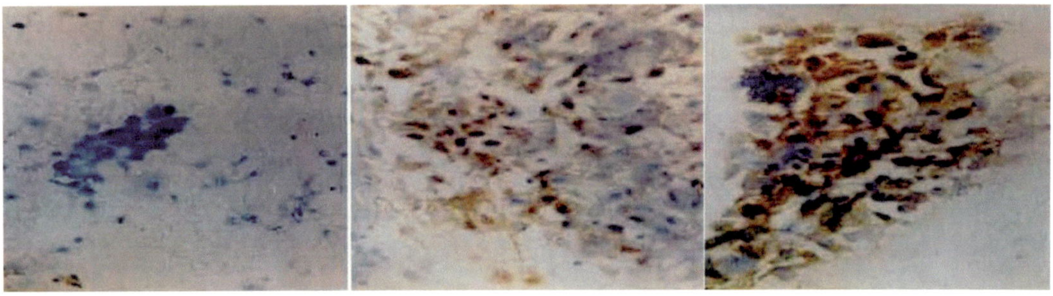

Fig. 3. Images of MIB-1 staining in Pap smears (40X)

In a study by Garzetti *et al.* (1996), MIB-1 immunostaining as an index of cellular proliferations in CIN and micro invasive carcinoma was analysed, with the aim to identify a relationship with the degree of dysplastic lesion and the risk of neoplastic progression. 41 cases of CIN, 23 cases of cervical condyloma, 22 of squamous metaplasia and 10 with micro invasive carcinoma were selected. It was shown that a) positive MIB-1 immunostaining increased progressively from squamous metaplasia to CIN and micro invasive carcinoma, ($p<0.001$) suggesting that neoplastic proliferation is associated with dysfunctional proliferation of cervical epithelium. b) Considering only CINs the MIB 1 index showed a significant increase with respect to CIN degrees, ($p<0.0001$). c) That there is a significant correlation between the MIB-1 index and CIN degree but not with respect to HPV DNA presence and d) that MIB-1 immunostaining might be useful for a clinical evaluation of mild and moderate dysplastic lesions. Gorstein et al in 2000 found that in cervical intraepithelial lesions associated with infection by HPV types 16 and 18, the expression of Ki 67 is greater than in lesions unrelated to viral presence.

Prior studies have suggested that Ki-67 (MIB-1) and p16 expression may be preferentially expressed in cervical neoplasia. However, a study conducted by Keating *et al.* in 2001, examined and compared the distribution of staining of these antigens in normal and reactive epithelial changes, diagnostically challenging cases (atypical metaplasia and atrophy) SIL, and high and low risk HPV, type specific SIL. Overall, a histologic diagnosis of SIL correlated strongly with these biomarkers used. Positive scores for Ki-67 and p16 were seen in 68.4% and 100% of LSILS and 94.7% and 100% of HSILs respectively.

P16 INK4a and Ki-67 biomarkers have been evaluated in conventional histopathological sections and more recently on Pap smears. However Akpolat ***et al.*** in 2004 evaluated the utility of P16 INK4a and Ki-67 staining on cell blocks prepared from residual thin layer cervicovaginal material. Results of cytological based thin prep Pap test were SCC (n=3), HSIL (n=27), LSIL (n=20), ASCUS (n=11), negative for malignancy (n=24). Results of cell blocks preparation were, SCC (n=2), HSIL (n=20), LSIL (n=30), negative for malignancy (n=32). In 62 cases (73%) the diagnosis made using cell blocks were in agreement with thin pap smears. The results indicate that cell blocks represent an additional reliable diagnostic tool in the evaluation of cervical samples[52]. Chisa Aoyama *et al.* in 2005 conducted a study to determine that histologic and immunohistochemical characteristics are useful for distinguishing neoplastic and non-neoplastic lesions. They classified atypical squamous lesion (ASL - a histologic diagnosis of unclear significance in the uterine cervix) (n=37) into neoplastic (n=19) and non-neoplastic (n=18) groups. They chose 7 histologic and IHC indicators to classify ASL. Mitosis, vertical nuclear growth pattern, no perinuclear halo, indistinct cytoplasmic border, primitive cells in the upper third of the squamous layer, p16+ cells in the upper 2/3 of squamous layer and Ki67 positive cells in upper 2/3 of squamous layer were significant indicators for neoplastic ASLs (5 or more of these 7 indicators). Out of 19 ASL, 16 had 5 or more of these indicators. Majority of non-neoplastic ASLs, 16/18 had 2 or fewer indicators.

In a study done by Goel *et al* in 2005, 49 adequate pap smears were stained for MIB-1 and PCNA. Out of 49 cases, 40 cases showed positive immunostaining with MIB-1 and PCNA. Proliferative labelling index of MIB-1 increased with ascending grades of CIN lesions to carcinoma. The highest proliferative index for MIB-1 was observed for the carcinoma group (PCNA-LI 39.200 ± 1.865; MIB–1 LI 35.300 ± 1.888). A significant positive correlation between ascending grades of SIL and LI of markers ($r=0.87$ for MIB-1 and $r=0.88$ for PCNA) was seen. This suggests that MIB-1 can be used as an adjunct to cytomorphological interpretation of conventional cervical Pap smear.

	Authors	Year	Number of cases	Results
1	Valasoulis et al	2011	95/LSIL smears	SS=41%;SP=86% PPV=62%;NPV=72%
2	Mendez et al		67/abnormal cytology	35.8% cases positive by p16 and associated with HPV
3	Samir et al	2011	188/pap smears	P16 correlates with increasing CIN grade
4	Balan et al	2010	20/LSIL, HSIL	P16 positive in 68% LSIL;84% CIN2;100%CIN3
5	Schmidt et al	2011	776/ASCUS, LSIL P16/Ki-67 dual stain cytology	SS=92.2% ASCUS; 94.2% LSIL SP=80.6% ASCUS;68% LSIL
6	Petry et al	2011	425/pap negative; HPV positive P16/Ki-67 dual stain cytology	25.4% positive; SS=91.9% for CIN2; 96.4% for CIN3 SP=82.1% for CIN2; 76.9%for CIN3
7	Alameda et al	2011	109/ frozen sections of ASCUS	SS=82.3%; SP=100%; NPV=94.5%; PPV=100% for HSIL
8	Passamonti et al	2011	91/ ASCUS;60 LSIL;36 ASCH;59 HSIL	46% ASCUS;53% LSIL
9	Srivastava et al	2010	63 /cervical biopsy and pap smears	P16 positive in increasing grades of CIN
10	Bolanca et al	2010	81/ cervical smears	33.3% of HPV positive cases showed p16 positivity
11	Oberg et al	2010	64/ LBC	86% agreement between ProEx C and p16

	Authors	Year	Number of cases	Results
12	Sung et al	2010	105/ ASC-H and ASC-US	P16 correlated significantly with SIL in ASC-H smears
13	Yu et al	2010	63 /cell blocks	HPV L1 and p16 expression increased with severity of cervical lesions
14.	Adamopoulou et al	2009	62 /abnormal pap smears and biopsies	P53, p16 and Bcl-2; SS=83.3%; SP=65.4%
15	Kurshumliu et al	2009	312/ pap smears	36.2% positive for p16
16	Haidopoulos et al	2009	62/abnormal pap smears	SS=100%; SP=76%; PPV=61%; NPV==100%
18	Dray *et al.*	2005	18/Biopsies 188/Thin pap smears	p16 +ve in HSIL, LSIL. -ve in inflammatory and reactive changes
20	Pientong *et al.*	2004	165/ pap smear 165/LBC	p16 +ve in 0/30, 21/40, 19/35, 30/30, 30/30 in normal, ASCUS, LSIL, HSIL, Ca.
21	Zielenskii *et al.*	2002	142/Biopsies of glandular neoplasia	All ACIS and ADCA were HPV positive therefore hr HPV testing is must in cervical cancer screening programme
22	Agoff *et al.*	2003	569/Biopsies	p16 and Ki67 correlated with cervical neoplasia and HPV
23	Klaes *et al.*	2002	194/Cervical biopsies	p16 improves the interobserver agreement in diagnosis of CIN

Table 1. Review of literature

LSIL, low grade squamous intraepithelial lesion; SS, sensitivity; SP, specificity; NPV, negative predictive value; PPV, positive predictive value; HPV, human Papilloma virus; CIN, cervical intraepithelial neoplasia; HSIL, high grade squamous intraepithelial lesion; ASCUS, atypical squamous cell of unknown significance; ASCH, atypical squamous cell cannot exclude high grade squamous intraepithelial neoplasia; LBC, liquid base cytology; ACIS, adenocarcinoma in situ; ADCA, adenocarcinoma

5. Conclusion

In a tropical country like India, any perimenopausal women presenting in gynaecological out patient department with any complaint is subjected to a single Pap smear test. However single Pap test is subject to suboptimal sensitivity limited reproducibility and many a times with high rate of false positive and false negative along with equivocal results. To compensate for the aforementioned deficiencies, a screening programme with repeated testing, and follow up of positive cases is warranted. Moreover, colposcopic performed biopsy is directed in any suspicious appearing acetowhite area. This subjects the patient to unnecessary surgical intervention. Therefore, additional diagnostic and prognostic markers for detection of cervical cancers precursors are required which could save the patients from surgical intervention and high screening cost associated with repeated testing.

Also, biomarkers that can help in screening, detection, diagnosis of the disease as well as predict the prognosis can aid the clinicians in correct management of the patients. P16 and MIB-1 are two such candidate markers that fit well in the above mentioned criteria. Through our study we have thus concluded that for LSIL, (because the sensitivity of the p16 marker is 80%), the marker should be evaluated together with MIB-1 or HPV test. For HSIL, the sensitivity and specificity of the p16 marker is 100% and thus it can be used as a stand-alone test. We also recommend that with a careful interpretation of immunostaining with morphological characteristic in the conventional Pap smears, the immunostaining with p16 and MIB-1 markers may be a diagnostic adjunct, reducing the need of tissue biopsy. This is simple, reliable and easily applicable in routine cytosmears. Having said this, there is still need of validation of these markers in a larger cohort and targeted population.

Acknowledgement: The author would like to acknowledge the help of the technical staff of the Department of Pathology, KGMU, Lucknow, India.

6. References

Adamopoulou M, Kalkani E, Charvalos E, Avgoustidis D, Haidopoulos D, Yapijakis C. Comparison of cytology, Colposcopy, HPV typing and biomarker analysis in cervical neoplasia. Anticancer Res. 2009 Aug; 29(8):3401-9.

Agoff et al. p16 expression correlates with degree of cervical neoplasia: A comparison of Ki67 expression and detection of high risk HPV types. Mod. Path. 2003; 16(7): 665-673.

Alameda F, Pijuan L, Lloveras B, Bellosillo B, Larrazabal F, Mancebo G, Muñoz R, Carreras R, Serrano S. The value of p16 in ASCUS cases: a retrospective study using frozen cytologic material. Diagn Cytopathol. 2011 Feb; 39(2):110-4.

AI Nafussi AI, Colquhoun MK. Mild cervical intraepithelial neoplasia (CIN-1)—a histological overdiagnosis. Histopathology 1990; 17:557–61.

Ansari L, Staebler A, Zaino R, Shah K, Ronnett B. Distinction of Endocervical and Endometrial Adenocarcinomas: Immunohistochemical p16 expression correlated with human Papilloma virus (HPV) DNA detection. Am J Surg Pathol 2004 Feb; 28(2): 160-167.

Akpolat I, Smith DA, Ramzy I, Chirala M, Mody DR. The utility of p16INK4a and Ki-67 staining on cell blocks prepared from residual thin-layer cervicovaginal material. Cancer.2004; 102(3):142-9.

Arbyn M, Bergeron C, Klinkhamer P, Martin-Hirsch P, Siebers AG, Bulten J. Liquid compared with conventional cervical cytology. A systematic review and meta-analysis. Obstet Gynecol 2008; 111:167–77.

Baak JPA, Kruse AJ, Robboy SJ, Janssen EAM, van Diermen B, Skaland I. Dynamic behavioural interpretation of cervical intraepithelial neoplasia with molecular markers. J Clin Pathol 2006;59: 1017–1028.

Balan R, Giuşcă S, Căruntu ID, Gheorghiță V, Neacşu D, Amălinei C. Immunochemical assessment of p16 and HPV L1 capsid protein in cervical squamous intraepithelial lesions. Rev Med Chir Soc Med Nat Iasi. 2010 Oct-Dec; 114(4):1118-24.

Bolanca IK, Sentija K, Simon SK, Kukura V, Vranes J. Estimating clinical outcome of HPV induced cervical lesions by combination of capsid protein L1 and p16INK4a protein detection. Coll Antropol. 2010 Mar;34(1):31-6.

Brinton LA, Reeves WC, Brenes MM et al. The male sexual factor in the etiology of cervical cancer among sexually monogamous women. Int J Cancer 1989;44:199.

Brinton LA, Schairer C, Haenszel W et al. Cigarette smoking and invasive cervical cancer. J Am Med Assoc 1986; 225: 3265

Broder S. From the National Institutes of Health. Rapid Communication—The Bethesda System for Reporting Cervical/Vaginal Cytologic Diagnoses—Report of the 1991 Bethesda Workshop. JAMA 1992;267:1892.

Brown DC, Gatter KC. Ki67 protein: the immaculate deception. Histopathology 2002; 40: 2-11.

Buckley CH, Butler EB, Fox H. Cervical Intraepithelial neoplasia. J Clin Pathol 1982; 35: 1-13.

Butterworth CE, Hatch KD, Macaluso M. Folate deficiency and cervical dysplasia. J Am Med Assoc 1992; 267: 528.

Cattoretti G, Becker MH, Key G. Monoclonal antibodies against recombinant parts of the Ki-67 antigen (MIB-1 and MIB-3) detects proliferating cells in microwave processed formalin fixed paraffin sections. J Pathol 1992, 168: 357-363.

Chisa Aoyama *et al.* Histologic and immunohistochemical characteristics of neoplastic and non-neoplastic subgroups of atypical squamous lesions of the uterine cervix. *Am J Clin Pathol.* 2005, 123: 699-706

Creagh T, Bridger JE, Kupek E, et al. Pathologist variation in reporting cervical borderline epithelial abnormalities and cervical intraepithelial neoplasia. J Clin Pathol 1995; 48:59–60.

Crook T, Wrede D, Vousden KH. p53 point mutation in HPV negative human cervical carcinoma cell lines. Oncogene 1991; 6:873.

Crum CP, Nuovo GJ. Genital papillomaviruses and related neoplasms. New York: Raven Press, 1991, pp. 64-83, 167-185.

Dray M, Russell P, Dalrymple C, Wallman N, Angus G, Leong A, Carter J, Cheerala B. p16 INK 4a as a complementary marker of high? grade intraepithelial lesions of the uterine cervix. I: Experience with squamous lesions in 189 consecutive biopsies. Taylor and Francis Issue 2005 April, 37(2): 112-124.

Fenoglio CM, Galloway DA, Crum CP et al. Herpes simplex virus and cervical neoplasia. In: Fenoglio CM, Wolff M, eds. Progress in surgical pathology. New York: Raven Press, 1982, pp. 45-82.

Garzetti GG, Ciavattini A, De Nictolis M, Lucarini G, Goteri G, Romanini C, Biagini G. MIB 1 immunostaining in cervical intraepithelial neoplasia: prognostic significance in mild and moderate lesions. Gynecol Obstet Invest. 1996; 42(4):261-6.

Gerdes J. Ki-67 and other proliferation markers useful for immunohistological diagnostic and prognostic evaluation in human malignancies. In: Osborn M, editor Seminars in Cancer Biology, 1990; Vol. I: 99-106.

Goel MM, Mehrotra A, Singh U, Gupta HP, Misra JC. MIB-1 and PCNA immunostaining as a diagnostic adjunct to cervical pap smear. Diagnostic Cytopathology 2005; Vol. 32(3).

Gorstein F: Precursor lesions of squamous cell carcinoma of the cervix: are there reliable predictors of biologic behaviour? Hum Pathol 2000; 31: 1339-1340.

Haidopoulos D, Partsinevelos GA, Vlachos GD, Rodolakis A, Markaki S, Voulgaris Z, Diakomanolis E, Antsaklis A. p16 INK4A is a strong biomarker for cervical intraepithelial neoplasia and invasive cervical carcinoma: a reappraisal. Reprod Sci. 2009 Jul; 16(7):685-93. Epub 2009 Apr 16.

Ham J, Dostatni N, Ganthier JM et al. The papillomavirus E2 protein: A factor with many talents. Trends Biochem Sci 1991; 16:440

Jemal A, Bray F, Melissa M, Ferlay J, Ward E, Forman D. Global Cancer Statistics; Ca Can J Clin 2011;61:69–90

Kalof AN, Evans MF, Summons-Arnold L, Beatty BG, Cooper K. p16INK4a immunoexpression and HPV in situ hybridization signal patterns: potential markers of high grade cervical intraepithelial neoplasia. Am J Surg Pathol 2005 May; 29(5): 674-679.

Keating JT, Cviko A, Riethdorf S, Riethdorf L, Quade BJ, Sun D, et al. Ki- 67, Cyclin E, and p16 INK4a Arc complimentary surrogate biomarkers for human papilloma virus - related cervical neoplasia. American Journal of Surgical Pathology 2001; 25:884-91

Klaes R, Friedrich T, Spitkovsky D, Ridder R, Rudy W, Petry U, et al. Over expression of p16 as a specific marker for dysplastic and neoplastic epithelial cells of the cervix uteri. Int J Cancer 2001; 92:276-84.

Klaes, Axel, Friedrich, Tibor, Ridder et al. p16 INK4A Immunohistochemistry improves interobserver agreement in the diagnosis of Cervical Intraepithelial neoplasia. Am. Jour. Surg. Pathol. 2002; 26(11).

Kurshumliu F, Thorns C, Gashi-Luci L. p16INK4A in routine practice as a marker of cervical epithelial neoplasia. Gynecol Oncol. 2009 Oct;115(1):127-31. Epub 2009 Jul 12.

Li J, Li FP, Blot WJ et al. Correlation between cancers of the uterine cervix and penis in China. J Natl Cancer Inst 1982;69: 1063.

Lorincz AT, Reid R, Jenson AB, Greenberg MD, Lancaster W, Kurman RJ et al. Human Papillomavirus infection of the cervix:relative risk associations of 15 common anogenital types. Obstet Gynecol 1992; 79:328-37.

McCluggage WG, Jenkins D. p16 immuno reactivity may assist in the distinction between endometrial and endocervical adenocarcinoma. Int J Gynaecol Pathol 2003 July; 22(3): 231-235.

Meisels A, Morin C. Human Papillomavirus and cancer of the uterine cervix. Gynecol Oncol 1981; 12: 111

Méndez M, Ferrández Izquierdo A. Detection of human papilloma virus (HPV) in liquid-based cervical samples. Correlation with protein p16INK4a expression]. Invest Clin. 2011 Mar; 52(1):3-14.

Munoz N, Bosch FX. Epidemiology of cervical cancer. In: Munoz N, Bosch FX, Jensen OM, eds. Human Papillomavirus and Cervical cancer. Lyon: IARC, 1989; p9

Murphy N, Ring M, Heffron CCBB, King B, Killalea AG, Hughes C, Martin CM, McGuinness E, Sheils O, O'Leary JJ. p16 INK4a, CDC6 and MCM5 : predictive biomarkers in cervical preinvasive neoplasia and cervical cancer. Jour Clin Pathol 2005, 58: 525-534.

Murphy N, Ring M, Killalea AG, Uhlmann V, Donovan MO, Mulcahy F, Turner M, McGuinness E, Griffin M, Martin C, Sheils O, Leary JJ. p16 INK4a as a marker for cervical dyskaryosis : CIN and cGIN in cervical biopsies and thin prep smears. J Clin Pathol 2003; 56: 56-63.

Negri G, Egarter-Vigl E, Kasal A, Romano F, Haitel A, Moan C. p16 INK4a is a useful marker for the diagnosis of Adenocarcinoma of the cervix uteri and its precursors. An Immunohistochemical study with immunocytochemical correlations. Am J Surg Pathol 2003; 27(2): 187-193.

Negri G, Vitadells F, Romano F et al. P16INK 4a expression and progression risk of low grade interepithelial nepolasia of the cervix uteri. Virchows Arch 2004; 445(6), 616-20.

Oberg TN, Kipp BR, Vrana JA, Bartholet MK, Fales CJ, Garcia R, McDonald AN, Rosas BL, Henry MR, Clayton AC. Comparison of p16INK4a and ProEx C immunostaining on cervical ThinPrep cytology and biopsy specimens. Diagn Cytopathol. 2010 Aug; 38(8):564-72.

Passamonti B, Gustinucci D, Recchia P, Bulletti S, Carlani A, Cesarini E, D'Amico MR, D'Angelo V, Di Dato E, Martinelli N, Malaspina M, Spita N. Expression of p16 in abnormal pap-tests as an indicator of CIN2+ lesions: a possible role in the low grade ASC/US and L/SIL (lg) cytologic lesions for screening prevention of uterine cervical tumours. Pathologica. 2010 Feb; 102(1):6-11.

Petry KU, Schmidt D, Scherbring S, Luyten A, Reinecke-Lüthge A, Bergeron C, Kommoss F, Löning T, Ordi J, Regauer S, Ridder R. Triaging Pap cytology negative, HPV positive cervical cancer screening results with p16/Ki-67 Dual-stained cytology. Gynecol Oncol. 2011 Jun 1; 121(3):505-9.

Pientong et al. Immunocytochemical staining of p16 protein conventional pap test and its association with human papiloma virus infection. Wiley Inter Science. 2004.

Reagen JW, Seidemann IL, Saracusa Y. Cellular morphology of carcinoma in situ and dysplasia or atypical hyperplasia of uterine cervix cancer. Cancer 1953; 6: 224-235

Sahebali J, Depuyde CF, Segars K, Moeneclacy L, Vercecken A, Marck E, Bogers E. p16 as an adjunct Marker in liquid-based cervical cytology. Br J Cancer 2004 108: 871-876.

Samir R, Asplund A, Tot T, Pekar G, Hellberg D. High-Risk HPV Infection and CIN Grade Correlates to the Expression of c-myc, CD4+, FHIT, E-cadherin, Ki-67, and p16INK4a. J Low Genit Tract Dis. 2011 May 7.

Sano T, Oyama T, Kashiwabara K, Fukuda T, Nakajima T. Expression status of p16 protein is associated with HPV oncogenic potential in cervical and genital lesions. Am J Pathol 1998; 153:1741-8.

Scheffner M, Takahashi T, Huibregtse JM et al. Interaction of the human papillomavirus type 16E6 on coprotein with wild-type and mutant human p53 proteins. J Virol 1992; 66:S100.

Scheffner M, Munger K, Huibregtse JM et al. Targeted degradation of the retinoblstoma protein by human Papillomavirus E7-E6 fusion proteins. EMBO J 1992; 11:2425.

Schmidt D, Bergeron C, Denton KJ, Ridder R; European CINtec Cytology Study Group. p16/ki-67 dual-stain cytology in the triage of ASCUS and LSIL papanicolaou cytology: res ults from the European equivocal or mildly abnormal Papanicolaou cytology study. Cancer Cytopathol. 2011 Jun 25;119(3):158-66.

Sherman ME, Schiffman MH, Lorinez AT, Manos MM, Scott DR, Kuman RJ, et al. Toward objective quality assurance in cervical cytopathology: Correlation of cytopathologic diagnoses with detection of high-risk human papillomavirus types. Am J Clin Pathol 1994; 102:182–7.

Solomon D, Davey D, Kurman R, Moriarty A, O'Connor D, Prey M, et al. The 2001 Bethesda System: terminology for reporting results of cervical cytology. JAMA 2002; 287:2114-9.

Spriggs AI, Butler EB, Evans DMD et al. Problems of cell nomenclature in cervical cytology smears. J Clin Pathol 1978; 31: 1226-1227.

Stoler MH, Schiffman M. Atypical Squamous Cells of Undetermined Significance-Low-grade Squamous Intraepithelial Lesion Triage Study (ALTS) Group. Interobserver reproducibility of cervical cytologic and histologic interpretations: realistic estimates from the ASCUS-LSIL Triage Study. JAMA 2001;285:1500–5.

Srivastava S. P16INK4A and MIB-1: an immunohistochemical expression in preneoplasia and neoplasia of the cervix. Indian J Pathol Microbiol. 2010 Jul-Sep;53(3):518-24

Stanley MA. Prognostic factors and new therapeutic approaches to cervical cancer. Virus Res 2002; 89: 241-248.

Sung CO, Kim SR, Oh YL, Song SY. The use of p16(INK4A) immunocytochemistry in "Atypical squamous cells which cannot exclude HSIL" compared with "Atypical squamous cells of undetermined significance" in liquid-based cervical smears. Diagn Cytopathol. 2010 Mar;38(3):168-71.

The 1988 Bethesda System for reporting cervical/ vaginal cytological diagnoses. National Cancer Institute Workshop. JAMA 1989; 262:931-4.

Tomita Y, Shirasawa H, Sekine H, Simizu B. Expression of the human papilloma virus type 6bL2 open reading frame in Escherichia coli : L2 β-galactosidase fusion proteins and their antigenic properties. Virology 1987; 158: 8-14.

Toro de Méndez M, Ferrández Izquierdo A. Detection of human papilloma virus (HPV) in liquid-based cervical samples. Correlation with protein p16INK4a expression].

Tringler B, Gup CJ, Singh M, Groshong S, Shroyer AL, Heinz DE, Shroyer KR. Evaluation of p16 and pRb expression in cervical squamous and glandular neoplasia. Hum Pathol 2004 Jun; 35(6): 689-96

Valasoulis G, Tsoumpou I, Founta C, Kyrgiou M, Dalkalitsis N, Nasioutziki M, Kassanos D, Paraskevaidis E, Karakitsos P. The role of p16(INK4a) immunostaining in the risk assessment of women with LSIL cytology: a prospective pragmatic study. Eur J Gynaecol Oncol. 2011;32(2):150-2.

Van Hoven KH, Rauondetta L, Kovatich AJ, Bibbo L. Quantitative image analysis of MIB I reactivity in inflammatory, hyperplastic and neoplastic endocervical lesions. Int J Gynecol Pathol. 1997; 16: 15-21.

Ward P, Coleman DV, Malcolm ADB. Regulatory Mechanisms of the papillomaviruses. Trends Genet 1989; 5:97.

WHO/ICO Information Centre on HPV and Cervical Cancer. Available from: http://www.who.int/hpv centre. [last cited on 2009 May 5]

World Health Organization. International Classification of Tumors No. 8. In: Ritton G, Christopherson WM Eds. Cytology of the female genital tract. Geneva: World Health Organization, 1973.

Wright TC Jr, Massad LS, Dunton CJ, Spitzer M, Wilkinson EJ, Solomon D, for the 2006 American Society for Colposcopy and Cervical Pathologysponsored consensus conference. 2006 Consensus guidelines for the management of women with abnormal cervical cancer screening tests. Am J Obstet Gynecol. 2007;197(4):346-355.

Yu L, Wang L, Zhong J, Chen S. Diagnostic value of p16INK4A, Ki-67, and human papillomavirus L1 capsid protein immunochemical staining on cell blocks from residual liquid-based gynecologic cytology specimens. Cancer Cytopathol. 2010 Feb 25;118(1):47-55.

Zielinski G, Snijders P, Rozendaal L, Daalmeijer N, Risse E, Voorhorst, Medijiwa N, Linden H, Schipper FA, Runsink AP, Meijer JLM. The presence of high risk-HPV combined with specific p53 and p16 INK4a expression patterns points to high-risk HPV as the main causative agent for adenocarcinoma in situ and adenocarcinoma of the cervix. Journal of Pathology 2003; 201: 535-543.

Zur-Hausen H. Human Papillomaviruses in the pathogenesis of anogenital cancer. Virology 1991;184:9.

Zur- Hausen H. Sexually transmitted diseases and oncogenesis. Abstracts of the Tenth International Meeting of the Society for STD research, Helsinki, Finland,1993, p1.

12

Cervical Intraepithelial Neoplasia (CIN) (Squamous Dysplasia)

Oguntayo Olanrewaju Adekunle
Department of Obstetric and Gynaecology, Ahmadu Bello University Teaching Hospital, Zaria Kaduna State Nigeria

1. Introduction

Cervical intraepithelial neoplasia (CIN) is a premalignant cervical disease that is also called cervical dysplasia or **cervical interstitial neoplasia** or cervical squamous intraepithelial lesions (CSIL).

The nomenclature in use in the past was mild, moderate, and severe dysplasia, these were the terms used to describe premalignant squamous cervical cellular changes. Although still in use by some, it has generally been replaced by the term Cervical Intraepithelia Neoplasia(CIN), which is used to describe histologic changes on the uterine cervix. The trend is now tending towards the use of Squamous Intraepithelia Lesions(SIL).

1.1 Definition

What is cervical intraepithelial Neoplasia-? It is a potentially premalignant transformation and abnormal growth (dysplasia) of squamous cells on the surface of the cervix.[Kumar etal 2007] CIN is not cancer, and is usually curable.[ACOG 2010] Most cases of CIN remain stable, or are eliminated by the host's immune system without intervention. However a small percentage of cases progress to become cervical cancer, usually cervical squamous cell carcinoma (SCC), if left untreated.[Agorastos et al 2005]

It can actually be defined as a spectrum of intraepithelial changes (dysplasia) with indistinct boundaries that begins with mild atypia and progresses through stages of more marked intraepithelial abnormalities to carcinoma in situ if untreated or managed. (UVA Health)

1.1.1 Dysplasia is a potentially reversible change characterized by an increase in mitotic rate, atypical cytologic features (size, shape, nuclear features) and abnormal organization (cellularity, differentiation, polarity) that fall short of invasive carcinoma (premalignant change).Dysplasia may progress to cancer and dysplastic changes may be found adjacent to foci of cancer.

1.2 Epidemiology

Population distribution of cervical intraepithelial neoplasia/dysplasia resembles the epidemiology of an infectious disease that is sexually transmitted. Multiple male sexual partners, early age at first sexual intercourse and male partner with multiple previous/current female sexual partners are very important risk factors.

1.3 Incidence

The estimated annual incidence in the United States of CIN among women who undergo cervical cancer screening is 4 percent for CIN 1 and 5 percent for CIN 2,3 [Agorastos et al 2005]. High grade lesions are typically diagnosed in women 25 to 35 years of age, while invasive cancer is more commonly diagnosed after the age of 40, typically 8 to 13 years after a diagnosis of a high grade lesion. Between 250,000 and 1 million American women are diagnosed with CIN annually. Women can develop CIN at any age, however, women generally develop it between the ages of 25 to 35.[Kumar etal 2007]

In developing Nations like Nigeria the mean age for cervical intraepithelial neoplasia (CIN) was 37.6 years. CIN I accounted for 3.6%, CIN II 0.8% and CIN III was only 0.4%.The combined prevalence was 48 per 1000.The peculiarity of the developing nations result is the poor uptake or use of screening methods(Oguntayo & Samaila).

In view of the fact that CIN is a premalignant or precursor of cervical cancer it is pertinent to briefly see the incidence and prevalence of this disease condition.

Cervical cancer is second only to breast cancer in its incidence world wide. Cancer registry data shows that that there are approximately 400,000 new cases of cervical cancer and 200,000 deaths from this disease every year (IARC 2001).

The incidence rate varies from country to country with eighty percent (80%) of the cases occurring in less developed countries. The reasons for this may lie in the socio economic conditions that prevail in these countries where facilities for family planning, obstetric and gynaecological health care are scarce and cervical screening programmes are virtually non existent. (IARC 2001).

The relative incidences of cervical intra-epithelial neoplasia (CIN) and invasive cervical cancer were studied in black and white patients at the academic hospitals of the University of the Orange Free State. A statistically high significant differences was found between black and white patients, with a higher incidence of invasive cervical cancer than stage III CIN (CIN III) in black patients and a higher incidence of CIN III than invasive cervical cancer in white patients (P=0,000092; 95% confidence interval -0,355 - -0,128). The time interval between the peak incidence of CIN III and that of invasive cervical cancer was found to be shorter in black than in white patients. These distressing findings emphasise the urgent need for a national cervical cytological screening programme to decrease the incidence of invasive cervical cancer (NEL1994)

2. Anatomy

2.1 Anatomy of the uterine cervix

The cervix is actually the lower, narrow portion of the uterus, connected to the uterine fundus by the uterine isthmus. Its name is derived from the Latin word for "neck." It is cylindrical or conical in shape. Its upper limit is considered to be the internal os, which is an anatomically and histologically ill-defined junction of the more muscular uterine body and the denser, more fibrous cervical stroma. The size and shape of the cervix varies widely with age, hormonal state, and parity. In parous women, the cervix is bulkier and the external os, or lowermost opening of the cervix into the vagina, appears wider and more slit-like and gaping than in nulliparous fig 2 women. Before childbearing, the external os is a small, circular opening at the center of the cervix fig 1. After the menopause it may narrow almost to a pin point fig 3. The portion of the cervix exterior to the external os is called the ectocervix. The passageway between the external os and the body of the uterus at the isthmus above is referred to as the endocervical canal. Its upper limit is the internal os.5

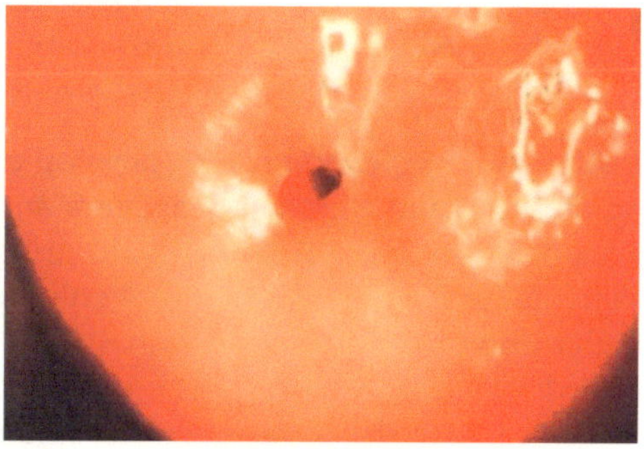

Fig. 1. The nulliparous cervix: note the small round os

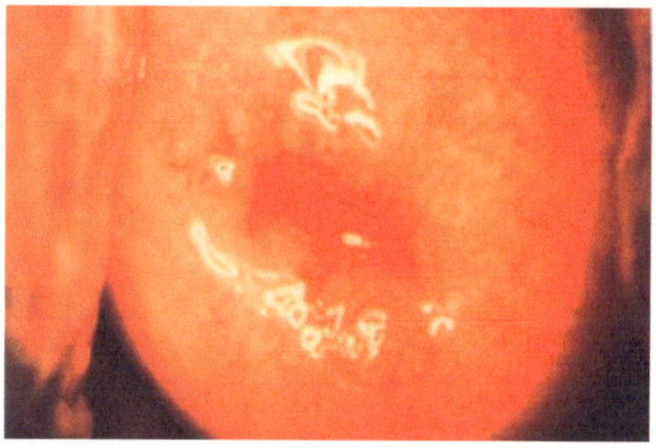

Fig. 2. Multiparous cervix

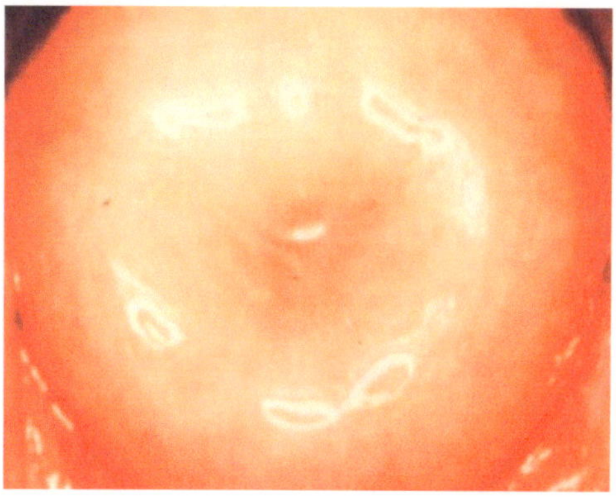

Fig. 3. Menopausal cervix

The canal itself shows a complex configuration of mucosal folds or plicae. These make cytologic screening and colposcopy of the endocervical tissues technically more difficult and less reliable than for the smoother and more accessible squamous epithelium of the ectocervix.(ASCCP 2011)

2.2 Embryology of the uterine cervix

Two paramesonephric ducts form from coelomic epithelium extending beside the mesonephric ducts. In the absence of Mullerian Inhibitory Factor these ducts proliferate and grow extending from the vaginal plate on the wall of the urogenital sinus to lie beside the developing ovary. The paired ducts begin to fuse from the vaginal plate end, forming the primordial body of the uterus and the unfused lateral arms form the uterine tubes.see fig 4

The picture bellow is the summary of the embryonic development of the uterine cervix and the second is showing the infantine uterus as it appears and this is an evidence that there are significant changes that do occur as the girl child grows fig 5.The main clinical reference to this is basically in the epithelia changes between pre pubertal and post pubertal period.The epithelia lining of the cervical canal (endocervix) is the columnar epithelium while that of external cervix (endocervix) is squamous epithelium. The squamo-columnar junction is located at the point where the squamous epithelium and the columnar epithelium meet. The location varies throughout a woman's life due to the process of metaplastic changes in the cervical epithelium which occur after puberty and in pregnancy.(Mark 2010)

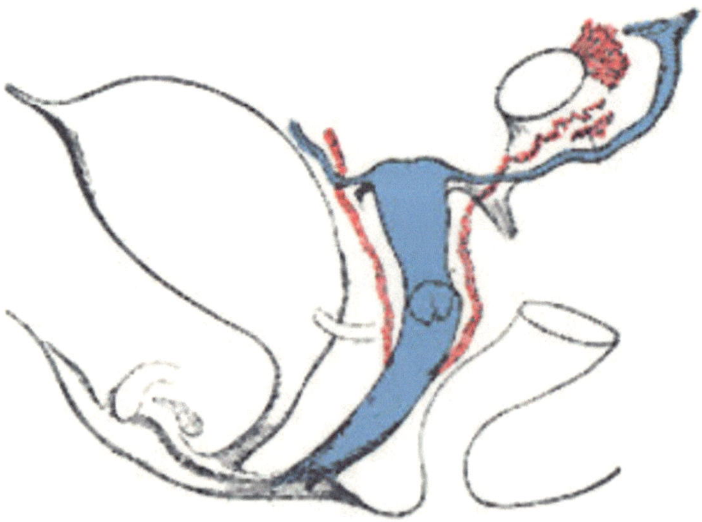

Fig. 4. Embryological Origin of the Uterus

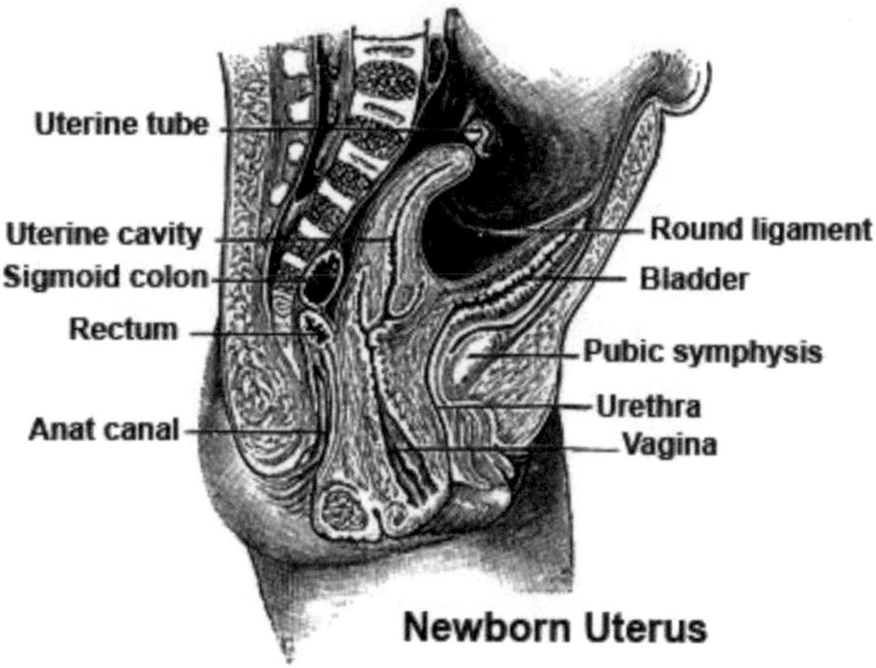

Fig. 5.

2.3 Cervix-normal histology

Most of the cervix is composed of fibromuscular tissue. The Epithelium is either squamous or columnar.

The endocervix is lined by columnar epithelium that secretes mucus this epithelium has complex infoldings that resemble glands or clefts on cross section and the mucosa rests on inconspicuous layer of reserve cells.

The ectocervix (exocervix)is covered by nonkeratinizing, stratified squamous epithelium, either native or metaplastic; has basal, midzone and superficial layers. A fter menopause and in prepubertal girls the superficial layer becomes atrophic with mainly basal and parabasal cells with high nucleo-cytoplasmic ratio that resembles dysplasia.

2.3.1 Squamocolumnar junction: where squamous and glandular (columnar) epithelium meets this a major land mark in cervical dyplasia,it is usually in exocervix.The nearby reserve cells are involved in squamous metaplasia, dysplasia and carcinoma.

2.3.2 Transformation zone: also called ectropion, between original squamocolumnar junction and border of **metaplastic squamous epithelium**; epidermalization and squamous differentiation of reserve cells transform this area to squamous epithelium; site of squamous cell carcinomas and dysplasia.

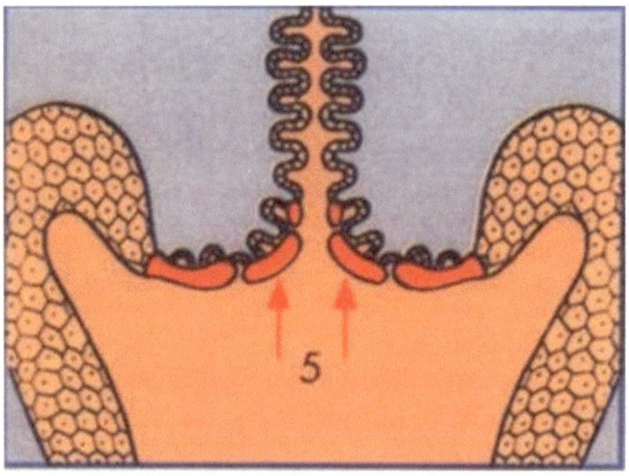

Metaplastic change of endocervical epithelium in the transformation zone

In the cervix a lot of metaplasia takes place which was what encouraged a lot of study to be conducted.

- Metaplasia is the name given to the process by which one fully differentiated type of epithelium changes into another.
- It is usually an adaptive change which occurs in reaction to longstanding (chronic) irritation of any kind, or in response to hormonal stimuli.
- Metaplastic change is reversible and theoretically transformed epithelium should revert to its original form after the stimulus is removed but this does not always happen.
- Metaplasia occurs at many body sites eg gastric mucosa, bladder,bronchi etc. The metaplastic process has been extensively studied in the cervix.

2.4 Physiology of metaplastic changes on the cervix

The metaplastic changes seen are related to the following:

Pre-Puberty, Post puberty, Pregnancy and Menopause.

Pre-puberty-From birth until puberty the endocervical epithelium is composed of columnar epithelium and the ectocervix of native squamous epithelium. The interface between the two is termed the original squamocolumnar junction.

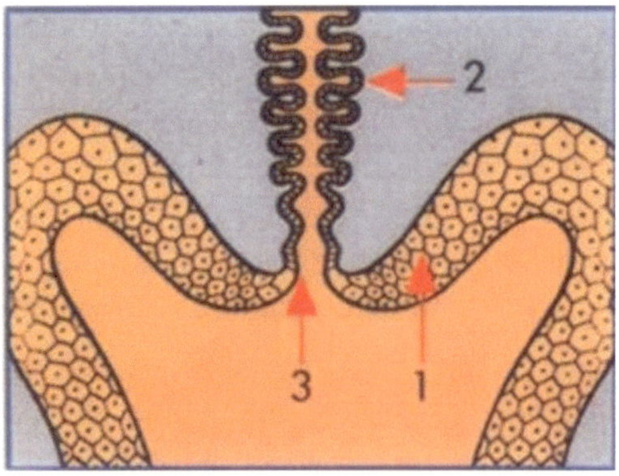

Squamocolumnar junction prior to puberty.

Puberty-During puberty and at the first pregnancy the cervix increases in volume in response to hormonal changes. The endocervical epithelium everts onto the ectocervix (portio vaginalis) exposing it to the acid pH of the vagina. This provides a stimulus for metaplastic change of the columnar epithelium.

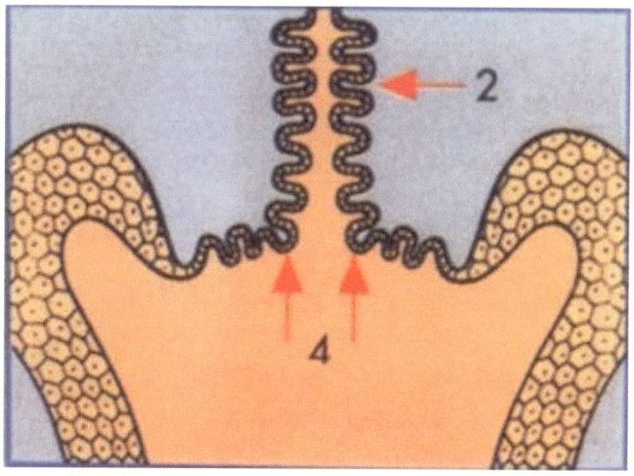

Eversion of the endocervical epithelium at puberty and first pregnancy

Menopause-The process of metaplasia is a patchy one: It starts initially in the crypts and at the tips of the endocervical villae which gradually fuse. Eventually the whole of the everted endocervical epithelium may be replaced by squamous epithelium.

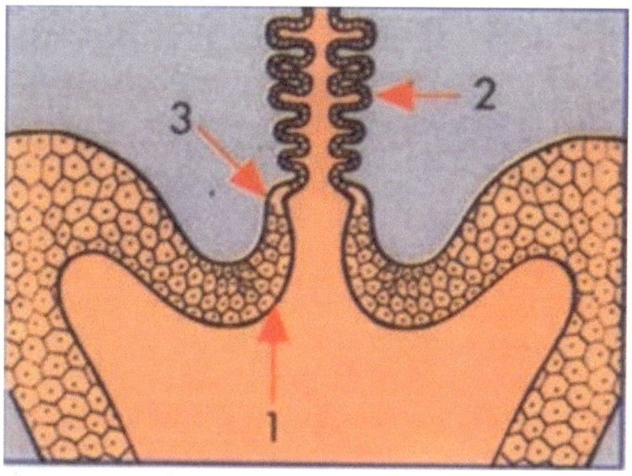

Relocation of SCJ in the endocervical canal after the menopause

Key:

- 1: native squamous epithelium
- 2: columnar epithelium of endocervix
- 3: squamocolumnar junction (SCJ)
- 4: Eversion of endocervical epithelium
- 5: Metaplastic change in transformation zone (Eurocytology 2011)

The Clinical significance of squamous metaplasia in the cervix is that, this area of the cervical epithelium has under gone metaplasia(Transformation zone) and all the immature metaplastic are susceptible to carcinogens.In view of the afore mentioned it is not surprising that most cervical cancers arise here.

2.4.1 Basal cells (reserve cells): cuboidal to low columnar with scant cytoplasm and round/oval nuclei; acquire eosinophilic cytoplasm as they mature; positive for low molecular weight keratin and estrogen receptor; negative for high molecular weight keratin and involucrin

2.4.2 Suprabasal cells: have variable amount of glycogen, detectable with Lugol/Schiller's test (application of iodine)

2.4.3 Glandular epithelium: positive for estrogen receptor.

3. Aetiology

3.1 Association of human papillomaviruses and cervical Intraepithelia neoplasia

Human papillomaviruses (HPV) are members of a family of viruses known as the Papovaviruses fig 5. They are epitheliotropic viruses which promote cell proliferation which results in the development of benign papillomatous lesions of the genital tract upper respiratory tract, digestive tracts and cutaneous lesions of the skin. More than 70 distinct HPV types have been identified as a result of molecular hybridisation of DNA extracted from condylomata or warty lesions from a variety of sites. Each virus type has a very restricted site of infection and viruses which occupy similar niches appear to be genetically related. Molecular hybridisation of anogenital warts and cervical biopsies have shown that about 30 of the 70 distinct types of HPV are confined to the female genital tract. (Eurocytology).

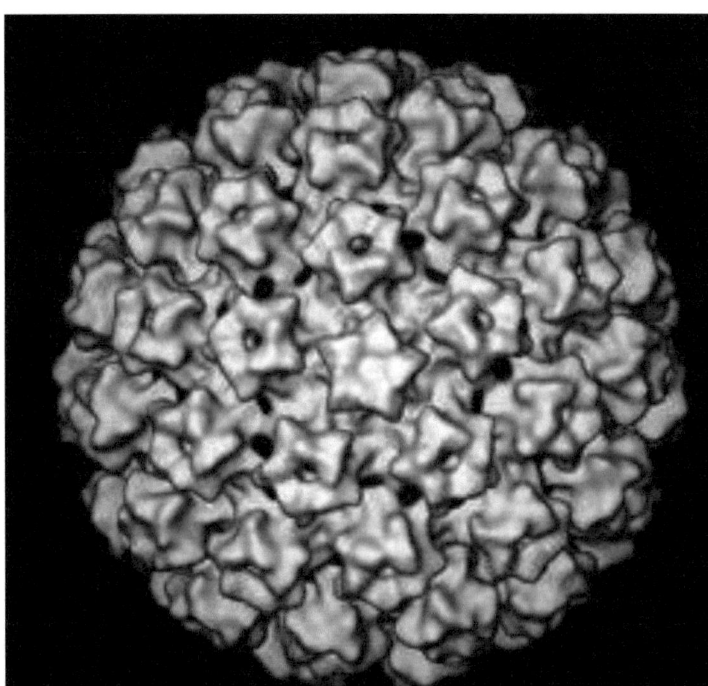

Fig. 6. Electronmicrograph of human papillomavirus (courtesy Eurocytology)

DNA analysis of anogenital warts,CIN and cervical cancerous tissue has shown that two groups of HPV can be identified in the female genital tract. One group of HPV is almost always associated with low grade CIN lesions and exophytic anogenital warts which have a *low risk* **of progressing to cervical cancer**. A second group of viruses is found most commonly in CIN2 and CIN3 which have a *high risk* **of developing into invasive cancer.**

3.1.1 HPV types found in the female genital tract

The major cause of CIN is chronic infection of the cervix with the sexually transmitted human papillomavirus (HPV), especially the high-risk HPV types 16 or 18(**viruses from the high risk group (HPV16 and HPV 18) have the ability to immortalise primary human keratinocytes** ***ie*** **extend their lifespan)** In comparison viruses from the low risk group (HPV-6 and HPV -11) do not extend the life span of transfected human cells which mature and die at the same rate as non infected cells fig 7. Similarly the low risk viruses perform poorly in experiments concerned with the malignant transformation of rodent cells in comparison to the high risk HPV types. Moreover, HPV-16 and HPV -18 infected human keratinocytes in raft culture (an organotypic culture medium) exhibit a differentiation pattern very similar to that seen in vivo in CIN.(Eurocytology). Over 100 types of HPV have been identified. About a dozen of these types appear to cause cervical dysplasia and may lead to the development of cervical cancer. Other types cause warts. Wikipedia,

High risk	
	16,18, 31, 33, 35, 39, 45, 51, 52, 56, 58, 59, 68 may lead to Invasive Cancer
Low risk	
	6, 11, 42, 44, 53, 54, 62, 66 may lead to condylomata

Fig. 7.

3.2 The viral DNA Integration

The viral DNA Integration is a consistent finding in all cancers harbouring the *high risk* virus types HPV16 and HPV18 and provides the **strongest evidence** that HPV16 and HPV18 play an important role in the development of cervical cancer. **HPV DNA is present in 90% of all cervical invasive cancer.**

It is not sufficient to say that simple infection with high risk HPV or even integration of HPV 16 /18 into the host cell nucleus is enough for malignant transformation of the cervical epithelium.Obviously Infection of the genital tract with HPV 16 is relatively common whereas invasive cancer is rare; and integration has been detected in some cases of genital warts and CIN lesions. A number of associated-factors have been proposed such as impaired immune response, persistence of virus, smoking and administration of steroid hormones (as oral contraceptives). Other genetic events such as loss of tumour suppressor genes and the activation of oncogenes may also play a role . Mutations in *ras ,fos* and other oncogenes have been detected in cervical cancer cell lines but their role *in vivo* is still to be determined.The knowledge of HPV infection has made a remarkable improvement in the screening,diagnosis,treatment,prevention and prognosis of cancer of the cervix.

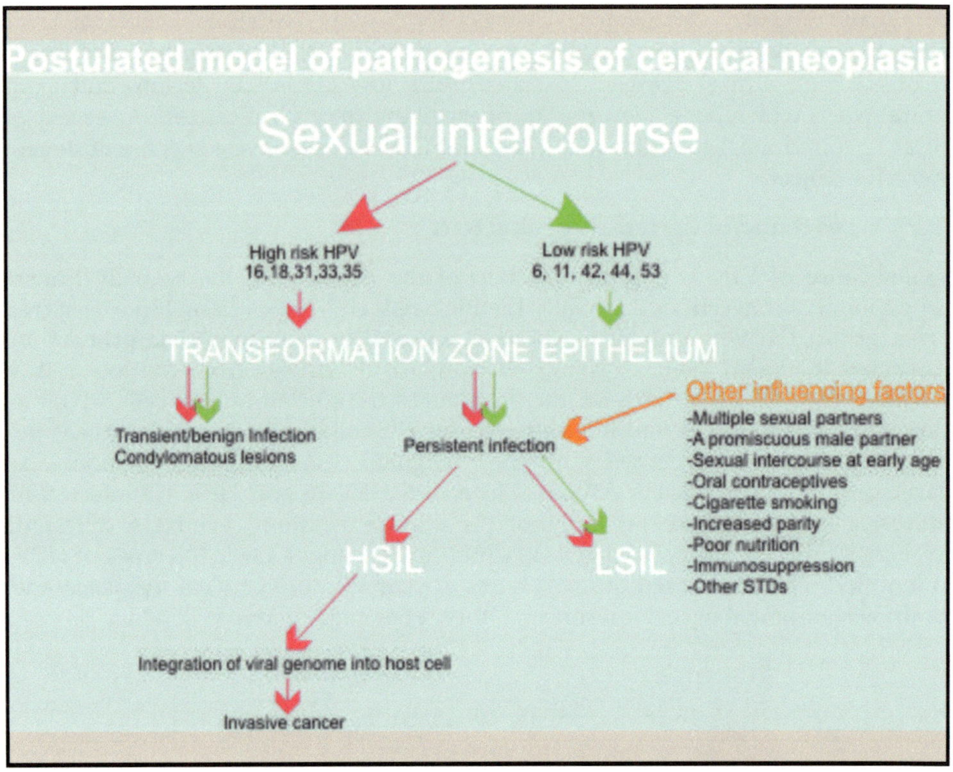

Fig. 8.

3.3 The host immune system and HPV

The host immunity plays a significant role in the control of this disease entity. The fact that HPV remains localised to cervix and vagina further indicates that local immune responses are sufficient in controlling and resolving HPV infection. Both cell mediated immunity and humoral immunity fig 8. Also immunosuppression has been implicated as an associated factor. The majority of infections are transient and not clinically evident with 70-90% of infections clearing within 12-30 months. This suggests that host immunity is generally able to clear HPV infection.

4. Histopathological features

4.1 Histo-pathological changes

Abnormal cellular proliferation, maturation and atypia characterize cervical intraepithelial neoplasia(CIN). Nuclear abnormality is the hallmark of CIN and includes hyperchromasia, pleomorphism, irregular borders, and abnormal chromatin distribution. These nuclear abnormalities persist throughout the epithelium irrespective of cytoplasmic maturation towards the surface. Mitotic rate is increased and abnormal mitotic figures may be seen.

Histologic grading of CIN is based on the proportion of the epithelium occupied by dysplastic cells. The epithelium is divided into thirds.

4.2 Grading

- **4.2.1 CIN 1** is considered a low grade lesion. It refers to mildly atypical cellular changes in the lower third (basal 1/3) of the epithelium (formerly called **mild dysplasia**/Abnormal cell growth). HPV viral cytopathic effect (koilocytotic atypia) is often present. This corresponds to infection with HPV, and typically will be cleared by immune response in a year or so, though can take several years to clear.
- **4.2.2 CIN 2** is considered a high grade lesion. It refers to moderately atypical cellular changes confined to the basal **two-thirds** of the epithelium (formerly called moderate dysplasia) with preservation of epithelial maturation.
- **4.2.3 CIN 3** is also considered a high grade lesion/Severe dysplasia. It refers to severely atypical cellular changes encompassing **greater than two-thirds** of the epithelial thickness, and includes full-thickness lesions (formerly called severe dysplasia or carcinoma in situ).

CIN 1 (mild dysplasia): Dysplastic cells occupy the lower third of the epithelium.fig 9

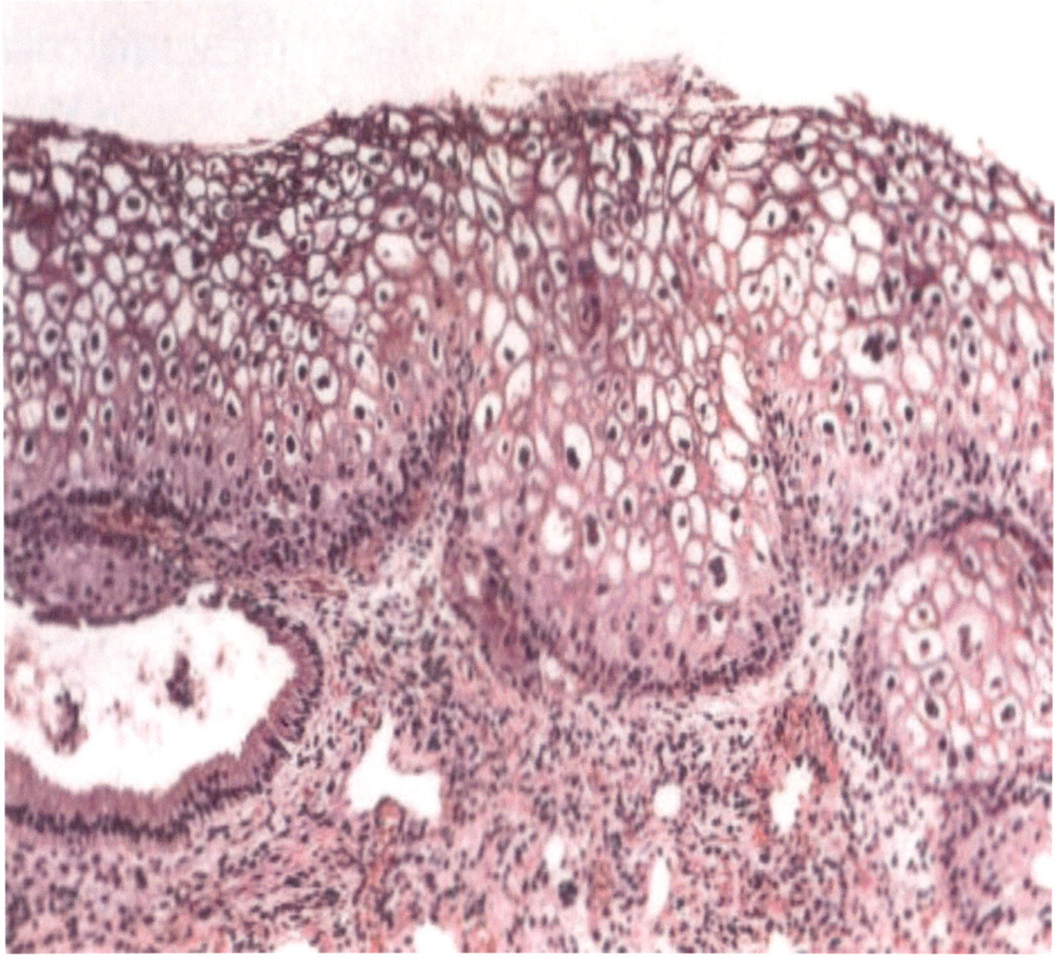

Fig. 9.

CIN 2 (moderate dysplasia): Dysplastic cells occupy up to the middle third of the epithelium. See fig 10.

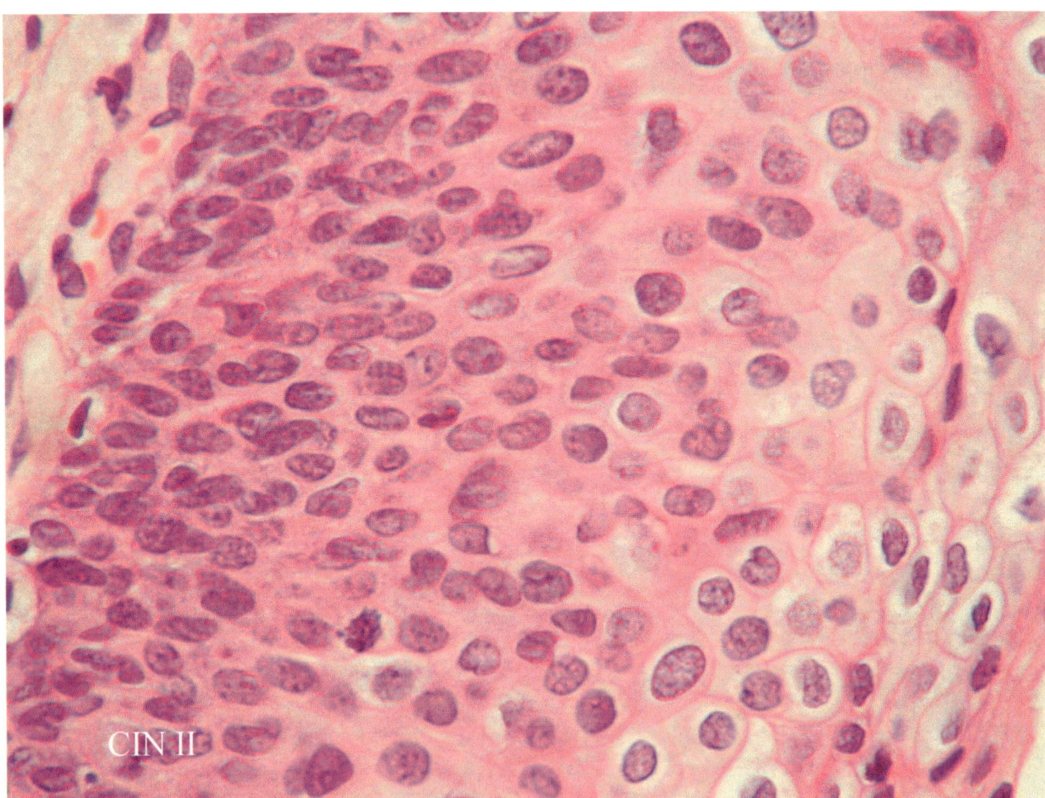

Fig. 10. CIN 2. Note superficial koilocytosis.

CIN 3 (severe dysplasia, carcinoma in situ): Dysplastic cells extend into the upper third and may occupy the full thickness of the epithelium.fig 11

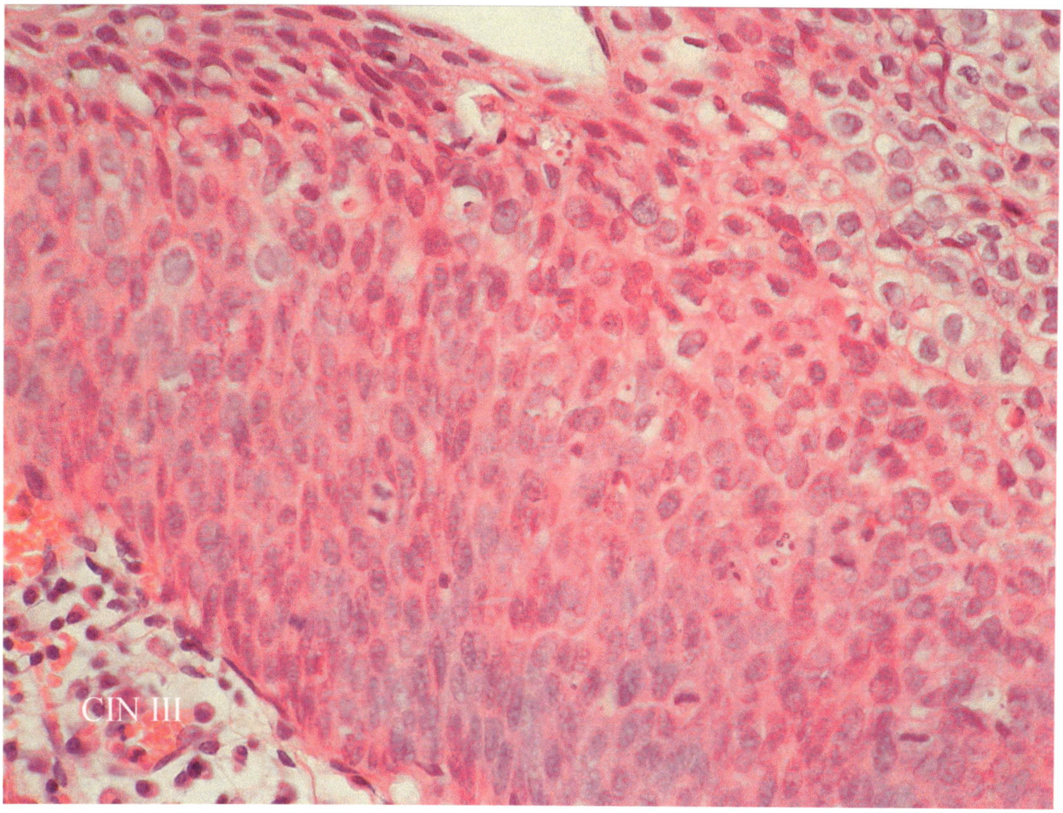

Fig. 11. CIN3. Note adjacent koilocytes (bottom right)

Cytologic grading of CIN also uses a three-tier system. However, the new Bethesda System for cytological diagnosis divides precursors of cervical squamous cell carcinoma into ***low-grade squamous intraepithelial lesion*** and ***high-grade intra-epithelial lesion***.

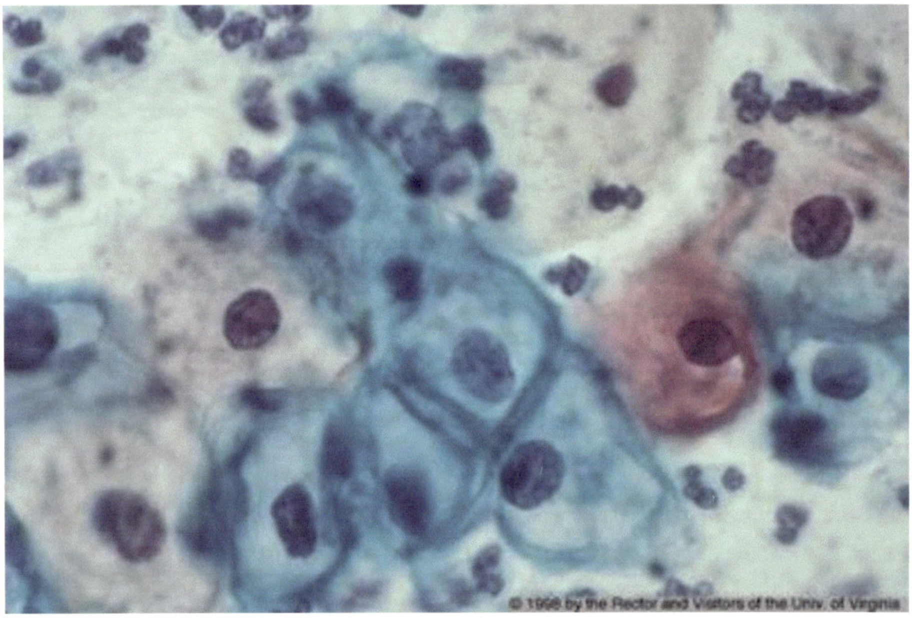

Fig. 12. Pap smear of CIN 1. Note large, dark nuclei, but also large amount of surrounding cytoplasm.

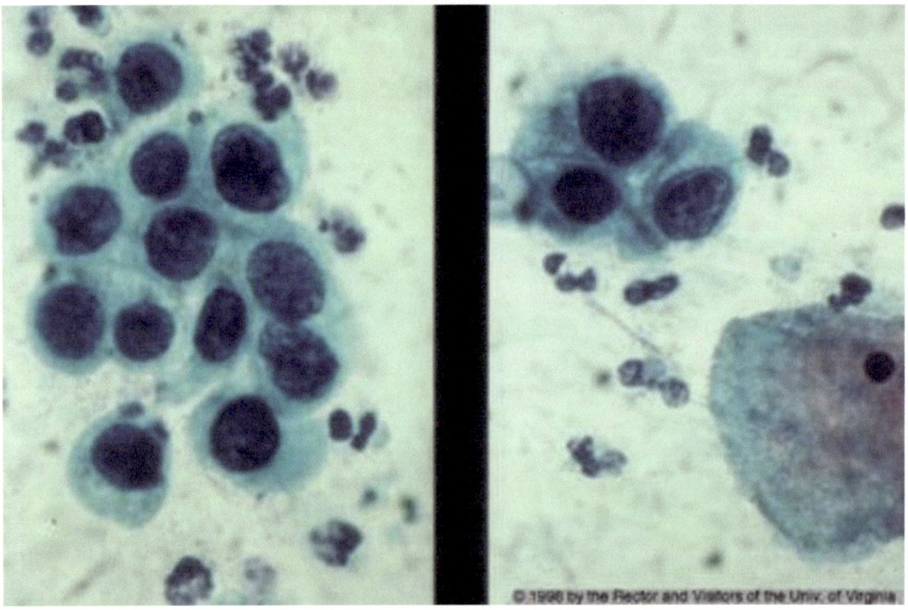

Fig. 13. Pap smear of CIN 3. Note large, dark nuclei with a lesser amount of surrounding cytoplasm. Compare to superficial cell (lower right hand corner).see fig 12 & 13

5. Clinical presentation

5.1 Clinical appearances

CIN lesions are characterized by the appearance of white patches on the cervix following application of acetic acid. Distinct vascular patterns can be seen on colposcopic examination of the cervix in high grade CIN. Lesions occur on the anterior lip twice as commonly as the posterior lip. They are found in the transformation zone and areas of squamous metaplasia in the endocervix and stop abruptly at the junction with the native portio squamous epithelium but can extend along the entire endocervical canal. In general, the portion of CIN on the portio surface is low grade (CIN 1) whereas the portion that extends into the endocervical canal is high grade (CIN 2 and 3).

5.2 Clinical behavior

CIN may regress (spontaneously, especially CIN1), persist or progress. If untreated, up to 16% of CIN1 will progress to CIN3 and up to 70% of CIN3 will progress to invasive squamous cell carcinoma in 1 to 20 years. It is not presently possible to predict which lesions will progress. However, the risk of progression to invasive cancer increases and the time required is shorter with increasing severity of the lesion.(UVa Health).

6. Screening

The aim of screening is to prevent the development of cancer. For screening to be effective, a disease should satisfy the following criteria.

Be common, serious and an important public health concern for the individual and the community.

The disease condition must have a long, latent interval in which pre-malignant change or occult cancer can be detected for the case of cancer of the cervix it is 10-15years.

The natural history of the disease, especially, its evolution from latency to disease should be adequately documented.

There should be effective treatment for pre-malignant change or condition.

The good news is that cervical cancer screening has satisfies the above criteria, especially with regards to developing countries where it really is a public health problem. Cervical screening has been shown to be effective in several countries.

Cervical cancer prevention efforts worldwide have focused on screening women at risk of the disease using Pap smears. Treating precancerous lesions has also prevents cervical cancer in many of the developed countries. In view of the afore mentioned cancer of the cervix is almost extinct in the developed nations,making it the 11th cancer in women and 2nd commonest in developing nations.

6.1 Coverage of the screening programme

It is recommended for all women; especially aged 20 – 64 are invited for screening.

It should be carried out every 3-5 years.

The screening is carried out every 3years in Women aged 45years and bellow.

Where as it is done every 5years in Women aged >45yrs.

Some other risk factors that have been found to be important in developing CIN that would benefit from screening includes☹(Kumar et al 2007)

- Women who become infected by a "high risk" types of HPV, such as 16, 18, 31, or 45
- Women who have had multiple sexual partners
- Women who smoke
- Women who are immunodeficient and Women who give birth before age 17years.

6.2 Screening technique/process

There are various types of screening test.AS was earlier discussed in this chapter cervical cancer is one of the cancers that has meet all the requirement for cancer screening.The methods that can be employed for this purpose includes,visual inspection using either Acetic acid or Lugos Iodine,Cytological analysis and Human papilloma virous immune assays.

6.2.1 Types of visual inspection test

Visual inspection with Acetic Acid or Visual Inspection with Lugols Iodine.The former is the one that is commonly use for ease of interpretation.

6.2.2 Visual inspection with acetic acid (VIA) can be done with the naked eye (also called cervicoscopy or direct visual inspection [DVI]), or with low magnification (also called gynoscopy, aided VI, or VIAM).

Visual Inspection with Acetic Acid (VIA)—It more relevant in the developing Nations.

Visual inspection with acetic acid (VIA) is an attractive screening method for early- phase cervical cancer in underdeveloped countries.It is an acceptable screening method for cervical cancer and seems to be an efficient and cost-effective method to detect high-level dysplasia.

6.3 Test performance: Sensitivity and specificity (Defn)

Sensitivity: The proportion of all those with disease that the test correctly identifies as positive.

Specificity: The proportion of all those without disease (normal) that the test correctly identifies as negative.

In the screening of cervical cancer, the sensitivity of VIA was high, whereas the corresponding specificity was only at an acceptable level. The Positive Predictive Value (PPV) and Negative Predictive Value of VIA were found to be high. In other words, the validity of VIA during early-phase screening is high in terms of sensitivity and acceptable for specificity and predictive values. (Ardahan et al).

6.4 Technique of VIA

Performing a vaginal speculum exam is the first step; then the health care provider applies dilute (3-5%) acetic acid (vinegar) to the cervix.

Abnormal tissue temporarily appears white when exposed to vinegar.

The cervix is viewed with the naked eye to identify color changes on the cervix.fig 14 & 15

Determining whether the test result is positive or negative for possible precancerous lesions or cancer and this based on the Aceto-white reactions.

VIA Category	Clinical Findings
Test-negative	No acetowhite lesions or faint acetowhite lesions; polyp, cervicitis, inflammation, Nabothian cysts.
Test-positive	Sharp, distinct, well-defined, dense (opaque/dull or oyster white) acetowhite areas—with or without raised margins touching the squamocolumnar junction (SCJ); leukoplakia and warts.
Suspicious for cancer	Clinically visible ulcerative, cauliflower-like growth or ulcer; oozing and/or bleeding on contact.fig 16

Negative VIA

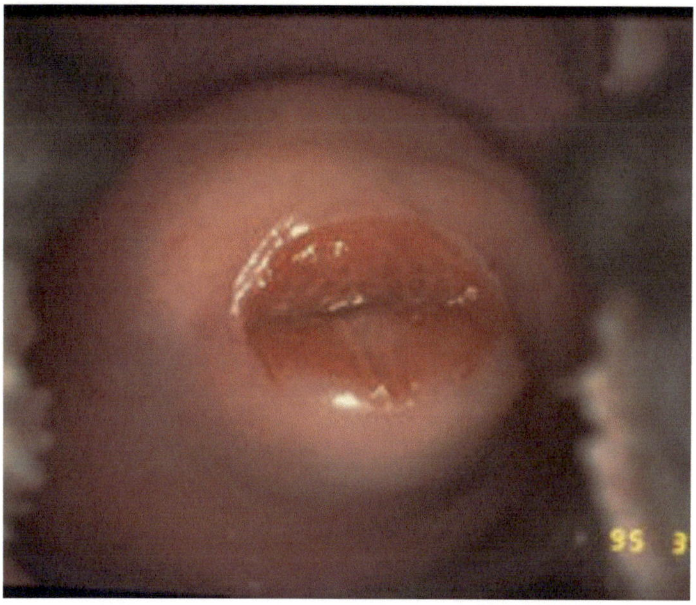

Fig. 14. Photo source: JHPIEGO

Positive VIA

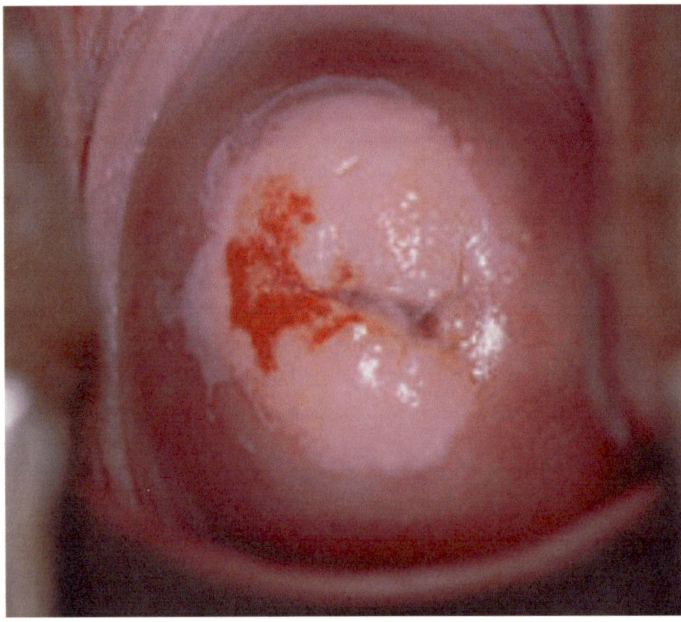

Fig. 15. Photo source: JHPIEGO

Suspicious Cancer

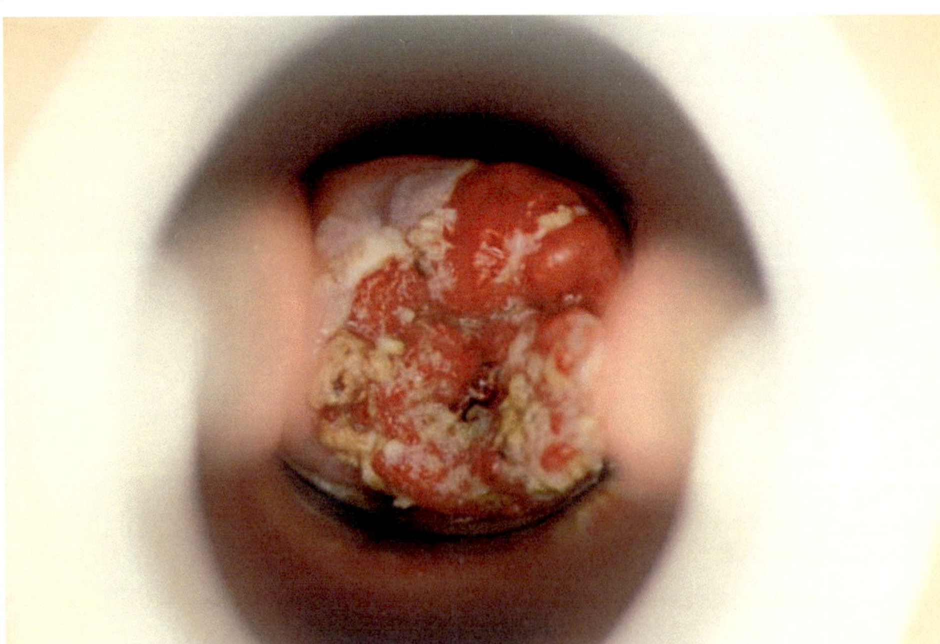

Fig. 16. Suspicion of carcinoma of the cervix. Photo source: PAHO, Jose Jeronimo

6.5 The advantages

It is Simple, easy-to-learn approach that is minimally reliant upon infrastructure.

It is not expensive to start-up and the sustaining costs is affordable.

Many types of health care providers can perform the procedure especially the middle cadre of health care providers.

The Test results are available immediately and as such the issue of follow up is out of the question.

Only requires a single visit.

It may be possible to integrate VIA screening into primary health care services and it will go along way to reduce the incidence and prevalence of carcinoma of the cervix.

There is a need for developing standard training methods and quality assurance measures.

This method isLikely to be less accurate among post-menopausal women caution in its interpretations.

6.6 Visual inspection with Lugol's iodine (VILI)

Visual inspection with Lugol's iodine (VILI), also known as Schiller's test, uses Lugol's iodine instead of acetic acid and it is based on colour change also.

6.7 Pap smear

The Pap test was developed by Dr George Papanicolaou an American anatomist in 1944. Pap test is used primarily as a tool for screening healthy women for preinvasive cervical cancer (CIN) and early invasive cancer.In as much as pap test is a screening tool,it could also be use to identify women at risk of cervical cancer. Women with early invasive cancer (FIGO Stage 1) are often unaware that they are harbouring the tumour as they are usually symptom free. Diagnosis and treatment of invasive cancer while it is still in the early stages of development signficantly improves the prognosis (chances of long term survival) of the patient.

It has been proven over time that the cervical smear may be negative even in the presence of an advanced invasive cervical cancer. This is because blood, inflammatory cells and necrotic debris from the cancer site frequently obscure the abnormal cells in the smear.

6.8 Specimen sampling

The sample for pap smear can be collected in three ways

6.8.1 a) liquid-based cytology (LBC) - using a cyto- brush a device which samples both endo and ectocervix. These can be used for preparing conventional smear. Some devices have been modified for the preparation of liquid based cytology (LBC) specimens

6.8.2 b) Papanicolaou (Pap) smear test uses a brush or the Ayres spatula to sample the ectocervix. Scraping the ectocervix with with a modified spatula (the Ayre spatula or a variation of it). This is the most widely used method in developing countries and some part of Europe for obtaining material for preparing conventional cervical smears

6.8.3 c) Using an endocervical brush to sample the endocervix this grossly inadequate and it is been discouraged.

Some of the items required for Pap smear.

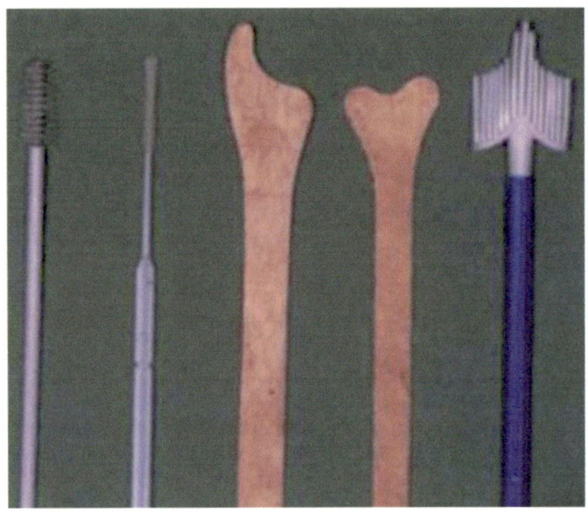

Fig. 17. Example of Fixatives

95% ethanol (for fixation)
80% isopropanol
95% denatured alcohol

Ayres/Cytobrush

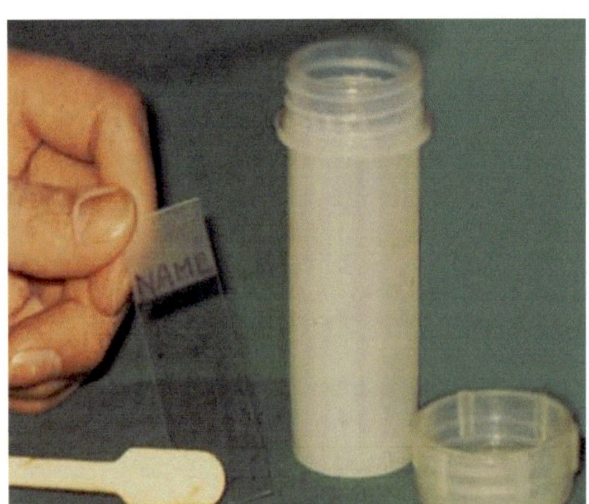

Fig. 18. Fixative Jar/Glass slide

6.8.4 The step by step approach of Pap test

1. A speculum must be inserted into vagina and the cervix clearly visualised.The cervical os should be located.
2. The sampling device(s) used should be selected according to the shape and size of the cervix and the location of the squamocolumnar junction. An Ayre spatula is suitable for sampling the cervix in a parous woman ; however a spatula and brush may be needed in a post menopausal woman where the squamocolumnar junction lies within the endocervical canal.fig 17
3. The pointed end of the spatula should be inserted into the cervical os in a nulliparous cervix and the rounded end of the spatula inserted into the patulous os of a parous woman. The device should be rotated 360 degrees to remove the cells from the region of the transformation zone, squamocolumnar junction and endocervical canal.
4. The material on the spatula or brush must be transferred immediately to a glass slide which has been previously labeled with the patient's name and date of birth.
5. The glass slide (fig 18) must be fixed immediately with an appropriate fixative (95%alcohol) and the slides transported to the cytology laboratory in a container for processing together with the corresponding cytology request form.
6. Samples taken for Liquid Based Cytology should be processed strictly in accordance with the manufacturers instructions. After sampling the cervix, the tip of the sampling device should be broken off into the transport medium in the container provided which should then be transported to the laboratory for processing if the Surepath method is being used. However if the Thinprep method is being used it is of the upmost importance that the tip of the sampling device is not included in the container.

Fixation must be immediate. The smear must not be allowed to dry before fixation.

Test Limitations as it relates to the sensitivity and specificity and technique of smear. There is no difference in specificity, but sensitivity is 12% better with LBC compared with the Pap smear, and its "inadequate rate" is only 1.6%, compared with mean of 9.1% with Pap smears(Sasieni P etal). Problems include:

- Variable sampling of appropriate cells from the cervix.
- Poor transfer of cellular material on to the glass slide.
- Sub-optimal preparation and fixation by the smear taker.

6.9 Smear reporting

It is widely acknowledged that the criteria and terminology used to interpret and report cervical smears differs country to country. This has led to problems of communication between cytopathologists , cytotechnologists and clinicians and makes it difficult for epidemiologists to make valid comparisons of the effectiveness of the different cervical screening programmes. The variability in terminology impedes meaningful discussion between laboratories and also affects patient management and the introduction of optimal methods of patient care.

We have the Following reporting methods:

- a) British Society: In the UK current reporting guidelines are based on those published by the British Society of Clinical Cytology (BSCC) in 1985
- These are currently under review and new guidelines are expected soon.

- b) American (Bethesda) system.: The system of terminology used in the United States
- First devised in 1988, being revised in 1991 and again in 2001
- A 2 -tier system which refers to :

Atypical Squamous Cells of undetermined significance **(ASC-US)**

Low grade Squamous intraepithelia neoplasia**(LSIL)**

High grade Squamous intraepithelial neoplasia**(HSIL)**

- Proposed new BSCC guidelines will bring it in line with the Bethesda system

Compare and contrast the two (British & American)

BSCC	BETHESDA
Inadequate	Unsatisfactory for evaluation
Borderline Nuclear Change	• ASC-US • ASC- cannot exclude high grade • Atypical glandular cells
Mild Dyskaryosis	LSIL
Moderate Dyskaryosis	HSIL
Severe Dyskaryosis	HSIL
Severe Dyskaryosis/?SCC	SCC
? Glandular Neoplasia	• Endocervical Ca in situ • Adenocarcinoma – Endocx., Endomet., Extrauterine, NOS

Fig. 19. Courtesy of Vanessa Jackson

7. Cytology report

7.1 Handling of cytology reports

- Women with normal smears are offered re-screening at the standard 3-5 year interval - follow the advice of your local laboratory. High risk individuals may be screened more frequently. Women with moderate or severe dyskaryotic tests need colposcopy ±biopsy. Women with borderline or mildly dyskaryotic smears are monitored at a reduced screening interval with persistent abnormalities (including persistently inadequate smears) needing colposcopy.

- Unsatisfactory - Repeat smear four weeks later.

7.1.1 Inadequate slide

An inadequate slide may occur as a result of insufficient smear, or when it is adequate it is obscured .As much as possible this should be avoided.

In phase of any abnormal cells, a result of inadequate should not be given rather the abnormality should be reported.

7.1.2 Management of inadequate smear

It is an indication for a Repeat smear

- If there is a recognisable infection present the patient should be treatmented before a repeat smear is done.
- After three consecutive inadequate samples, their is a need to refer such for colposcopic assessment.

7.1.3 Negative

There should be enough cellular material to cover 1/3 of the slide before a pronouncement or report of a negative smear. The report actually makes the woman to be confident that she is not at risk of any dysplasia for a period of three years.

- In atrophic smears, where the cellular material is comprised of parabasal sheets, 10% of the slide can be considered adequate.
- There are no official guidelines for LBC samples.

It is possible that 15,000 cells will be the standard for adequacy.

7.1.4 Management of negative slides

We should give a recommendation of routine recall to our clients. They should be encouraged to adhere to this recommendation:

- Women Age 25-45 should be advised to repeat there smear *every* three *years.* While those above 45years to 65 should have smear every five years.

Exceptions: There are exceptions to the above stated rules or recommendation.

Any patient with Clinical symptoms which are suggestive of immune surpression or are immune compromise or have been diagnosed to have immune compromised disease such as HIV positive women or women on immune suppressive drugs as in patients with renal transplant should have a repeat smear every year/12 *months*

The other exception is for those women who may have had the following conditions in the past : Post coital bleeding (PCB),Post menopausal bleeding(PMB),and friable cervix

All patients on follow up for previous abnormal smears are candidate for repeat based on the findings.

7.1.5 Reporting of infections

The presence of specific infections may be reported based on the histological features of such infections: Such as

- Candida
- Trichomonas - with advice to culture before treatment
- Herpes Simplex Virus - referral for counselling should be advised
- Actinomyces - like organisms
- Follicular Cervicitis - report in younger women

It is advisable that additional investigations towards definitive diagnosis must be pursued before embarking on treatment.

7.1.6 Follow up of patients on treatment

The Follow-up of women who have been treated for CIN is very crucial to ensure that there is no progression of the disease condition.

- CIN1 - repeat smears at 6months, 12months and 2years this is the schedule if the smear is persistently negative.
- CIN2 and above -This categories of patients require annual smears for 10 years of follow up.
- CGIN(Cervical Glandular Intraepithelia Neoplasia) - are at greater risk of recurrent disease so they are recommended to have smears every 6months for 2years,then annually for 10 years

Follow-up of women with low grade smears but normal colposcopy and no biopsy - require a repeat smear at 6 months, 6 months , 12 months, then return to normal recall

Follow-up of women after hysterectomy for CIN or SCC :

Where there was complete excision and the margins were clear of dysplastic cells, vault smears should be carried out at 6 months and 18 months before recall can be cancelled as no further smears are required.

In the case of women with incomplete or uncertain excision at hysterectomy, they would require follow-up as for women with CIN2 or above.

In women who have been exposed to radiotherapy as an adjuvant therapy, Smears are not advised in this group of women.

7.1.7 Borderline nuclear change

This is a "holding" category where there is genuine doubt as to whether or not a smear is abnormal. The nuclear changes are not typical and convincing of cervical dyskaryosis and as such it can not be labelled as negative.

Borderline nuclear change is used when wart virus changes are seen on the smear, without dyskaryosis.

It can also be used when severe inflammatory changes exist on the smear, which can sometimes appear almost dyskaryotic.

When interpretation of the smear is difficult e.g. as it is in poor handling or fixing and or staining process (such as due to air drying)

7.1.8 Management of borderline nuclear change

The smear should be repeated at 6 months, interval for 1year and 12 months later. - If all are negative, normal recall can be resumed.

If in the course of the follow up, there are a maximum of 3 reports of borderline nuclear change in the follow-up period, referral for colposcopy is advised.

At any point in time One report of borderline glandular cells requires immediate referral for further evaluation..

In difficult cases, where there is concern that high grade disease may be present, immediate referral can be recommended.

8.1 CIN I/Low sil management

CIN I/Low SIL correlates to Nucleus occupying up to 1/2 of the area of the cell(Nucleocytoplasmic ratio of half)

8.1.1 Management of mild dyskaryosis

It is advisable that she should have a colposcopy done,in centres where this facilities are not available, "it remains acceptable to recommend a repeat test".

If the repeat smear is the same diagnosis (mild dyskaryosis) then a referral must be advised.

8.2.1 CINII/High SIL

8.2.2 Cytological features

CIN II/High SIL correlates to Nucleus occupying up to ½ to 2/3 of the area of the cell(Nucleocytoplasmic ratio of ½ to 2/3)

The Chromatin pattern is usually more abnormal compare to CIN I

If a smear is obviously dyskaryotic, but difficult to grade e.g. because there are too few cells or they are poorly preserved, it is recommended that they be coded as moderate.

8.2.3 Management of moderate dyskaryosis

All patients with moderate dyskaryosis should be referred for colposcopy.

8.3.1 CIN III/ High SIL

8.3.2 Cytological features

CIN III/High SIL correlates to Nucleus occupying more than 2/3 of the area of the cell(Nucleocytoplasmic ratio greater than 2/3).The nucleus may have a bizarre shape.

The Chromatin pattern is usually more abnormal compare to CIN I

8.3.3 Management of severe dyskaryosis/CIN III/High SIL

Referral for colposcopy is the standard approach of management.This will include tissue biopsy for histology.

8.4.1 Invasive squamous carcinoma

8.4.2 Cytological features

The histological features are essentially that of Bizarre nuclear changes and keratinisation.

Diathesis is also a notable findings in this patients.

8.4.3 Management of invasive squamous carcinoma

In this case an URGENT referral for colposcopy and tissue diagnosis is advised.

9. Treatment of cervical intra-epithelia neoplasia

9.1 Low grade lesions

In the treatment of this disease entity a colposcopy,with or without a repeat smear,and or tissue biopsy is an essential requirement as stated above. The uses of additional investigative tools are very essential in the treatment of this condition. The time interval between diagnosis and treatment can be very crucial

The option of treatment range between Cryotherapy, cold coagulation,Laser agglutination therapy and Electrocautery. A lot of caution must be applied to avert over treatment especially in young women who are still desirous of conception (over treatment can cause fertility problems).

The follow up schedule as stated above and the patient should be encouraged to adhere to this to achieve the desired goal of screening.

9.2 High grade lesions

The additional investigations include Colposcopy, repeat smear and tissue biopsy is important toward establishing a diagnosis,because the treatment involved is usually irreversible. Such definitive treatment includes ablative procedures and amputation surgeries.

The definitive treatments include Cold coagulation,Lletz, laser agglutination therapy, electrcautery, knife cone biopsy and trachelectomy.

9.3 Summary of indication for colposcopy examinations

The under listed are the patient that would benefit from colposcopy

- Following 3 consecutive inadequate smears.
- Women with clinical symptoms e.g. PMB, friable cervix
- Post menopausal women with unexplained endometrial cells
- Women with genital warts.
- Persistent borderline smears (maximum 3)
- One report of borderline nuclear change in glandular cells.
- After 3 abnormal smear results (any grade) in a 10 year period.
- One report of mild dyskaryosis.

- One report of moderate dyskaryosis.
- One report of severe dyskaryosis.
- One report of ? invasive SCC.
- One report of ? glandular neoplasia.
- A report of mild or worse in women on follow-up for treated CIN

10. Human immunosuppressive virus and cervical intra-epithelia neoplasia

This is actually of more relevance in the developing nations. It's a major scourge of our time that needs to be address at all time and at every given opportunity.

Follow up in CIN cases is done closely in HIV-positive women: treatment of CIN I has a high failure rate in these women, but it has a relatively low rate of progression (Robert Finn 2011).

HIV-infected women were 3.7 times more likely to develop CIN than HIV-uninfected women. These results highlight the importance of regular cervical cytological screening for HIV-Infected women.(Wright)

The interplay between HIV infection, HPV infection and CIN/cervical cancer is complex (see Box 34.1). Cervical dysplasia and possibly invasive cervical cancer are more prevalent in HIV-positive women. The latter has a higher rate of HPV infections which are strongly associated with high-grade SIL and invasive cervical cancer.(Sun et al 1997) Immune suppression is the factor predisposing HIV positive women to HPV infections fig 20. CIN is commoner in HIV infected women with a lower CD4 count or AIDS. (Sun et al 1995) have suggested that the presence of immunosuppression shifts the ratio of latent: clinically expressed HPV infection from 8:1 in the general population to 3:1 in HIV-positive women with CD4 >500/µL and to 1:1 when CD4<200/µL. Linking the US AIDS and Cancer Registry, the observed cervical cancer cases in HIV infected women were up to 9 folds higher than the expected number of cases but the likelihood of cervical cancer is not related to the CD4 count. (mbulaiteye et al2003).

The screening process for the HIV positive patients differs significantly based on the prelude of our discussion and as such the have the following schedules:

Pelvic examination and Pap smear are repeated six months after the baseline.(Anderson 2005) If both times are normal, cervical screening is then performed every twelve months alongside with careful vulval, vaginal and anal inspections. There is no specific CD4 threshold under which the frequency of Pap smear would need to be increased, though this may be considered in cases of(Anderson 2005)

a. Previous abnormal Pap smear
b. HPV infection
c. Symptomatic HIV disease
d. CD4 counts <200/µL
e. Post-treatment for CIN

Other forms of screening may be employed in the management of those who are positive for HIV. *HPV-DNA* has recently been introduced as one form of screening. As there is a high incidence of HPV infection in HIV patient and most HIV patients with abnormal smear will ultimately need colposcopy evaluation (to rule out CIN and cervical cancer), the use of HPV-DNA in the triage for colposcopy is of limited value and it is not cost effective. On the other hand, despite the higher incidence of cervical abnormality in HIV infected patients, *colposcopy* is not generally recommended for primary cervical screening (Anderson et al 2005) but indicated when pap smear reveals epithelial cell abnormality.

Box 34.1 Relationship between HIV, HPV and CIN/cervical cancer

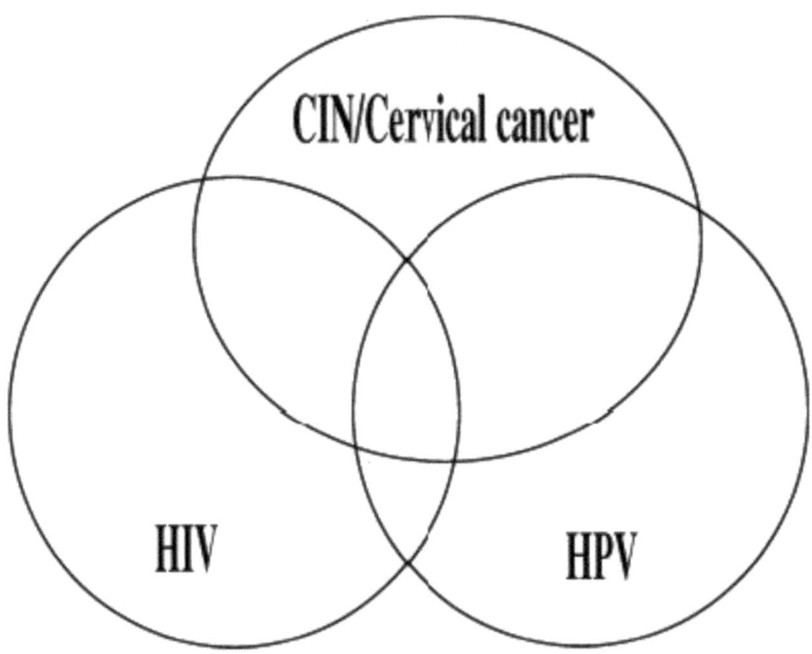

Fig. 20. (Courtesy Siu-Keung LAM) Relationship Between HIV,HPV & CIN 1

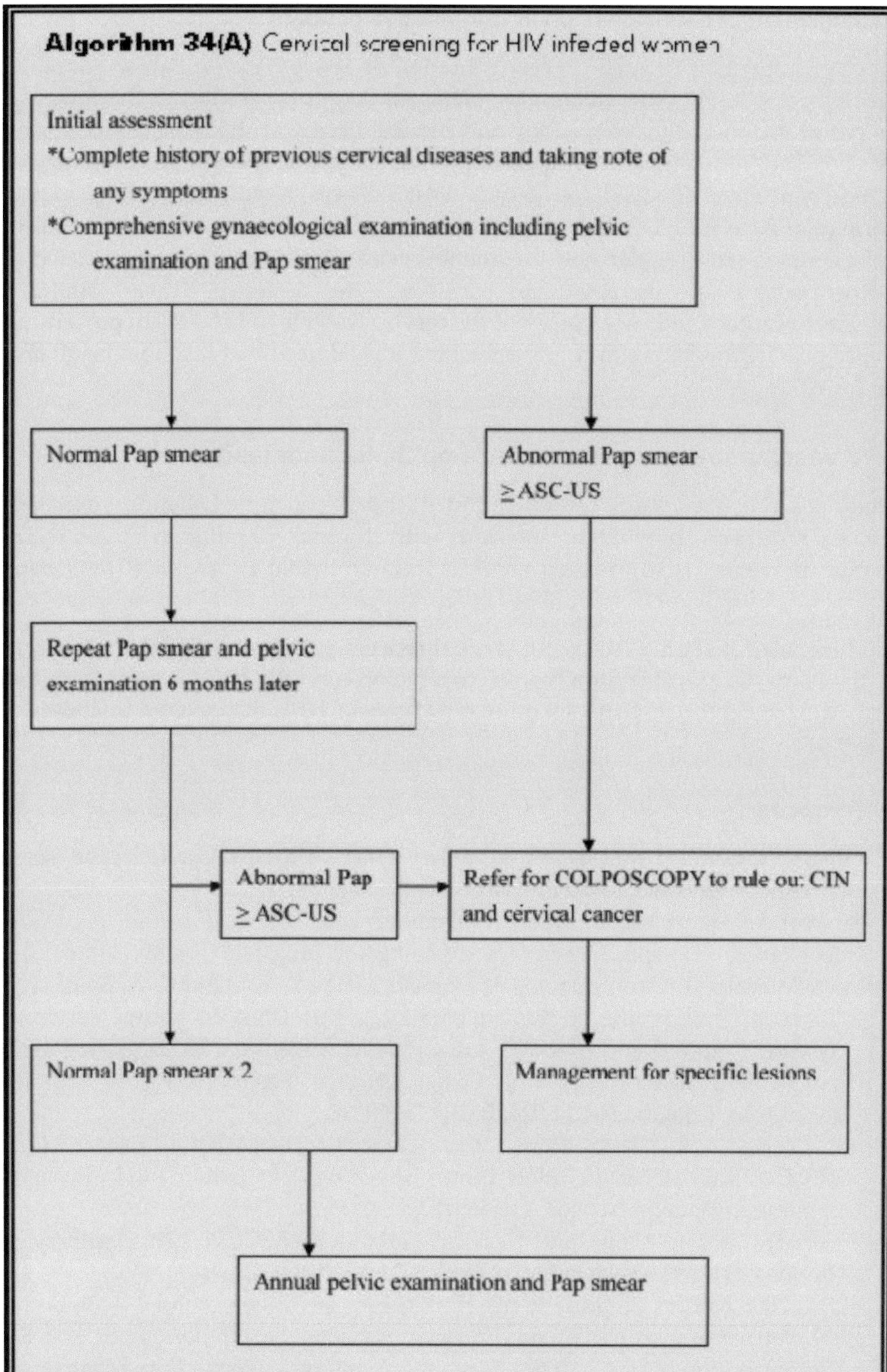

Fig. 21. (Courtesy of Siu-Keung LAM)

10.1 Management of cervical lesion in HIV positive patients

HIV-infected patients with ASC-US cervical lesion or above once on Pap smear should be referred for colposcopy. At a colposcopy clinic, thorough evaluation of the lower genital tract is performed including colposcopy and cervical biopsy at the most suspicious area to rule out CIN and/or malignancy. If there is no HGSIL, patients are followed up regularly in the colposcopy clinic. If HGSIL is found, most patients require large loop excision of transformation zone (LLETZ), to reduce the chance of progression to cervical cancer. This has to be coupled with regular post-treatment cervical smear surveillance as stated above. The other forms of therapy that can be use includes, Laser agglutination therapy,Electrocautery and cone biopsy of the cervix. The role of HAART in preventing CIN recurrence post treatment is still controversial,but it is adviced that it should be given.(**Siu-Keung LAM)**

11. HPV vaccination and cervical intra-epithelia neoplasia

In a randomised control study (double blinded) it was concluded that, In young women who have not been previously infected with human papillomavirus-16 (HPV16), vaccination prevents HPV16-related cervical intra-epithelial neoplasia (CIN).(Mao et al 2006).

It should be noted that only 75% of all cervical cancers are caused the HPV viruses 16 and 18,it is therefore still possible for a woman to develop cervical cancer even though they are immunised. This is because there are other sero types of HPV not covered by those vaccine in the market.

12. References

ACCP. Visual screening approaches: (October 2002). Promising alternative screening strategies. Cervical Cancer Prevention Fact Sheet.

ACCP & World Health Organization. November 2003 Cervical cancer prevention in developing countries: A review of screening and programmatic strategies.

Agorastos T, Miliaras D, Lambropoulos A, Chrisafi S, Kotsis A, Manthos A, Bontis J (2005). "Detection and typing of human papillomavirus DNA in uterine cervices with coexistent grade I and grade III intraepithelial neoplasia: biologic progression or independent lesions?". *Eur J Obstet Gynecol Reprod Biol* 121 (1): 99–103. doi:10.1016/j.ejogrb.2004.11.024. PMID 15949888.

American College of Obstetricians and Gynecologists.(ACOG) Obstet Gynecol. 2010;Cervical cancer in adolescents: screening, evaluation, and management. Committee Opinion No. 463. 116:469–72.

America Society for colposcopy and Cervical Pathology (ASCCP) 2011 Anatomy of the Uterine Cervix.The society for the lower Genital Tract disease.

Anderson JR. 2005 edition. A guide to the clinical care of women with HIV-. Published by US Department of Health and Human Services, Health Resources and Service Administration, HIV/AIDS Bureau. Available from http://hab.hrsa.gov/ publications/womencare05.

Ardahan, Melek PhD, RN; Temel, Ayla Bayik PhD, RN. March/April 2011 Visual Inspection With Acetic Acid in Cervical Cancer Screening

Cancer Nursing: Volume 34 - Issue 2 - pp 158-163doi: 10.1097/NCC.0b013e3181efe69f Articles.

Barbara G,2011 Cervical Intraepithelia Neoplasia in Up to Date Marketing Professionals.

Dina.R. Eurocytology 5th-10th September 2011 Hammersmith AdvancedClinical Cytopathology Course Held at Imperial College- HammersmithHospital campus - Commonwealth Building.

IARC(International Agency for Research on Cancer) 2001 An Introduction to Cervical Intraepithelial Neoplasia (CIN)charpter 2.

Kumar, V; Abbas, A K.; Fausto, N; & Mitchell, R N. (2007). Robbins Basic Pathology (8th ed.). Saunders Elsevier. pp. 718–721. ISBN 978-1-4160-2973-1. ^Cervical Dysplasia: Overview, Risk Factors.

Mao C, Koutsky LA, Ault KA, et al. 2006 Efficacy of human papillomavirus-16 vaccine to prevent cervical intraepithelial neoplasia. Obstet Gynecol; 107:18-27.

Mark H (2010)UNSW Embryology of Genital System - Female Uterus

Mbulaiteye SM, Biggar RJ, Goedert JJ, Engels EA. 2003 Immune deficiency and risk for malignancy among persons with AIDS. J Acquir Immune Defic Syndr;32:527-33.

NEL J. T.; DE LANGE L. ; MEIRING P. J. ; DE WET J. I.1994 Cervical intra-epithelial neoplasia and invasive cervical cancer in black and white patients ; SAMJ. South African medical journal ISSN 0256-9574 CODEN SAMJAF , vol. 84, no1, pp. 18-19 (16 ref.)

Oguntayo O A and Samaila .M O A Prevalence of Cervical Intraepithelia Neoplasia in Zaria,Annals of African Medicine Vol 9,No 3;2010:194-5.

Robert Finn 2011Follow CIN closely in HIV-positive women: .(Gynecology): An article from: OB GYN News [HTML] [Digital.

Sasieni P, Adams J (1999 May):Effect of screening on cervical cancer mortality in England and Wales: analysis of trends with an age period cohort model;*BMJ* 8;318(7193):1244-5.

Siu-Keung LAM CERVICAL NEOPLASIA IN HIV/AIDS.

Sun XW, Ellerbrock TV, Lungu O, Chiasson MA, Bush TJ, Wright TC Jr. 1995 Human papillomavirus infection in human immunodeficiency virus-seropositive women. Obstet Gynecol;85(5 Pt 1):680-6.

Sun XW, Kuhn L, Ellerbrock TV, Chiasson MA, Bush TJ, Wright TC Jr. 1997 Human papillomavirus infection in women infected with the human immunodeficiency virus. N Engl J Med;337:1343-9.

UVa Health 2006 Pathology Thread IV. *Premalignant and Malignant Neoplasms* University of Virginia School of Medicine. Department of Patholo PO Box 800214 System www.med-ed.virginia.edu/courses/path/gyn/cervix4.cfm -

Vanessa Jackson 2006 CERVICAL CYTOLOGY REPORTING AND TERMINOLOGY AND MANAGEMENT OF ABNORMAL SMEARS Advanced Biomedical Scientist Practitioner Leeds Teaching Hospitals NHS Trust.

Wright TC, Ellerbrock TV, Chiasson MA, Williamson J, Sun X, Bush TJ 1995 Jan 29-Feb 2 Incidence and risk factors for cervical intraepithelial neoplasia (CIN) in HIV-infected women.; National Conference on Human Retroviruses and Related Infections. *Program Abstr Second Natl Conf Hum Retrovir Relat Infect Natl Conf Hum Retrovir Relat Infect 2nd Wash DC;* 90. Columbia University and NYC Department of Health, NY.

Wart From Wikipedia, the free encyclopedia www.facebook.com/pages/Warts/110511208977959

Wright TC Jr, Cox JT, Massad LS, Twiggs LB, Wilkinson EJ; 2002 ASCCP-Sponsored Consensus Conference. 2001 Consensus Guidelines for the management of women with cervical cytological abnormalities. JAMA;287:2120-9.

13

AKNA as Genetic Risk Factor for Cervical Intraepithelial Neoplasia and Cervical Cancer

Kirvis Torres-Poveda, Ana I. Burguete-García, Margarita Bahena-Román, Alfredo Lagunas-Martínez and Vicente Madrid-Marina
Division of Chronic Infection Diseases and Cancer, Centro de Investigación Sobre Enfermedades Infecciosas, Instituto Nacional de Salud Pública, Cuernavaca, Morelos, Mexico

1. Introduction

Cervical cancer (CC) is the second most common cancer among women worldwide. The highest incidence rates of CC are reported in Central and South America, East Africa, South and Southeast Asia and Melanesia. In 2005 there were, according to WHO projections, more than 500, 000 new cases and 274, 000 deaths from CC (WHO, 2007). This is due to the fact that the majority of women in the world do not have access to cervical screening, which can prevent up to 75% of CC cases (Ferlay et al., 2001). Predictions based on the passive growth of the population and the increase in life expectancy say that the expected number of CC cases in 2020 will increase by 40% worldwide, corresponding to 56% in developing countries and 11% in the developed parts of the world (Ferlay et al., 2001).

The development of CC is preceded by a series of cellular abnormalities characterized by cytological and histological changes in cytoplasm maturation and nuclear irregularities. The disease starts as an atypical proliferation of epithelial cells that invade epithelial thickness and degenerate into more serious injuries that invade the stroma. The development of precancerous lesions of the cervix involves several events: exposure to a high-risk Human Papilloma Virus (HR-HPV) causes an initial infection of the squamous epithelium in the transformation zone, followed by morphological and biological alterations of the HPV infected cells (Walboomers et al., 1999).

As the understanding of the natural history of the disease has improved, the classification of these lesions has received different names: PAP I to V, moderate dysplasia, severe carcinoma in situ, cervical intraepithelial neoplasia (CIN) I, II, III, low grade squamous intraepithelial lesions (LSIL) and high grade squamous intraepithelial lesions (HSIL). Microscopically, the evolution of the lesion is characterized by the differentiation of epithelial cells that proliferate and invade the epithelial tissue. Progression is described in terms of increase in the degree of dysplasia (mild, moderate, severe) and carcinoma in situ (El-Ghobashy et al., 2005). Early lesions are now considered manifestations of HPV infection, which are characterized by the presence of nuclear changes and cell proliferation of the epithelium. These cellular abnormalities tend to regress spontaneously, but some of these lesions, particularly those caused by highly oncogenic HPV (16, 18, 31, 33, 35, 45, 56, 58) can modify the thickness of the epithelium and the disease (Nobbenhuis et al., 2001). LSIL and CIN II, have a diploid or polyploid DNA content, which correlates with their tendency to reverse. In contrast, CIN III is often aneuploid, has a greater degree of cellular atypia and is more likely to persist, or progress (Grubisi¢ et al., 2009).

The causal role of HPV in CIN and CC has been firmly established biologically and epidemiologically (Walboomers et al., 1999). Current meta-analysis of the literature shows that the most common HPV types worldwide, in descending order of frequency, are HPV 16, 18, 45, 31, 33, 52, 58 and 35. These are responsible for about 90% of all CC worldwide. The distribution is very similar to that of pre-invasive HSIL (Muñoz et al., 2004; Smith et al., 2007). Since the main route of transmission of genital HPV is sexual, certain patterns of sexual behavior (age of onset of sexual activity, number of sexual partners and sexual behavior of the couple) are associated with an increased risk of infection with genital HPV. But persistent infection with HR-HPV is necessary for carcinogenesis, and cofactors such as multiparity, prolonged use of oral contraceptives, smoking and co-infection with HIV, enhance the progression of infection to cancer (Almonte et al., 2008).

HPVs are species-specific and induce epithelial or fibroepithelial proliferations of benign skin and mucosa in humans and in several animal species. These viruses have a specific tropism for squamous epithelial cells and their production cycle only happens in these cells. HPV infection begins in the basal cells, which are mitotically active. After infection, the virus can lie dormant, replicate and produce infectious particles or become integrated into the cellular genome. Productive infection is divided into several stages depending on the state of differentiation of the epithelial cells. The full cycle that includes viral DNA synthesis, production of viral capsid proteins and assembly of virions, occurs selectively in terminally differentiated keratinocytes (Doorbar, 2006). The basal layer cells proliferate; despite containing HPV DNA, they appear to be very active in the expression of some viral proteins. Apparently, there are cellular factors that negatively regulate viral transcription in these cells.

This regulation is released when the infected cells migrate upward from the epithelium in the granular layer, where they undergo differentiation until they can no longer divide. First, transcription of early and late viral genes is activated in these cells, viral proteins are then synthesized and viral particles are assembled in some superficial cells (Longworth et al., 2004). Although most HPV infections are transient and subclinical, progression is strongly associated with HPV persistence. This process often leads to viral breakthrough in the E1/E2 regions and integration of viral DNA into the cell. The rupture releases the viral E6/E7 promoters and increases the expression of these transformer genes (Moody et al., 2010; Ghittoni et al., 2010). Infection with a HR-HPV acts as a trigger for the cascade of events in which the mechanisms of repair or correction of cell replication, mediated by p53 and retinoblastoma protein (Rb) are altered. Thus, the cell cycle is controlled by the virus, which triggers cellular changes that culminate in the transformation and immortalization of epithelial cells, thus establishing conditions for the start of cancer (Pim & Banks, 2010).

Most HPV infections are transient and intermittent. Epidemiological studies have shown that HPV clearance in healthy, immune competent individuals, takes 8 to 12 months (Woodman et al., 2007). Cohort studies have shown that the continued presence of HR-HPV is necessary for the development, maintenance and progression of HSIL (Ho et al., 1998; Bory et al., 2002; Muñoz et al., 2003; Dalstein et al., 2003; Cuschieri et al., 2005). To establish a persistent infection, HPVs gain access to mitotically active basal-layer keratinocytes, where low-copy replication begins. The viral DNA persists as a nuclear episome in infected cells. In the non-productive stage of infection, HPVs replicate at low copy number in mitotically active basal layer cells within stratified epithelia (Howley, 1996). HPV genomes can persist in proliferating keratinocytes for years or decades. This persistent phase of the viral lifecycle is characterized by detectable levels of viral genome, but the absence of virus production (Stubenrauch & Laimins, 1999), which is most likely a strategy to evade immune surveillance. So, there are two well-defined phenomena in the development of neoplasia - first, there is an alteration in the cellular immune response that allows the persistence of the virus for many years (Walboomers et al., 1999; Nobbenhuis et al., 2001) and second, the phenomena of transformation in epithelial cells produced by oncogenic virus proteins (E6 and E7) through degradation of p53 and pRb (Scheffner et al., 1990; Boyer et al., 1996) and alteration in the expression of proto-oncogenes such as c-Myc and Ras (Marangoz et al., 1999).

Genetic factors intrinsic to the host immune system play a role in susceptibility and/or resistance to the development of CC. Genetic factors associated with CC are polymorphisms in genes coding for tumor necrosis factor alpha (TNF-α) (Wilson et al., 1997; Kirkpatrick et al., 2004), matrix metallopeptidase 1 (Lai et al., 2005), p53 (Dokianakis et al., 2000; Makni et al., 2000), Human Leukocyte Antigen-HLA (Apple et al., 1994; Hildesheim & Wand, 2002) and Fas (Lai et al., 2003). In a complete genome scan in families with more than one child with CC, it was found that in the long arm of chromosome 9 there is a susceptibility locus for the development of cervical carcinoma. In this locus, candidate genes could be potentially involved in genetic predisposition to this disease (Engelmark et al., 2006). Genes such as IKBKAP, PTPN3, TSCOT, AMBP, *akna*, TNFSF15, TNFSF8 and DEC1, have important roles in the development of the immune response.

Among these is the *akna* gene, which is located in band 32 (9q32) on chromosome 9 (HGNC: 24108) and consists of 24 exons (http://www.ncbi.nlm.nih.gov/gene/80709) (Figure 1A). Up to 9 different *akna* transcripts have been identified, resulting from alternative promoter usage, splicing and poly-adenylation. Of the 9 reported transcripts, the 3.1 kb F1 transcript has been functionally tested by our research group (Sims et al., 2005; Perales et al., 2010).

The AKNA protein encoded by this gene is a nuclear protein consisting of 633 amino acids with an approximate weight of 63 kDa. AKNA contains an AT-hook motif of nine amino acids, RTRGRPADS (arginine, threonine, arginine, glycine, arginine, proline, alanine, aspartic acid, serine), which satisfies the consensus requirements of an AT hook DNA-binding motif. The AT-hook is a small motif with a typical sequence signature, in which the tripeptide GRP (Gly^{58}, Arg^{59} and Pro^{60}) is the centre of the DNA-binding domain (Siddiqa et al; 2011). Besides, AKNA contains multiple PEST protein-cleavage motifs, which have been shown to target proteins of rapid turnover (Chevallier, 1993; Siddiqa et al., 2001) and has three domains located in the PEST regions: Leu10-Thr43, H149-Ser171, and P616-T63. These regions are sites of protein degradation so AKNA is considered to have a short half-life (Siddiqa et al., 2001) (Figure 1B).

It has been demonstrated that AKNA expresses at least nine transcripts, some of which are expressed in a tissue-specific manner, reflecting its functional diversity. Besides, several of these transcripts are predicted to encode proteins of 155, 137, 100 and 70 kDa. However, only two isoforms (70 and 100 kDa) are expressed in B- and T- cell lines, and both bind to the promoters of the costimulatory molecules of the immune response - CD40 and CD40L (CD40 ligand) (Sims et al; 2005). It has been shown that PEST-dependent cleavage of AKNA is key to its DNA binding function, because in the absence of the PEST-dependent cleavage, the expression of AKNA alone is not sufficient to induce CD40 expression (Sims et al., 2005; Ma et al., 2011).

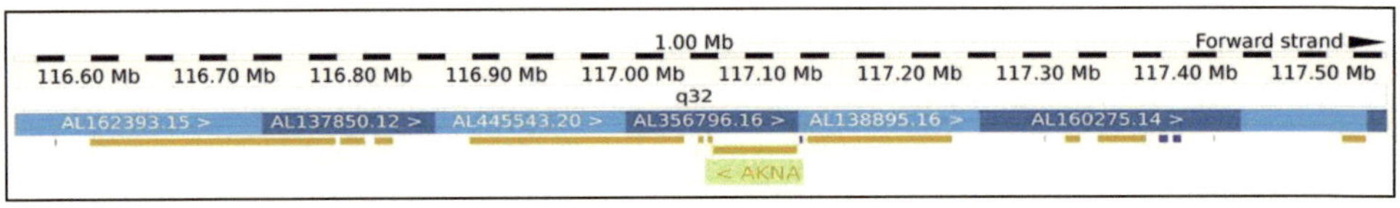

Fig. 1A. Akna gene localized in chromosome 9Q32

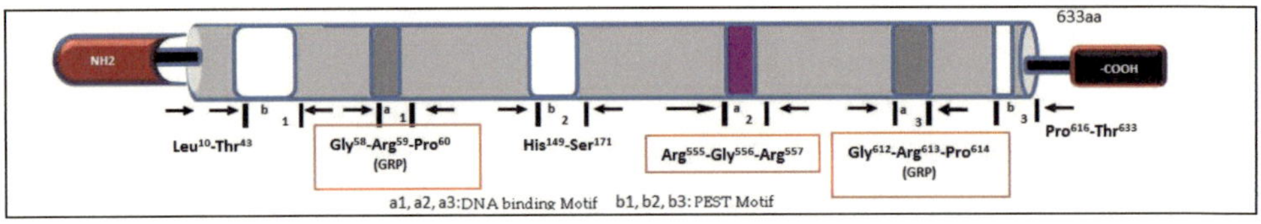

Fig. 1B. Protein at-hook-containning transcription factor

AT-hook proteins have been mainly recognized within the high mobility group A (HMGA) family, which includes chromatin remodeling proteins that coordinate transcriptional complexes to regulate gene expression (Cui & Leng, 2007). However, non-HMG AT-hook proteins have been identified and characterized. Among these, proteins with AT-hook-like motifs (ALMs) have been found to be capable of binding A/T-rich gene targets and regulating their transcription (Senthilkumar & Mishra, 2009; Gordon et al., 2010). In keeping with this notion, the human AKNA gene is a non-HMG transcription factor, which contains N- and C- terminus AT-hook motifs (Siddiqa et al., 2001; Sims et al., 2005). In addition, the AT-hook motif is considered to be the key to upregulation of expression of immune system co-activator molecules, since it has been shown to be directly involved in inducing the expression of molecules belonging to the TNFR family members. AKNA is mainly expressed in secondary lymphoid organs; it is expressed by germinal centre B lymphocytes during B-lymphocyte differentiation and by natural killer (NK) cells and dendritic cells (Siddiqa et al., 2001). AKNA binds the A/T-rich regulatory elements of the CD40 and CD40L promoters (a key receptor-ligand pair that is critical for antigen-dependent B cell development) and induces its expression (Siddiqa et al., 2001).

Thus, in this chapter we will discuss the findings of our research group with respect to the immune response against HPV, CIN and CC, and associated genetic factors of susceptibility to the disease that we found in population studies, particularly the *akna* gene.

2. Immune response against HPV & CIN

In the HPV cycle in keratinocytes, mature virions are shed from the epithelial surface of infected keratinocytes. HPV infection is poorly immunogenic because it is productive (produces no characteristic local inflammation) and during infection there is little presentation of viral antigens to the immune system by professional antigen presenting cells, both locally and systemically (Feller et al., 2010). There is no significant evidence in the literature of inflammation being a risk factor for lesion progression, as observed in several tumor models. On the contrary, the inflammatory infiltrate in patients with established lesions seems to display anti-inflammatory or suppressor characteristics, like the absence of inducible NO synthase (iNOS) expression by macrophages (Mazibrada et al., 2008) and indoleamina2′3′-deoxigenase expression by dendritic cells (Kobayashi et al., 2008).

Interestingly, the number of infiltrating macrophages seems to increase in correlation with lesion grade (Hammes et al., 2007; Kobayashi et al., 2008; Mazibrada et al., 2008). T lymphocytes also infiltrate cervical HPV associated lesions, where the phenotype, abundance and balance between different populations are important in determining the fate of lesions or tumors (Piersma et al., 2004; van der Burg, 2007; Woo et al., 2008). Cellular immune response plays an important role in the control and course of HPV infection; this response varies depending on the degree of injury and the oncogenic potential of HPV. There is evidence that HPV interferes with cell cycle control, secondary to the accumulation of genetic abnormalities; this accounts for viral persistence and the progression of lesions. In many patients secondary factors, such as inadequate immune response, play an important role (Riethmuller & Seilles, 2000).

At the cervical level, after infection of epithelial cells by HPV, a non-specific response is triggered accompanied by chemoattraction of neutrophils, activation of macrophages, activation of NK, natural antibodies and complement system; this is a first defensive barrier of specific immunity. Reticular cells of Langerhans (RCL) and some keratinocytes act as antigen presenting cells (APCs). RCLs are immature dendritic cells of myeloid origin residing in the squamous epithelium, including genital mucosa. RCL recognize the viral particles, capture antigens by micropinocytosis or mannose receptors, process captured proteins and transform them into immunogenic peptides, start the activation process (which includes a surface antigen polypeptide chain with HLA class II, CD40 and B7), migrate to local lymph nodes and present viral peptides to T cells in the context of the major histocompatibility complex (MHC) and costimulatory molecules (CD80, CD86 and CD40). Thus, native lymphocytes are activated and direct their differentiation into effector cells, initiating the antigen-specific immune response (Stern, 2008).

During a primary immune response, depending on the microenvironment and the signals received from certain cytokines, naive $CD4^{+}$ T cells can differentiate into three to four major subsets of Th cells, with distinct patterns of cytokine secretion that drive different types of immune responses (Seder et al., 2003; Weaver et al., 2006). Briefly, IFN-γ and Interleukin (IL)-12 induce differentiation of Th1 cells to produce more IFN-γ, which enhances the clearance of viruses and the proliferation of specific CD8 cytotoxic T lymphocytes (CTL); on the contrary, if the local context does not express IL-12, it promotes the Th2 pathway which induces activation and expansion of B cells; these evolve, differentiating into plasma cells producing antibodies to viral proteins and inducing the expression of interleukins type IL-4, IL-5, IL-6 and IL-10 (Stern, 2008). The mediators of cell-mediated immunity against HPV infected cells and some tumors are CTL, which eliminate virally infected cells by means of antigen-specific, cell-mediated citotoxicity. Additionally, CD4+ T helper cells participate in the control of these processes. Under certain conditions, the Tumor Growth Factor Beta (TGF-β1) or IL-10 alone drives regulatory CD4+ T cell (Treg) differentiation which regulates immune responses by several distinct mechanisms (Damoiseaux, 2006; Robertson & Hasenkrug, 2006). Thus, together with CTL, the only Th subset that is desirable in pre-malignant CC lesions is that of Th1 cells, as IFN-γ favors immune responses against viral infections.

The natural history of these tumors is long and includes the following steps: infection, persistent infection, viral genome integration into the host cell genome, genomic alterations, immortalization and transformation of epithelial cells. During all these steps, evasion of the immune system is an obligatory feature. The immune evasion mechanisms displayed by the infected cells include absence of cell death (Tindle, 2002), blocking of type I Interferon signaling and reduction of antigen presentation by MHC-I (Ashrafi et al., 2005; Stern, 2008).

2.1 Cellular immune response

Local cellular immune response detected in SIL is characterized by a moderate infiltrate and a decreased inverted Th/Tc (CD4/CD8) ratio, with decreased proliferative capacity (Santin et al., 2001). An imbalance in the pattern of cytokines, as by an increase in type II interleukin (IL-4, IL-10, suppressing the cellular immune response) and a concomitant reduction in interleukin type I [(IL-2, gamma interferon (IFN-γ)], has been reported in women with SIL and CC (Giannini et al., 1998; Clerici et al., 1998; Bor-Ching et al., 2001). Anti-tumor immunity in CC is activated by Th1 cytokines and inhibited by Th2 cytokines. Cytokines such as IL-4, IL-12, IL-10 and/or TGF-β1, produced by various cell types (macrophages, dendritic cells and keratinocytes) have been involved in the suppression of cellular immune response (Giannini et al., 1998).

The pattern of cytokines and their expression in women with CC biopsies has been analyzed. 80% of the tumors express low levels of mRNA of CD4 T lymphocytes and high levels of CD8 CTL. Most tumors express the mRNA of IL-4 and IL-10 and 100% of them express the mRNA of TGF-β1 and IFN-γ. None of the tumors express the IL-12 mRNA, IL-6 mRNA or TNF-α (Alcocer et al., 2006). Immunohistochemical analysis of tumors has demonstrated the presence of IL-10 in tumor cells and cell koilocytes, but not in infiltrating lymphocytes, suggesting that the cells producing IL-10 can be transformed by HPV. On the other hand, a correlation has been found between the immunostaining of IL-10 protein, the level of mRNA IL-10 expression and the supernatants of HPV transformed cell lines expressing IL-10 and TGF-β1 (Alcocer et al., 2006). These findings show a predominant expression of immunosuppressive cytokines, which help to downregulate tumor specific immune response in the tumor microenvironment (Alcocer et al., 2006).

In a recent study, the functionality of peripheral blood T lymphocytes (PBL) and tumor-infiltrating lymphocytes (TIL) of women with SIL and CC was assessed, including proliferation, mRNA expression of IL-2, IFN-γ, IL-4, IL-10 and TGF-β1, as well as the expression of CD3ζ. Using immunohistochemistry, we have seen that TIL is distributed in the stroma more than in epithelium in advanced stages of the disease where CD8 CTL prevail. PBL stimulated with phytohemagglutinin in patients with CC, proliferate less than in SIL patients and healthy subjects. Also, a significant difference is observed in the PBL stimulated with anti-CD3, between patients with CC and healthy subjects. This shows that women with CC have a poor proliferative PBL response and a lack of response to TIL (Díaz et al., 2009).

Antigen recognition of cells with cytotoxic capacity is mediated by receptors. In T cells, these are called T-cell receptors (TCR), which consist of a heterodimer of $\alpha\beta/\gamma\delta$ chains and four ε, δ, γ, ε chains, which together are recognized as TcR-CD3. These receptors are in turn associated with two "zeta" strings which are responsible for the transmission of activation signals within the cell. Zeta chains are also present in the receptor for NK cell antigens. Molecular studies have shown a decreased expression of the dimer formed by the zeta chain, in both T cells and NK cells, contributing to the inefficiency of the effector mechanisms of lymphocytic infiltrate present in the lesions. It has been demonstrated that there is a decreased expression of CD3-zeta chain in patients with CC and CIN (Kono et al., 1996; Shondel et al., 2007), and that suppression *in vivo* can be the result of a circulating factor (Shondel et al., 2007). We found that IL-10 and TGF-ß1 produced by HPV-transformed cells are responsible for CD3-zeta suppression in CC patients (Diaz et al., 2009). These processes are regulated by local factors derived from tumor cells.

As there is an imbalance of cytokines in the microenvironment of these lesions, this affects the transcriptional level. Lymphocytic infiltrate present in the cervical lesions reflects an ineffective immune response (De-Gruijl et al., 1999). A significant correlation between low lymphocyte proliferation and decreased mRNA expression of CD3ζ has been reported in T lymphocytes stimulated with anti-CD3, indicating that T cell function decreases with the progression of CC (Díaz et al., 2009). These changes result in a loss of control of certain HPV 16-18 genes and deregulation in the mechanisms of antigen presentation. Thus, the expression of HLA antigens is reduced or absent (Wang et al., 2002) and there is partial or total absence of Langerhans cells, considered to be they key antigen-presenting immune response against the tumor (Hachisuga et al., 2001).

2.1.1 Role of AKNA in immune response

Proteins containing AT hooks bind A/T-rich DNA through a nine amino-acid motif and are thought to co-regulate transcription by modifying the architecture of DNA, thereby enhancing the accessibility of promoters to transcription factors (Reeves & Nissen, 1990; Friedmann et al., 1993). AKNA is a human AT-hook protein that directly binds the A/T-rich regulatory elements of CD40 and CD40L promoters and coordinately regulates their expression. Consistent with its function, AKNA is a nuclear protein that contains multiple PEST protein-cleavage motifs, which are common in regulatory proteins with high turnover rates (Chevaillier, 1993).

AKNA is mainly expressed by B and T lymphocytes, NK cells and dendritic cells. During B-lymphocyte differentiation, AKNA is mainly expressed by germinal centre B lymphocytes, a stage in which receptor and ligand interactions are crucial for B-lymphocyte maturation (Berek et al., 1991; Liu et al., 1991; Jacob & Kelsoe, 1992; McHeyzer-Williams et al., 1993; Clark & Ledbetter, 1994; MacLennan, 1994; Arpin et al., 1995; Liu et al., 1996). These findings show that an AT-hook molecule can coordinately regulate the expression of a key receptor and its ligand, and point towards a molecular mechanism that explains homotypic cell interactions (Siddiga et al., 2001).

Human AKNA is a transcription factor with N- and C- terminus AT-hook motifs (Siddiga et al., 2001; Sims et al., 2005). Thus, it is possible that AKNA expression plays a role in mechanisms that, if altered, could result in systemic and potentially fatal disorders. Human AKNA is encoded by a single gene located within the FRA9E region of chromosome 9q32 (Sims et al., 2005), a common fragile site (CFS) linked to loss-of-function mutations that often lead to inflammatory and neoplastic diseases (Thye et al., 2003; Landvik et al., 2009; Savas et al., 2009). Based on this reasoning, two independent gene-targeting mouse models were engineered to assess *in vivo* the physiological significance of *akna* gene expression. It was found that the phenotypes resulting from the deletion of the putative C-terminus ALM sequence (AKNA KO) or disruption of AKNA's exon 3 (AKNA KO2) were by and large similar: a) mice died prematurely at neonatal age; b) probable causes of sudden death included acute inflammatory reactions and alveolar destruction; c) triggering of the observed inflammation appeared to be pathogen-induced; d) systemic neutrophil mobilization and alveolar infiltration were routinely observed and; e) concerted activation of neutrophil-specific chemokine, cytokine and proteolytic enzyme expression seemed to be the norm. The central goal of the AKNA function was provided and supports the hypothesis that AKNA expression plays an important role in the mechanisms that regulate the magnitude of inflammatory responses to pathogens (Ma et al., 2011).

It was reported that deletion of murine *akna* gene results in small, frail mice that die suddenly at 10 days of life. Besides, AKNA KO mice present systemic inflammation, predominantly in the lungs, that is accompanied by enhanced leukocyte infiltration (mainly neutrophils) and alveolar destruction. Because AKNA functions as an AT-hook transcription factor, Ma and colleagues investigated expression of genes related to neutrophil function and found a significant enrichment in genes encoding inflammatory cytokines (IL-1β, IFN-γ), inflammatory proteins [neutrophilic granule protein (NGP), cathelin-related antimicrobial peptide (CRAMP), S100A8/9] and proteases (matrix metalloprotease-9; MMP-9), which are implicated in alveolar damage. Given that AKNA deficiency results in an increase of MMP-9, IL-1β, IFN-γ, NGP, and CRAMP S100A9 gene expression, it is possible that AKNA functions as a multi-faceted transcriptional repressor that can coordinately temper pathway-specific gene transcription (Ma et al., 2011; Moliterno & Resar, 2011).

It has been suggested that AKNA´s function is necessary to regulate the magnitude of pathogen-elicited neutrophil activation, proliferation and tissue infiltration by coordinately restricting autocrine/paracrine cytokine and chemokine. This implies that when AKNA is productively expressed, neutrophil reactions are increased to neutralize and destroy pathogens. However, loss of AKNA expression could exacerbate neutrophil activation and cause irreparable tissue damage. This hypothesis is in tune with the enhanced MMP-9, IL-1β, IFN-γ, and NGP expression and the resulting lethal syndrome associated with AKNA deficiency, in which transcriptional repression is seemingly lost (Ma et al., 2011). It is interesting to note that a significantly decreased expression of AKNA in CD4+ T cells has been reported in active patients with Vogt-Koyanagi-Harada Syndrome (VKH, a systemic autoimmune disease). It is unknown whether a decreased AKNA could play a role in VKH syndrome via downregulation of CD40 and CD40L (Mao et al., 2011). In conclusion, it will be interesting to determine if loss-of-function mutations, polymorphisms or epigenetic alterations in *akna* contribute to myeloid function, inflammation and neoplastic transformation.

2.1.2 Evasion of immune surveillance

There is evidence of CIN regression to normal epithelium and it has been suggested that cellular immune response is responsible for HPV clearance (Woo et al., 2010). The cellular immune response mechanisms against HPV are similar to other responses used against viral infection. However, sometimes these mechanisms fail; allow HPV persistence and tumor development. There are several mechanisms for immune response evasion; however, three operate in HPV-infected women: 1) the expression of immunesuppressor cytokines such as, IL-10 and TGF-β1; 2) Fas ligand expression in HPV-transformed cells, and 3) the presence of Treg cells (de Gruijl et al., 1999; Bor-Ching et al., 2001; Alcocer et al., 2006) which are associated with HPV persistence (Molling et al., 2007) and CIN development (Scott et al., 2009). The presence of immune suppressor cytokines in HPV-CIN patient sera has been demonstrated (Clerici et al., 1997).

It is well known that IL-10 and TGF-β1 expression are initiated at the onset of HPV infection and increase as the disease progresses. This allows us to postulate IL-10 as an HPV escape mechanism of the cellular immune response (Bermúdez-Morales et al., 2008). IL-10 and TGF-β1 are expressed in HPV-transformed cells and are induced by HPV E2, E6 and E7 proteins (Bor-Ching et al., 2001; Peralta et al., 2006; Bermúdez et al., 2011).

A susceptibility factor for the development of CC is an alteration of the immune response in patients. This immunosuppression produces a decrease of CTL and NK activation, cells that play an important role in tumor cell elimination. Consequently, HPV-transformed cells do not express antigen presenting molecules, HLA class I and II, an effect mediated by IL-10 and TGF-β1 and by the presence of Treg (Keating et al., 1995; Ploegh, 1998; Nakamura et al., 2007). IL-10 and TGF-β1 also decrease CD3ζ chain expression of the T-cell antigen receptor (Díaz et al., 2009; Patel & Chiplunkar, 2009), which is responsible for antigen recognition. Additionally, it is well known that there are infiltrating T-lymphocytes in CIN and CC, predominantly CD8 CTL; however, these lymphocytes have a low proliferation rate and the absence of costimulatory molecules of cellular immune response. Thus, there is no activation of CTL and no elimination of neoplastic cells (Alcocer et al., 2006; Díaz et al., 2009).

2.2 Humoral immune response

Regarding the humoral response, variability has been reported in antibody titers, regardless of the high levels of circulating immune complexes, especially in those patients with tumors in advanced stages. In early lesions, high levels of IgG antibodies against HPV oncogenic proteins E6/E7 and E4 have been observed, as a result of greater antigenic stimulation, with a decreased IgG1/IgG2 ratio; this is a reflection of the Th1/Th2 imbalance (Matsumoto et al., 1999; Pedroza-Saavedra et al., 2000). In advanced tumors, higher titers of IgA and IgM decrease proportionally as the disease progresses, perhaps due to an impaired immune system (Baay et al., 1997).

3. Genetic susceptibility and AKNA polymorphisms

3.1 Cancer genetic susceptibility

Scientific advances have enabled us to predict susceptibility to developing diverse diseases, including breast, ovarian, and other cancers like CC. With this new knowledge we are able to identify, in a specific population, who are at greater risk of developing a disease.

Cancer is a complex disease that should be considered as a genetic disease. In this respect, genetic factors are not considered to be a direct cause of disease but, in combination with environmental factors, have effects on the resistance or susceptibility to diseases as cancer. Furthermore, cancer risk assessment includes the collection and interpretation of multiple factors that contribute to carcinogenesis. These factors include personal and family health history, reproductive history and hormone use, environmental risk factors such as HPV infection and lifestyle habits associated with cancer risk, as well as any genetic/genomic information (Jenkins, 2009) (Figure 2).

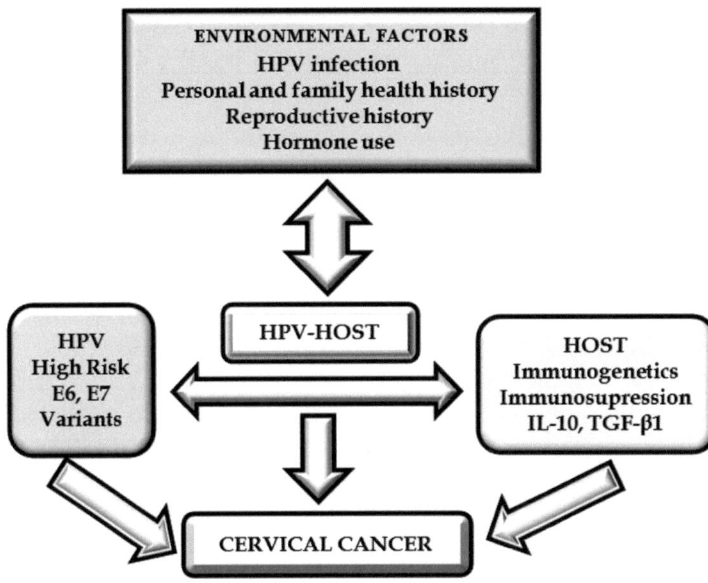

Fig. 2. Factors affecting the persistence of HPV infection and cervical cancer onset

A number of mechanisms leading to cancer have been identified through the discovery of structural alterations of genes called oncogenes and tumour suppressor genes. Somatic and germinal mutations are rare but play a determinant role in the emergence of cancer, while common and frequent variations (polymorphisms) play a role in cancer susceptibility and in the effects of anticancer drugs (efficacy and toxicity)(Robert, 2010; Hildesheim & Wand, 2002).

The susceptibility of a woman to developing CC is largely attributed to the type of HPV infecting the cervix and the persistent HPV infections associated with a high viral load; these are considered to be the major risk factors for persistent cervical lesions (Schlecht et al., 2003; de Araujo Souza & Villa, 2003). Persistence of infections by HR-HPV types is the single greatest risk factor for malignant progression. Although prophylactic vaccines have been developed that target HR-HPV types, there is a continuing need to better understand the virus-host interactions that underlie persistent benign infection and progression to cancer (Bodily & Laimins, 2011). Even though HPV is considered to be a necessary but not sufficient cause for CC, the hereditary component has been reported and several studies indicate that genetic background of the host is important for CC susceptibility and for the carcinogenic process. (de Araujo Souza & Villa, 2003; Hemminki et al., 1999; Magnusson et al., 2000; Wank & Thomssen, 1991).

To study the genetic background and to explore the differences in individual cancer susceptibility, a recent focus of research efforts has been on SNPs (single nucleotide polymorphisms). SNPs are the most common known form of human genetic variation and are defined as stable single-base substitutions with a frequency of greater than 1% in at least one population (Taylor et al., 2001; Meyer et al., 2008). For cancer research, the focus has been on SNPs that alter the function or expression of a gene, to attempt to explain observed associations with a pathogenic mechanism. Indeed, genetic polymorphisms in functionally critical genes such as immune response genes have been suggested as risk factors for the development of a variety of cancers including CC (Taylor et al., 2001; Milam et al., 2007). There are several reports about genes related to immune response (e.g. MHC genes), cytokine genes, genes involved with cancer development (e.g. p53) and CC susceptibility (Glew et al., 1992; Haukin et al., 2002; Sierra-Torres et al., 2003).

Concerning HLA polymorphisms and the risk of CC, discordant results have often been observed among different populations, where the most consistent reports are for the DRB1*13 and DRB1*0603 alleles as a protection factor with OR 0.3-0.4 (Hildesheim & Wand, 2002; Apple et al., 1994; Maciag et al., 2002) and increasing risk for the DQB1*03 and DRB1∗1501-DQB1∗0602 with OR 2.9 and for the DRB1∗0301-DQB1∗0201 haplotype, which was associated with a two-fold reduction in risk for transient and persistent HPV infections. DRB1∗1102-DQB1∗0301 showed a lower risk effect only for persistence. DRB1∗1602-DQB1∗0502 and DRB1∗0807-DQB1∗0402 were associated with seven- and three-fold increases in risk for persistence, respectively (Hildesheim & Wand, 2002; Apple et al., 1994; Maciag et al., 2002). More recently, a study of CC cases that were HPV-16 positive and controls, carried out in Mexican population, showed consistent results of association between the HLA-DRB1*15 (OR, 3.9; 95 % CI, 1.6-10.2) and the DRB1*15 DQB1*0602 haplotype (OR, 4.1; 95 % CI, 1.4-12.7) in CC cases, compared with the control group. Also for the HLA class I, the haplotypes HLA-A2-B44-DR4-DQ*0302, HLA-A24-B35-DR16-DQ*0301 and HLA-A2-B40-DR4-DQ*0302 showed a positive association with CC (OR> 1), while HLA-A2-B39-DR4-DQ*0302, HLA-A24-B35-DR4-DQ*0302 and HLA-A68-B40-DR4-DQ*0302 showed a negative association (OR <1) (Hernández et al., 2009).

Also TNF-α has been implicated in direct and indirect control of HPV infection through induction of apoptosis and stimulation of inflammatory responses. Two types of polymorphism have been described in TNF-α gene. One involves several polymorphisms in the TNF-α promoter region, including SNPs at positions -76, -161, -237, -243, -308 (G→A), -375, -568, -572, -575, -857 and -863; the second involves SNPs in DNA microsatellites (Martin et al., 2006). Evidence suggests that the GG genotype of SNP G/T at position -308 in the TNF-α promoter region, has been associated with CC precursor lesions (Kirkpatrick et al., 2004). Other TNF-α SNPs with reported associations with CC include -237, -572, -857 and –863, and haplotype analysis has again strengthened these regions as potential targets for determination of CC susceptibility. The other TNF-α polymorphisms associated with CC are the microsatellite polymorphisms TNF-α2, TNF-α8 and TNF-α11, with significant associations between CIN I and the TNF-α8 allele, CIN III and the TNF-α2 allele in patients who are HPV-18 positive, and TNF-α11 with HPV-16 infection and CIN, in combination with HLA DQB allele (Martin et al., 2006).

Also, p53 polymorphism in codon 72 has been associated with CC. It has been observed that the p53 variants differ biochemically from each other and that the p53-Arg is more susceptible to HPV E6-mediated degradation than the proline variant (Madeleine et al, 2002; Beckman et al., 1994). Furthermore, Storey et al., have shown that individuals who were homozygous for the arginine allele had a seven times higher persistence of HPV associated to CC than heterozygous proline/arginine women (Storey et al., 1998). However, similar analyses performed in other populations did not confirm the association between such polymorphism of the p53 gene and the risk of developing HPV-associated lesions (Minaguchi et al., 1998; Hildesheim et al., 1998). Beside MHC and p53 polymorphism, polymorphisms in cytokine genes can influence immune responses to HPV infection, possibly modifying risks of CC. (Kirkpatrick et al., 2004; Howell & Rose, 2006; Bidwell et al., 1999; Haukin et al., 2002; Stanczuk et al., 2002; Matsumoto et al., 2010).

IL-10 and TGF-β1 polymorphisms have also been reported in diverse populations. G allele of SNP (A/G) at position -1082 in interleukin-10 promoter region, has been associated with high levels of IL-10, which increases with disease severity ($p<0.001$) (Farzaneh et al., 2006; Singh et al., 2009; Matsumoto et al., 2010). On the other hand, CC patients with -509TT showed marginal low risk for stage I cancer ($p = 0.04$, OR = 0.95, 95% CI = 0.91-0.99) but -509TT genotype of TGF-β1 was associated with increased risk for stage II cancer ($p = 0.07$, OR = 3.13, 95% CI = 0.87-11.14) (Singh et al., 2009).

3.2 AKNA polymorphism

A number of genetic susceptibility factors have been proposed, but with the exception of the HLA class II, have not shown consistent results among studies. The first genome-wide linkage scan was performed using 278 affected sib-pairs to identify loci involved in susceptibility to CC. This study found that 9q32 contains the susceptibility locus for CC, and some of these candidate genes are potentially involved in the genetic predisposition to this disease; among these genes is *akna* (Engelmark et al., 2006).

AKNA is a transcriptional factor that is involved in lymphocyte maturation and in the up-regulation of signaling molecules, such as CD40L (Siddiqa et al., 2001; Sims et al., 2005). Even though the precise molecular mechanisms for AKNA function have not been defined, AT-hook transcription factors have emerged as multifaceted regulators that can activate or repress broad A/T-rich gene networks. Thus, alterations of AT-hook genes could affect the transcription of multiple genes causing global cell dysfunction which could mediate DNA bending and chromatin rearrangement (Cairns et al., 1999; Ma et al., 2011).

Although functional data concerning AKNA are scarce, sequences of *akna* genes deposited in the GenBank databases are increasing. SNP analysis in the Genecard site (http://www.genecards.org/), at the 313 SNPs, reported that, for all *akna* genes, only 11 of them are coding non- synonyms. Among all the SNPs reported for *akna*, SNP (rs3748178) involving the transition G/A, at nucleotide 114189600(-) of chromosome 9 (accession no. AK024431) (Ota et al., 2004), appears to be functionally relevant. This mutation produces an R to Q amino acid change at codon 1119 (protein accession NP_110394). Such R/Q mutation occurs at an important AT-hook DNA binding motif within the highly conserved core that has a typical sequence pattern centered around a glycine-arginine-proline (GRP) tripeptide (codons 1118-1120). This short conserved sequence is relevant because it is necessary to bind DNA (Aravind & Landsman, 1998). The importance of producing a GQP core motif, instead of a GRP, is because glutamine lacks the positive charge that arginine has and thus potentially affects its DNA-binding capacity (Reeves & Nissen, 1990; Huth et al., 1997).

The AT-hook motif interacts directly with the minor groove of DNA in AT rich regions. Although some sequence specificity is present in the AT hook itself, and this may affect the main function of this motif (which is to anchor to the proteins in the minor groove of the DNA, near sequences targeted by other regions of the AT hook proteins), it is probably dependent on the spacing between successively interacting AT-hooks and their binding sites may be crucial for conformational changes of the DNA (Huth et al., 1997; Aravind & Landsman, 1998). A SNP at codon 1119 of the *akna* gene, yields a potentially relevant amino acid change (R1119Q) located at the DNA binding AT-hook motif; the AT hook may serve as a contact which affects the specificity and affinity of the DNA binding protein (Figure 3).

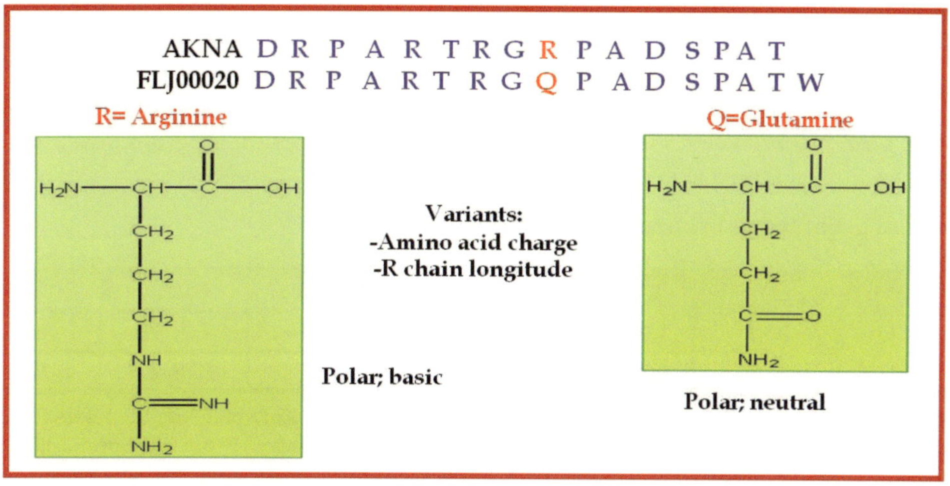

Fig. 3. AT-hook akna polymorphism (rs3748178)

Recently, we examined the frequency of Arginine (R) or Glutamine (Q) 1119 alleles of the *akna* gene in 47 HPV-positive biopsies from Mexican women with cervical lesions, with diagnoses of 21 CIN and 26 CC, as well as in 50 healthy controls without cervical lesions and with HPV-negative status (194 alleles in total). Genomic DNA was amplified by PCR and examined by restriction fragment length polymorphism (RFLP) analysis (Perales et al., 2010). We observed that the frequencies of genotypes in all studied 97 allele pairs were: R/R= 0.597, R/Q= 0.278, Q/Q= 0.123 and the individual frequencies of the R and Q alleles were 0.737 and 0.262, respectively. Q/Q homozygozity was present in 8.33% of healthy controls, 16.67% of CIN and 75% of CC patients. The distribution of the different genotypes in the three study groups showed a statistically significant difference by Fisher's exact test (Perales et al., 2010) (Figure 4).

This study, using a bivariate analysis with a model of multinomial logistic regression, with respective confidence intervals of 95% (IC 95%), showed that these differences were highly significant for the presence of Q/Q in CC (p= 0.01, OR= 3.66, 95%CI: 1.35- 9.94); there was a strong association between the homozygote phenotype Q/Q and the severity of the cervical lesions (Perales et al., 2010). These data support the importance of the genomic region where *akna* is located (Table 1).

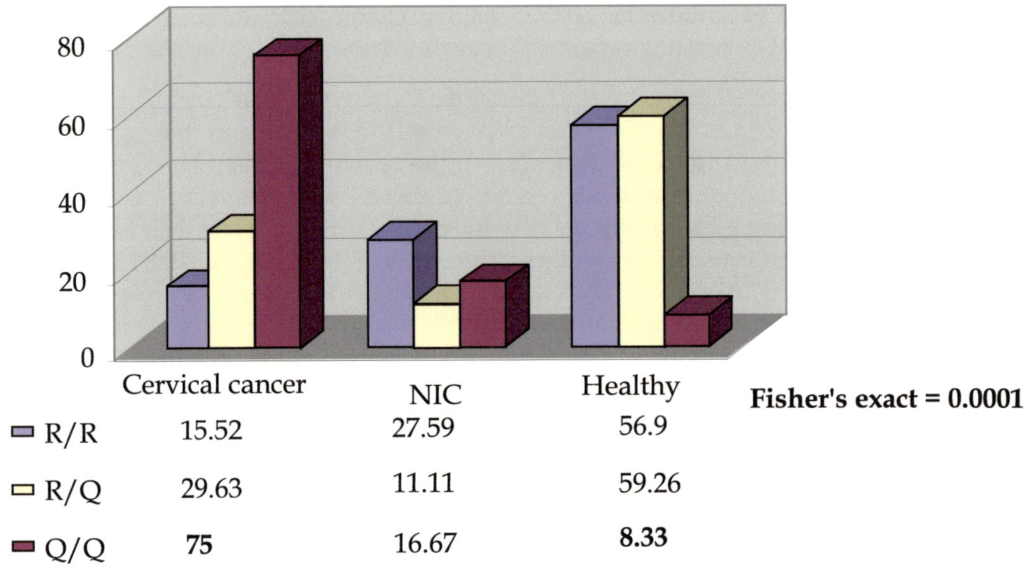

akna genotype distribution, Modified from Perales G, et al,. Biomarkers, 2010

Fig. 4. *akna* genotype distribution

	ORc	CI 95%	P value	ORa	CI95%	P value
CACU	**3.66**	**1.35, 9.94**	**0.01**	**4.22**	**1.3, 13**	**0.01**
NIC	**0.6**	**0.18, 1.93**	**0.39**	**0.61**	**0.18, 2.0**	**0.42**

CI, confidence interval; CIN, cervical intraepithelial neoplasia; Multinomial logistic regression: ORc, unadjusted odds ratio; ORa, adjusted OR by age. Modified from Perales G, et al,. Biomarkers, 2010

Table 1. Risk of Cervical cancer associated with Q/Q *akna* genotype

The AT-hook *akna* motif studied in this work is present in all reported *akna* isoforms except in the C1 and C2 isoforms (Sims et al., 2005). Therefore, the relevance of our observation is valid for the wide range of isoforms potentially expressed by the *akna* gene (Sims et al., 2005). The observed frequencies of *akna* Q/Q genotype in this group of 194 studied chromosomes, and the demonstration of a statistically significant association between a mutation in the *akna* gene (that results in an R-Q amino acid change) and susceptibility to CC, is of high relevance to biological knowledge of the development of CC. Whether this mutation contributes to an alteration of AKNA protein structure and immune function, and to CC development, is under investigation (Perales et al., 2010).

4. Conclusions and perspectives

HPV infection has two different cycles, the productive cycle and the transforming cycle. In the productive cycle of HPV, which occurs in keratinocytes, mature virions are shed from the epithelial surface of infected keratinocytes. HPV infection is poorly immunogenic because it is productive (produces no characteristic local inflammation) and during infection there is little presentation of viral antigens to the immune system by professional antigen-presenting cells, both locally and systemically. In some cases, HPV infection produces a non-inflammatory reaction. There is no adequate cellular immune response, due to excessive secretion of immunosuppressor cytokines, essentially IL-10, which produces a reduction of antigen-presenting and co-stimulatory molecules, and hence no recognition by the surrounding CD8 CTL. The AKNA transcription factor that induces the expression of stimulatory molecules, such as CD40 and CD40L, may play an important role in regulating the immune response against HPV. We found a genetic variant of the *akna* gene that has high frequency in patients with CC. Consequently, we believe that this genetic variant plays an important role, as a risk factor in CC development; the absence of AKNA protein may play an important role in the immune response against HPV. Thus, at the cervical level, after infection of epithelial cells by HPV, a nonspecific response is triggered that is accompanied by chemoattraction of neutrophils. Therefore, this interesting information about *akna*-KO raises important questions and further avenues for biomedical research. For instance, the enrichment of AKNA in wild-type neutrophils, and excess neutrophil counts in the absence of AKNA, suggests that this protein is important in the negative regulation of myeloid differentiation or neutrophil survival. It is of high relevance to determine whether loss-of-function mutations, polymorphisms or epigenetic alterations in *akna* contribute to myeloid diseases, such as myeloproliferative neoplasias, and CC. In conclusion, AKNA appears to be an important genetic factor associated with the progression of CC and genes regulated by this transcription factor could be involved in the resistance to CC progression.

5. References

[1] Alcocer-González, JM., Berumen, J., Tamez-Guerra, R., Bermúdez-Morales, VH., Peralta-Zaragoza, O., Hernández-Pando, R., Moreno, J., Gariglio, P., & Madrid-Marina, (2006). In vivo expression of immunosuppressive cytokines in human papillomavirus-transformed cancer cells. *Viral Immunology,* 19. 3, (July 2006), pp. (481-491), ISSN 1557-8976 (Electronic).

[2] Almonte, M., Albero, G., Molano, M., Carcamo, C., García, PJ., & Pérez G, (2008). Risk factors for human papillomavirus exposure and co-factors for cervical cancer in Latin America and the Caribbean. *Vaccine,* 26. Suppl 11, (August 2008), pp. (L16-36), ISSN 1873-2518 (Electronic).

[3] Apple, RJ., Erlich, HA., Klitz, W., Manos, MM., Becker, TM., & Wheeler, CM, (1994). HLA DR-DQ associations with cervical carcinoma show papilomavirus-type specificity. *Nature Genetics,* 6. 2, (February 1994), pp. (157-162), ISSN 1546-1718 (Electronic).

[4] Aravind, L., & Landsman, D., (1998). AT-hook motifs identified in a wide variety of DNA-binding protein. *Nucleic Acids Research,* 26. 19, (Octubre 1998), pp. (4413-21), ISSN 1362-4962 (Electronic).

[5] Arpin, C., Déchanet, J., Van Kooten, C., Merville, P., Grouard, G., Brière, F., Banchereau, J., Liu, YJ., (1995). Generation of memory B cells and plasma cells in vitro. *Science,* 268. 5211, (May 1995), pp. (720-722), ISSN 1095-9203 (Electronic).

[6] Ashrafi, GH., Haghshenas, MR., Marchetti, B., O'Brien, PM., & Campo, MS., (2005) E5 protein of human papillomavirus type 16 selectively downregulates surface HLA class I. *International Journal of Cancer,* 113. 2, (January 2005), pp. (276-283), ISSN 1097-0215 (Electronic).

[7] Baay, MF., Duk, JM., Groenier, KH., Burger, MP., de Bruijn, HW., Hollema, H., Stolz, E., & Herbrink, P, (1997). Relation between HPV-16 serology and clinico-pathological

data in cervical carcinoma patients: Prognostic value of anti E6 and/or anti E7 antibodies. *Cancer Immunology and Immunotherapy,* 44. 4, (June 1997), pp. (211-213), ISSN 1432-0851 (Electronic).

[8] Beckman, G., Birgander, R., Sjalander, A., Saha, N., Holmberg, PA., Kivela A., & Beckman, L., (1994). Is p53 polymorphism maintained by natural selection? *Human Heredity*, 44. 5, (September 1994), pp. (266–270), ISSN 1423-0062 (Electronic).

[9] Berek, C., Berger, A., & Apel, M., (1991). Maturation of the immune response in germinal centers. *Cell*, 67. 6, (December 1991), pp. (1121-1129), ISSN 1097-4172 (Electronic).

[10] Bermúdez-Morales, VH., Burguete, AI., Gutiérrez, ML., Alcocer-González, JM., & Madrid-Marina, V, (2008). Correlation between IL-10 expression & human papillomavirus infection in cervical cancer. A mechanism for immune response escape. *Cancer Investigation*, 26. 10, (December 2008), pp. (1037–1043), ISSN 1532-4192 (Electronic).

[11] Bermúdez-Morales, VH., Peralta-Zaragoza, O., Moreno, J., Alcocer-González, JM., & Madrid-Marina, V, (2011). IL-10 expression is regulated by HPV E2 protein in cervical cancer cells. *Molecular Medicine Reports*, 4. 2, (Marzo 2011), pp. (369-375), ISSN 1791-3004 (Electronic).

[12] Bidwell, J., Keen, L., Gallagher, G., Kimberly, R., Huizinga, T., McDermott, MF., Oksenberg, J., McNicholl, J., Pociot, F., Hardt, C., & D'Alfonso, S., (1999). Cytokine gene polymorphism in human disease: on line databases. *Genes and Immunity*, 1. 1, (September 1999), pp. (3-19), ISSN 1476-5470 (Electronic).

[13] Bodily, J & Laimins, LA., (2011). Persistence of human papillomavirus infection: keys to malignant progression. Trends in Microbiology, 19. 1, (January 2011), pp. (33-39), ISSN 1878-4380 (Electronic).

[14] Bor-Ching, S., Rong-Hwa, L, Huang-Chung, L., Hong-Nerng, H., Su-Ming, H., & Su-Cheng, H, (2001). Predominant Th2/Tc2 polarity of tumor-infiltrating lymphocytes in human cervical cancer. *Journal of immunology*, 167. 5, (September 2001), pp. (2972-2978), ISSN 1550-6606 (Electronic).

[15] Bory, JP., Cucherousset, J., Lorenzato, M., Gabriel, R., Quereux, C., Birembaut, P., & Clavel, C, (2002). Recurrent human papillomavirus infection detected with the hybrid capture 2 assay selects women with normal cervical smears at risk for developing low grade cervical lesions: a longitudinal study of 3091 women. *International Journal of Cancer*, 102. 5, (December 2002), pp. (519–25), ISSN 1097-0215 (Electronic).

[16] Boyer, SN., Wazer, DE., & Band, V, (1996). E7 protein of human papilloma virus-16 induces degradation of retinoblastoma protein through the ubiquitin–proteasome pathway. *Cancer Research*, 56. 20, (October 1996), pp. (4620–4624), ISSN 1538-7445 (Electronic).

[17] Cairns, B., Schlinchter, A., Erdjument, B., Tempst, P., Kornberg, R., & Winston, F, (1999). Two functionally distinct forms of the RSC nucleosome-remodeling complex, containing essential AT-hook, BAH, and bromodomains. *Molecular Cell*, 4. 5, (November 1999), pp. (715-723), ISSN 1097-4164 (Electronic).

[18] Chevalier, P., (1993). PEST sequences in nuclear proteins. *The International Journal of Biochemistry, 25. 4, (*April 1993), pp. (479-482), ISSN 0020-711X (Print).

[19] Clark, EA & Ledbetter, JA., (1994). How B and T cells talk to each other. *Nature*, 367. 6462, (February 1994), pp. (425-428), ISSN 1476-4687 (Electronic).

[20] Clerici, M., Merola, M., Ferrario, E., Trabattoni, D., Villa, ML., Stefanon, B., Venzon, DJ., Shearer GM., De Palo, G., & Clerici, E, (1997). Cytokine production patterns in cervical intraepithelial neoplasia: association with human papillomavirus infection. *Journal of the National Cancer Institute, 89.* 3, (February 1997), pp. (245–250), ISSN 1460-2105 (Electronic).

[21] Clerici, M., Gene, MS., & Clerici, E, (1998). Cytoquine dysregulation in invasive cervical carcinoma and other human neoplasias: time to consider the Th1/Th2 Paradigm. *Journal of the National Cancer Institute,* 90. 4, (February 1998), pp. (261-263), ISSN 1460-2105 (Electronic).

[22] Cui, T & Leng, F., (2007). Specific recognition of AT-rich DNA sequences by the mammalian high mobility group protein AT-hook 2: a SELEX study. *Biochemistry,* 46. 45, (November 2007), pp. (13059-13066), ISSN 1520-4995 (Electronic).

[23] Cuschieri, KS., Cubie, HA., Whitley, MW., Gilkison, G., Arends, MJ., Graham, C., & McGoogan, E, (2005). Persistent high risk HPV infection associated with development of cervical neoplasia in a prospective population study. *Journal of clinical pathology,* 58. 9, (September 2005), pp. (946–950), ISSN 1472-4146 (Electronic).

[24] Dalstein, V., Riethmuller, D., Prétet, JL., Le, Bail., Carval, K., Sautière, JL., Carbillet, JP., Kantelip, B., Schaal, JP., & Mougin, C., (2003). Persistence and load of high-risk HPV are predictors for development of high-grade cervical lesions: A longitudinal French cohort study. *Intermational Journal of Cancer,* 106. 3, (September 2009), pp. (396-403), ISSN 1097-0215 (Electronic).

[25] Damoiseaux, J., (2006). Regulatory T cells: back to the future. *The Netherlands Journal of Medicine,* 64. 1, (January 2006), pp. (4-9), ISSN 1872-9061 (Electronic).

[26] de Araujo Souza, PS & Villa, LL., (2003). Genetic susceptibility to infection with human papillomavirus and development of cervical cancer in women in Brazil. *Mutation Research,* 544. 2-3, (November 2003), pp. (375–383), ISSN 1873-135X (Electronic).

[27] De-Gruijl, TD., Bontkes, HJ., Peccatori, F., Gallee, MP., Helmerhorst, TJ., Verheijen, RHH., Aarbiou, J., Mulder, WM., Walboomers, JM., Meijer, CJ., van de Vange, N., & Scheper, RJ., (1999). Expression of CD3-zeta on T-cell sin primary cervical carcinoma and in metastasis-positive and negative pelvic lymph nodes. *British Journal of Cancer,* 79. 7-8, (March 1999), pp. (1127-1132), ISSN 1532-1827 (Electronic).

[28] Díaz-Benítez, CE., Navarro-Fuentes, KR., Flores-Sosa, JA., Juárez-Díaz, J., Uribe-Salas, FJ., Román-Basaure, E., González-Mena, LE., Alonso de Ruíz, P., López-Estrada, G., Lagunas-Martínez, A., Bermúdez-Morales, VH., Alcocer-González, JM., Martínez-Barnetche, J., Hernández-Pando, R., Rosenstein, Y., Moreno, J., & Madrid-Marina, V., (2009). CD3ζ expression and T cell proliferation are inhibited by TGF-β1 and IL-10 in cervical cancer patients. *Journal of Clinical Immunology,* 29. 4, (July 2009), pp. (532–544), ISSN 1573-2592 (Electronic).

[29] Dokianakis, D., & Spandidos, D., (2000). p53 Codon 72 polymorphism as a risk factor in the development of HPV-associated cervical cancer. *Molecular Cell Biology Research Communications,* 3. 2, (February 2000), pp. (111–114), ISSN 1522-4732 (Electronic).

[30] Doorbar J., (2006). Molecular biology of human papillomavirus infection and cervical cancer. *Clinical Science,* 110. 5, (May 2006), pp. (525-541), ISSN 0009-9287 (Print).

[31] El-Ghobashy, AA., Shaaban, AM., Herod, J., & Herrington, CS., (2005). The pathology and management of endocervical glandular neoplasia. *International Journal of Gynecological Cancer*, 15. 4, (July 2005), pp. (583-592), ISSN 1525-1438 (Electronic).

[32] Engelmark, MT., Ivansson, EL., Magnusson, JJ., Gustavsson, IM., Beskow, AH., Magnusson, PK., & Gyllensten, UB., (2006). Identification of susceptibility loci for cervical carcinoma by genome scan of affected sib-pairs. *Human Molecular Genetics*, 15. 22, (November 2006), pp. (3351–3360), ISSN 1460-2083 (Electronic).

[33] Farzaneh, F., Roberts, S., Mandal, D., Ollier, B., Winters, U., Kitchener, HC., & Brabin, L., (2006). The IL-10 -1082G polymorphism is associated with clearance of HPV infection. *British journal of obstetrics and gynaecology*, 113. 8, (August 2006), pp. (961-964), ISSN 0306-5456 (Print).

[34] Feller, L., Wood, NH., Khammissa, RA., Chikte, UM., Meyerov, R., & Lemmer, J., (2010). HPV modulation of host immune responses. *South African Dental Association*, 65. 6, (July 2010), pp. (266-268), ISSN 1029-4864 (Print).

[35] Ferlay, J., Bray, F., Pisani, P., & Parkin, DM., (2001). GLOBOCAN 2000: Cancer Incidence, Mortality and Prevalence Worldwide. Versión 1.0. IARC Cancer Base N.o 5. Lyon: IARC Press. Retrieved from http://www-dep.iarc.fr/globocan/globocan.htm.

[36] Friedmann, M., Holth, LT., Zoghbi, HY., & Reeves, R., (1993). Organization, inducible-expression and chromosome localization of the human HMG-I(Y) nonhistone protein gene. *Nucleic Acids Research*, 21. 18, (September 1993), pp. (4259-4267), ISSN 1362-4962 (Electronic).

[37] Giannini, SL., Al-Saleh, W., Piron, H., Jacobs, N., Doyen, J., Boniver, J., & Delvenne, P., (1998). Cytokine expresion in squamous intraepithelial lesions of the uterine cervix : implications for the generation of local inmunosuppression. *Clinical and Experimental Immunology*, 113. 2, (August 1998), pp. (183-189), ISSN 1365-2249 (Electronic).

[38] Ghittoni, R., Accardi, R., Hasan, U., Gheit, T., Sylla, B., & Tommasino, M., (2010). The biological properties of E6 and E7 oncoproteins from human Papillomaviruses. *Virus Genes*, 40. 1, (February 2010), pp. (1-13), ISSN 1572-994X (Electronic).

[39] Glew, SS., Stern, PL., Davidson JA., & Dyer, PA., (1992). HLA antigens and cervical carcinoma. *Nature* 356. 6364, (March 1992), pp. (22), ISSN 1476-4687 (Electronic).

[40] Gordon, BR., Li, Y., Wang, L., Sintsova, A., van Bakel, H., Tian, S., Navarre, WW., Xia, B., & Liu, J., (2010). Lsr2 is a nucleoid-associated protein that targets AT-rich sequences and virulence genes in Mycobacterium tuberculosis. *Proceedings of the National Academy of Sciences of the United States of America*, 107. 11, (March 2010), pp. (5154-5159), ISSN 1091-6490 (Electronic.

[41] Grubisi¢, G., Klari¢, P., Jokanovi¢, L., Soljaci¢-Vranes, H., Grbavac, I., & Bolanca, I., (2009). Diagnostic approach for precancerous and early invasive cancerous lesions of the uterine cervix. *Collegium antropologicum*, 33. 4, (December 2009), pp. (1431-1436), ISSN 0350-6134 (Print).

[42] Hachisuga, T., Fukuda, K., & Kawarabayashi, T., (2001). Local immune response in squamous cell carcinoma of the uterine cervix. *Gynecologic and Obstetric Investigation*, 52. 1, (July 2001), pp. (3-8), ISSN 1423-002X (Electronic).

[43] Hammes, LS., Tekmal, RR., Naud, P., Edelweiss, MI., Kirma, N., Valente, PT., Syrjänen, KJ., & Cunha-Filho, JS., (2007). Macrophages, inflammation and risk of cervical

intraepithelial neoplasia (CIN) progression-clinicopathological correlation. *Gynecologic Oncology*, 105. 1, (April 2007), pp. (157-165), ISSN 1095-6859 (Electronic).

[44] Haukin, N., Bidwell, JL., Smith, AJ., Keen, LJ., Gallagher, G., Kimberly, R., Huizinga, T., McDermott, MF., Oksenberg, J., McNicholl, J., Pociot, F., Hardt, C., & D'Alfonso, S., (2002). Cytokine gene polymorphism in human disease: on line databases. Supplement 2. *Genes and Inmunity*, 3. 6, (September 2002), pp. (313-330), ISSN 1476-5470 (Electronic).

[45] Hemminki, K., Dong, C., & Vaittinen, P., (1999). Familial risks in cervical cancer: is there a hereditary component? *International Journal of Cancer*, 82. 6, (September 1999), pp. (775–781), ISSN), ISSN 1097-0215 (Electronic).

[46] Hernández-Hernández, DM,. Cerda-Flores, RM., Juárez-Cedillo, T., Granados-Arriola, J., Vargas-Alarcón, G., Apresa-García, T., Alvarado-Cabrero, I., García-Carrancá, A., Salcedo-Vargas, M., & Mohar-Betancourt, A., (2009). Human leukocyte antigens I and II haplotypes associated with human papillomavirus 16-positive invasive cervical cancer in Mexican women. *International Journal of Gynecological Cancer*, 19. 6, (August 2009), pp. (1099-10106), ISSN 1525-1438 (Electronic).

[47] Hildesheim, A., Schiffman, M., Brinton, LA., Fraumeni, JF Jr., Herrero, R., Bratti, MC., Schwartz, P., Mortel, R., Barnes, W., Greenberg, M., Mcgowan, L., Scott, DR., Martin, M., Herrera, JE., & Carrington, M., (1998). p53 polymorphism and risk of cervical cancer. *Nature*, 396. 6711, (December 1998), pp. (531–532), ISSN 1476-4687 (Electronic).

[48] Hildesheim, A., & Wand, SS., (2002). Host and viral genetics & risk of cervical cancer: a review. Virus Research, 89. 2, (November 2002), pp. (229-240), ISSN 1872-7492 (Electronic).

[49] Ho, GY., Bierman, R., Beardsley, L., Chang, CJ., & Burk, RD., (1998). Natural history of cervicovaginal papilloma virus infection in young women. *The New England Journal of Medicine*, 338. 7, (February 1998), pp. (423–428), ISSN 1533-4406 (Electronic).

[50] Howley, PM., (1996) Virology. 2nd edition ed. Philadelphia, Pa.: Lippincott-Raven Publishers; Papillomavirinae: the viruses and their replication, pp. (2045-2076).

[51] Howell, WM & Rose-Zerilli, MJ., (2006). Interleukin-10 polymorphisms, cancer susceptibility and prognosis. *Familial Cancer*, 5. 2, (July 2006), pp. (143-149), ISSN 1573-7292 (Electronic).

[52] Huth, J., Bewley, C., Nissen, M., Evans, J., Reeves, R., Gronenborn, A., & Clore, G., (1997). The solution structure of an HMG-I(Y)-DNA complex defines a new architectural minor groove binding motif. *Nature Structural Biology*, 4. 8, (August 1997), pp. (657-665), ISSN 1072-8368 (Print).

[53] Jacob, J & Kelsoe, G., (1992). In situ studies of the primary immune response to (4-hydroxy-3-nitrophenyl)acetyl. II. A common clonal origin for periarteriolar lymphoid sheath-associated foci and germinal centers. , 176. 3, (September 1992), pp. (679-687), ISSN1540-9538 (Electronic).

[54] Jenkins JF. (Ed(s)). *(2009). Consensus Panel on Genetic/Genomic Nursing Competencies, Essentials of genetic and genomic nursing: competencies, curricula guidelines, and outcome indicators,* American Nurses Association, Silver Spring, MD (Ed 2), ISBN-13: 978-1-55810-263-7 ISBN-10: 1-55810: American Nurses Association.

[55] Keating, PJ., Cromme, FV., Duggan-Keen, M., Snijers, PJ., Walboomers, JM., Hunter, RD., Dyer, PA., & Stern, PL., (1995). Frequency of down-regulation of individual

HLA-A and B alleles in cervical carcinomas in relation to TAP-1 expression. *British Journal of Cancer*, 72. 2, (August 1995), pp. (405-411), ISSN 1532-1827 (Electronic).

[56] Kirkpatrick, A., Bidwell, J., van den Brule, A., Meiler, C., Pawad, J., & Glew S., (2004). TNFα polymorphism frequencies in HPV-associated cervical dysplasia. *Gynecologic Oncology*, 92. 2, (February 2004), pp. (675–679), ISSN 1095-6859 (Electronic).

[57] Kobayashi, A., Weinberg, V., Darragh, T., & Smith-McCunne, K., (2008). Evolving immunosuppressive microenvironment during human cervical carcinogenesis. *Mucosal Immunology*, 1. 5, (September 2008), pp. (412-420), ISSN 1935-3456 (Electronic).

[58] Kono, K., Ressing, ME., Brandt, RM., Melief, CJ., Potkul, RK., Andersson, B., Petersson, M., Kast, WM., & Kiessling, R., (1996). Decreased expression of signal-transducing zeta chain in peripheral T cells and natural killer cells in patients with cervical cancer. *Clinical Cancer Research*, 2. 11, (November 1996), pp. (1825-1828), ISSN 1078-0432 (Print).

[59] Landvik, NE., Hart, K., Skaug, V., Stangeland, LB., Haugen, A., & Zienolddiny, S., (2009). A specific interleukin-1B haplotype correlates with high levels of IL1B mRNA in the lung and increased risk of non-small cell lung cancer. *Carcinogenesis*, 30. 7, (July 2009), pp. (1186-1192), ISSN 1460-2180 (Electronic).

[60] Lai, H., Sytwu, H., Sun, C., Yu, C., Liu, H., Chang, C., & Chu, T., (2003). Single Nucleotide Polymorphism at Fas promoter is associates with Cervical Carcinogenesis. *International Journal of Cancer*, 103. 2, (January 2003), pp. (221–225), ISSN 1097-0215 (Electronic).

[61] Lai, HC., Chu, CM., Lin, YW., Chang, CC., Nieh, S., Yu, MH., & Chu, TY., (2005). Matrix metalloproteinase 1 gene polymorphism as a prognostic predictor of invasive cervical cancer. *Gynecologic Oncology*, 96. 2, (February 2005), pp. (314-319), ISSN 1095-6859 (Electronic).

[62] Liu, YJ., Zhang, J., Lane, PJ., Chan, EY., & MacLennan, IC., (1991). Sites of specific B cell activation in primary and secondary responses to T cell-dependent and T cell-independent antigens. *European Journal of Immunology*, 21. 12, (December 1991), pp. (2951-2962), ISSN 1521-4141 (Electronic).

[63] Liu, YJ., Malisan, F., de Bouteiller, O., Guret, C., Lebecque, S., Banchereau, J., Mills, FC., Max, EE., & Martinez-Valdez, H., (1996). Within germinal centers, isotype switching of immunoglobulin genes occurs after the onset of somatic mutation. *Immunity*, 4. 3, (March 1996), pp. (241-250), ISSN1097-4180 (Electronic).

[64] Longworth, MS., & Laimins, LA., (2004). Pathogenesis of human papillomaviruses in differentiating epithelia. *Microbiology and Molecular Biology Reviews*, 68. 2, (June 2004), pp. (362-372), ISSN 1098-5557 (Electronic).

[65] Ma, W., Ortiz-Quintero, B., Rangel, R., McKeller, MR., Herrera-Rodríguez, S., Castillo, EF., Schluns, KS., Hall, M., Zhang, H., Suh, WK., Okada, H., Mak, TW., Zhou, Y., Blackburn, MR., & Martínez-Valdez, H., (2011). Coordinate activation of inflammatory gene networks, alveolar destruction and neonatal death in AKNA deficient mice. *Cell Research*, Epub ahead of print (May 2011), pp. (1-14), ISSN 1748-7838 (Electronic).

[66] Maciag, PC., Schlecht, NF., Souza, PS., Rohan, TE., Franco, EL., & Villa, LL., (2002). Polymorphisms of the human leukocyte antigen *DRB1* and *DQB1* genes and the

natural history of human papillomavirus infection. *Journal of infectious diseases*, 186. 2, (July 2002), pp. (164–172), ISSN 1537-6613 (Electronic).

[67] MacLennan, IC., (1994). Germinal centers. *Annual Review of Immunology*, 12, (July 1994), pp. (117-139), ISSN 1545-3278 (Electronic).

[68] Madeleine, MM., Brumback, B., Cushing-Haugen, KL., Schwartz, SM., Daling, JR., Smith, AG., Nelson, JL., Porter, P., Shera, KA., McDougall, JK., & Galloway, DA., (2002). Human leukocyte antigen class II and cervical cancer risk: a population-based study. *Journal of infectious diseases*, 186. 11, (December 2002), pp. (1565–1574), ISSN 1537-6613 (Electronic).

[69] Makni, H., Franco, E., Kaiano, J., Villa, L., Labrecque, S., Dudley, R., Storey, A., & Matlashewski, G., (2000). p53 polymorphism in codon 72 and risk of human papilloma virus-induced cervical cancer: effect of inter-laboratory variation. *International Journal of Cancer*, 87. 4, (August 2000), pp. (528–533), ISSN ISSN 1097-0215 (Electronic).

[70] Magnusson, PK., Lichtenstein, P., & Gyllensten UB., (2000). Heritability of cervical tumours. *International Journal of Cancer*, 88. 5, (December 2000), pp. (698–701), ISSN ISSN 1097-0215 (Electronic)

[71] Mao, L., Yang, P., Hou, S., Li, F., & Kijlstra, A., (2011). Label-Free proteomics reveals decreased expression of CD18 and AKNA in peripheral CD4+ T Cells from patients with Vogt-Koyanagi-Harada Syndrome. *Plos One*, 6. 1, (January 2011), pp. (e14616), ISSN 1932-6203 (Electronic).

[72] Marangoz, S & Güllü, IH., (1999). Expression of ras, c-myc, and p53 proteins in cervical intraepithelial neoplasia. *Cancer*, 85. 12, (June 1999), pp. (2668-2669), ISSN 1097-0142 (Electronic).

[73] Martin, CM., Astbury, K., & O'Leary, JJ., (2006). Molecular profiling of cervical neoplasia. *Expert Review of Molecular Diagnostics*, 6. 2, (March 2006), pp. (217-229), ISSN 1744-8352 (Electronic)

[74] Matsumoto, K., Yoshikawa, H., Yasugi, T., Nakagawa, S., Kawana, K., Nozawa, S., Hoshiai, H., Shiromizu, K., Kanda, T., & Taketani, Y., (1999). Balance of IgG subclasses toward human papillomatype 16 (HPV 16) L1-capside is a possible predictor for the regression of HPV16-positivecervical intraepithelial neoplasia. *Biochemical and Biophysical Research Communications*, 258. 1, (April 1999), pp. (128-131), ISSN 1090-2104 (Electronic).

[75] Matsumoto, K., Oki, A., Satoh, T., Okada, S., Minaguchi, T., Onuki, M., Ochi, H., Nakao, S., Sakurai, M., Abe, A., Hamada, H., & Yoshikawa, H., (2010). Interleukin-10 -1082 gene polymorphism and susceptibility to cervical cancer among Japanese women. *Japanese Journal of Clinical Oncology*, 40. 11, (November 2010), pp. (1113-1116), ISSN 1465-3621 (Electronic).

[76] Mazibrada, J., Rittà, M., Mondini, M., De Andrea, M., Azzimonti, B., Borgogna, C., Ciotti, M., Orlando, A., Surico, N., Chiusa, L., Landolfo, M., & Gariglio, M., (2008). Interaction between inflammation and angiogenesis during different stages of cervical carcinogenesis. *Gynecologic Oncology*, 108. 1, (January 2008), pp. (112-120), ISSN 1095-6859 (Electronic).

[77] McHeyzer-Williams, MG., McLean, MJ., Lalor, PA., & Nossal, GJ., (1993). Antigen-driven B cell differentiation in vivo. *The Journal of experimental medicine*, 178. 1, (July 1993), pp. (295-307), ISSN 1540-9538 (Electronic).

[78] Meyer, LA., Westin, SN., Lu, KH, & Milam, MR., (2008). Genetic polymorphisms and endometrial cancer risk. *Expert Review of Anticancer Therapy*, 8. 7, (July 2008), pp. (1159-1167), ISSN 1744-8328 (Electronic).

[79] Milam, MR., Gu, J., Yang, H., Celestino, J., Wu, W., Horwitz, IB., Lacour, RA., Westin, SN., Gershenson, DM., Wu, X., & Lu, KH., (2007). STK15 F31I polymorphism is associated with increased uterine cancer risk: a pilot study. *Gynecologic Oncology*, 107. 1, (October 2007), pp. (71-74), ISSN 1095-6859 (Electronic).

[80] Minaguchi, T., Kanamori, Y., Matsushima, M., Yoshikawa, H., Taketani, Y., & Nakamura, Y., (1998). No evidence of correlation between polymorphism at codon 72 of p53 and risk of cervical cancer in Japanese patients with human papillomavirus 16/18 infection. *Cancer Research*, 58. 20, (October 1998), pp. (4585–4586), ISSN 1538-7445 (Electronic).

[81] Moliterno, AR & Resar, LMS., (2011). AKNA: Another AT-hook transcription factor "hooking-up" with inflamation. *Cell Research*, Epub ahead of print (June 2011), pp. (1-3), ISSN 1748-7838 (Electronic).

[82] Molling, JW., de Gruijl, TD., Glim, J., Moreno, M., Rozendaal, L., Meijer, CJ., van den Eertwegh, AJ., Scheper, RJ., von Blomberg, ME., & Bontkes, HJ., (2007). CD4(+)CD25hi regulatory T-cell frequency correlates with persistence of human papillomavirus type 16 and T helper cell responses in patients with cervical intraepithelial neoplasia. International Journal of Cancer, 121. 8, (October 2007), pp. (1749-1755), ISSN 1097-0215 (Electronic).

[83] Moody, CA & Laimins, LA., (2010). Human papillomavirus oncoproteins: Pathways to transformation. *Nature reviews Cancer*, 10. 8, (August 2010), pp. (550-560), ISSN 1474-1768 (Electronic)

[84] Muñoz, N., Bosch, FX., de Sanjosé, S., Herrero, R., Castellsagué, X., Shah, KV., Snijders, PJ., Meijer, CJ., & International Agency for Research on Cancer Multicenter Cervical Cancer Study Group., (2003). Epidemiologic classification of human papillomavirus types associated with cervical cancer. *The New England Journal of Medicine*, 348. 6, (February 2003), pp. (518–527), ISSN 1533-4406 (Electronic).

[85] Muñoz, N., Bosch, FX., Castellsagué, X., Díaz, M., de Sanjosé, S., Hammouda, D., Shah, KV., & Meijer, CJ., (2004). Against which human papillomavirus types shall we vaccinate and screen? The international perspective. *International Journal of Cancer*, 111. 2, (August 2004), pp. (278-285), ISSN 1097-0215 (Electronic).

[86] Nakamura, T., Shima, T., Saeki, A., Hidaka, T., Nakashima, A., Takikawa, O., & Saito, S., (2007). Expression of indoleamine 2, 3-dioxygenase and the recruitment of Foxp3-expressing regulatory T cells in the development and progression of uterine cervical cancer. *Cancer Science*, 98. 6, (June 2007), pp. (874-881), ISSN 1349-7006 (Electronic).

[87] Nobbenhuis, ME., Helmerhorst, TJ., van den Brule, AJ., Rozendaal, L., Woorhorst, FJ., Bezemer, PD., Verheijen, RH., & Meijer, CJ., (2001). Cytological regression and clearance of high-risk human papilomavirus in women with an abnormal cervical smear. *Lancet*, 358. 9295, (November 2001), pp. (1782-1783), ISSN 1474-547X (Electronic).

[88] Ota T, Suzuki Y, Nishikawa T, Otsuki T, Sugiyama T, Irie R, Wakamatsu A, Hayashi K, Sato H, Nagai K, & others., (2004). Complete sequencing and characterization of

21,243 full-length human cDNAs. *Nature Genetics*, 36. 1, (January 2004), pp. (40–45), ISSN 1546-1718 (Electronic).

[89] Patel, S & Chiplunkar, S., (2009). Host immune responses to cervical cancer. *Current Opinion in Obstetrics & Gynecology*, 21. 1, (February 2009), pp. (54-59), ISSN 1473-656X (Electronic).

[90] Pedroza-Saavedra, A., Cruz, A., Esquivel, F., De La Torre, F., Berumen, J., Gariglio, P., & Gutiérrez, L., (2000). High prevalence of serum antibodies to Ras and type 16 E4 proteins of human papillomavirus in patients with precancerous lesions of the uterine cervix. *Archives of Virology*, 145. 3, (July 2000), pp. (603-623), ISSN 1432-8798 (Electronic).

[91] Perales, G., Burguete-García, AI., Dimas, J., Bahena-Román, M., Bermúdez-Morales, VH., Moreno, J & Madrid-Marina., (2010). V. A polymorphism in the AT-hook motif of the transcriptional regulador AKNA is a risk factor for cervical cancer. *Biomarkers*, 15. 5, (August 2010), pp. (470-474), ISSN 1366-5804 (Electronic).

[92] Peralta-Zaragoza O, Bermúdez-Morales V, Gutiérrez-Xicotencatl L, Alcocer-González, J., Recillas-Targa, F., & Madrid-Marina, V., (2006). E6 and E7 oncoproteins from human papillomavirus type 16 induce activation of human transforming growth factor beta1 promoter throughout Sp1 recognition sequence. *Viral Immunology*, 19. 3, (July 2006), pp. (468-480), ISSN 1557-8976 (Electronic).

[93] Piersma, SJ., Jordanova, ES., van Poelgeest, MI., Kwappenberg, KM., van der Hulst, JM., Drijfhout, JW., Melief, CJ., Kenter, GG., Fleuren, GJ., Offringa, R., & van der Burg, SH., (2004). High number of intraepithelial CD8+ tumor-infiltrating lymphocytes is associated with the absence of lymph node metastases in patients with large early-stage cervical cancer. *Cancer Research*, 67. 1, (January 2007), pp. (354-361), ISSN 1538-7445 (Electronic).

[94] Pim D & Banks L., (2010). Interaction of viral oncoproteins with cellular target molecules: infection with high-risk vs low-risk human papillomaviruses. *Acta Pathologica, Microbiologica, et Immunologica Scandinavica*, 118, 6-7, (June 2010), pp. (471-493), ISSN 1600-0463 (Electronic).

[95] Ploegh, HL., (1998). Viral strategies of immune evasion. *Science*, 280. 5361, (April 1998), pp. (248-253), ISSN 1095-9203 (Electronic).

[96] Reeves, R & Nissen, MS., (1990). The A.T-DNA-binding domain of mammalian high mobility group I chromosomal proteins. A novel peptide motif for recognizing DNA structure. *The Journal of Biological Chemistry*, 265. 15, (May 1990), pp. (8573-8582), ISSN 1083-351X (Electronic).

[97] Reeves, R., (2010). Nuclear functions of the HMG proteins. BBA *International Journal of Biochemistry and Biophysics*, 1799. 1-2, (January 2010), pp. (3-14), ISSN 0006-3002 (Print).

[98] Riethmuller, D & Seilles, E., (2000). Inmunity of the female genital tract mucosa and mechanisms of papillomavirus evasion. *Journal de Gynécologie, Obstétrique et Biologie de la Reproduction*, 29. 8, (July 2000), pp. (729-740), ISSN 0368-2315 (Print).

[99] Robert, J., (2010). Gene polymorphisms. Bull Cancer, 97. 11, (November 2010), pp. (1253-1264), ISSN 1769-6917 (Electronic).

[100] Robertson, SJ & Hasenkrug, KJ., (2006). The role of virus-induced regulatory T cells in immunopathology. *Springer Seminars in Immunopathology*, 28. 1, (August 2006), pp. (51-62), ISSN 1432-2196 (Electronic).

[101] Santin, AD., Ravaggi, A., Bellone, S., Pecorelli, S., Cannon, M., Parham, GP., & Hermonat PL., (2001). Tumor-infiltring lymphocytes contain higher numbers of type1 cytoquine expressors and DR+ T cells compared with Lymphocytes from tumor drainig lymph nodes and peripheral blood in patients with cancer of the uterine cervix. *Gynecologic Oncology,* 81. 3, (June 2001), pp. (424-432), ISSN 1095-6859 (Electronic).

[102] Savas, S & Liu, G., (2009). Genetic variations as cancer prognostic markers: review and update. *Human Mutations,* 30. 10, (October 2009), pp. (1369-1377), ISSN 1098-1004 (Electronic).

[103] Scheffner, M., Werness, BA., Huibregtse, JM., Levine, AJ., & Howley, PM., (1990). The E6 oncoprotein encoded by human papillomavirus types 16 and 18 promotes the degradation of p53. *Cell,* 63. 6, (December 1990), pp. (1129–1136), ISSN 1097-4172 (Electronic).

[104] Schlecht, NF., Trevisan, A., Duarte-Franco, E., Rohan, TE., Ferenczy, A., Villa, LL., & Franco, EL., (2003). Viral load as a predictor of the risk of cervical intraepithelial neoplasia, *International Journal of Cancer,* 103. 4, (February 2003), pp. (519–524), ISSN 1097-0215 (Electronic).

[105] Scott, ME., Ma, Y., Kuzmich, L., & Moscicki, AB., (2009). Diminished IFN-gamma and IL-10 and elevated Foxp3 mRNA expression in the cervix are associated with CIN 2 or 3. *International Journal of Cancer,* 124. 6, (March 2009), pp. (1379-1383), ISSN 1097-0215 (Electronic).

[106] Seder, RA & Ahmed, R., (2003). Similarities and differences in CD4+ and CD8+ effector and memory T cell generation. *Nature Immunology,* 4. 9, (September 2003), pp. (835-842), ISSN 1529-2916 (Electronic).

[107] Senthilkumar, R & Mishra, RK., (2009). Novel motifs distinguish multiple homologues of Polycomb in vertebrates: expansion and diversification of the epigenetic toolkit. *BMC Genomics,* 10. (November 2009), pp. (549), ISSN 1471-2164 (Electronic).

[108] Shondel, SM., Helm, CW., Gercel-Taylor, C., & Taylor, DD., (2007). Differential expression of T-cell CD3-zeta chains in patients with cervical dysplasia before and after treatment. *International Journal of Gynecological Cancer,* 17. 6, (November 2007), pp. (1278-1282), ISSN 1525-1438 (Electronic).

[109] Siddiqa, A., Sims-Mourtada, JC., Guzmán-Rojas, L, Rangel, R., Guret, C., Madrid-Marina, V., Sun, Y., & Martínez-Valdez, H., (2001). Regulation of CD40 and CD40 ligand by the AT-hook transcription factor AKNA. *Nature,* 410. 6826, (March 2001), pp. (383–387), ISSN 1476-4687 (Electronic).

[110] Sierra-Torres, CH., Au, WW., Arrastia, CD., Cajas-Salazar, N., Robazetti, SC., Payne, DA., & Tyring, SK., (2003). Polymorphisms for chemical metabolizing genes and risk for cervical neoplasia. *Environmental and Molecular Mutagenesis,* 41. 1, (July 2003), pp. (69–76), ISSN 1098-2280 (Electronic).

[111] Singh, H., Jain, M., & Mittal, B., (2009). Role of TGF-beta1 (-509C>T) promoter polymorphism in susceptibility to cervical cancer. *Oncology Research,* 18. 1, (July 2009), pp. (41-45), ISSN 0965-0407 (Print).

[112] Sims-Mourtada, JC., Bruce, S., Mckeller, MR., Rangel, R., Guzmán-Rojas, L., Cain, K., López, C., Zimonjic, DB., Popescu, NC., Gordon, J., Wilkinson, MF., & Martínez-Valdez, H., (2005). The Human AKNA Gene Expresses Multiple Transcripts and Protein Isoforms as a Result of Alternative Promoter Usage, Splicing, and

Polyadenylation. *DNA and Cell Biology*, 24. 5, (May 2005), pp. (325-338), ISSN 1557-7430 (Electronic).

[113] Smith, JS., Lindsay, L., Hoots, B., Keys, J., Franceschi, S., Winer, R., & Clifford, GM., (2007). Human papillomavirus type distribution in invasive cervical cancer and high-grade cervical lesions: a meta-analysis update. *International Journal of Cancer*, 121. 3, (August 2007), pp. (621-632), ISSN 1097-0215 (Electronic).

[114] Stanczuk, GA., Tswana, SA., Bergstrom, S., & Sibanda, EN., (2002). Polymorphism in codons 10 and 25 of the transforming growth factor-beta 1 (TGF-beta1) gene in patients with invasive squamous cell carcinoma of the uterine cervix. *European Journal of Immunogenetics*, 29. 5, (October 2002), pp. (417-421), ISSN 1365-2370 (Electronic).

[115] Stern, PT., (2008). Natural immune control of HPV infection, In: *Vaccines for the prevention of cervical cancer.* Peter L Stern, Henry C Kitchener, pp. (57-65), Oxford University Press, ISBN 978-0-19-954345-8, New York.

[116] Storey, A., Thomas, M., Kalita, A., Harwood, C., Gardiol, D., Mantovani, F., Breuer, J., Leigh, IM., Matlashewski, G., & Banks, L., (1998). Role of a p53 polymorphism in the development of human papillomavirus-associated cancer. *Nature*, 393. 6682, (May 1998), pp. (229–234), ISSN 1476-4687 (Electronic).

[117] Stubenrauch, F & Laimins, LA., (1999). Human papillomavirus life cycle: active and latent phases. *Seminars in Cancer Biology*, 9. 6, (December 1999), pp. (379–386), ISSN 1096-3650 (Electronic).

[118] Taylor, JG., Choi, EH., Foster, CB., & Chanock, SJ., (2001). Using genetic variation to study human disease. *Trends in Molecular Medicine*, 7. 11, (November 2001), pp. (507-512), ISSN 1471-499X (Electronic).

[119] Thye, T., Burchard, GD., Nilius, M., Muller-Myhsok, B., & Horstmann, RD., (2003). Genomewide linkage analysis identifies polymorphism in the human interferon-gamma receptor affecting Helicobacter pylori infection. *American Journal of Human Genetics*, 72. 2, (February 2003), pp. (448-453), 1537-6605 (Electronic).

[120] Tindle, RW., (2002). Immune evasion in human papillomavirus-associated cervical cancer. *Nature Reviews Cancer*, 2. 1, (January 2002), pp. (59-65), ISSN 1474-1768 (Electronic).

[121] van der Burg, SH., Piersma, SJ., de Jong, A., van der Hulst, JM., Kwappenberg, KM., van den Hende, M., Welters, MJ., Van Rood, JJ., Fleuren, GJ., Melief, CJ., Kenter, GG., & Offringa, R., (2007). Association of cervical cancer with the presence of CD4+ regulatory T cells specific for human papillomavirus antigens. *Proceedings of the National Academy of Sciences of the United States of America*, 104. 29, (July 2007), pp. (12087-12092), ISSN 1091-6490 (Electronic).

[122] Walboomers, JM., Jacobs, MV., Manos, MM., Bosch, FX., Kummer, JA., Shah, KV., Snijders, PJ., Peto, J., Meijer, CJ., & Muñoz, N., (1999). Human papilomavirus is a necessary cause of invasive cervical cancer worldwide. *The Journal of Pathology*, 189. 1, (September 1999), pp. (12-19), ISSN 1096-9896 (Electronic).

[123] Wang, SS., Hildesheim, A., Gao, X., Schiffman, M., Herrero, R., Bratti, MC., Sherman, ME., Barnes, WA., Greenberg, MD., McGowan, L., Mortel, R., Schwartz, PE., Zaino, RJ., Glass, AG., Burk, RD., Karacki, P., & Carrington, M., (2002). Human leukocyte antigen class I alleles and cervical neoplasia no heterozygote advantage. *Cancer*

Epidemiology, Biomarkers and Prevention, 11. 4, (April 2002), pp. (419-420), ISSN 1538-7755 (Electronic).

[124] Wank, R & Thomssen, C., (1991). High risk of squamous cell carcinoma of the cervix for women with HLA-DQw3. *Nature,* 352. 6337, (August 1991), pp. (723–725), ISSN 1476-4687 (Electronic).

[125] Weaver, CT., Harrington, LE., Mangan, PR., Gavrieli, M., & Murphy, KM., (2006). Th17: an effector CD4 T cell lineage with regulatory T cell ties. *Immunity,* 24. 6, (June 2006), pp. (677-688), ISSN 1097-4180 (Electronic).

[126] World Health Organization., 2007. *Integración de la atención sanitaria para la salud sexual y reproductiva y las enfermedades crónicas. Control integral del CaCU.* Guía de prácticas esenciales, pp. 281.

[127] Wilson, A., Symons, J., McDowell, T., McDevitt, HO., & Duff, G., (1997). Effects of a polymorphism in the human tumor necrosis factor a promoter on transcriptional activation. *Proceedings of the National Academy of Sciences of the United States of America,* 94. 7, (April 1997), pp. (3195–3199), ISSN 1091-6490 (Electronic).

[128] Woo, YL., Sterling, J., Damay, I., Coleman, N., Crawford, R., van der Burg, SH., & Stanley, M., (2008) Characterising the local immune responses in cervical intraepithelial neoplasia: a crosssectional and longitudinal analysis. *British Journal of Obstetrics and Gynaecology,* 115. 13, (December 2008), pp. (1616-1621), ISSN 1471-0528 (Electronic).

[129] Woo, YL., van den Hende, M., Sterling, JC., Coleman, N., Crawford, RA., Kwappenberg, KM., Stanley, MA., & van der Burg, SH., (2010). A prospective study on the natural course of low-grade squamous intraepithelial lesions and the presence of HPV16 E2-, E6- and E7-specific T-cell responses. *International Journal of Cancer,* 126. 1, (January 2010), pp. (133-141), ISSN 1097-0215 (Electronic).

[130] Woodman, CB., Collins, SI., & Young, LS., (2007). The natural history of cervical HPV infection: unresolved issues. *Nature Reviews Cancer,* 7. 1, (January 2007), pp. (11-22), ISSN 1474-1768 (Electronic).

14

Cervical Glandular Intraepithelial Neoplasia (CGIN)

Narges Izadi-Mood, Soheila Sarmadi and Kambiz Sotoudeh
Department of Pathology
Tehran University of Medical Sciences,
Iran

1. Introduction

Invasive adenocarcinoma is the second most common malignancy of cervix (after squamous cell carcinoma) and accounts for about 15–25% of all cervical cancers (Hopkins & Morley, 1991). The pre-invasive lesion of the adenocarcinoma of cervix which diagnosed as a spectrum of changes has been named cervical glandular intraepithelial neoplasia (CGIN). Over the past several decades, the incidence of cervical adenocarcinoma as well as its relative proportion to squamous cell carcinoma has been increasing. In 1950s and 1960s, adenocarcinoma accounted for only 5% of all invasive cancers of cervix, however it was increased and responsible for 10-22% in 1990s (Hopkins & Morley,1991; McCluggage,2000; Zaino, 2000, 2002; Wang et al.,2004; Leminen et al.,1990).

This increment may be representing both a real and an apparent increase due to a reduction in the number of invasive cervical squamous carcinomas as a consequence of organized screening programs. There also may be due to better recognition of adenocarcinoma and dysplastic endocervical glandular lesions by pathologists and appreciation of the fact that some poorly differentiated carcinomas may be glandular rather than squamous in type (revealed by the use of ancillary staining), therefore favors a real increase in the incidence of adenocarcinoma in women below 35–40 years of age (McCluggage, 2000).

The pre-invasive lesions of cervical adenocarcinoma are a heterogeneous group with various histomorphological patterns which may be confused with a wide range of non-neoplastic glandular lesions; therefore it is imperative to recognizing these presumed precursors as well as knowledge of their differential diagnosis.

This chapter focuses on an overview of the different terminology, various histopathological features, ancillary diagnostic techniques, and practical diagnostic approach to cervical glandular intraepithelial neoplasia.

2. Precursors glandular lesion of the uterine cervix

2.1 Definition

Cervical glandular intraepithelial neoplasia (CGIN) is a spectrum of presumed pre-invasive (or preneoplastic) cervical glandular lesion. The term 'presumed pre-invasive' is used because there is some controversy as to whether these lesions, especially at the lower end of the spectrum, progress to adenocarcinoma (McCluggage, 2000). The concept of histological recognizable pre-invasive form of adenocarcinoma was at first suggested by Friedell and McKay in 1953. They have proposed that like other organs such as breast, stomach, bronchus, skin and also squamous cell carcinoma of cervix, adenocarcinoma of cervix could have these precursor lesions. Subsequent investigation was renewed interest in characterizing precursor lesions of invasive adenocarcinoma with intent to invoke a unifying theory of a common subcolumnar reserve cell for all types of cervical cancer or to categorize lesions in a fashion analogous to precursors of squamous cell carcinoma of the cervix (Zaino, 2002; Christopherson, 1979). Smedts et al. had reported that cervical intraepithelial neoplasia (CIN), combined adenocarcinoma in situ (AIS) / CIN, and a part of the solitary AIS lesions share a common, marker phenotype comparable with that endocervical reserve cells, which is indicate of a common origin. However, a second group of solitary AIS lesions with an endocervical phenotype possibly originate from a luminal type progenitor cells, within the endocervix (Smedts et al., 2010). Although endocervical adenocarcinoma in situ (AIS) is a known precursor of invasive adenocarcinoma, there is no universally accepted precursor lesion of AIS itself (Ioffe et al., 2003).

2.2 Classification and terminology of pre-invasive cervical glandular lesions

There is no consensus about the terminology using for the classification of pre-invasive endocervical glandular lesions. The term of adenocarcinoma in situ (AIS) as a precursor lesion of adenocarcinoma of uterine cervix was first described by Friedell and McKay in 1953 and most subsequent studies used this terminology (Friedell & Mckay, 1953). Other terms used to describe pre-invasive endocervical glandular lesions include *endocervical glandular dysplasia, cervical intraepithelial glandular neoplasia, cervical glandular atypia, endocervical columnar cell intraepithelial neoplasia* and *atypical endocervical hyperplasia.*

The International Society of Gynecological Pathologists under the auspices of the World Health Organization (WHO) included categories of glandular atypia, atypical hyperplasia (glandular dysplasia), adenocarcinoma in situ and invasive adenocarcinoma in its classification (McCluggage, 2000; Kurman, 2010).

In WHO classification, 3 categories were introduced: *1-Glandular atypia:* which refers to nonneoplastic changes often associated with inflammation; *2-Atypical hyperplasia (glandular dysplasia):* which refers to intraepithelial glandular neoplasia that is less severe than AIS and *3- AIS* (Kurman,2010).

Cervical glandular intraepithelial neoplasia (CGIN) : which is a three-tier grading system *(CGIN 1, 2 and 3)*similar to that used for pre-invasive cervical squamous lesions, that originally has been introduced by Gloor and Hurlimann (Gloor & Hurlimann,1986).This three-tier grading system was performed according to cytohistological criteria including nuclear abnormality, presence of mitosis, amount of intracellular mucin and architectural abnormality. Following this grading a new terminology was introduced by a working party of the Royal College of Pathologists and the NHS Cervical Screening Program in the Britain (NHS Cervical Screening Programme [NHSCSP], 1999). Because of difficulties in three-tier grading, particularly the distinction between CGIN 1 and 2, most authors therefore recognize only two grades of CGIN, termed high grade and low grade CGIN. This does not mean that

CGIN is a two stage disease but reflects the fact that differentiation into three grades is probably poorly reproducible. Alternatively high grade and low grade CGIN may be designated as AIS and glandular dysplasia, respectively (McCluggage, 2000).

The Silverberg group (Ioffe et al.,2003) introduced the Silverberg scoring system for assessment of the endocervical glandular lesions that is designed to aid in diagnosis and to bring about better inter- and intra observer agreement in this difficult area (McCluggage, 2000; Liang et al.,2007). This scoring scheme is based on 3 separately graded components: nuclear stratification, nuclear atypia, and mitoses/apoptosis. The scores for which are added to result in the total score equivalent to a diagnostic category: benign (score = 0-3), endocervical glandular dysplasia (score = 4-5), and adenocarcinoma in situ (score = 6-9) (Table 1) (Ioffe et al., 2003).

Stratification
-None = 0
-Mild = 1
-Moderate = 2
-Up to the luminal surface = 3
Nuclear atypia
-As normal = 0
- Small (size of normal) or slightly enlarged uniform nuclei, minimal hyperchromasia, little dispolarity, no nucleoli = 1
-Nuclear enlargement (up to 3 × normal), moderate anisocytosis, moderate hyperchromasia, moderate dispolarity, occasional small nucleoli = 2
-Large nuclei (>3 × normal), marked anisocytosis, marked hyperchromasia, severe dispolarity, frequent prominent nucleoli = 3
Mitoses and apoptosis
[In two most active glands, number per gland (average between two glands)]
-None= 0
-Less than 0.5 per gland = 1
-0.6–3.0 per gland = 2
- >3.0 per gland = 3
Total score
0–3 = benign
4–5 = endocervical glandular dysplasia (EGD)
6–9 = adenocarcinoma in situ (AIS)

Table 1. Silverberg group's scoring system for assessment of the endocervical glandular lesions

2.3 Pathogenesis

Among a variety of factors investigated, including the absence of a prior Pap smear, number of sexual partners, age at first intercourse, history of genital infections, obesity, and tobacco use, two conditions have emerged as potential risk factors in the development of cervical adenocarcinoma: Human Papilloma Virus (HPV) infection and oral contraceptive (OCP) use (Zaino,2000). But from different descriptive epidemiological observations, it has been suggested that adenocarcinoma may differ in pathogenetic mechanisms and that its etiology should be investigated with reference to hormonal, rather than infectious, aspects (Parazzini et al., 1988). Ursin et al. reported that the highest risk was for oral contraceptive use for more than 12 years. No additional increased risk was found for early age at start of oral contraceptive use, use before age 20 or before first pregnancy, time since first use, time since last use, or particular formulations, once total duration of use had been accounted for (Ursin et al., 1994).But in the study by Parazzini et al., oral contraceptive use was not related to the risk of adenocarcinoma of the cervix (Parazzini et al., 1988; Madeleine et al., 2001).

Although morphologic evidence of productive HPV infection is generally limited to squamous or transitional epithelium, now overwhelming data supports the high frequency of HPV infection in both AIS and invasive adenocarcinoma (Madeleine et al., 2001; Bulk et al., 2006). In early 1980s wart viruses were not found in many of the in situ and invasive adenocarcinoma of the cervix, but with more sensitive techniques, HPV type 16, 31, and more frequently 18, have been identified in 80% and more of adenocarcinoma and adenosquamous carcinoma (Zaino, 2000). Recent studies have shown that HPV type 18 and 16 are the most common types which are detected in 43% and 23% of CGIN, respectively (Zielinski et al.,2003; Pirog et al.,2000).

2.4 Clinical signs and colposcopic features

The early diagnosis of glandular lesions still represents a real challenge for clinicians, who are likely to miss the lesions because of the absence of clinical indicators, normal cytology, or cytology suggestive of squamous disease and/or because of unfamiliarity with the diseases newly delineated colposcopic presentations.

For identifying pre-invasive cervical glandular lesions, colposcopy has not been helpful since colposcopic features of AIS and early adenocarcinoma are widely seen as known nonspecific and also this is because the disease only slightly changes the surface contour and because the neoplastic "glands "are often buried beneath the surface (Campion, 2010; Wright, 2002).

Usually most glandular lesions lie within or close to the transformation zone. While the majority of squamous lesions are usually visible by colposcopic examination, AIS may locate proximally, involving the endocervix, or may lie under the metaplastic epithelium or placed in an abnormal transformation zone and thus be out of colposcopic view (Campion, 2010; Wright, 2002).

Because of AIS coexists with high grade CIN in 30%-70% of cases and the location of the lesion, the abnormal smear will frequently predicate only the squamous lesion (van Aspert-van Erp et al.,2004). In mixed conditions that AIS and squamous cell lesions are concomitantly present, cytologic examination may only exhibiting squamous abnormality that mislead the colposcopist to look exclusively for a squamous lesion and to be satisfied upon finding it. Furthermore, the colposcopic biopsy may confirm the squamous lesion, with AIS being detected only on a subsequent wide excision or within a hysterectomy specimen. Diagnostic excisional biopsy must be always performed when AIS is found on punch biopsy or when AIS is suspected cytologically or colposcopically but not proven histologically (Campion, 2010).

Commonly colposcopic diagnosis of glandular lesions is less than satisfactory because have no specific appearance and mostly mimic the other lesions.

However, to overcome this problem a new set of colposcopic criteria has been recommended for differentiation between glandular lesion and metaplasia, condyloma, squamous intraepithelial neoplasia and squamous cell carcinoma.

The criteria are:

- Lesion locatied over columnar epithelium, not contiguous with the squamocolumnar junction;
- Large "gland" or crypt openings;
- Papillary structure;
- Budding;
- Patchy red and white coloration;
- Waste-thread, tendril, root, and character-writing blood vessels;
- Single or multiple dots produced at tips of papillary projection by looped vessels (Wright, 2002; Ostör et al., 1984).

Some features can be used to eliminate a lesion from consideration, such as punctuation and true mosaic pattern (which are present only in squamous intraepithelial lesions) and corkscrew vessels (which are associated only with invasive squamous disease).

Although many colposcopically recognized features are common to a variety of diseases, paying attention to surface contour and vascular configurations can greatly help the colposcopist discover glandular disease when it is present and differentiate it from other conditions (Wright, 2002).

2.5 Morphological features

2.5.1 Histopathological features of cervical glandular intraepithelial neoplasia (CGIN)

Adenocarcinoma in situ (AIS) of the cervix has no distinguishing clinical and colposcopic features, and because it is rare, pathologists may not be familiar with its microscopic appearances. It is easily overlooked since it may be focal and because it is frequently associated with cervical intraepithelial neoplasia (CIN), which is more impressive. There is little information about its natural history (Ostör et al., 1984).

Although there are several proposed classifications and terminologies used for describing CGINs, in most of them the morphologic criteria are nearly the same with small differences, set them in a wide spectrum between the reactive/benign lesions and invasive carcinoma in two extremities of classification.

By using these diagnostic criteria, identification of high grade lesion has been more reproducible than low grade , but most often the diagnosis of low grade lesion resulted in a confusing state of affairs for pathologists and clinicians. In most instances high grade CGIN (HCGIN) is diagnosed more often than low grade CGIN (LCGIN) in contrast to some earlier studies that reported low grade CGIN was more common (Brown, 1986).

There is a popular misconception among pathologists and gynecologists that CGIN often occurs in upper parts of the endocervical canal. However, in most, but not all cases, CGIN occurs close to the transformation zone (McCluggage, 2003). CGIN is commonly associated with a concomitant squamous intraepithelial lesion and may affect the surface epithelium and/or endocervical crypts, usually in the region of the transformation zone (Bekkers et al., 2003).

Another popular misconception is that skip lesions are extremely common in CGIN. Skip lesions undoubtedly do occur but these are relatively uncommon, probably occurring in up to 15% of patients (McCluggage, 2003).

Both high and low grades CGIN are characterized by a combination of cytological and architectural features. These features are more pronounced in high grade CGIN but not all are necessarily present in a given case of CGIN (McCluggage, 2000).

The recognition of low grade CGIN is more problematic and this lesion easily underdiagnosed by pathologists. Low grade CGIN has many overlapping features with reactive changes. Dysplastic changes in low grade CGIN are not fulfill the diagnosis of high grade CGIN and qualitatively less severe than high grade CGIN. The most common changes are: glands composed of pseudostratified cells that slightly loss their polarity, with large and hyperchromatic nuclei and minimal mitosis and apoptotic bodies. Usually stroma lacks any inflammatory or reactive changes (NHSCSP, 1999) (Figure 1- A and B).

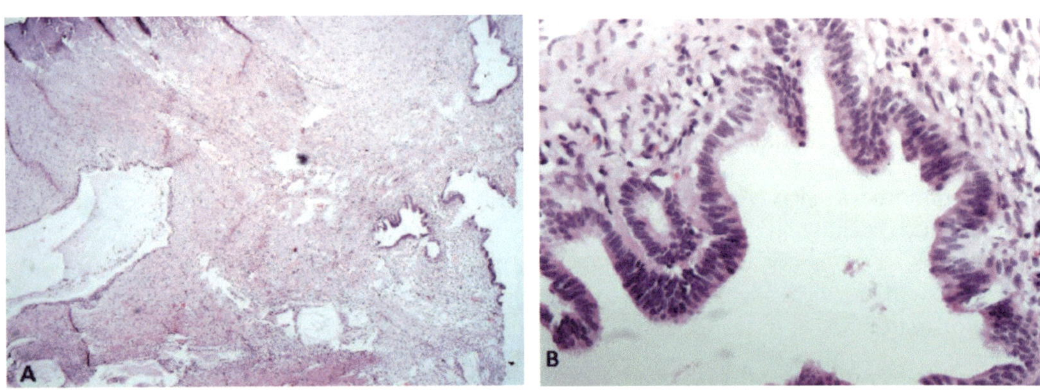

Fig. 1. LCGIN. **A,** Normal crypt in the left comparable with darker epithelium of LCGIN in the right in low magnification. **B,** Partially pseudostratified epithelium, crowded nuclei, and occasional mitotic figures are seen in higher magnification.

In high grade CGIN which abruptly begins beside the normal columnar cells (Figure 2- A and B) dysplastic changes are more severe and characterized by usually crowded glands (Figure 2- C) with various architectural patterns like budding and branching (Figure 2- D), exophytic papillae (Figure 3-A), intraluminal papillary projections (Figure 3-B) , micropapillae (Figure 3-C) and cribriform (Figure 4-A and B) , that composed of atypical cells that variably loss their cytoplasmic mucin, and display large pleomorphic hyperchromatic nuclei with lack of polarity and easily finding mitoses and apoptotic bodies (Figure 4- C and D)(For detailed definition of histopathological features see Table 2).Glands are commonly surrounded by a compact stroma (NHSCSP, 1999).

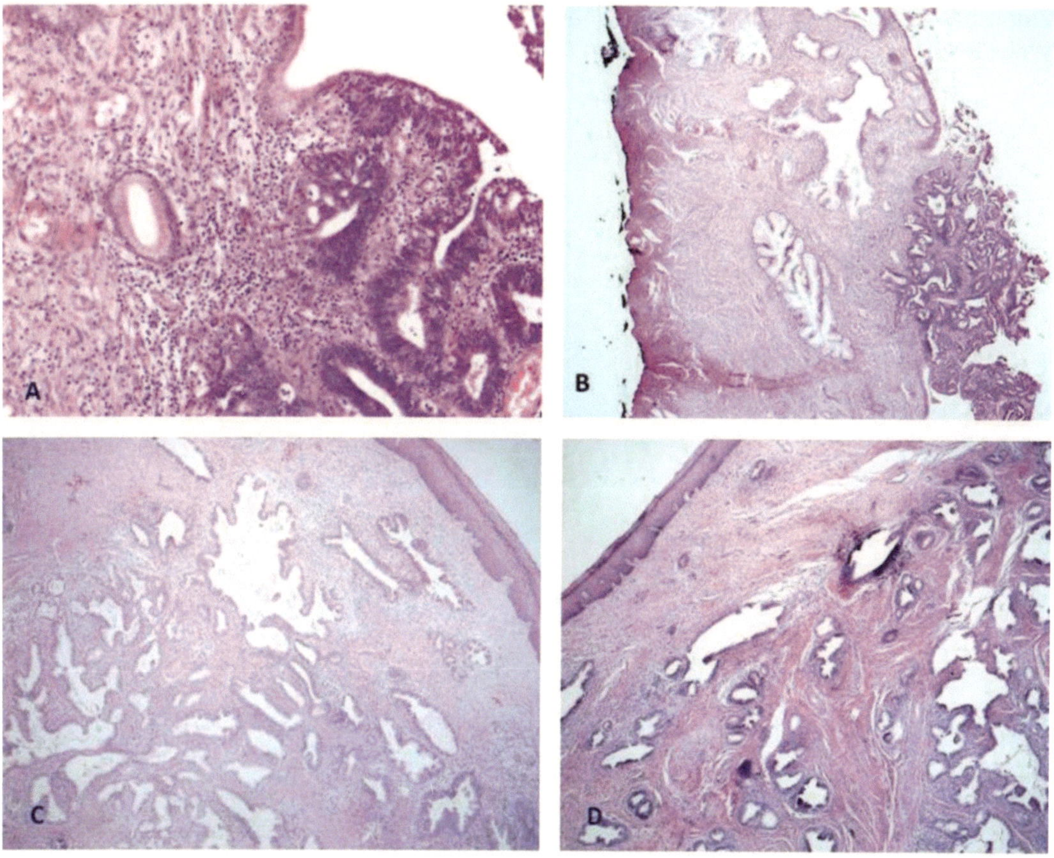

Fig. 2. HCGIN. **A,** Abrupt transition from normal endocervical columnar epithelium (top & left) to the stratified epithelium of the CGIN (right). **B,** Abrupt transition from normal endocervical columnar epithelium (top) to the stratified epithelium of the CGIN (center). **C,** A cluster of closely packed glands with branching, out-pouching and occasional in-folding. **D,** A cluster of glands with branching (irregular contour).

High grade CGIN displays three common histological subtypes: endocervical, endometrioid and intestinal as well as several uncommon subtypes: serous, clear cell, adenosquamous, villoglandular and tubal (McCluggage, 2000; Zaino, 2000).

Among them the endocervical HCGIN (alone or admixed with other types) is the most common type which mimic the normal endocervical glands. In contrast to endocervical type that small to moderate amount of cytoplasmic mucin present in luminal side of atypical cell, in endometrioid HCGIN which cells mimic the proliferative endometrial cells, their eosinophilic cytoplasm lack any mucin. Another characteristic feature in this type is significant nuclear pseudostratification. Intestinal HCGIN is recognized by its prominent goblet cell and occasional neuroendocrine or paneth cells. There is no evidence that behavior of the different subtypes of HCGIN is significantly differed (McCluggage, 2000; Zaino,2000,2002; Wang et al., 2004; Gloor & Hurlimann,1986; NHSCSP, 1999; Brown & Wells,1986; Gloor & Ruzicka,1982; Kurian & al-Nafussi,1999).

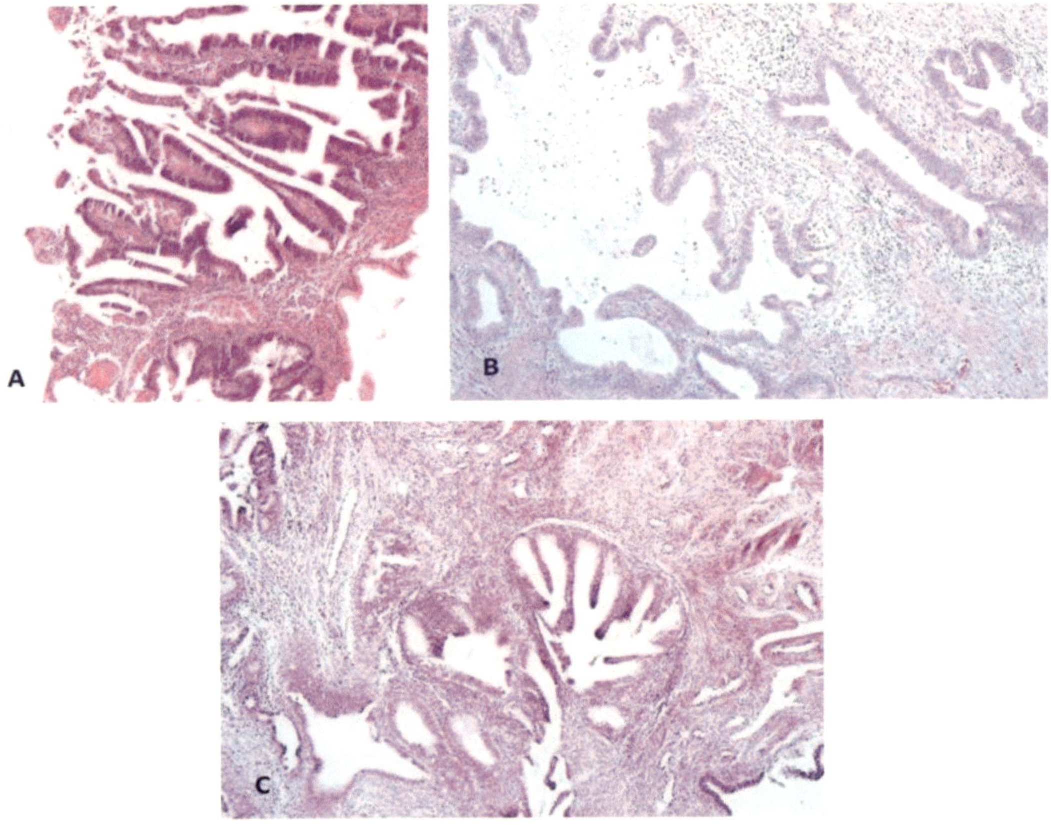

Fig. 3. HCGIN. **A,** Simple exophytic papillary pattern with thin delicate stromal stalk.
B, Infolding of epithelium into the glandular lumina with supporting stroma.
C, Intraluminal exuberance and delicate micropapillary projection with no supporting stroma.

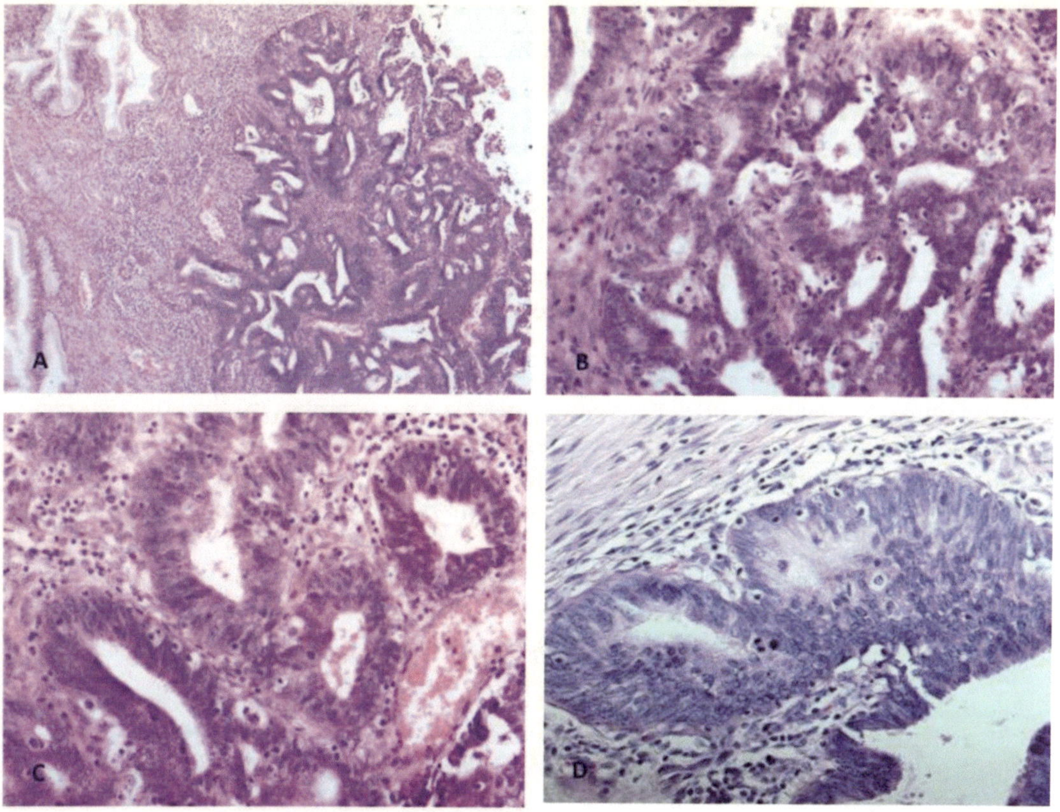

Fig. 4. HCGIN. **A,** Macroglands with secondary or multiple generation of bridging subdividing the lumen into smaller glandular spaces; no stroma supports the bridging cells (low power). **B,** Macroglands with secondary or multiple generation of bridging subdividing the lumen into smaller glandular spaces; no stroma support the bridging cells (High power). **C,** Nuclear stratification (loss of mucin secretion); nuclear hyperchromasia with mitotic activity and apoptotic bodies. **D,** Nuclear Stratification; loss of nuclear polarity with mitotic activity and apoptotic bodies.

2.5.2 Cervical cytology

The diagnostic category and the terminology of atypical glandular cell (AGC), has been widely used since it was first established at the 2001 Bethesda convention (Covell et al., 2003). Before 2001, AGC within The Bethesda System (TBS) were mentioned as atypical glandular cells of undetermined significance (AGUS). The incidence of endocervical adenocarcinoma has increased steadily over the past two decades (Hopkins & Morley, 1991). Since TBS was introduced, the diagnosis of AGC has risen and now accounts for 0.17–1.83% of all cervical smears (Nasu et al., 1993). The term AGC applies to glandular cells that demonstrate changes beyond those typical of benign reactive processes but lack sufficient features for a diagnosis of adenocarcinoma. Generally, the origin of AGCs, endocervical or endometrial, can be distinguished based on the larger nuclear size and more abundant cytoplasm of endocervical cells (Solomon et al., 1998).

Definition of architectural features
-Glandular crowding: A cluster of closely packed glands. **-Glandular budding:** Glands out-pouching into the surrounding stroma to produce "finger-in-glove" pattern. **-Glandular branching:** Glands with multiple out-pouching and irregular counters. **-Villoglandular /exophytic papillae:** Simple branching exophytic papillary pattern with thin delicate stromal stalk,reminds of villous adenoma of the GI tract. **-Intraluminal papillary projections:** Infolding of epithelium into the glandular lumina with supporting stroma which creates a cribriform-like pattern. **-Micropapillae pattern:** Intraluminal exuberance and delicate micropapillary projection with no supporting stroma. **-Cribriform pattern:** Macroglands with secondary or multiple generation of bridging subdividing the lumen into smaller glandular spaces; no stroma support the bridging cells.
Definition of cytological features
-Abrupt junction between the normal columnar epithelium and the CGIN: Partially affected epithelial lining by CGIN with sharp demarcation between normal epithelium and CGIN. **-Intestinal metaplasia /goblet cell formation:** A form of intestinal metaplasia, exhibits goblet cells and even paneth or neuroendocrine cells. **-Loss of mucin secretion in cells of endocervical type:** Reduction or complete absence of intracellular mucin. **-Nuclear stratification:** Pseudostratified up to stratified epithelium in reciprocal reduction in cytoplasmic mucin with or without loss of nuclear palisading and polarity. **-Nuclear changes:** Enlarged, elongated, pleomorphic and hyperchromatic nuclei with granular dense and evenly or abnormal dispersion of nuclear chromatin and presence of prominent nuclei. **-Mitotic activity**: Presence of juxtaluminal and increased numbers of mitotic figures (normal/ or abnormal). **-Apoptosis (apoptotic bodies):** Markedly condensed homogenous nuclei (with or without nuclear fragmentation) often associated with densly eosinophilic cytoplasm.

Table 2. Definition of various architectural and cytological features of CGIN

The Bethesda System (TBS) recommends subclassification of AGC into the categories of *"favor endocervical origin"*, *"favor endometrial origin"* and *"not otherwise specified (NOS)"*. Favor endocervical origin lesions are further classified into the categories of *"favor neoplastic"* and *"favor NOS"* (Covell et al., 2003). However, subclassification of AGC has yet to be proved clinically effective, and although The Bethesda Committee and many others have studied cytologic criteria important in subclassification, these criteria have not been tested vigorously. The rates of AGC (reported as AGUS before 2001) quoted in the literature vary from 0.095% to 1.83% (Nasu et al., 1993; Mood et al. , 2006; Marques et al.,2011; Tam et al.,2003; Scheiden et al.,2004; Pecorelli et al., 2009).

According to TBS 2001, cytological features of subcategorized AGC is as follow:

In atypical endocervical cells (NOS) (Figure 5-A and B):

- Cells occur in sheets and strips with some crowding and nuclear overlap.

- Nuclear enlargement, up to three to five times the area of normal endocervical nuclei, may be seen.
- Some variation in nuclear size and shape is present.
- Mild hyperchromasia is frequently evident.
- Nucleoli may be present.
- Mitotic figures are rare. Cytoplasm may be fairly abundant, but the nuclear /cytoplasmic (N/C) ratio is increased.
- Distinct cell borders often are discernible.

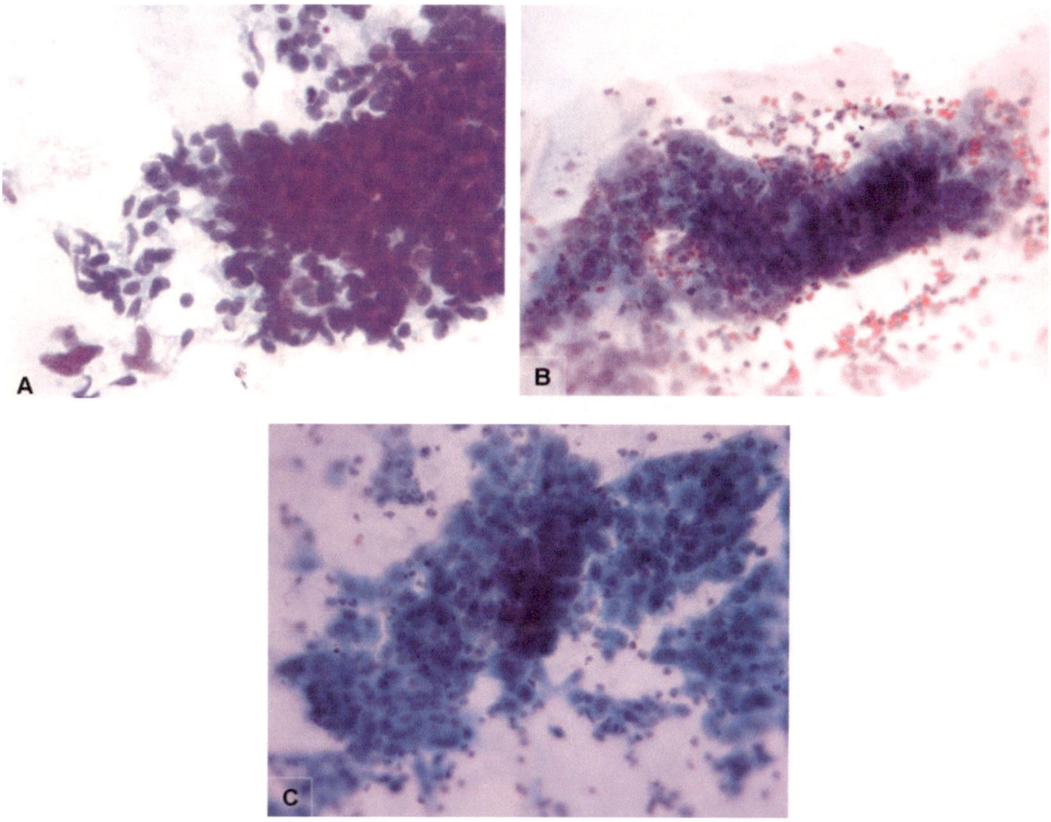

Fig. 5. **A**, Atypical endocervical cells (NOS) .A sheet of endocervical cells with some crowding and nuclear overlap. **B**, Atypical endocervical cells (NOS). Strip of endocrvical cells with stratification, elongation of nuclei, nuclear enlargment and hyperchromasia . **C**, Atypical endocervical cells, (favor neoplastic). A sheet of endocervical cells with crowding and nuclear overlap shows increased nuclear/cytoplasmic ratios.The quantity of cytoplasm is diminished, and cell borders are ill defined.

In liquid-based preparation groups are more rounded and three dimensional with piled-up of cells, making individual cells in the center difficult to visualize.

In atypical endocervical cells, (favor neoplastic) (Figure 5-C) alongside above mentioned features, added cytological features incorporated:

- Cell morphology, either quantitatively or qualitatively, falls just short of an interpretation of endocervical adenicarcinoma in situ or invasive adenocarcinoma.
- Rare cell groups may show rosetting or feathering
- Nuclei are enlarged with some hyperchromasia
- Occasional mitosis may be seen.
- Nuclear/cytoplasmic ratios are increased, quantity of cytoplasm is diminished, and cell borders may be ill defined.

In liquid-based preparation groups may be three dimensional, thick, with layers of cells obscuring central nuclear detail.

It is important that the interpretation of "atypical glandular cells" (AGC) should be qualified, if possible, to indicate whether the cells are thought to be endocervical or endometrial origin. If the origin of the cells cannot be determined, the generic "glandular" term is used. Atypical endocervical cells should be further qualified when a particular entity, including neoplasia, is favored.

AIS is often identified in cytological specimens as abundant abnormal cells, typically with columnar configuration, single cells, two-dimensional sheets, or three-dimensional clusters and syncytial aggregates with nuclear crowding and overlap, without an accompanying tumor diathesis. Characteristic features of glandular differentiation include rosette formation, nuclear feathering ,and palisading (Figure 6-A and B).

In liquid-based preparation three-dimensional clusters are common. Chromatin is more open (vesicular) with irregular distribution and parachromatin clearing (Covell et al., 2003).

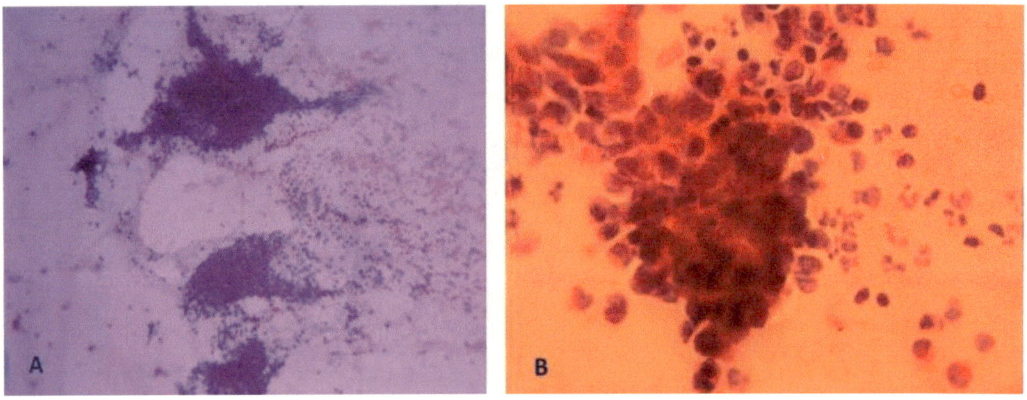

Fig. 6. Adenocarcinoma in situ. **A,** Abundant abnormal cells, typically with columnar configuration, single cells, two-dimensional sheets, or three-dimensional clusters and syncytial aggregates with nuclear crowding and overlap. **B,** Characteristic rosette formation in glandular differentiation.

2.5.3 Differential diagnosis

2.5.3.1 Invasive adenocarcinoma

The most important differential diagnosis of CGIN is microinvasive and invasive adenocarcinoma.

By definition the concept of microinvasive adenocarcinoma (MIA) is the same as microinvasive squamous cell carcinoma and represents an invasive adenocarcinoma with limited depth of stromal invasion up to 5 millimeters (Pecorelli et al., 2009). Despite plenty data about its squamous counterpart, MIA is suffering from a reliable cytological and histological diagnostic criteria as well as information about its prognosis and management. While diagnosis of early stromal invasion in squamous cell carcinoma (SCC) is relatively simple and easy, however, identifying early invasion in high grade CGIN may be extremely difficult or even impossible (McCluggage, 2000; Zaino, 2000; NHSCSP, 1999,Nucci,2002). High grade CGIN should be limited to the normal glandular field but problems occur when closely packed, architecturally abnormal glands are lined by dysplastic epithelium which fulfils the criteria for a diagnosis of high grade CGIN (McCluggage, 2000; Zaino, 2000; Nucci, 2002).

MIA characterized by effacement of normal glandular tissue by irregular atypical glands that extends beyond the deepest normal crypt associated with a stromal reactivity of desmoplastic, infiltration of chronic inflammatory cells or edematous type.

There are two certain features that identify the presence of invasion in endocervical adenocarcinoma (1) Individual cells or incomplete glands (Figure 7-A and B) lined by cytologically malignant-appearing cells at a stromal interface and (2) malignant appearing glands surrounded by a host response (Figure 7-C). It is important to determine that the glands are lined by cytologically malignant-appearing cells, because endocervicitis, microglandular hyperplasia, and ruptured mucin-filled glands all may have incomplete glands that at times may be associated with a host response of dense inflammation and, occasionally, edema or fibrosis. Unfortunately, many adenocarcinomas do not display these two changes yet are invasive. It should be noted that infiltration of chronic inflammatory cells around the CGIN may also be present and result in a confusing and complex status (McCluggage, 2000; Zaino, 2000; Nucci, 2002).

Additional features that are not entirely specific may help to identify invasion in other cases including:

(1) Architecturally complex, branching, or small glands, which grow confluently or in a labyrinthine pattern; (2) A cribriform growth pattern of malignant-appearing epithelium devoid of stroma within a single gland profile; (3) The presence of glands below the deep margin of normal glands; and (4) The presence of early stromal infiltration from glands involved by HCGIN of small buds of cells, often with a squamoid appearance (McCluggage, 2000; Zaino, 2000; Nucci, 2002).

Large masses of densely packed architecturally complex glands with luminal bridges and a cribriform growth pattern strongly suggest invasion. More difficult is the assessment of the "deep margin" of normal glands. Although it is stated that endocervical glands should be confined to the inner third of the cervix and less than 1 cm deep, benign glands in various patterns including nabothian cysts, tunnel clusters, laminar endocervical hyperplasia, deep endocervical glands, and mesonephric duct remnants may be found deeper in the stroma on occasion. Pathologists should, wherever possible, make every effort to make this distinction, but it is recognized that there will be cases in which the pathologist remains uncertain as to whether a lesion is invasive or not, even after the mandatory examination of many levels. This must be stated in the report (McCluggage, 2000, 2003; Zaino, 2000; NHSCSP, 1999; Nucci, 2002).

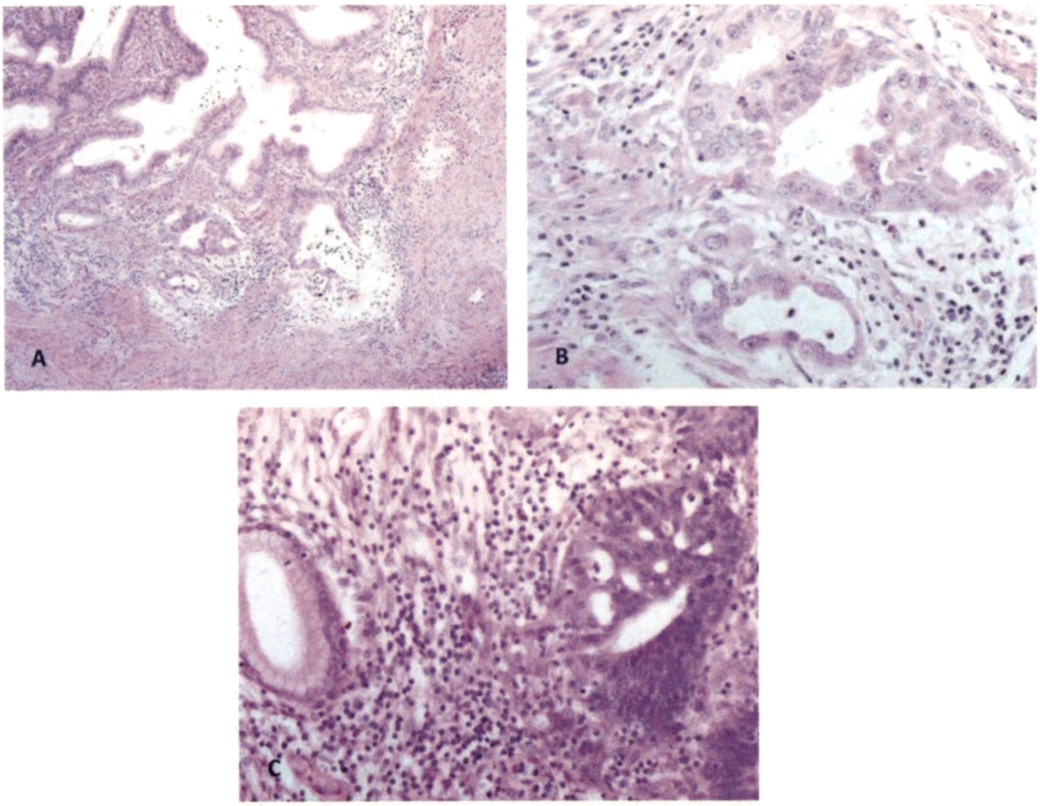

Fig. 7. Microinvasive adenocarcinoma. **A,** Individual cells and incomplete glands beneath the crypt surronded by edematous stroma and lymphocytic infiltration (low power). **B,** Individual cells and incomplete glands beneath the crypt surrounded by edematous stroma and lymphocytic infiltration (High power).Note the severe degree of cytological atypia. The nuclei are pleomorphic, there is loss of nuclear polarity and several nuclei contain large nucleoli. Cell above the incomplete gland has copious eosinophilic cytoplasm. **C,** A cribriform macrogland with cells in the lower right part with copious eosinophilic cytoplasm should arouse a suspicion that invasion may be present. Note normal gland in the left.

2.5.3.2 Tuboendometrioid metaplasia and Endometriosis

Tuboendometrioid metaplasia (TEM) is very common within the cervix and the most common lesion to be misdiagnosed as CGIN (McCluggage, 2000). It usually develops after cervical biopsy or diathermy, but may also occur in the absence of any surgical intervention. In TEM, the normal endocervical surface or crypt epithelium replaced by tubal or endometrioid cell type or by a population of cubo-columnar cells with regular, oval to round, darkly staining, hyperchromatic basal nuclei and high nuclear/cytoplasmic ratios; some of the cells may be ciliated (Figure 8- A and B). Tubal metaplsia usually involves a single gland or a few glands near the squamocolumnar junction and is not associated with inflammation.

Mitoses are uncommon except when estrogenic proliferative activity is present. Nuclear pleomorphism and atypical mitoses are absent (NHSCSP, 1999). A helpful clue to the diagnosis is the presence of cilia on the luminal border of some of the cells.

Occasionally invasive cervical adenocarcinoma may also contain ciliated cells, thus it is not need to overemphasize that the presence of cilia in the cervix does not unequivocally denote a benign process.

Ancillary techniques, such as the use of proliferation markers, have been used with some success in attempting to distinguish TEM and other benign glandular lesions from CGIN. These are discussed in detail later (McCluggage, 2000).

Endometriosis, which is characterized by the presence of endometrial-type glands set in an endometrial stroma, most commonly occurs in the region of the external cervical os or in the lower endocervical canal (Figure 9-A and B).

At colposcopy it appears as a hemorrhagic lesion. Regular bleeding may lead to stromal fibrosis and stenosis of the external cervical os. It can usually be easily recognized histologically and, if active, is most commonly approximately in phase with the intrauterine endometrium (NHSCSP, 1999) (Figure 9-C).

Cervical endometriosis not associated with TEM may have either a superficial or deep location. Deep cervical endometriosis is often associated with pelvic endometriosis and generally causes no problems in diagnosis. However, superficial endometriosis may be mistaken for CGIN (Tam et al., 2003). The presence of endometrial type stroma is a clue to the diagnosis but this is often significantly obscured by accompanying inflammation or hemorrhage and rarely by smooth muscle metaplasia. Particularly in young women there may be considerable mitotic activity when estrogen induced proliferative activity is present (McCluggage, 2000) (Figure 9-D).

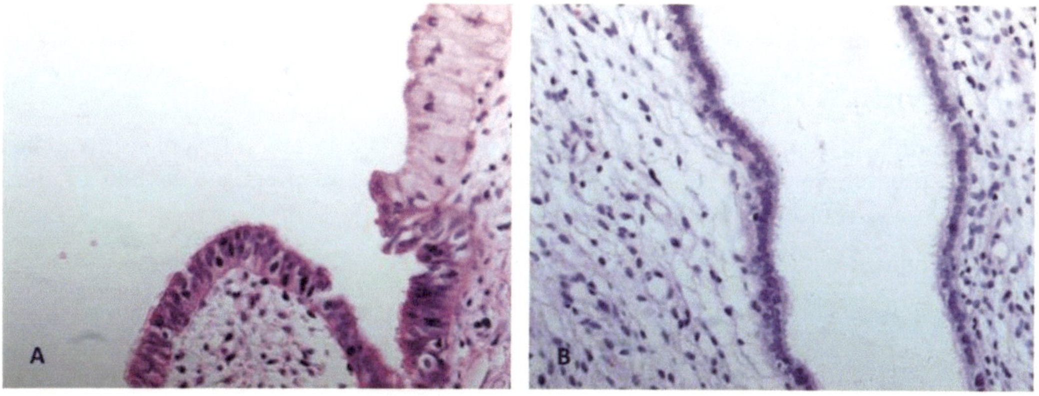

Fig. 8. **A,** Tubal metaplasia. Note abrupt transition between the mucus-secreting endocervical cells and the ciliated cells. **B,** Tuboendometrioid metaplasia (TEM). The normal endocervical crypt epithelium replaced by a population of cubo-columnar cells with regular, oval to round, darkly staining, hyperchromatic basal nuclei and high nuclear/cytoplasmic ratios; some of the cells may be ciliated.

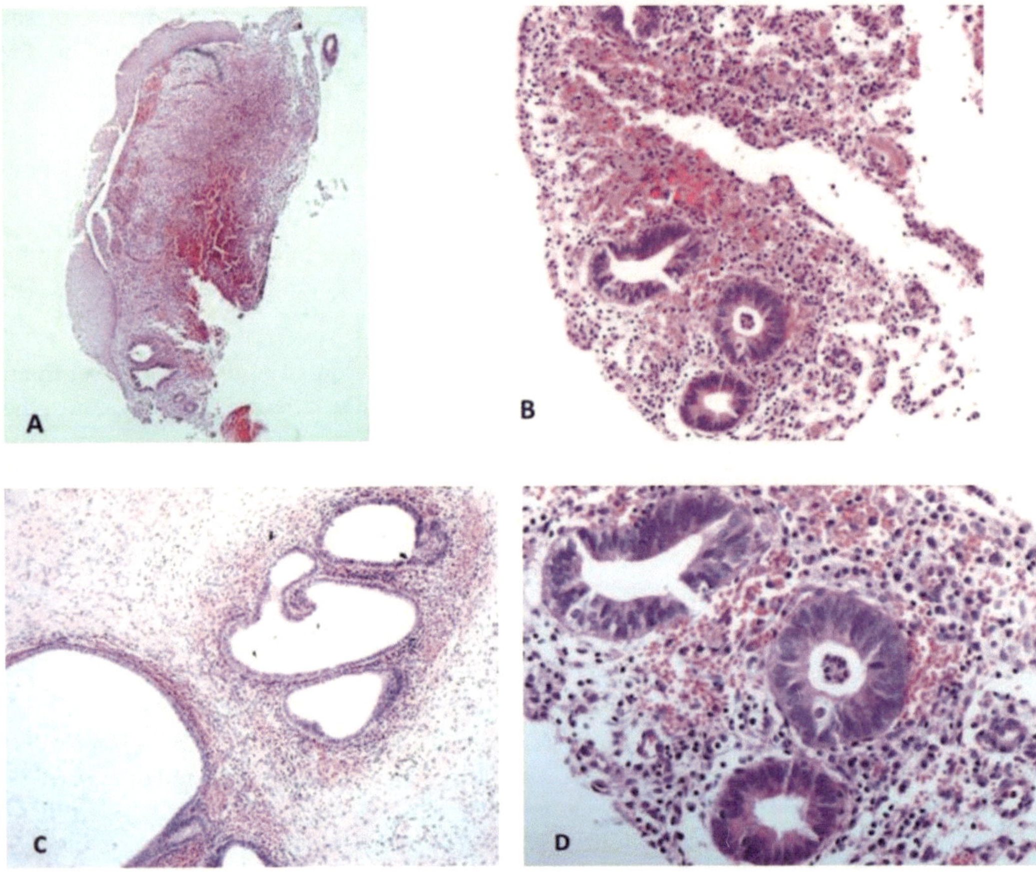

Fig. 9. Endometriosis. **A,** Presence of endometrial-type glands set in an endometrial stroma beneath the squamous epithelium (low power). **B,** High power view. **C,** Subnuclear vacuoles in active endometriosis. **D,** Note mitotic activity in estrogen induced proliferative activity.

2.5.3.3 Microglandular hyperplasia

Microglandular hyperplasia or microglandular adenosis is a common lesion, seems to be a result of progesterone effects, and most commonly found in pregnant women or those receiving oral contraceptives or progestines.

In gross findings is often polypoid and may be unifocal or multifocal (Fig. 10- A).

Early lesions may show sessile. Microscopically, it is characterized by the presence of closely packed small glandular structures lined by cuboidal epithelial cells with vesicular nuclei. Mitotic figures are uncommon, but may be found, and there is often prominent subnuclear and supranuclear vacuolation. There may be associated with reserve cell hyperplasia and immature squamous metaplasia and there is often a striking neutrophilic infiltrate (Figure 10- B and C).

Signet ring like cells may be seen. Typical or atypical forms of microglandular hyperplasia may be mistaken for CGIN or clear cell carcinoma. The suspicion of malignancy may be heightened when microglandular hyperplasia results in a polypoid mass. CGIN and clear cell carcinoma generally have a higher mitotic rate than microglandular hyperplasia, atypical mitoses are often seen and nuclei are not vesicular (McCluggage, 2000; Zaino, 2000, 2002; NHSCSP, 1999; Ostör, 2000, Nucci, 2003).

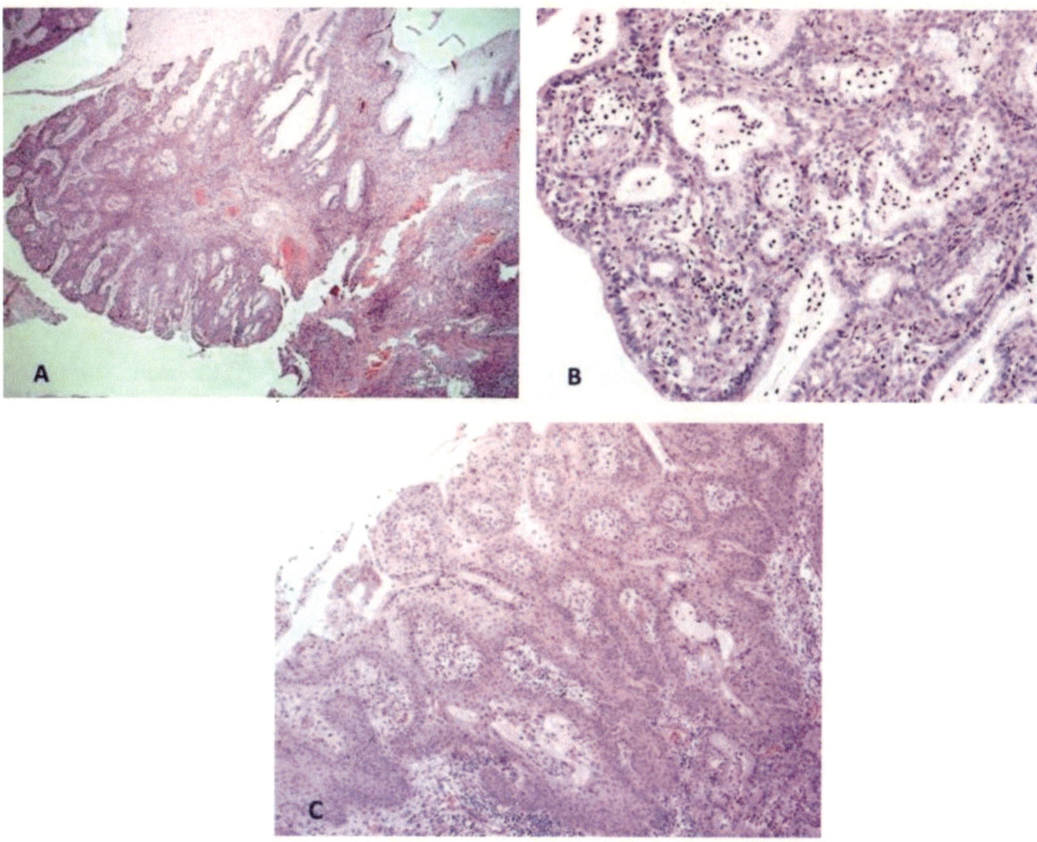

Fig. 10. Microglandular hyperplasia. **A,** Polypoid configuration (low power). **B,** Note small size glands and neutrophilic infiltration. **C,** Reserve cell hyperplasia and immature squamous metaplasia.

2.5.3.4 Tunnel clusters

Tunnel clusters are benign, relatively rare, endocervical lesions which are most common in multigravid patients. This has led some to suggest that they are a result of subinvolution of endocervical glands following pregnancy. Tunnel clusters are characterized by a lobular arrangement of closely packed, often dilated endocervical glands. The lining epithelium is of mucinous type but is often compressed and attenuated and filled by mucinous eosinophilic secretions. Nuclear pleomorphism and mitotic figures are absent and the lesion is always an incidental finding. Two histological types have been described. In type A there is little or no dilatation of glands whereas type B is characterized by marked glandular dilatation (Figure 11).

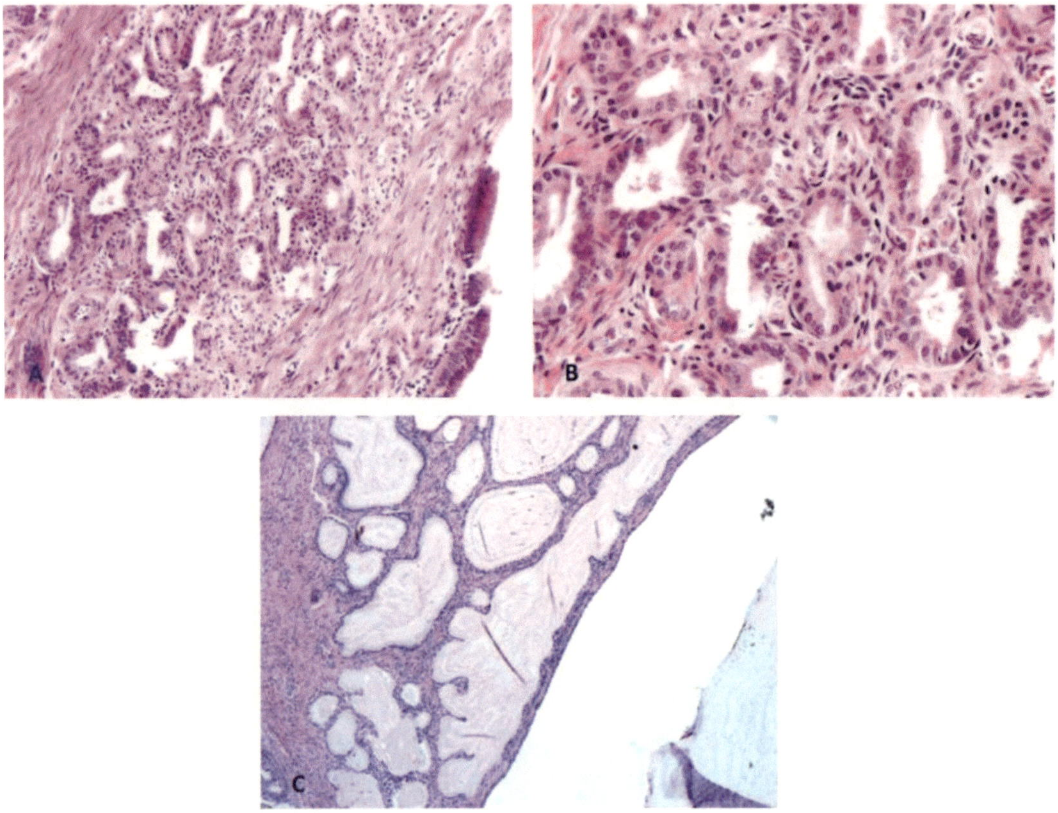

Fig. 11. Tunnel clusters. **A,** Type A. Closely packed endocervical glands (Low power). **B,** Type A. (High power). **C,** Type B. Closely packed, dilated endocervical glands.

Although malignancy, especially minimal deviation adenocarcinoma (or adenoma malignum), may be considered, this is not a significant problem and once the characteristic histological features of tunnel clusters are known, they are easily appreciated (McCluggage, 2000; Zaino, 2000, 2002; NHSCSP, 1999; Ostör, 2000, Nucci, 2003).

2.5.3.5 Reactive glandular atypia

This very common category, including atypia as a result of inflammation, tissue repair, and response to irradiation, may mimic adenocarcinoma. Inflammation and tissue repair may result in lacelike masses of glandular cells with enlarged, pleomorphic nuclei and prominent nucleoli. Typically, the epithelium lining the glands is not stratified. The presence of a dense inflammatory infiltrate, frequently extending into the epithelium, often coupled with loss of polarity and acquisition of abundant, polygonal cytoplasm, assists in the recognition of the presence as reactive. Isolated multinucleated endocervical cells are common (Figure 12).

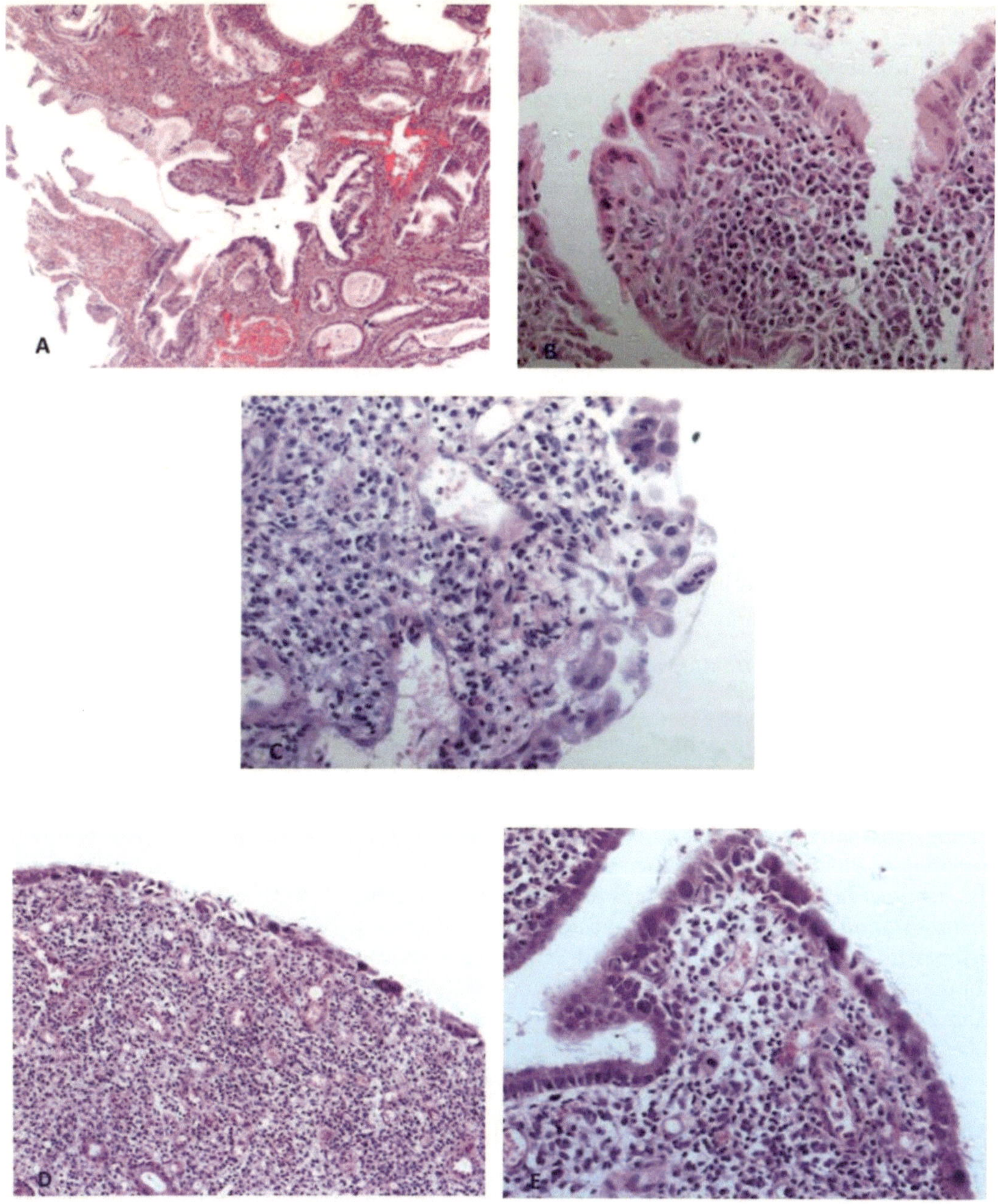

Fig. 12. Reactive glandular atypia. **A,** Note loss of polarity in a part of crypt lining produce abrupt transition and darker area between normal and reactive epithelium. **B,** Note enlarged, pleomorphic nuclei in endocervical epithelium. **C,** Dense inflammatory infiltrate, extending into the epithelium, coupled with loss of polarity.Enlarged, pleomorphic nuclei in endocervical epithelium and dense inflammatory infiltrate in the stroma. **D,** (Low power). **E,** (High power).

Reactive atypia is generally differentiate from CGIN by the lack of epithelial stratification, degenerative or reactive type changes in nuclear chromatin rather than granular hyperchromasia, and a paucity of mitotic activity and apoptotic bodies. Papillary endocervicitis is a specific form of tissue response characterized by relatively short edematous papillae, often containing lymphoid aggregates, covered by a simple columnar epithelium displaying nuclear changes of reactive cells. In contrast, radiation may result in glands being lined by large columnar or cuboidal cells with very large, hyperchromatic nuclei, but the chromatin is usually smudged and mitoses are rare. A clue to the reactive nature is that the abrupt transition to normal endocervix commonly seen in CGIN is not present (McCluggage, 2000; Zaino, 2000, 2002; NHSCSP, 1999).

2.5.3.6 Arias-Stella reaction

The Arias-Stella reaction is an incidental finding in about 10% of pregnant women. This reaction may involve endocervical glands as well as cervical endometriosis during pregnancy. The histological appearances of cells with enlarged pleomorphic nuclei and abundant vacuolated clear or eosinophilic cytoplasm are well known but may be misdiagnosed as CGIN or clear cell carcinoma. The fact that this lesion is focal and associated with the history of pregnancy facilitates the diagnosis. Mitotic figures are uncommon but may occur in the Arias-Stella reaction and indeed the presence of abnormal mitotic figures has been described in the Arias-Stella reaction involving endometrial glands (McCluggage, 2000; Zaino, 2000, 2002; NHSCSP, 1999).

2.5.3.7 Mesonephric remnants and hyperplasia

Mesonephric remnants take place in up to 22% of cervices. Their occurrence varies with the type of specimen because they are seldom seen in biopsy specimens, but are relatively common in conization and hysterectomy specimens in which deep portions of the cervix are routinely examined. The mesonephric or Wolffian ducts commonly persist as small remnants usually located in the lateral walls of the vagina or cervix, in the broad ligament, and in the hilus of the ovary. Microscopic lobules frequently surround a central duct within the deep cervical stroma. The acini are lined by cuboidal cells with oval, bland nuclei and scant to moderate quantities of eosinophilic cytoplasm. Mucin is not present in the cytoplasm, but a dense, periodic acid-Schiff (PAS)-positive, luminal secretory product is common. Hyperplasia typically is an incidental finding (McCluggage, 2000; Zaino, 2000, 2002; NHSCSP, 1999).

2.5.4 Ancillary techniques for distinction of pre-invasive lesions from benign mimics

Although the histological features of cervical glandular intraepithelial neoplasia are well described, but a wide variety of benign endocervical glandular lesions may be confused with CGIN and even invasive cervical adenocarcinoma. Many of these benign mimics are rare and in everyday practice the lesions most likely to be confused with CGIN are tuboendometrial metaplasia (TEM) and endometriosis. TEM is extremely common in the cervix, especially after loop or cone biopsy or some other operative procedure. The presence of cilia is a useful diagnostic clue to TEM, but these may be absent or inconspicuous, especially in cases showing endometrioid differentiation. Moreover, cervical TEM, especially when associated with a previous operative procedure, may have an altered stroma, raising the possibility of a desmoplastic reaction. Endometriosis within the superficial cervix may also cause diagnostic problems, especially when the characteristic stroma is inconspicuous. Fibrosis, caused by previous episodes of hemorrhage, may result in consideration of a desmoplastic stromal reaction (McCluggage, 2003).

While tuboendometrial metaplasia and endometriosis are especially likely to be misdiagnosed as cervical glandular intraepithelial neoplasia, microglandular hyperplasia (MGH) is more likely to be mistaken for an invasive adenocarcinoma, usually clear cell adenocarcinoma. A diagnosis of low-grade CGIN (LCGIN) especially is poorly reproducible and, in many institutions, this diagnosis is rarely, if ever, made in the absence of high-grade cervical glandular intraepithelial neoplasia (Cameron et al., 2002).

Microglandular hyperplasia is also common within the cervix. Although most cases are easily recognized, atypical features may be found, including the presence of signet ring cells, stromal hyalinization, or a lace-like growth pattern. These features may cause confusion with invasive cervical adenocarcinoma, especially of the clear cell type (McCluggage, 2003).

Immunohistochemical staining using a panel of antibodies, namely- MIB1, bcl2, and p16 - may be extremely useful in problematic cases in distinguishing these benign mimics from high grade CGIN (HCGIN) or invasive adenocarcinoma; although it has been emphasized that careful morphological examination is the mainstay of diagnosis (Cameron et al., 2002). The proliferation marker MIB1, which reacts with the Ki-67 antigen, has been shown to be a useful adjunct to histology in distinguishing HCGIN from benign mimics. A proliferation index of > 30% is generally indicative of HCGIN, whereas most cases of TEM, endometriosis, and MGH exhibit a proliferation index of < 10%. However, there may be some overlap, with occasional cases of HCGIN also exhibiting a proliferation index of < 10%. In addition, in some studies occasional benign lesions have exhibited a proliferation index of up to 50% (Nucci, 2002; Ostör et al., 2000).

In general, however, there are great differences in the MIB1 index between TEM, endometriosis, and HCGIN. Characteristically, many positive nuclei are present in HCGIN, with only scattered immunoreactivity in benign lesions. Immunohistochemical staining for bcl2 may also be useful in distinguishing TEM and endometriosis from HCGIN. Some studies have shown that cervical TEM and endometriosis (but not MGH) show consistent cytoplasmic expression of bcl2 (Cameron et al., 2002; McCluggage, 2002, 1997). Most cases of CGIN are negative. Why cervical TEM and endometriosis should exhibit positive staining for bcl2 is not certain but interestingly there is strong positive staining of normal fallopian tube epithelial cells and of proliferative endometrium with antibodies to bcl2. Of course, TEM and endometriosis are morphologically similar to normal fallopian tube and normal proliferative endometrium, respectively.

Also CD10 is a useful marker for confirming the presence of endometrial stroma and in establishing a diagnosis of endometriosis; however, this is of limited value in the cervix since a rim of CD10 reactive stromal cells surrounds normal endocervical glands (McCluggage, 2003).

In the distinction of benign mimics from HCGIN, p16 staining may also be of value. Some studies have shown overexpression of p16 in high grade cervical squamous intraepithelial lesions and in low grade lesions associated with high risk Human Papilloma Virus (HPV) types, p16 overexpression seems to be related to the presence of high risk HPV types (McCluggage et al., 2003; Pavlakis et al.,2006; Li et al.,2007; Riethdorf et al.,2002). Cameron et al. have founded a consistent positive staining of HCGIN (involving 100% of cells) with antibodies to p16. In contrast, cells of MGH were negative (Cameron et al., 2002). Staining of TEM and endometriosis was common but this was always focal and completely different to the pattern of immunoreactivity found in HCGIN. Thus, the combination of p16, MIB1, and bcl2 may be extremely useful in separating these benign mimics from HCGIN (McCluggage, 2003; Scheiden et al., 2004).

The diffuse distribution of p16 immunostaining in HPV 16/18 positive glandular neoplasms support a strong association with HPV infection and indicates that this biomarker mainly discriminate AIS from benign mimics (Riethdorf et al. , 2002). The situation with LCGIN has not been well studied and further work is necessary to ascertain whether these antibodies are of value in the separation of LCGIN from benign mimics. It is stressed that, in all cases, these antibodies are only of ancillary use and that careful morphological examination remains the cornerstone of diagnosis.

Immunohistochemical staining with carcinoembryonic antigen (CEA) has been reported to be of value in the separation of neoplastic endocervical glandular lesions and benign mimics (McCluggage, 2003). Diffuse cytoplasmic staining is usually present in neoplastic but not in benign lesions. However, as minimal deviation adenocarcinoma (MDA) is the neoplastic lesion most likely to be confused with benign lesions and as cytoplasmic staining with CEA may be focal and may not be present on a small biopsy, the value is limited. Conversely, normal endocervical epithelium may show luminal CEA positivity and some benign lesions, especially microglandular adenosis, may show cytoplasmic positivity, usually confined to areas of immature squamous metaplasia or reserve cell hyperplasia (McCluggage, 2003).

Other studies have found that a combination of CEA, MIB1, and p53 staining is useful in discriminating between benign and malignant endocervical glandular lesions (McCluggage, 2003; Pavlakis et al. , 2006). Polacarz et al. have shown *myc* immunostaining seemed to be a powerful discriminator between normal cervical glandular epithelium and epithelium show in intraepithelial changes or overt malignant changes. Apical cytoplasmic *myc* localisation thus seemed to be specific for CGIN and invasive adenocarcinoma of the cervix (Polacarz et al., 1991).

Other studies have evaluated the use of silver stained nucleolar organiser regions (AgNORs) in the separation of high grade CGIN and adenocarcinoma from benign histological mimics. In one study, significant differences in AgNOR counts were found between microglandular hyperplasia and HCGIN (McCluggage, 2000). However, the counting of AgNORs is laborious and time-consuming and is probably of less value than the use of proliferation markers.

In a recent study by Li et al.,their findings demonstrate significant expression of insulin-like growth factor-II mRNA-binding protein 3 (IMP3)and p16INK4a in adenocarcinoma in situ as compared to benign endocervical glands, suggesting that expression of these biomarkers may be helpful in the distinction of adenocarcinoma in situ from benign endocervical glands, particularly in difficult borderline cases (Li et al.,2007).

Findings of Little et al. study demonstrate that cyclin D1 can be included within an immunohistochemical panel to aid in the distinction between reactive cervical glandular lesions and adenocarcinoma in situ. The localized distribution of staining within invasive lesions suggests that cyclin D1 up-regulation has a specific role during the progression of some endocervical adenocarcinomas (Little & Stewart, 2010).

As result, immunohistochemical staining using a panel of antibodies may be very practical in problematic cases in distinguishing these benign mimics from high grade CGIN (HCGIN) or invasive adenocarcinoma; although it has been emphasized that careful morphological examination is the basis of diagnosis.

2.5.5 Approach to the diagnosis of cervical glandular intraepithelial neoplasia (CGIN) and pathological reporting

The approach to the diagnosis of CGIN is outlined below and is based on our experience and review of published article.

1. Generally speaking, the frequency of CGIN is low, and pathologists may rarely encounter to such a lesion in daily practice. Therefore in every case of cervical biopsy, it is rational to be aware of CGIN and its mimics and consider them in differential diagnosis.
2. Combination of invasive and pre-invasive lesions of squamous and glandular epithelium is a common event which has been reported in 30% to 70% of CGIN. Usually in low power examination, changes in a stratified squamous epithelium are more eye-catching and one may missed the concomitant glandular lesion. To prevent such a pitfall, we recommend to carefully examining the glandular epithelium architecturally and cytologically with low and high power field microscopy, especially when the lining of the canal and the glandular one had been replaced by a darker epithelium in each cervical specimen (Gloor & Ruzicka, 1982).
3. The next step is attention to any change in architectural pattern of endocervical glandular epithelium, including glandular branching, budding, crowding, infolding, villoglandular and cribriform, which is easily recognized even in low power microscopic examination. It is essential to emphasize that normal cleft and glands of endocervical epithelium can be variable in size and shape and may be mistaken for CGIN yet minimal deviation of adenocarcinoma. However comparison of the suspicious glands with uninquestionably benign ones in the vicinity may provide guidance and attention to the following points should help to exclude CGIN or carcinoma: absence of cytologic atypia, desmoplastic response and marked variation in size and shape of endocervical glands. However, regardless of presence, these criteria have not solved the difficulty in diagnosis, and this may require the examination of additional tissue (e.g. Cervical cone).
4. Even though some cytological features including stratification, mucin depletion and abrupt junction between normal and abnormal columnar epithelium, can be recognized in low power microscopic examination, emergence of a darker epithelium which indicate replacement of normal epithelium by stratified epithelium may be helpful.
5. As mentioned before, architectural pattern may be associated with benign conditions (cervicitis, tubal metaplasia, endometriosis, tunnel clusters and etc) or invasive adenocarcinoma and then must be combined with cytological features. The cytological features are nuclear changes, apoptotic bodies, mitotic figures and intestinal metaplasia can be evaluated exactly by x10, x 40 microscopic power examinations. Because many of cytological features may be associated with benign reactive changes or metaplastic condition; pathologist must be aware and combined cytological and architectural features for final diagnosis. High N/C ratio of the columnar epithelium in some metaplastic conditions can mimic endocervical or tubal type of AIS. Increased mitotic index (MI) especially atypical mitosis is a clue in the diagnosis of CGIN. The average MI of CGIN is intermediate between benign condition and invasive adenocarcinoma (Moritani et al.,

2002). Although mitosis is uncommon in benign condition, it is occasionally seen in endometriosis, estrogen consumption, and in the repair process (NHSCSP, 1999).

6. Apoptotic bodies are useful in establishing a diagnosis of CGIN, although they may not be prominent in all cases. Apoptotic body is a constant feature of HCGIN and the increase number of apoptotic bodies was significantly higher than in nonspecific endocervical glandular lesions (Moritani et al., 2002).
7. Most cases of CGIN are of usual endocervical type. However, other rare variants have been described. An endometrioid variant of CGIN has been reported. However, this is rare (if it occurs at all) and most cases diagnosed as such are probably cases of usual endocervical-type CGIN with scant intracytoplasmic mucin. An intestinal variant of HCGIN exists and is not uncommon. This is characterized by the presence of goblet cells and less commonly paneth or neuroendocrine cells (McCluggage, 2003). These microscopic features are along with Gloor study that was named CGIN type B alongside all other mentioned above features that described as CGIN type A (Pirog et al., 2000). It is doubtful whether intestinal differentiation in endocervical glands ever occurs without coexistent CGIN or invasive adenocarcinoma. Benign intestinal metaplasia involving endocervical glands has been described, but it is probably an extremely rare phenomenon, if it occurs at all, and the presence of goblet cells almost always indicates CGIN (Ioffe, 2003).

In regard to above mentioned approach the following points are emphasized in histological reporting of CGIN because these factors would influence the management:

1. Lesion location: exocervical, endocervical or both
2. Tridimensional lesion geometry: linear length of lesion and underlying crypt involvement depth. Clearly, there is no consensus in the acceptable depth of involvement. Ostor study revealed the depth of crypt involvement (measured from the surface) varied from 1.5 to 4 mm with an average of 2.6mm.The length of extent as measured horizontally in single section ranged from 0.5 to 30mm, with an average of 7mm.The width of the lesion (as determined from the number of blocks involved) ranged from 0.5 mm to 25 mm, with an average of 12 mm. From these parameters hypothetical tumor volumes could be calculated, the smallest being 0.25mm^3, and the largest 1,500 mm^3.The average tumor volume was 313 mm^3 (Ostör et al.,1984).
3. Potentional for AIS to be buried under metaplstic or dysplastic epithelium
4. Presence of squamous component (Colgan & Lickrish, 1990)
5. Possibly multifocal lesions and skip lesions
6. Possibly multicentric lesions (more than one quadrant involvement) or circumferential extent (Sheets, 2002)
7. Specimen margin status (post excision)

2.6 Biological behavior/management

It is beyond the scope of this chapter to discuss in detail the management of CGIN but it is clear that in those who wish to preserve their fertility (HCGIN and early invasive adenocarcinoma often occur in young women), local excision with careful pathological examination and free margins combined with close cytological follow up may be used for treatment. After completion of childbearing , hysterectomy is necessary because of the paucity of data concerning the long-term natural history of CGIN (Ostör, 2000; Sheets, 2002; Zhao et al., 2009).

3. Conclusion

There is a real increase in the incidence of malignant and premalignant endocervical glandular lesions, which are thus arrogant increasing importance in diagnostic surgical pathology but the frequency of CGIN is low, and pathologists may rarely encounter to such a lesion in daily practice. Therefore in every case of cervical biopsy, it is rational to be aware of CGIN and its mimics and consider them in differential diagnosis. In most, but not all, cases CGIN occurs close to the transformation zone and there is often an associated squamous intraepithelial lesion. CGIN can be confused with a wide variety of benign endocervical glandular lesions and even invasive cervical adenocarcinoma. CGIN should be classified as low grade or high grade CGIN. High grade CGIN is alternatively known as AIS and Low grade CGIN is alternatively known as glandular dysplasia. High grade CGIN is a vigorous diagnosis but distinction from early invasive adenocarcinoma may be difficult and Low grade CGIN may be underdiagnosed by pathologists. A combination of architectural and cytological features is necessary for diagnosis of CGIN. Immunohistochemical staining using a panel of antibodies may be useful in difficult cases in distinctive benign mimics from high grade CGIN or invasive carcinoma , although it is stressed that careful morphological examination is the basis of diagnosis.

4. Acknowledgment

The authors would like to thank Dr. Sanaz Sanii for preparing the proposal text.

5. Common abbreviations

AIS: Adenocarcinoma in situ
CGIN: Cervical glandular intraepithelial neoplasia
CIN: Cervical intraepithelial neoplasia
HCGIN: High grade CGIN
LCGIN: Low grade CGIN
MGH: Microglandular hyperplasia
MIA: Microinvasive adenocarcinoma
SCC: Squamous cell carcinoma
TBS: The Bethesda System
TEM: Tuboendometrioid metaplasia

6. Referrences

Bekkers, R. L., Bulten, J., Wiersma-van Tilburg, A., Mravunac, M., Schijf, C. P., Massuger, L. F., et al. (2003). Coexisting high-grade glandular and squamous cervical lesions and human papillomavirus infections. *Br J Cancer, 89*(5), 886-890.

Brown, L. J., & Wells, M. (1986). Cervical glandular atypia associated with squamous intraepithelial neoplasia: a premalignant lesion? *J Clin Pathol, 39*(1), 22-28.

Bulk, S., Berkhof, J., Bulkmans, N. W., Zielinski, G. D., Rozendaal, L., van Kemenade, F. J., et al. (2006). Preferential risk of HPV16 for squamous cell carcinoma and of HPV18 for adenocarcinoma of the cervix compared to women with normal cytology in The Netherlands. *Br J Cancer, 94*(1), 171-175.

Cameron, R. I., Maxwell, P., Jenkins, D., & McCluggage, W. G. (2002). Immunohistochemical staining with MIB1, bcl2 and p16 assists in the distinction of cervical glandular intraepithelial neoplasia from tubo-endometrial metaplasia, endometriosis and microglandular hyperplasia. *Histopathology, 41*(4), 313-321.

Campion M.J.(2010). Preinvasive disease, in: *Berek & Hacker Gynecologic Oncology,* Berek J.S. & Hacker N.F, (Ed.), pp. 3132-414, LWW, ISBN 0781795125, Philadelphia ,USA.

Christopherson, W. M., Nealon, N., & Gray, L. A., Sr. (1979). Noninvasive precursor lesions of adenocarcinoma and mixed adenosquamous carcinoma of the cervix uteri. *Cancer, 44*(3), 975-983.

Colgan, T. J., & Lickrish, G. M. (1990). The topography and invasive potential of cervical adenocarcinoma in situ, with and without associated squamous dysplasia. *Gynecol Oncol, 36*(2), 246-249.

Covell J.L.,Wilbur D.C.,Guidos B.,Lee K.R.,Chieng D.C.,Mody D.R. (2003). Epithelial abnormalities: glandular. In: *The Bethesda System for Reporting Cervical Cytology,* Solomon D., Nayar R.,(Eds). pp. 123-141. Spriger. ISBN 0387403582, New York, USA.

Friedell, G. H., & Mc, K. D. (1953). Adenocarcinoma in situ of the endocervix. *Cancer, 6*(5), 887-897.

Gloor, E., & Ruzicka, J. (1982). Morphology of adenocarcinoma in situ of the uterine cervix: a study of 14 cases. *Cancer, 49*(2), 294-302.

Gloor, E., & Hurlimann, J. (1986). Cervical intraepithelial glandular neoplasia (adenocarcinoma in situ and glandular dysplasia). A correlative study of 23 cases with histologic grading, histochemical analysis of mucins, and immunohistochemical determination of the affinity for four lectins. *Cancer, 58*(6), 1272-1280.

Histopathology Reporting in Cervical Screening.(1999). *NHSCSP Publication.* No 10. April 1999.

Hopkins, M. P., & Morley, G. W. (1991). A comparison of adenocarcinoma and squamous cell carcinoma of the cervix. *Obstet Gynecol, 77*(6), 912-917.

Ioffe, O. B., Sagae, S., Moritani, S., Dahmoush, L., Chen, T. T., & Silverberg, S. G. (2003). Symposium part 3: Should pathologists diagnose endocervical preneoplastic lesions "less than" adenocarcinoma in situ?: Point. *Int J Gynecol Pathol, 22*(1), 18-21.

Kurian, K., & al-Nafussi, A. (1999). Relation of cervical glandular intraepithelial neoplasia to microinvasive and invasive adenocarcinoma of the uterine cervix: a study of 121 cases. *J Clin Pathol, 52*(2), 112-117.

Kurman RJ, Ronnett BM, Sherman ME, Wilkinson EJ. (2010).*Tumours of the cervix, vagina and vulva. Atlas of tumor pathology,* 4th series, Fascicle 13 ,American Registry of Pathology,1-933477-11-3. Washington,DC

Leminen, A., Paavonen, J., Forss, M., Wahlstrom, T., & Vesterinen, E. (1990). Adenocarcinoma of the uterine cervix. *Cancer, 65*(1), 53-59.

Li, C., Rock, K. L., Woda, B. A., Jiang, Z., Fraire, A. E., & Dresser, K. (2007). IMP3 is a novel biomarker for adenocarcinoma in situ of the uterine cervix: an immunohistochemical study in comparison with p16(INK4a) expression. *Mod Pathol, 20*(2), 242-247.

Liang, J., Mittal, K. R., Wei, J. J., Yee, H., Chiriboga, L., & Shukla, P. (2007). Utility of p16INK4a, CEA, Ki67, P53 and ER/PR in the differential diagnosis of benign, premalignant, and malignant glandular lesions of the uterine cervix and their relationship with Silverberg scoring system for endocervical glandular lesions. *Int J Gynecol Pathol, 26*(1), 71-75.

Little, L., & Stewart, C. J. Cyclin D1 immunoreactivity in normal endocervix and diagnostic value in reactive and neoplastic endocervical lesions. *Mod Pathol, 23*(4), 611-618.

Madeleine, M. M., Daling, J. R., Schwartz, S. M., Shera, K., McKnight, B., Carter, J. J., et al. (2001). Human papillomavirus and long-term oral contraceptive use increase the risk of adenocarcinoma in situ of the cervix. *Cancer Epidemiol Biomarkers Prev, 10*(3), 171-177.

Marques, J. P., Costa, L. B., Pinto, A. P., Lima, A. F., Duarte, M. E., Barbosa, A. P., et al. Atypical glandular cells and cervical cancer: systematic review. *Rev Assoc Med Bras, 57*(2), 234-238.

McCluggage, G., McBride, H., Maxwell, P., & Bharucha, H. (1997). Immunohistochemical detection of p53 and bcl-2 proteins in neoplastic and non-neoplastic endocervical glandular lesions. *Int J Gynecol Pathol, 16*(1), 22-27.

McCluggage, W. G., & Maxwell, P. (2002). bcl-2 and p21 immunostaining of cervical tubo-endometrial metaplasia. *Histopathology, 40*(1), 107-108.

McCluggage, W. G., Oliva, E., Herrington, C. S., McBride, H., & Young, R. H. (2003). CD10 and calretinin staining of endocervical glandular lesions, endocervical stroma and endometrioid adenocarcinomas of the uterine corpus: CD10 positivity is characteristic of, but not specific for, mesonephric lesions and is not specific for endometrial stroma. *Histopathology, 43*(2), 144-150.

McCluggage, W. G. (2003). Endocervical glandular lesions: controversial aspects and ancillary techniques. *J Clin Pathol, 56*(3), 164-173.

McCluggage, W. G. (2007). Immunohistochemistry as a diagnostic aid in cervical pathology. *Pathology, 39*(1), 97-111.

Mood, N. I., Eftekhar, Z., Haratian, A., Saeedi, L., Rahimi-Moghaddam, P., & Yarandi, F. (2006). A cytohistologic study of atypical glandular cells detected in cervical smears during cervical screening tests in Iran. *Int J Gynecol Cancer, 16*(1), 257-261.

Moritani, S., Ioffe, O. B., Sagae, S., Dahmoush, L., Silverberg, S. G., & Hattori, T. (2002). Mitotic activity and apoptosis in endocervical glandular lesions. *Int J Gynecol Pathol, 21*(2), 125-133.

Nasu, I., Meurer, W., & Fu, Y. S. (1993). Endocervical glandular atypia and adenocarcinoma: a correlation of cytology and histology. *Int J Gynecol Pathol, 12*(3), 208-218.

Nucci, M. R. (2002). Symposium part III: tumor-like glandular lesions of the uterine cervix. *Int J Gynecol Pathol, 21*(4), 347-359.

Ostor, A. G., Pagano, R., Davoren, R. A., Fortune, D. W., Chanen, W., & Rome, R. (1984). Adenocarcinoma in situ of the cervix. *Int J Gynecol Pathol, 3*(2), 179-190.

Ostor, A. G. (2000). Early invasive adenocarcinoma of the uterine cervix. *Int J Gynecol Pathol, 19*(1), 29-38.

Parazzini, F., La Vecchia, C., Negri, E., Fasoli, M., & Cecchetti, G. (1988). Risk factors for adenocarcinoma of the cervix: a case-control study. *Br J Cancer, 57*(2), 201-204.

Pavlakis, K., Messini, I., Athanassiadou, S., Kyrodimou, E., Pandazopoulou, A., Vrekoussis, T., et al. (2006). Endocervical glandular lesions: a diagnostic approach combining a semi-quantitative scoring method to the expression of CEA, MIB-1 and p16. *Gynecol Oncol, 103*(3), 971-976.

Pecorelli, S. (2009). Revised FIGO staging for carcinoma of the vulva, cervix, and endometrium. *Int J Gynaecol Obstet, 105*(2), 103-104.

Pirog, E. C., Kleter, B., Olgac, S., Bobkiewicz, P., Lindeman, J., Quint, W. G., et al. (2000). Prevalence of human papillomavirus DNA in different histological subtypes of cervical adenocarcinoma. *Am J Pathol, 157*(4), 1055-1062.

Pirog, E. C., Isacson, C., Szabolcs, M. J., Kleter, B., Quint, W., & Richart, R. M. (2002). Proliferative activity of benign and neoplastic endocervical epithelium and correlation with HPV DNA detection. *Int J Gynecol Pathol, 21*(1), 22-26.

Polacarz, S. V., Darne, J., Sheridan, E. G., Ginsberg, R., & Sharp, F. (1991). Endocervical carcinoma and precursor lesions: c-myc expression and the demonstration of field changes. *J Clin Pathol, 44*(11), 896-899.

Riethdorf, L., Riethdorf, S., Lee, K. R., Cviko, A., Loning, T., & Crum, C. P. (2002). Human papillomaviruses, expression of p16, and early endocervical glandular neoplasia. *Hum Pathol, 33*(9), 899-904.

Scheiden, R., Wagener, C., Knolle, U., Dippel, W., & Capesius, C. (2004). Atypical glandular cells in conventional cervical smears: incidence and follow-up. *BMC Cancer, 4*, 37.

Sheets, E. E. (2002). Management of adenocarcinoma in situ, micro-invasive, and early stage adenocarcinoma of the cervix. *Curr Opin Obstet Gynecol, 14*(1), 53-57.

Smedts, F., Ramaekers, F. C., & Hopman, A. H. The two faces of cervical adenocarcinoma in situ. *Int J Gynecol Pathol, 29*(4), 378-385.

Solomon, D., Frable, W. J., Vooijs, G. P., Wilbur, D. C., Amma, N. S., Collins, R. J., et al. (1998). ASCUS and AGUS criteria. International Academy of Cytology Task Force summary. Diagnostic Cytology Towards the 21st Century: An International Expert Conference and Tutorial. *Acta Cytol, 42*(1), 16-24.

Tam, K. F., Cheung, A. N., Liu, K. L., Ng, T. Y., Pun, T. C., Chan, Y. M., et al. (2003). A retrospective review on atypical glandular cells of undetermined significance (AGUS) using the Bethesda 2001 classification. *Gynecol Oncol, 91*(3), 603-607.

Ursin, G., Peters, R. K., Henderson, B. E., d'Ablaing, G., 3rd, Monroe, K. R., & Pike, M. C. (1994). Oral contraceptive use and adenocarcinoma of cervix. *Lancet, 344*(8934), 1390-1394.

van Aspert-van Erp, A. J., Smedts, F. M., & Vooijs, G. P. (2004). Severe cervical glandular cell lesions with coexisting squamous cell lesions. *Cancer, 102*(4), 218-227.

Wang, S. S., Sherman, M. E., Hildesheim, A., Lacey, J. V., Jr., & Devesa, S. (2004). Cervical adenocarcinoma and squamous cell carcinoma incidence trends among white women and black women in the United States for 1976-2000. *Cancer, 100*(5), 1035-1044.

Wells, M., & Brown, L. J. (2002). Symposium part IV: investigative approaches to endocervical pathology. *Int J Gynecol Pathol, 21*(4), 360-367.

Wright V.C. (2002). Colposcopic features of cervical adenocarcinoma in situ and adenocarcinoma and management of preinvasive disease. In: *Colposcopy Principles and Practice*. Apgar B.S., Brotzaman G.L. & Spitzer M. (Ed.).pp.301-303. Saunders. ISBN 1416034056. Philadelphia, USA

Zaino, R. J. (2000). Glandular lesions of the uterine cervix. *Mod Pathol, 13*(3), 261-274.

Zaino, R. J. (2002). Symposium part I: adenocarcinoma in situ, glandular dysplasia, and early invasive adenocarcinoma of the uterine cervix. *Int J Gynecol Pathol, 21*(4), 314-326.

Zhao, C., Florea, A., Onisko, A., & Austin, R. M. (2009). Histologic follow-up results in 662 patients with Pap test findings of atypical glandular cells: results from a large academic womens hospital laboratory employing sensitive screening methods. *Gynecol Oncol, 114*(3), 383-389.

Zielinski, G. D., Snijders, P. J., Rozendaal, L., Daalmeijer, N. F., Risse, E. K., Voorhorst, F. J., et al. (2003). The presence of high-risk HPV combined with specific p53 and p16INK4a expression patterns points to high-risk HPV as the main causative agent for adenocarcinoma in situ and adenocarcinoma of the cervix. *J Pathol, 201*(4), 535-543.

15

The Role of the Pap Smear Diagnosis: Atypical Glandular Cells (AGC)

Chiung-Ru Lai[1,2], Chih-Yi Hsu[1,2] and Anna Fen-Yau Li [1,2]
[1]*Department of Pathology and Laboratory Medicine, Taipei Veterans General Hospital,*
[2]*School of Medicine, National Yang-Ming University, Taipei, Taiwan*

1. Introduction

Glandular lesions of the female genital tract have always been a challenge for pathologists. The precise cytological diagnosis of these lesions is difficult because of their inherent complexity, as well as the lack of experience of many cytopathologists in this field.

The term atypical glandular cells of undetermined significance (AGUS) was first introduced at the 1988 Bethesda Conference (National Cancer Institute Workshop, 1989) and defined as morphologic changes in glandular cells beyond those suggestive a benign reactive process, but insufficient for the interpretation of adenocarcinoma. In the 2001 Bethesda System (TBS 2001) (Solomon, 2002), the term has been changed to better reflect current knowledge and understanding of glandular neoplasia. The category has been defined and renamed "atypical glandular cells" (AGC), with the subclassifications "not otherwise specified" (AGC-NOS) and "favor neoplastic" (AGC-FN). The cell type of origin, endocervical or endometrial, should be addressed whenever possible. Adenocarcinoma in situ has been separated as another distinct category of diagnosis.

In 2006, the American Society for Colposcopy and Cervical Pathology (ASCCP) released consensus guidelines for the management guidelines for the management of AGC (Wright, 2007). The guidelines emphasized combined colposcopy and endocervical sampling was recommended for all women across all subcategories of AGC, with the addition of endometrial sampling for women over 35. So, since 2006, more comprehensive evaluations were applied for these women. Recent studies concerning the follow-up outcomes of AGC revealed more patients with precancerous or malignant diseases of different sites ranging from the exo-cervix, endocervix, endometrium, fallopian tube, ovary and even extra-genital organs (Behtash, 2007; Duska, 1998; Jeng, 2003; Koonings, 2001; Lai, 2008; Manetta, 1999; Mood, 2006; Soofer, 2000). Since the introduction of Pap smear screening, the incidence of cervical squamous cell carcinoma has been dramatically declined but the relative incidence of glandular cancer has been increased. However, the sensitivity of detecting cervical glandular precancerous or cancer lesions is much less than that of the squamous lesions making cervical glandular cancer prevention remains a challenge and problem to be solved

(Koss, 1989; Wingo, 2003). So, our ability to recognize and diagnose AGC-NOS or AGC-FN is very important. After correct triage of patients with AGC Pap smears, early treatment of these lesions may be achieved. The protective effects of cytologic screening for glandular lesions can be then improved.

In our previous study (Lai, 2008), it supported the view that a diagnosis of AGC is clinically significant by the 2001 Bethesda System, especially the AGC-FN category. The subclassification of AGC is important and demanded in the diagnosis of Pap smears. Addressing the cell origin of endometrium, although being found no statistically significant difference, it showed a more common significant pathology outcome. Since then, we still followed the 2001 Bethesda System to subclassify and address the cell origin in AGC Pap smears. As to management protocol, we strongly recommend following the ASCCP consensus guidelines. In the current retrospective study of 9 years experience, histological follow-up results obtained and paired to the corresponding cytology interpretation, and the results further enhanced the importance of the role of the Pap smear diagnosis of AGC in screening and diagnosing the precancerous and cancer lesions.

2. Materials and methods

A retrospective review of the archives of the Department of Pathology, Taipei Veterans General Hospital, from January 2002 to December 2010 identified 234 smears diagnosed as AGC with at least 6 months follow-up. All of the Pap smears since January 2002 were diagnosed and classified according to the 2001 Bethesda System criteria at the time of diagnosis. If cellular findings suggestive of endometrial glandular or stromal cells were noted, the description of "endometrial origin" would be made in the space of "educational notes and suggestion" in the cytologic report. An adequate evaluation for AGC Pap smears suggested by the ASCCP included a colposcopy with or without cervical biopsy, endocervical curettage and an endometrial sampling, especially in those patients in whom endometrial origin was addressed in the Pap test. In addition, those patients who received other diagnostic or treatment procedures such as conization, loop electrosurgical excision procedure (LEEP) or hysterectomy were also included in this study. The most abnormal histology was considered to be the outcome. Patients who failed to receive the management described even with multiple repeated pap smears were excluded in the evaluation.

The clinical information of patient, such as age, menopausal status, hormonal replacement therapy status, tamoxifen use status, and presence of abnormal bleeding were collected from medical record. Pathology findings of endometrial biopsy were categorized as benign, precursors (high grade squamous intra-epithelial lesion, endocervical adenocarcinoma in situ, endometrial atypical complex hyperplasia), and malignant. The precursors and malignant pathology results are defined as abnormal pathology. Based on cyto-histological and available clinical data, we made meticulous description of the cytological findings including atypical glandular cells themselves and the background pattern and statistical analyses on the different subclassifications of AGC by using Chi-square test and multivariate logistic regression. A P value <0.05 was considered to be statistically significant.

3. Results

3.1 Pathology results

From a total of 228,451 cervicovaginal cytologic specimens within a 9-year period from January 2002 to December 2010, a total of 234 (0.1%) AGC Pap smears were identified. The age distribution ranged from 27 to 93 years (median 49). All were conventional Pap smears and primarily carried out for cervical cancer screening. 190 of 234 (81%) cases with adequate histologic evaluation were included in this study. (Table 1)

AGC subtype	Number	Histologic follow-up (%)
AGC-NOS	197	157 (80%)
AGC-FN	37	33 (89%)
Total	234	190 (81%)

AGC: atypical glandular cells
AGC-NOS: atypical glandular cells, not otherwise specified
AGC-FN: atypical glandular cells, favor neoplastic

Table 1. Histologic follow-up rates by AGC subtype

Adequate initial evaluation for AGC Pap smears suggested by the ASCCP included a colposcopy with or without cervical biopsy, endocervical curettage and an endometrial sampling, especially in those patients endometrial origin was addressed in the Pap test. Abnormal histology of precursors and invasive lesions were found in 76 patients (40%) (Table 2) Final pathology results included 37 endometrial adenocarcinomas, 6 endocervical adenocarcinomas, 1 cervical squamous cell carcinoma, 1 endometrial malignant mixed Mullerian tumor (MMMT), 3 ovarian carcinomas, 3 colon-rectal adenocarcinomas, 1 fallopian tube adenocarcinoma, 4 endocervical adenocarcinoma in situ, 2 endocervical glandular dysplasia, 6 high grade squamous intraepithelial lesion (HSIL), and 11 endometrial complex hyperplasia. Invasive diseases, accounting for 28% (53 of 190) were much more common than precursors, 12% (23 of 190). All of the patients with significant pathology received definitive treatment, including complete staging surgery for those harboring invasive neoplastic diseases.

There were 83 smears sub-classified as AGC-NOS; 75 as AGC-NOS, endometrial origin (EM); 21 as AGC-N, endometrial origin (EM); 11 as AGC-N. The subgroup of AGC-N, EM had the highest rate of abnormal pathology, followed by AGC-NOS, EM, AGC-N and AGC-NOS; 18 of 21 (86%), 30 of 75 (40%), 4 of 11 (36%) and 24 of 83 (29%), respectively. The difference was significant. ($P<0.001$) Women with AGC-N were more likely to have significant pathology (22 in 32 (69%)) compared with those with AGC-NOS (54 in 158 (34%)). It was statistically significant. ($P<0.001$) The endometrial origin addressed cases had more abnormal pathology results than those not being addressed, 48 of 96 (50%) v.s. 28 of 94 (30%). ($P=0.004$) (Table 3)

Histologic results	Cases (%)
Benign	114 (60%)
Abnormal	76 (40%)
Invasive lesions	53 (28%)
Cervical cancer	7
Adenocarcinoma	6
Squamous cell carcinoma	1
Endometrial cancer	38
Adenocarcinoma	37
Malignant mixed Müllerian tumor	1
Extra-uterine malignancies	8
Ovary carcinoma	3
Rectal cancer	4
Tubal carcinoma	1
Precursor lesions	23 (12%)
Endocervical glandular dysplasia	2
Endocervical adenocarcinoma in situ	4
High grade squamous intraepithelial lesion	6
Endometrial complex hyperplasia (including atypical)	11

Table 2. Final Histologic results of 190 patients with AGC Pap smears

	N	Benign	Abnormal	*P*
Diagnostic category				
AGC-NOS, EM	75	45 (60%)	30 (40%)	<0.001[1]
AGC-NOS	83	59 (71%)	24 (29%)	
AGC-FN, EM	21	3 (14%)	18 (86%)	
AGC-FN	11	7 (64%)	4 (36%)	
EM				
Address	96	48 (50%)	48 (50%)	0.004[1]
Not address	94	66 (70%)	28 (30%)	
Favor neoplastic				
Yes	32	10 (31%)	22(69%)	<0.001[1]
No	158	104 (66%)	54 (34%)	
Total cases	190	114 (60%)	76 (40%)	

[1]chi-square test
EM: endometrial origin

Table 3. Abnormal histologic results in different AGC subtypes

3.2 Cytologic findings and differential diagnoses

Degenerative atypical endometrial glandular cells admixed with endometrial debris indicated endometrial origin, The endometrial debris distributed along the smearing direction (Figure 1-3) was characterized by watery diatheses, foamy histiocytes, degenerative necrotic debris and phagocytosis (Figure 4). Some or all of the above findings were observed in 1 fallopian tube adenocarcinoma , 25 endometrial adenocarcinomas and 1 MMMT but none of the cervical lesions and other extra-uterine cancers.

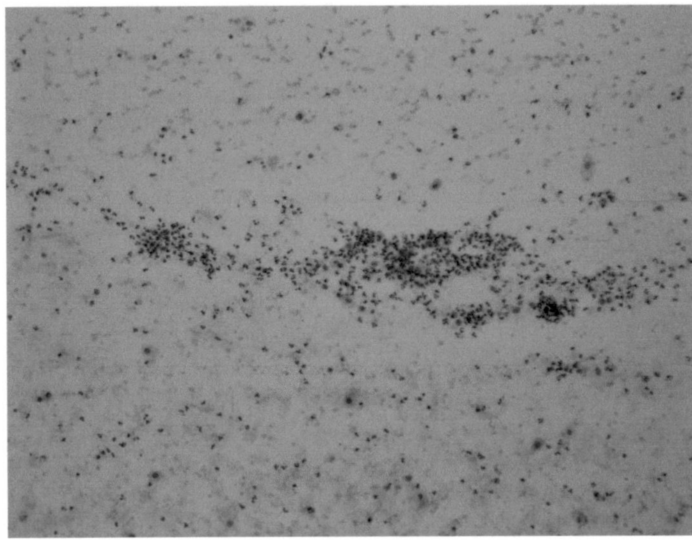

Fig. 1. The endometrial debris distributed along the smearing direction in the background. (Papanicolaou stain, 100x)

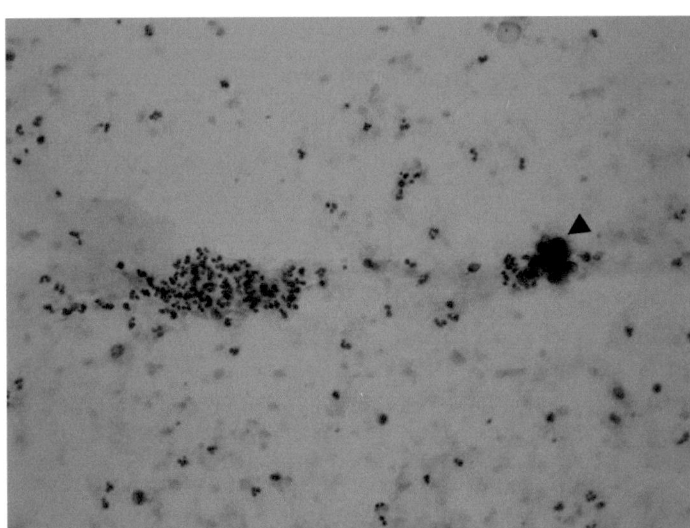

Fig. 2. Degenerative atypical endometrial glandular cells, favor neoplastic (arrow head), admixed with endometrial debris. The final pathology turned out to be an endometrioid adenocarcinoma, grade II. (Papanicolaou stain, 200x)

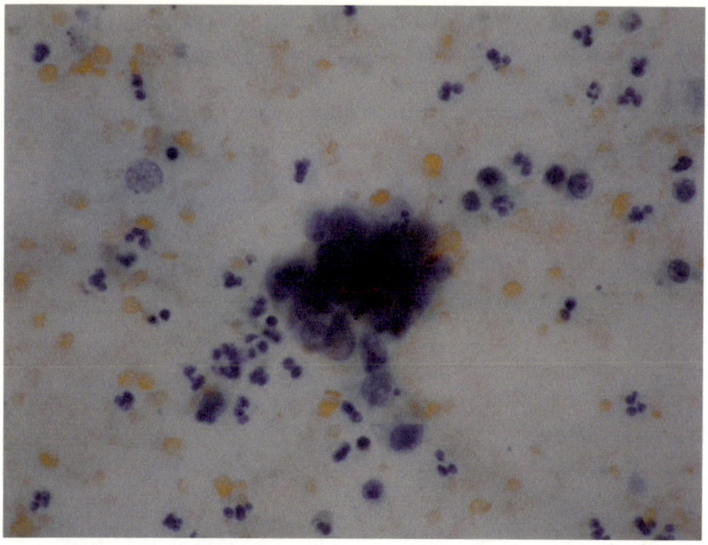

Fig. 3. The higher magnification showed tight cluster of atypical endometrial glandular cells with degeneration, high N/C ratio, three-dimensional structure, and small faint nucleoli. These features fall short of diagnosing an adenocarcinoma directly, either in quantity or quality. (Papanicolaou stain, 400x)

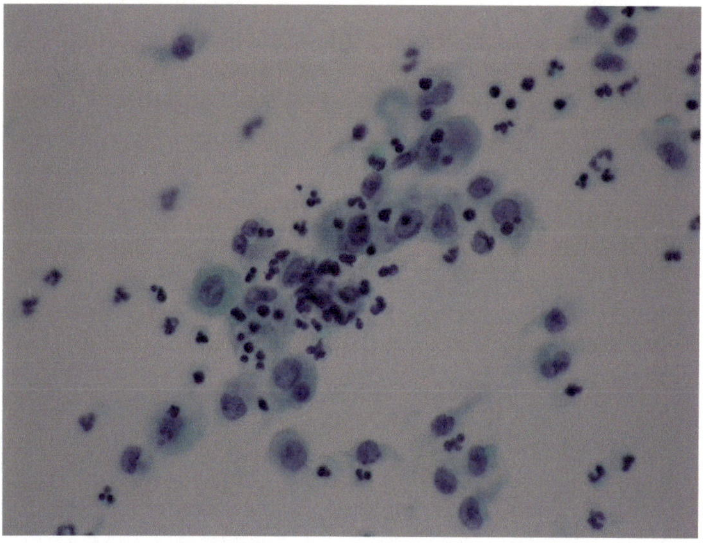

Fig. 4. The endometrial debris was characterized by watery diatheses, foamy histiocytes, degenerative necrotic debris and phagocytosis. It was very specific for endometrial lesions. (Papanicolaou stain, 400x)

The distribution pattern, along the smearing direction, was very characteristic for this kind of debris indicating shedding from endometrium instead of endocervix. However, it would disappear in the fluid-based preparations. In addition, mucin substance was always absent in the endometrial debris. On the contrary, we noticed that a characteristic finding consisting of necrosis and a mucinous background resembling the pattern seen in ileal conduit urine was an indicator suggestive of endocervical adenocarcinoma (Figure 5-8).

This feature was seen in 3 of the 6 endocervical adenocarcinomas but none of the other cancers.

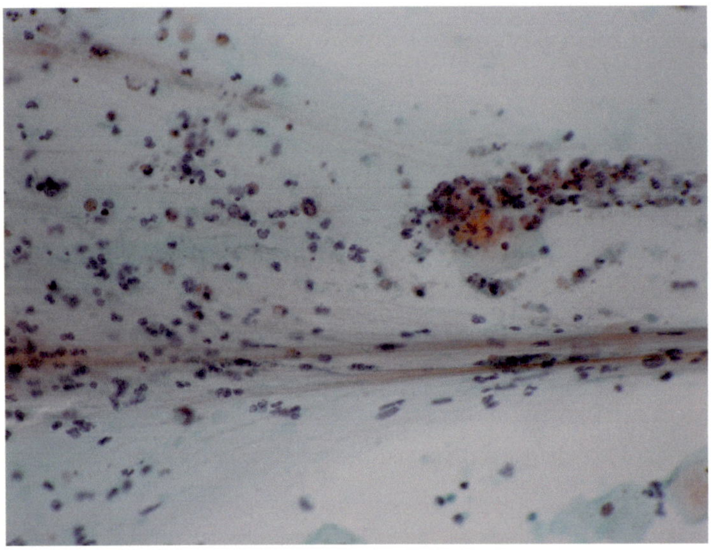

Fig. 5. Background of mucin streaks admixed with necrotic mucous cells resembling those of an ileal conduit urine specimen. (Papanicolaou stain, 200x)

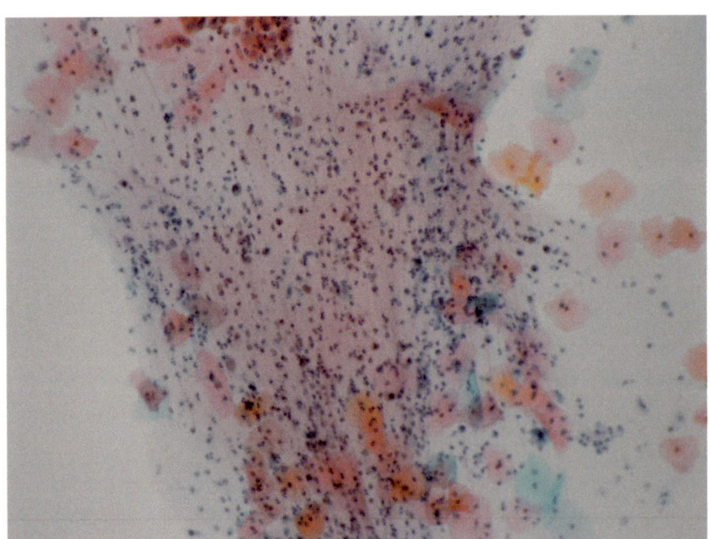

Fig. 6. Background mucin streaks are very thick and have characteristic color and distribution. (Papanicolaou stain, 100x)

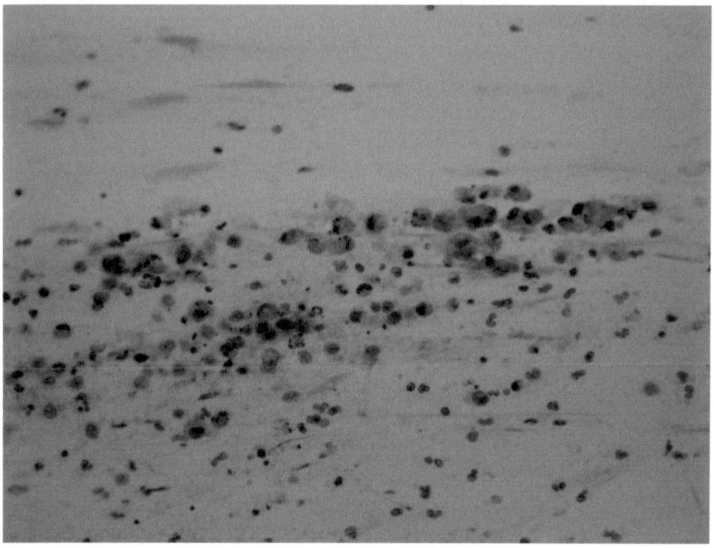

Fig. 7. Ileal conduit urine like features contained abundant degenerative glandular mucous cells and debris. (Papanicolaou stain, 200x)

Recognizing this dirty mucin background would be very important in the interpretation of AGC Pap smears and helped the clinicians successfully found the primary site of cancers.

Endometrial debris admixed with atypical endometrial glandular cells would be seen not only in the cancer patients but also in benign lesions, such as endometrial polyp and intra-uterine contraceptive device (Figure 9-10). Clinical information is very important to avoid over diagnosis.

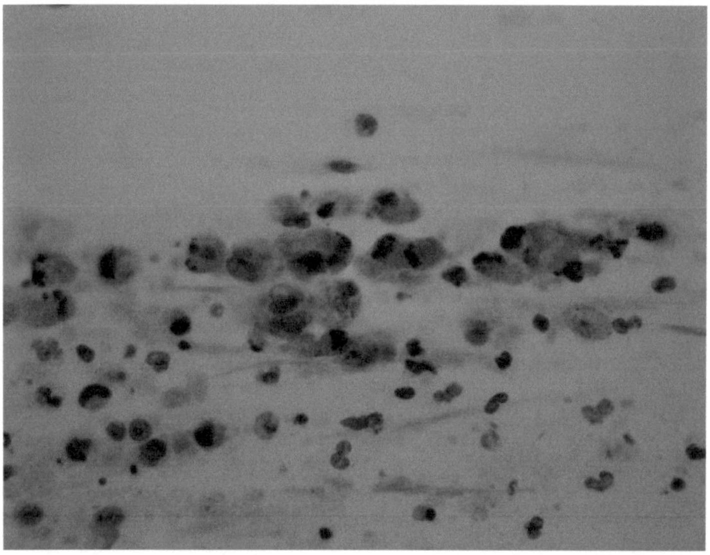

Fig. 8. These degenerative mucous cells had small eccentric hyperchromatic nuclei and abundant mucous cytoplasm indicating mucinous glandular origin. (Papanicolaou stain, 400x)

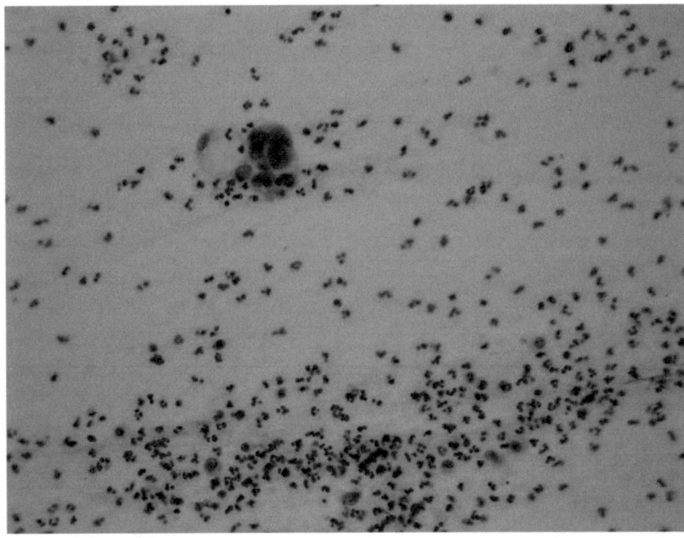

Fig. 9. Degenerative atypical endometrial glandular cells and endometrial debris were noted in a smear of patient with intra-uterine contraceptive device (IUD). Originally, the diagnosis of AGC-NOS, EM was given without knowing the IUD situation. (Papanicolaou stain, 200x)

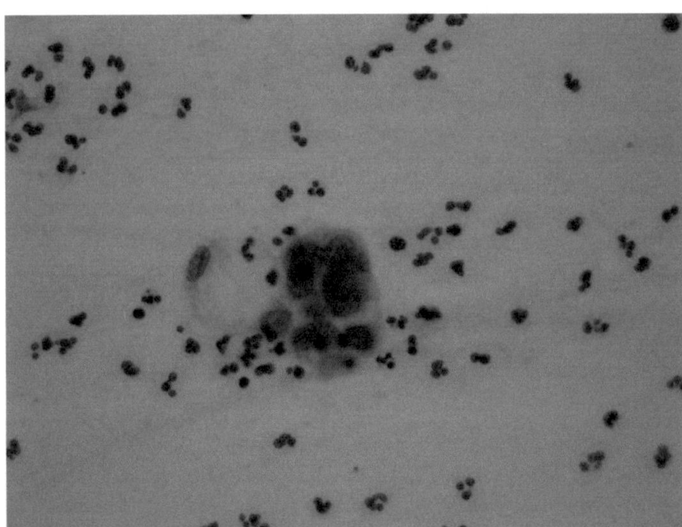

Fig. 10. Higher magnification showed small three-dimensional group of endometrial glandular cells with characteristic cytoplasmic vacuolation and slightly enlarged hyperchromatic nuclei. (Papanicolaou stain, 400x)

The major differential diagnoses of atypical endocervical glandular cells include adenocarcinoma in situ (Figure 11), tubal metaplasia (Figure 12) and lower uterine segment cells (Figure 13). When the lesion is adequately sampled and the abnormal cells are well visualized both quantitatively and qualitatively, the diagnosis will be no problem in most circumstances. Otherwise, these look-alike entities should be taken into the list of differential diagnoses.

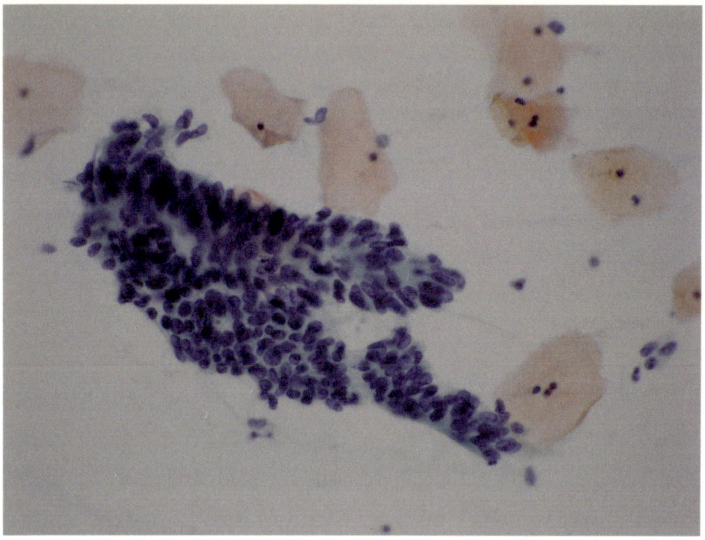

Fig. 11. Super-crowded endocervical glandular cells presenting pseudostratification and feathering edge. The nuclei are elongated and hyperchromatic with high N/C ratio.

Nucleoli are absent. However, only two fragments were seen. The diagnosis of AGC-FN was made. Final histology proved to be endocervical adenocarcinoma in situ. (Papanicolaou stain, 200x)

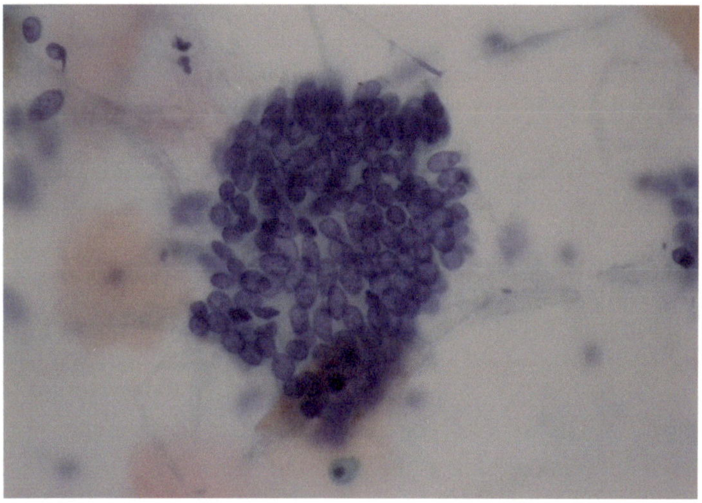

Fig. 12. Tubal metaplasia can closely mimic adenocarcinoma in situ. However, on close inspection, the abnormalities, such as crowding, nuclear elongation, hyperchromasia, and stratification are less severe. Locating terminal bars or cilia can help in confirmation, but they could not be identified in the smear we examined. The original diagnosis for this case was AGC-NOS, endocervical origin. (Papanicolaou stain, 400x)

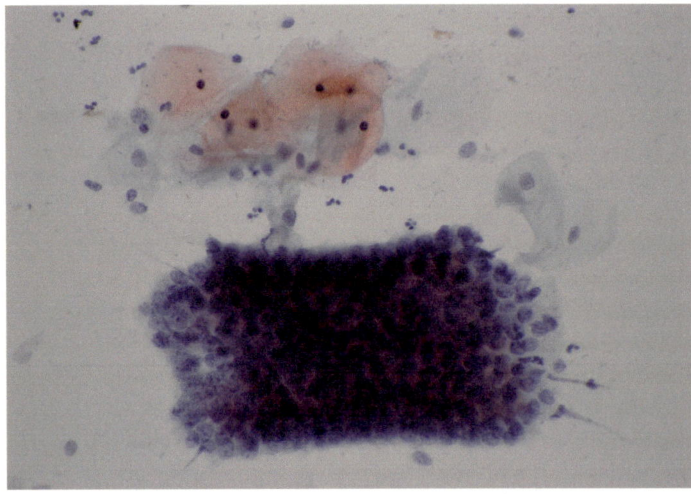

Fig. 13. Lower uterine segment cells were composed of tightly packed uniform glandular cells in crowded honeycomb appearance. A stromal element is usually present in the surrounding area, which is an aid in the differential diagnosis. However, the stromal component is absent in the present case, the original diagnosis was AGC-NOS, cell origin also not otherwise specified. (Papanicolaou stain, 400x)

4. Discussion

The TBS was first introduced in 1988 for reporting cervical/vaginal cytology findings (National Cancer Institute Workshop, 1989). Revisions were made in 2001 to improve its sensitivity and specificity. In terms of categories of atypical glandular cells, In the 1988 version these cells were defined as "atypical glandular cells of undetermined significance (AGUS)". In the current 2001 version (Solomon, 2002), this nomenclature has changed to "atypical glandular cells, not otherwise specified (AGC-NOS)" and "atypical glandular cells, favor neoplastic (AGC-FN). Subclassification of cell origin (endocervical, endometrial, or not otherwise specified) should be done whenever possible. The TBS 2001 reporting system was proved to be better for detecting underlying gynecological lesions, including precursors and invasive malignant diseases in many reports (Behtash, 2007; Duska, 1998; Jeng, 2003; Koonings, 2001; Lai, 2008; Manetta, 1999; Mood, 2006; Soofer, 2000). The incidence of abnormal pathology ranged from 8.2% to 53%. Most studies defined abnormal pathology as precursors and invasive malignant diseases. Low grade squamous intra-epithelial lesions (LSIL) were excluded. The invasive malignancies may originate not only from uterine cervix and corpus but also extra-uterine organs, such as fallopian tube, ovary, colon and rectum. In this current report, we found that endometrial cancer was by far the most common malignant disease, 38 in 53 cases (72%), diagnosed in the AGC smears (Table 2). This was the highest data ever reported. The reason may be that since our previous observation of the importance of endometrial debris (Lai, 2008), the screeners paid much attention to this kind of cytology findings. The sensitivity of reporting endometrial debris increased and then detected more endometrial cancers.

The concept of subclassification of AGC to NOS and FN categories as an important predictor for the risk of abnormal pathology was further supported in the current study (Table 3). The subgroup of AGC-N, EM had the highest rate of abnormal pathology, followed by AGC-NOS, EM, AGC-N and AGC-NOS; 18 of 21 (86%), 30 of 75 (40%), 4 of 11 (36%) and 24 of 83 (29%), respectively. The difference was significant. ($P<0.001$) Women with AGC-N were more likely to have significant pathology (22 in 32 (69%)) compared with those with AGC-NOS (54 in 158 (34%)). It was statistically significant. ($P<0.001$) The results were in accordance with other previous studies (Adhya, 2009; Behtash, 2007; Sawangsang, 2011; Westin, 2008; Zhao, 2009). They also confirmed the high risk nature of AGC smears. They have consistently demonstrated that the rate of abnormal pathology was significantly high if the AGC smears further classified as favoring neoplasia (41%-70%).

Since we have observed the importance of endometrial debris in our previous report (Lai, 2008), in the current study, only endometrial origin smears were calculated separately in order to strengthen the importance of this factor. The endocervical and not otherwise specified origins were counted together. The subgroup of AGC-N, EM had the highest rate of abnormal pathology, followed by AGC-NOS, EM, AGC-N and AGC-NOS; 18 of 21 (86%), 30 of 75 (40%), 4 of 11 (36%) and 24 of 83 (29%), respectively. The difference was significant. ($P<0.001$) The endometrial origin addressed cases had more abnormal pathology results than those not being addressed, 48 of 96 (50%) v.s. 28 of 94 (30%). ($P=0.004$) (Table 3) The results further confirmed the importance of cell origin of AGC, especially the endometrial origin. The predictive value of background endometrial debris such as histiocytes for endometrial pathology in Pap smears has been a subject of controversy. Some studies have suggested a significant finding but the others didn't (Iavazzo, 2008; Koss, 1962; Nassar, 2003; Ng, 1974; Nguyen, 1998; Wen, 2003). The controversy is understandable, because the biopsy rate and the yield of endometrial neoplasm in these patients were relatively low in the past. According to Browne's study (Browne, 2005), they found a 5-fold increase in the frequency with which endometrial cells were reported after the implementation of the TBS 2001. This then resulted in 25.2% of biopsies, a 1.3 fold increase in the overall number of tissue proof. Our another study (Lai, in press) of the importance of endometrial debris also revealed similar results. It showed that even in the absence of AGC, the presence of endometrial debris rather than the menopausal status was more related to the rate of biopsy procedure and a malignant pathology result. Degenerative necrotic debris is a significant risk factor for endometrial pathology, regardless of the presence or absence of AGC. Although the cervical screening program is not designed to detect endometrial lesions, early detection of any such cases is possible and is a bonus to be beneficial for these patients by identifying the significant degenerative endometrial debris in the Pap smears. Finally, another characteristic dirty mucinous background cytomorphology indicating endocervical adenocarcinoma observed in our series, being limited number of cases at present, will be continuously studied to investigate its sensitivity and specificity.

5. Conclusion

In the current study, AGC smears were associated with a high prevalence of abnormal pathology, including precursors and malignant diseases. Furthermore, the results of separations between "not otherwise specified" v.s. "favor neoplastic' and "endometrial origin" was statistically significant. Endometrial cancers were the most common neoplasm in the AGC patients. The above findings supported the TBS 2001 for subcategories of AGC and subclassifications of cell origins and the appropriate management algorithm of the guidelines of ASCCP 2006.

6. References

Adhya, A.K., Mahesha, V., Srinivasan, R., Nijhawan, R., Rajwanshi, A., Suri, V., & Dhaliwal, L.K. (2009). Atypical glandular cells in cervical smears: histological correlation and a suggested plan of management based on age of the patient in a low-resource setting, *Cytopathology*, Vol. 20, No. 6, (December 2009), pp. 375-379, ISSN 1365-2303

Behtash, N., Nazari, Z., Fakhrejahani, F., Khafaf, A., & Azar, E.G. (2007). Clinical and histological significance of atypical glandular cell on Pap smear, *Australian and New Zealand Journal of Obstetrics and Gynaecology*, Vol. 47, No. 1, (February 2007), pp. 46-49, ISSN 0004-8666

Browne, T.J., Genest, D.R., & Cibas, E.S. (2005). The clinical significance of benign-appearing endometrial cells on a Papanicolaou test in women 40 years or older, *American Journal of Clinical Pathology*, Vol. 124, No. 6, (January 2006), pp. 834-837, ISSN 0002-9173

Duska, L.R., Flynn, C.F., Chen, A., Whall-Strojwas, D., & Goodman, A. (1998). Clinical evaluation of atypical glandular cells of undetermined significance on cervical cytology, *Obstetrics and Gynecology*, Vol. 91, No. 2, (February 1998), pp. 278-282, ISSN 0029-7844

Iavazzo, C., Kalmantis, K., Ntziora, F., Balakitsas, N., & Paschalinopoulos, D. (2008). Detection of large histiocytes in pap smears: role in the prediction of endometrial pathology?, *Bratislavske Lekarske Listy*, Vol. 109, No. 11, (February 2009), pp. 497-498, ISSN 0006-9248

Jeng, C.J., Liang, H.S., Wang, T.Y., Shen, J., Yang, Y.C., & Tzeng, C.R. (2003). Cytologic and histologic review of atypical glandular cells (AGC) detected during cervical cytology screening, *Int J Gynecol Cancer*, Vol. 13, No. 4, (August 2003), pp. 518-521, ISSN 1048-891X

Koonings, P.P., & Price, J.H. (2001). Evaluation of atypical glandular cells of undetermined significance: is age important?, *American Journal of Obstetrics and Gynecology*, Vol. 184, No. 7, (June 2001), pp. 1457-1459; discussion 1459-1461, ISSN 0002-9378

Koss, L.G. (1989). The Papanicolaou test for cervical cancer detection. A triumph and a tragedy, *JAMA*, Vol. 261, No. 5, (February 1989), pp. 737-743, ISSN 0098-7484

Koss, L.G., & Durfee, G.R. (1962). Cytologic diagnosis of endometrial carcinoma. Result of ten years of experience, *Acta Cytologica*, Vol. 6, No., (November 1962), pp. 519-531, ISSN 0001-5547

Lai, C.R., Hsu, C.Y., Tsay, S.H., & Li, A.F. (2008). Clinical significance of atypical glandular cells by the 2001 Bethesda System in cytohistologic correlation, *Acta Cytologica*, Vol. 52, No. 5, (October 2008), pp. 563-567, ISSN 0001-5547

Lai, C.R., Hsu, C.Y., & Li, A.F. (in press). Degenerative necrotic endometrial debris in Pap smear: The role in the prediction of endometrial pathology, American Journal of Clinical Pathology , (in press), ISSN: 0002-9173

Manetta, A., Keefe, K., Lin, F., Ahdoot, D., & Kaleb, V. (1999). Atypical glandular cells of undetermined significance in cervical cytologic findings, *American Journal of Obstetrics and Gynecology*, Vol. 180, No. 4, (April 1999), pp. 883-888, ISSN 0002-9378

Mood, N.I., Eftekhar, Z., Haratian, A., Saeedi, L., Rahimi-Moghaddam, P., & Yarandi, F. (2006). A cytohistologic study of atypical glandular cells detected in cervical smears during cervical screening tests in Iran, *Int J Gynecol Cancer*, Vol. 16, No. 1, (February 2006), pp. 257-261, ISSN 1048-891X

Nassar, A., Fleisher, S.R., & Nasuti, J.F. (2003). Value of histiocyte detection in Pap smears for predicting endometrial pathology. An institutional experience, *Acta Cytologica*, Vol. 47, No. 5, (October 2003), pp. 762-767, ISSN 0001-5547

National Cancer Institute Workshop (1989). The 1988 Bethesda System for reporting cervical/vaginal cytological diagnoses. , *JAMA*, Vol. 262, No. 7, (August 1989), pp. 931-934, ISSN 0098-7484

Ng, A.B., Reagan, J.W., Hawliczek, S., & Wentz, B.W. (1974). Significance of endometrial cells in the detection of endometrial carcinoma and its precursors, *Acta Cytologica*, Vol. 18, No. 5, (September 1974), pp. 356-361, ISSN 0001-5547

Nguyen, T.N., Bourdeau, J.L., Ferenczy, A., & Franco, E.L. (1998). Clinical significance of histiocytes in the detection of endometrial adenocarcinoma and hyperplasia, *Diagnostic Cytopathology*, Vol. 19, No. 2, (August 1998), pp. 89-93, ISSN 8755-1039

Sawangsang, P., Sae-Teng, C., Suprasert, P., Srisomboon, J., Khunamornpong, S., & Kietpeerakool, C. (2011). Clinical significance of atypical glandular cells on Pap smears: Experience from a region with a high incidence of cervical cancer, *Journal of Obstetrics and Gynaecology Research*, Vol. 37, No. 6, (June 2011), pp. 496-500, ISSN 1341-8076

Solomon, D., Davey, D., Kurman, R., Moriarty, A., O'Connor, D., Prey, M., Raab, S., Sherman, M., Wilbur, D., Wright, T., Jr., & Young, N. (2002). The 2001 Bethesda System: terminology for reporting results of cervical cytology, *JAMA*, Vol. 287, No. 16, (April 2002), pp. 2114-2119, ISSN 0098-7484

Soofer, S.B., & Sidawy, M.K. (2000). Atypical glandular cells of undetermined significance: clinically significant lesions and means of patient follow-up, *Cancer*, Vol. 90, No. 4, (August 2000), pp. 207-214, ISSN 0008-543X

Wen, P., Abramovich, C.M., Wang, N., Knop, N., Mansbacher, S., & Abdul-Karim, F.W. (2003). Significance of histiocytes on otherwise-normal cervical smears from postmenopausal women. A retrospective study of 108 cases, *Acta Cytologica*, Vol. 47, No. 2, (April 2003), pp. 135-140, ISSN 0001-5547

Westin, M.C., Derchain, S.F., Rabelo-Santos, S.H., Angelo-Andrade, L.A., Sarian, L.O., Oliveira, E., & Zeferino, L.C. (2008). Atypical glandular cells and adenocarcinoma in situ according to the Bethesda 2001 classification: cytohistological correlation and clinical implications, *European Journal of Obstetrics, Gynecology, and Reproductive Biology*, Vol. 139, No. 1, (July 2007), pp. 79-85, ISSN 0301-2115

Wingo, P.A., Cardinez, C.J., Landis, S.H., Greenlee, R.T., Ries, L.A., Anderson, R.N., & Thun, M.J. (2003). Long-term trends in cancer mortality in the United States, 1930-1998, *Cancer*, Vol. 97, No. 12 Suppl, (June 2003), pp. 3133-3275, ISSN 0008-543X

Wright, T.C., Jr., Massad, L.S., Dunton, C.J., Spitzer, M., Wilkinson, E.J., & Solomon, D. (2007). 2006 consensus guidelines for the management of women with abnormal cervical screening tests, *J Low Genit Tract Dis*, Vol. 11, No. 4, (October 2007), pp. 201-222, ISSN 1089-2591

Zhao, C., Florea, A., Onisko, A., & Austin, R.M. (2009). Histologic follow-up results in 662 patients with Pap test findings of atypical glandular cells: results from a large academic womens hospital laboratory employing sensitive screening methods, *Gynecologic Oncology*, Vol. 114, No. 3, (September 2009), pp. 383-389, ISSN 1095-6859

16

Cytology of Cervical Intraepithelial Glandular Lesions

Ana Ovanin-Rakić
*Department of Gynecologic Cytology,
Department of Gynecologic and Perinatal Pathology, Zagreb,
Croatia*

1. Introduction

Cytology of the cervix has been properly recognized and accepted in the detection and follow-up of squamous intraepithelial lesions, whereas its role in endocervical cylindrical epithelium is less well defined. Glandular lesions of the cervix uteri have been showing a rising incidence for the last 20 years, especially among young women (Nieminen et al.1995). This trend could be attributed to several factors: better diagnosis with more appropriate techniques of sampling and specimen preparation for both cytological and histological analysis, better recognition of precursor lesions, changes in nomenclature, evolving methods of treatment and an improved understanding of morphological features, having all led to the development of criteria for the diagnosis of early dysplastic lesions. Another reason for the observed rise is the increased prevalence of these lesions.

As the major purpose of the Papanicolaou smear tests is the earliest possible diagnosis of cervical cancer and its precursors, both cervix and endocervix must be adequately sampled as the most common sites of these lesions. The best time for obtaining a smear is midcycle, i.e., two weeks after the first day of the last menses. Ideally, the woman should not have had intercourse, used douches, vaginal medication, or vaginal contraceptives 48 hours prior to obtaining a smear. It is vital that detailed clinical information be provided to the cytology laboratory. This information should include: date of the last menstrual period, results of previous Papanicolaou smears, history of fertility treatments or hormone therapy, history of abnormal bleeding, usage of intrauterine contraceptive devices, history of malignancy of female genitalia, of hysterectomy, radiation, and the results of any previous cervical biopsy.

The accuracy of clinical cytology relies to a large extent on sucessful sampling in obtaining the Papanicolaou smear and on its proper fixation and staining. A specimen from the cervicovaginal area that has been satisfactorily obtained and prepared for microscopic examination exhibits an abundance of well-preserved and meticulously stained diagnostic cellular material that remains preserved for indefinite slide storage and later review.

Glandular lesions are frequently detected in histology of cytologically diagnosed squamous intraepithelial lesions (SIL).

Cytological criteria for the identification of glandular intraepithelial lesions (GIL) have not yet been fully articulated, especially for the precursors of adenocarcinoma in situ (AIS), and these lesions may frequently remain unrecognized. Documenting the sequence of neoplastic events in the endocervix poses problems, except for its lowest segment, because the endocervical canal cannot be visualized by colposcopy and, therefore, cytological sampling cannot be targeted. Also, in spite of numerous efforts, morphological recognition of sequential abnormalities of endocervical cells is much more difficult than in squamous cells (Lee, 1999). Primary factors that contributed to either screening errors or diagnostic errors in AIS were insufficient quantities of material or poorly preserved abnormal material and aggregates of glandular cells. (Ruba et al., 2004).

2. Classification

By analogy to squamous cell cervical cancer precursors that demonstrate a wide spectrum of histological changes, some authors have proposed parallel classification schemas for endocervical adenocarcinoma precursors that include lesions with a lesser degree of abnormality than AIS. Such low grade putative glandular precursor lesions were termed endocervical dysplasia (Bousfield et al., 1980), cervical intraepithelial glandular neoplasia - CIGN (Gloor & Hurlimann, 1986), endocervical columnar cell intraepithelial neoplasia - ECCTN (van Aspert - van Erp et al., 1995), low grade glandular intraepithelial lesion - LGIL (DiTomasso et al., 1996), endocervical glandular dysplasia - EGD (Casper et al., 1997), endocervical glandular atypia - EGA (Goldstin et al., 1998), and cervical glandular intraepithelial neoplasia Low grade - L-CGIN (Kurian & al-Nafussi, 1999). We prefer the term glandular intraepithelial lesion (GIL) grade 1 and 2.

In contrast to squamous intraepithelial lesions with identifiable subgroups, in the case of glandular epithelium only adenocarcinoma in situ, included in the NCI Bethesda 2001 cytological classification, has been recognized. (http://bethesda 2001 .cancer.gov)

A uniform classification of cervical cytology findings known as Zagreb 1990 (Audy-Jurkovic et al., 1992) and developed by combining the original 1988 Bethesda System (TBS) classification (NCI, 1989) and our previous classification (Audy-Jurkovic et al., 1986) has been used in Croatia since 1990. As the TBS has been supplemented and/or modified on several occasions since its introduction (NCI, 1993 2001; Kurman & Solomon, 1994), we considered it plausible to revise our classification accordingly, i.e. by modifying and/or supplementing points of dispute noted over the past years, and by harmonizing it with the NCI Bethesda System 2001.

The current classification, **Zagreb 2002**, has been introduced as a new uniform classification system of cervical cytology findings used in Croatia (Fig. 1) (Ovanin-Rakic et al., 2003).

General classification consists of two groups, **"negative"**, for intraepithelial or invasive lesions, and **"abnormal cells"**, the latter referring to all cell alterations that are morphologically consistent with intraepithelial or invasive malignant lesions. The "negative" group refers to findings which are within normal limits, cell alterations associated with particular reactive and reparatory reactions, and with the presence of cells indicative of certain risks (e.g., findings of endometrial cells of benign appearance beyond the cycle or in the postmenopausal period).

COMPLETED BY GYNECOLOGIST

Name ____ Date of birth ____ City ____
Address ____ Tel./Fax/e-mail ____ Date ____
Health unit ____ Patient's number ____

Parity	Menstrual cycle	First day of LMP	Postmenopausis	Sample	Identification number	Laboratory number

Contraceptives: □ hormones □ IUD □ other □ without
Previous diagnostic-therapeutic procedures
Cytological diagnosis ____
Histological diagnosis ____
Other ____
Therapy ____

Sample: □ V □ C □ E □ Vulva □

Supravital analysis
L 1 2 3
□ Gardnerella vag.
□ Trichomonas vag.
□ Fungi
□........................

□ Colposcopy
□ Endocervicoscopy
Date:

Clinical diagnosis
□ Within normal limits
□ Other
Clinical remarks:

Gynecologist's Signature

SPECIMEN ADEQUACY

- □ **Satisfactory for interpretation**
- □ **Unsatisfactory for interpretation**
  - □ Specimen rejected/not processed
  - □ Specimen examined, but evaluation of epithelial abnormality is not possible
- Comments for the specimen adequacy:
  - □ Incorrect label
  - □ Broken slide
  - □ Poorly fixation or inadequately preserved
  - □ Scant cellularity
  - □ No endocervical cells
  - □ Obscuring inflammation
  - □ Obscuring blood
  - □ Thick areas
  - □ Presence of foreign material
  - □ Other: ____

GENERAL CATEGORIZATION

- □ **Negative for Intraepithelial Lesion or Malignancy**
- □ **Abnormal cells** (See descriptive diagnosis)

DESCRIPTIVE DIAGNOSIS

MICROORGANISMS

- □ Bacillus vaginalis
- □ Mixed flora
- □ Fungi
- □ Trichomonas
- □ Actinomyces
- □ Gardnerella vaginalis
- □ Chlamydia trachomatis
- □ Cellular changes associated with HSV
- □ Cellular changes associated with HPV
- □ Other: ____

Other non-neoplastic changes

- □ **Reactive cellular changes associated with:**
  - □ Inflammation
  - □ Radiation
  - □ IUD
  - □ Other: ____
- □ **Reparation**
- □ **Reserve cells**
- □ **Parakeratosis** □ **Diskeratosis** □ **Hyperkeratosis**
- □ **Glandular cells post hysterectomy**
- □ **Endometrial cells**
  - □ out of phase in menstrual patient □ in Postmenopausis
- □ **Cytohormonal status incompatible with age & anamnesis**
- □ **Other**

Abnormal cells

- □ **Squamous cells**
  - □ Atypical squamous cells (ASC)
    - □ Of undetermined significance (ASC-US)
    - □ Cannot exclude HSIL (ASC-H)
    - □ Cannot exclude invasion
  - □ Squamous intraepithelial lesion (SIL)
    - □ Dysplasia levis → CIN I → □ low-grade SIL
    - □ Dysplasia media → CIN II → □ high-grade SIL
    - □ Dysplasia gravis, □ Carcinoma in situ > CIN III → □ high-grade SIL
    - □ Plus: cellular changes associated with HPV
    - □ Cannot exclude early invasion
  - □ Carcinoma planocellulare

V | C | E

- □ **Glandular cells**
  - □ Atypical glandular cells
    - □ Favor reactive
    - □ Favor intraepithelial lesion
    - □ Favor invasive lesion
  - □ Adenocarcinoma in situ (AIS)
  - □ Adenocarcinoma

Origin:
- □ Endocervical
- □ Endometrial
- □ Ekstrauterine
- □ Not otherwise specified

V | C | E

- □ **Atypical cells of undetermined significance** ____
- □ **Other malignant neoplasm** ____

RECOMONDATION

- □ Repeat Smear
- □ Repeat after therapy
- □ Repeat in 4 months
- □ Repeat in 6 months
- □ Regular control
- □ Colposcopy
- □ Histology
- □ Further examination
- □ Other

RECOMONDATION:

Admitted: Replied: Cytotechnologist's Signature: Cytologist's Signature:

Fig. 1. Uniform classification of cytological findings of cervix uteri "Zagreb 2002", modification of the "Zagreb 1990" and "NCI Bethesda System 2001"

Unlike NCI 2001, we have kept the term **"diagnosis"** instead of "interpretation/finding result". Descriptive diagnosis contains the subgroups of **"microorganisms"** (microorganisms that can be identified directly or on the basis of a specific cytopathic effect); **"other non-neoplastic findings"** (reactive cell alterations, reparatory epithelium, reserve cells, parakeratosis, dyskeratosis, hyperkeratosis, post-hysterectomy cylindrical cells, endometrial cells beyond the cycle or in the postmenopausal period, and cytohormonal status inconsistent with age and/or history), and **"abnormal cells"** (squamous, glandular, abnormal cells of undetermined significance, and other malignant neoplasms).

In the **Zagreb 2002** classification, like in the NCI 2001, glandular lesions have been divided into three categories: **"atypical glandular cells"** (AGC), **"adenocarcinoma *in situ*"** (AIS), and **"adenocarcinoma"**. In the case of squamous epithelium, and unlike in NCI 2001, AGC have been divided into three subgroups, instead of two:

- favor reactive - cell alterations that are more pronounced than benign reactive ones but quantitatively and qualitatively less pronounced than those in intraepithelial lesions;
- favor intraepithelial (GIL1,GIL2) - cell alterations of low to moderate severity, without inflammatory cell changes, and/or suggestive of AIS, without definite criteria;
- favor invasive - cell alterations suggestive of invasive lesions, where differential cytological diagnosis cannot be made, mostly due to poor specimen preparation.

The group of adenocarcinoma in situ requires the establishment of well defined criteria.

The group of adenocarcinoma invasivum has not been modified relative to previous classifications.

For any group or subgroup of abnormal glandular cells, it is crucial to identify the origin of cylindrical epithelium whenever possible, as it is of great importance for further diagnostic and therapeutic procedures. At the end of the report, the cytologist provides the clinician with instructions on how to improve the quality of cervicovaginal smears, with guidelines on further procedures for a particular cytological finding. These instructions are in line with the current diagnostic-therapeutic protocols in use in Croatia (Ljubojevic et al., 2001).

Assessment of specimen adequacy is one of the substantial qualitative components of a finding. All criteria advocated by NCI Bethesda System 2001 (NCI, 1989,1993, 2001; Solomon et al., 2002) have been incorporated into our classification system. Information on the components of the transformation zone, i.e. finding of endocervical cylindrical epithelial cells, improves overall specimen quality thereby stimulating efforts to obtain an optimal specimen. However, the absence of such information is by no means a reason for a repeat smear (Pajtler & Audy-Jurkovic, 2002).

Cytodiagnosis of cervical cylindrical epithelial lesions lags behind the cytodiagnosis of squamous epithelial lesions both in terms of screening and differential diagnosis. The Australian (Roberts et al., 2000) modification of TBS (NCI, 1989) for glandular lesions points to the risks in the presence of high-grade abnormalities, thus resulting in more appropriate recommendations and protocols.

Cytological diagnosis of adenocarcinoma in situ of endocervical cylindrical epithelium as a separate entity was only included in the NCI Bethesda System 2001 classification, whereas dysplasia of endocervical cylindrical epithelium as an AIS precursor is still considered cytologically and histologically to be an inadequately defined entity (Zanino, 2000) and has not been included in the classification (NCI, 2001).

In most cases, morphological characteristics allow for differentiation between atypical endometrial cells and endocervical cells (Chieng & Cangiarella, 2003).

The proposed **Zagreb** classification, with amended and/or supplemented points of dispute identified in previous classifications, is uniform for Croatia. It allows for both internal and external performance quality control, along with appropriate reproducibility of cervical cytology relative to terminology adopted worldwide.

3. Epidemiology

The prevalence of AIS is not known, but is considerably lower than the prevalence of SIL. In the Surveillance Epidemiology End Results (SEER) public database, which contains data from patients entered into the database between 1973 and 1995 (Plaxe & Saltzstein, 1999), the ratio of in situ and invasive lesions is 1:3 for glandular and 5.25:1 for squamous lesions.

The rate of dysplasia of endocervical cylindrical epithelium is 16-fold that of AIS. and the mean age at diagnosis for endocervical glandular dysplasia is 37 (Brown & Wells, 1986).

The mean age at diagnosis of women with AIS in the SEER registry is 38.8, , and it is 51.7 for invasive adenocarcinoma (AI) of the cervix.

The median age of patients in our study (Ovanin-Rakic et al., 2010) was 40, which is comparable to 41, reported in the literature (Kurian & al-Nafussi, 1999), and was slightly higher than the averages from other studies (Shin et al., 2002).

Patients diagnosed with mild glandular lesions (GIL1) are on the average 10 years younger than those with the invasive disease. The mean age of AIS patients is about 13 years younger than in those with AI of the cervix. The age differnce between AIS and AI patients suggests the former to be a precursor lesion. It takes about 13 years for the AIS as an adenocarcinoma precursor to progress to AI. Such a long period of carcinogenesis recorded for lesions of endocervical cylindrical epithelium provides opportunities for their early detection and results in the reduction of incidence of AI. Additional support for implicating AIS as precursor of AI comes from several reports which had cytological or histological evidence of AIS appearing 2 - 8 years before detection of the invasive lesions (Boon et al., 1981).

Epidemiological risk factors for cervical adenocarcinoma include those that correlate with the risk of acquiring Human Papillomavirus (HPV) infections, such as multiple sexual partners and engaging in sexual intercourse at an early age. In addition, adenocarcinoma was also found to be associated with obesity and with the prolonged use of oral contraceptives.

Recent trials evaluating the efficacy of virus-like particle vaccines in the prevention of persistent infection with HPV-16 and HPV-18 in young women have been shown to be highly effective.

4. Etiology

In a series of initial cervical swabs, minimal to severe atypias of cylindrical epithelium were detected in 50% of cases with squamous epithelial lesions (Pacey & Ng, 1997), pointing to common etiological factors.

The incidence of coexisting squamous lesions was 74.8% in our study (Ovanin-Rakic, 2010), comparable to the 41 - 76.7% reported in the literature (Im et al.,1995; Shin et al., 2002).

The etiology of squamous cell carcinoma of the cervix, the most common type of cervical malignancy, is linked to infection with oncogenic types of HPV, but the pathogenesis of adenocarcinoma is less well understood. Pirog et al., 2000, detected a very high prevalence of HPV DNA in cervical adenocarcinoma relative to most previous reports. The relative difficulty in detecting HPV DNA in adenocarcinoma, in contrast to squamous cell carcinomas, may be attributed to lower viral load in glandular lesions as compared to squamous lesions. Premalignant and malignant squamous lesions, in particular those associated with HPV 16, contain a large number of episomal viral particles, in addition to integrated HPV sequences (Stoler et al., 1992). Glandular epithelium does not support productive viral infection, and HPV DNA in endocervical neoplasms (notably HPV 18) is usually present in integrated form (Park et al., 1997).

Associations between endocervical glandular atypia (dysplasia) and HPV are more contraversial. In the original study by Tase et al., 1989, only 2 of 36 cases of endocervical dysplasia contained HPV DNA. However, another study (Higgins et al., 1992) reported that 94% were associated with HPV DNA and 75% were associated with HPV 18.

5. Clinical features and management

Most patients diagnosed with GIL are free from clinical symptoms, thus a lesion is detected by cytology on routine swab sampling ("PAP" smears), or by histology (endocervical curettage - ECC, biopsy specimen, conization specimen, loop excision, hysterectomy material) on examination for SIL, or during operative procedure for myoma. (Ovanin-Rakic et al., 2010) In women who are symptomatic, the most common complaint is abnormal vaginal bleeding, either postcoital, postmenopausal, or out of phase. In intraepithelial glandular lesions, the portion is of normal macroscopic appearance and colposcopic images have long been considered nonspecific. However, some authors state that characteristic vascular changes are found in glandular lesions (Singer & Monaghan, 2000). Cytology has a very prominent and responsible role in detection of these lesions.

The anatomical distribution of AIS showed that AIS involved both surface and gland epithelia, a variable number of quadrants, glands beneath the transformation zone in about two thirds of cases, was multifocal only occasionally, and extend up the endocervical canal for a variable distance up to 30mm (Bertrand et al., 1987; Im et al., 1995). Several reports suggest that women of childbearing age may safely be followed after cold-knife conisation with minimal risk provided that the margins are negative. The cone should be cylindrical, encompassing the entire transformation zone if possible, and the sampling depth of endocervical glands should be 5mm from the canal.

It should extend parallel to the endocervical canal for at least 25mm before a 90-degree turn toward the endocervical canal (Bertrand et al., 1987). If the diagnosis is established with a loop excision, even with negative margins, a cold-knife conisation should be performed. After the completion of childbearing, a hysterectomy is recommended because of the paucity of data concerning the long-term history of AIS. In those women for whom childbearing is not important, simple hysterectomy in the face of negative margins is acceptable (Östör et al., 2000; Shin et al., 2002). Some reports indicated that a deep surgical excision with negative margins might be sufficient treatment for some women. (Azodi et al., 1999).

The treatment of glandular leasons is more difficult than that of their squmous counterparts because of the younger age at diagnosis. Managemant of fertility is often an issue, with strong desire for conservation of the uterus. Careful documentation of discussions regarding the risk of conservative management is important as well as documentation of the need for hysterectomy once the childbearing is completed.

6. Cytological features

The interpretation of observed cells requires meticulous scientific training, dedication and experience. Reaching a definitive diagnosis utilizing cells that have desquamated freely from epithelial surfaces or cells that have been forcibly removed from various tissues, demands detailed examination of all available evidence. One of the most important aspects of cytological interpretation is the acquisition of comprehensive knowledge of the normal environment of the tissue to be examined. This knowledge has to take into account the diverse physiological as well as pathological settings that would normally be found in that particular tissue. Without such detailed understanding, the exercise of cytological interpretation can become a trap for a novice. In order to recognize the cytological appearance of endocervical glandular neoplasia with maximal sensitivity and specificity, a solid understanding of normal and variant normal morphology of the cells is necessary.

6.1 Normal columnar cells

The columnar epithelial cells characteristically have basally placed nuclei and tall, uniform, finely granular cytoplasm filled with mucinous droplets. The cells lining the luminal surface have been termed "picket cells" because of their resemblance to a picket fence. It is not known whether regeneration occurs from the underlying subcolumnar reserve cells.

The nuclei of endocervical cells are finely granular and of approximately the **same size as the nuclei of intermediate squamous cells**. The nuclei tend to form dence, dark, nipple-like protrusion that usually appears as a homogeneous extension of the nucleus into the adjacent cytoplasm. The remainder of the nucleus is usually less dense and has a normal appearance. (Boon ME & Gray W, 2003) .

6.1.1 Endocervical reserve cells

Rarely seen, endocervical reserve cells are young, endocervical, parabasal cells in close contact with the basement membrane.

They have multipotential differentiation and may be seen in sheets or in loose clusters of single cells. (Fig.6.1.1.1.) Their cytoplasm is adequate to scanty, cyanophilic and finely vacuolated. Their round to oval nuclei are centrally located, with fine, uniformly distributed chromatin. Small, round chromocenters are often multiple. Mitoses are occasionally seen and have no significance (Naib, 1996).

Fig. 6.1.1.1. Loose clusters of normal endocervical reserve sells. The mitotic figure has little diagnostic significance. (Papanicolaou x100, and x400).

6.1.2 Ciliated endocervical cells

Ciliated endocervical cells are the result of direct traumatic exfoliation. They can be single, in tight clusters, in small sheets, or in palisade formations when viewed from the side and honeycomb-like in appearance when their apical ends are in focus. Their size varies, but their shape is fairly constant, cylindrical or pyramidal. When a cell is well preserved, delicate pink cilia are attached to this lavender or red terminal bar or plate. (Fig.6.1.2.1.) This terminal bar can persist even after the cilia have been lost through degeneration. Their length varies according to the original position of the exfoliated cell in relation to the axes of the endocervical canal. The cytoplasm is elongated, with a semitransparent, lacy appearance and cytoplasmic borders that are thin and distinct, in contrast to those found in other types of endocervical cells. They stain darker than the pale mucus-producing endocervical cells. (Naib, 1996; Boon & Gray, 2003).

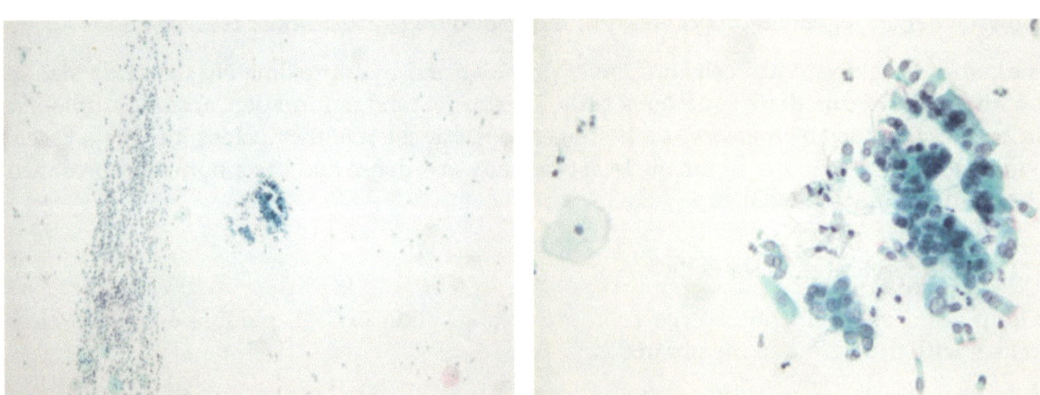

Fig. 6.1.2.1. Ciliated endocervical cells. Note the multincleation (Papanicolaou x100, x400).

Depending on the stage of maturation of the cell and its function, the nuclei are centrally placed or close to the apical cellular end, in contrast to the position of the nuclei in nonciliated cells. These nuclei are round or oval in shape and vary moderately in size. Their chromatin is finely granular and uniformly distributed. The nuclear borders are even and smooth, and they often merge with the cytoplasmic membrane on both sides. When multiple, the nuclei may overlap with little moulding.

Occasionally, nonsecretory cells with cilia are observed, the main function of which appears to relate to the distribution and mobilization of endocervical mucus. Rare, small, dark, nipple like protrusions may be seen in the nuclei of mature or reserve endocervical cells.

Detached ciliary tufts or ciliocytophthoria in cervicovaginal smears, are a very rare event and cannot be correlated with time of cycle or age of patient.(Fig.6.1.2.2.)

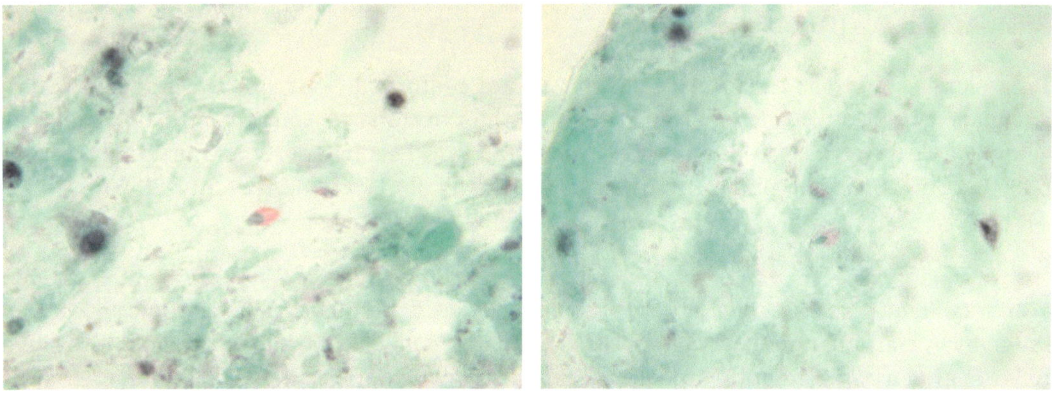

Fig. 6.1.2.2. Ciliocitophthoria. (Papanicolaou x1000).

6.1.3 Nonciliated endocervical cells

Nonciliated endocervical cells occur as single cells, in clusters, or in palisade formations and with a honeycomb-like appearance. (Fig.6.1.3.1.; Fig.6.1.3.2.)

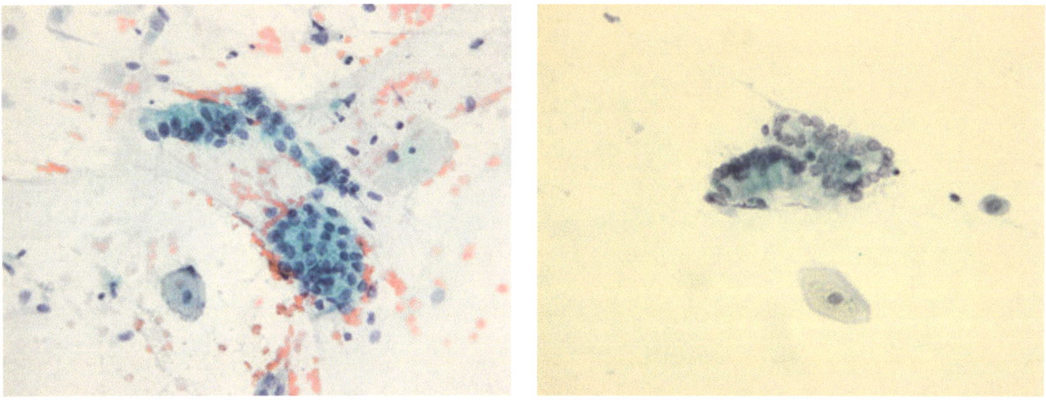

Fig. 6.1.3.1. Group of nonciciliated endocervical cells in sheet, palisade and rosettes. Note the same size nuclei of columnar and intermediate squamous cells. (Papanicolaou x400)

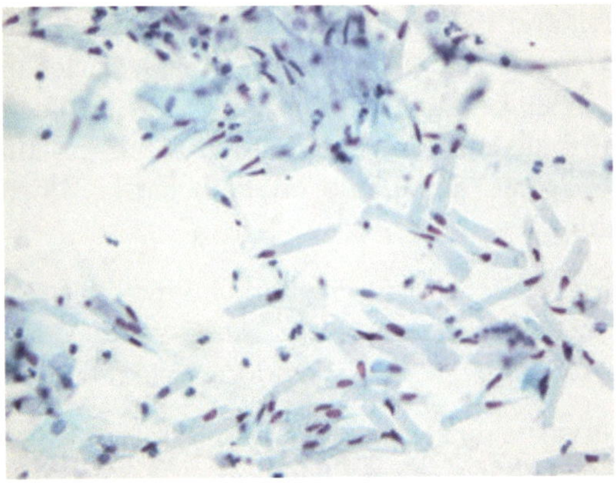

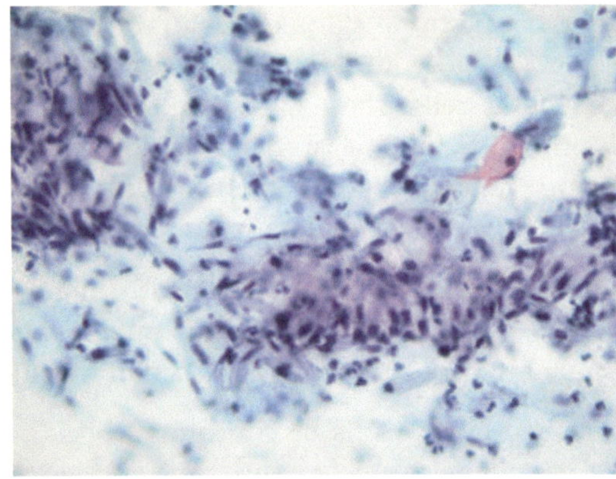

Fig. 6.1.3.2. Nonciliated singly, in cluster and palisade formation; very distended endocervical cells (Papanicolaou x400).

These long, columnar cells vary in size and are uniform in shape and elongated. Their adequate cytoplasm is narrow, and their borders are sharp, smooth, and delicate. The cytoplasm is semitransparent and finely vacuolated, and stains poorly and unevenly as pale blue. In some, fine acidophilic granules can be seen (Naib, 1996; Boon & Gray, 2003)

6.1.4 Secretory endocervical cells

Secretory endocervical cells are found in increased number with chronic irritation, pregnancy, glandular endocervical polyps, or intake of various hormones and contraceptive pills. They vary in size and exfoliate singly or in clusters. (Fig.6.1.4.1). Their shape varies from round to triangular. Their cytoplasm is usually distended by single or multiple small or large secretory vacuoles.

When degenerated, they may contain numerous, large, healthy polymorphonuclear cells. The borders of the cytoplasm are often indistinct, thin, and very delicate. Because of the fragility of the cytoplasm, it is common to find numerous stripped nuclei with only a wisp of transparent cytoplasm still attached in strands of thick cervical mucus in the smear.

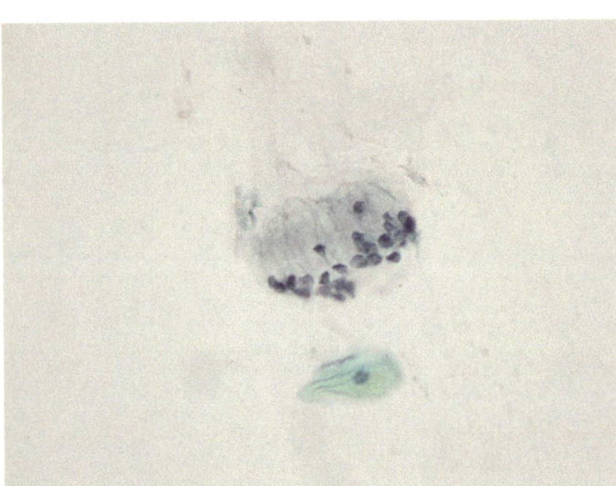

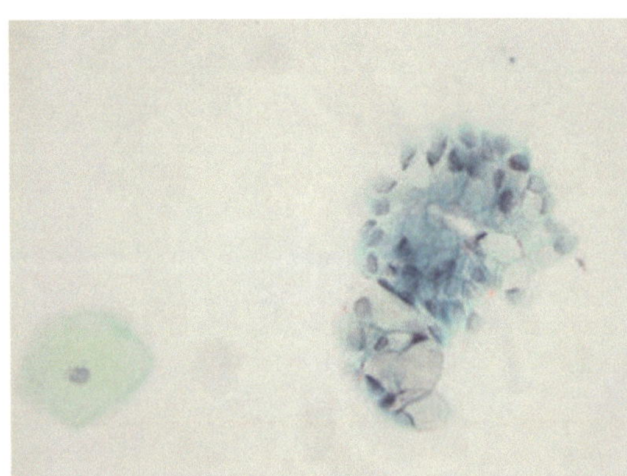

Fig. 6.1.4.1. Secretory endocervical cells in palisade and rosette formation.(Papanicolaou x400)

The nucleoli may be prominent, spherical in shape, and variable in number. Multinucleation is common, especially in cases of hormonal hyperplasia and chronic or acute cervicitis.

The nuclei are often enlarged, oval-to crescent-shaped, and eccentrically situated toward the narrow end of the cell as the result of the cell's displacement by the secretory vacuols.

The size of the nucleus may vary in diameter. The nuclear membrane is often fuzzy. The chromatin is coarsely clumped and has tendency to condense toward the nuclear membrane. Some of the nuclei may, in cases of hyper secretion, appear almost completely pyknotic with an extreme crescent-like shape. (Fig.6.1.4.2.)

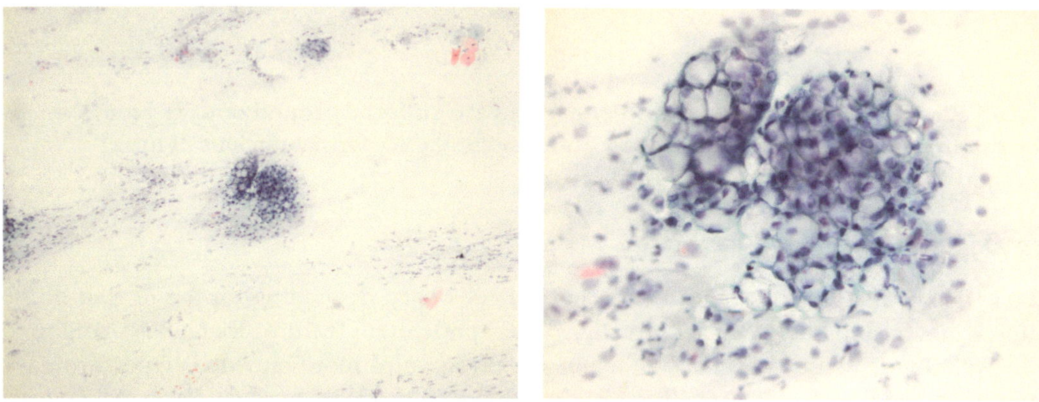

Fig. 6.1.4.2. Groups of secretory endocervical cells. Note the cytoplasmic secretory vacuoles. (Papanicolaou x100, and x400)

6.1.5 Endocervical stripped nuclei

Endocervical stripped nuclei, so-called bare, or naked, which often have a wisp of cytoplasm still attached, are commonly seen in smears from postmenopausal or pregnant women or from women with an endocervical ectropion.

These nuclei are uniformly round or oval but may vary moderately in size. Their nuclear membrane is regular and sharp with a small sign of degeneration. The chromatin pattern is uniform and finely granular with occasional clumping, similar to the normal nucleus of intact endocervical cell. (Fig.6.1.5.1.)

Condensation of the chromatin material toward the nuclear rim, pseudo hyperchromatism, or a clear, bland chromatic pattern may occur as a result of cellular degeneration. Occasional, single, small, central, reddish nucleoli can be seen in better-preserved naked nuclei.

These stripped nuclei should not be confused with poorly differentiated small-cell squamous carcinoma. Both may vary in size, but the shape of the endocervical nuclei is regular, with a smooth nuclear membrane, with chromatin finely granular, and uniformly distributed.

The cytological diagnosis of atypia should never be rendered from stripped nuclei alone.

An examination of better-preserved cells with intact cytoplasm is necessary. (Naib, 1996; Boon & Gray, 2003).

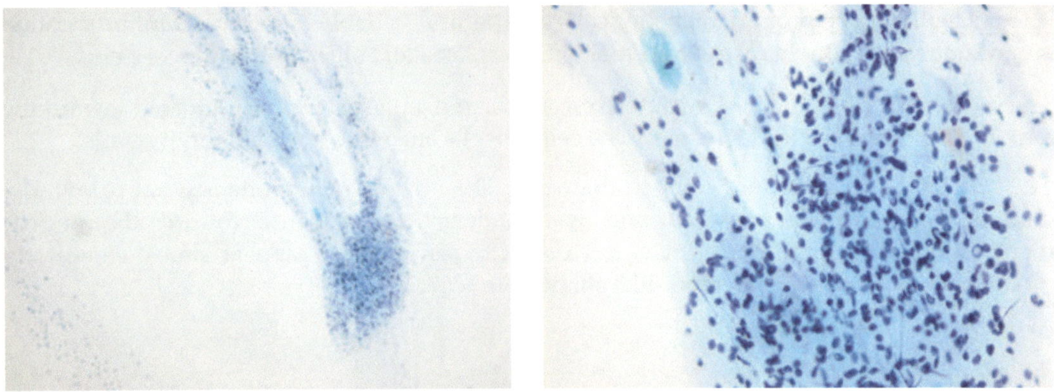

Fig. 6.1.5.1. "Stripped nuclei" of endocervical cells are uniformly round or oval. Note the chromatin pattern is uniform and finely granular similar to normal nucleus of intact endocervical cell. (Papanicolaou x 100, x 400)

6.2 Atypical Glandular Cells (AGC)

The cytologic features of atypical endocervical cells vary depending on the degree of the underlying histopathologic abnormality. The particular feature that may confound interpretation in these specimens is, again the presence of more crowded hyperchromatic groupings and the lack of spreading out that occurs in the making of conventional smears. This can lead to difficulty in identifying key nuclear and cytoplasmic features that could have otherwise made the interpretation more definitive, either toward benign/reactive or neoplastic. (Solomon, 2002; Chieng & Cangiarella, 2003; Waddell, 2003; Willson & Jones, 2004) .

6.2.1 Atypical Glandular Cells (AGC) favouring reactive process

These include endocervical cells from dense two- or three-dimensional aggregates, or sheets and palisades that have minor degrees of nucleolar overlapping. However, the changes may be reactive changes due to inflammation or trauma, as well as reflecting the earliest stages of GIL.(Fig.6.2.1.1.)

There is an increased number of intensely stained endocervical cells. Their abundant cytoplasm is dense, acidophilic, or overdistended by large secretory vacuoles, often containing well-preserved leukocytes or mucus secretions. Their nuclei are enlarged, with a smooth nuclear membrane and coarsely granular chromatin that is uniformly distributed and nucleolar feathering can be seen at the periphery of the cellular aggregates.

There is overlap between the nuclear features which may be seen in extreme inflammatory changes, and those which may be seen in some examples of glandular intraepithelial lesions.

(Fig.6.2.1.2.) They differ by regular distribution of their clumped chromatin and their smooth nuclear membrane. The nucleoli may be prominent, massive, spherical, and usually single, but they may vary in number.

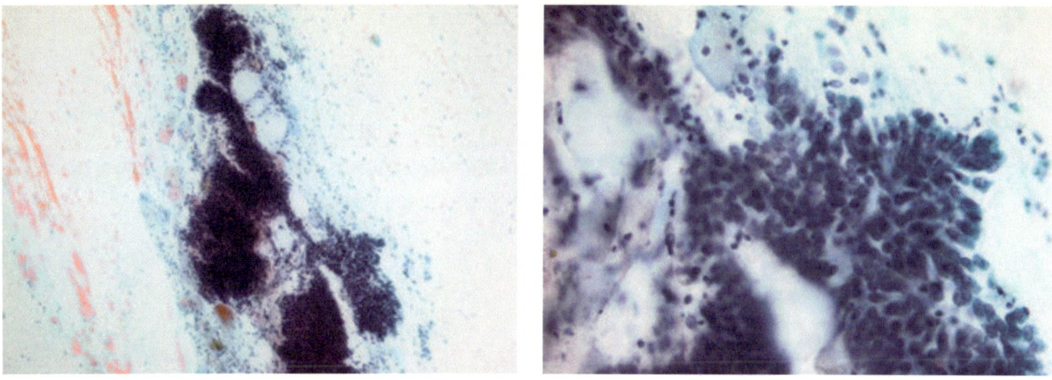

Fig. 6.2.1.1. Crowded sheets of endocervical cells. The nuclei are overlapping and hyperchromatic, but show only a mild variation in size within the sheet.

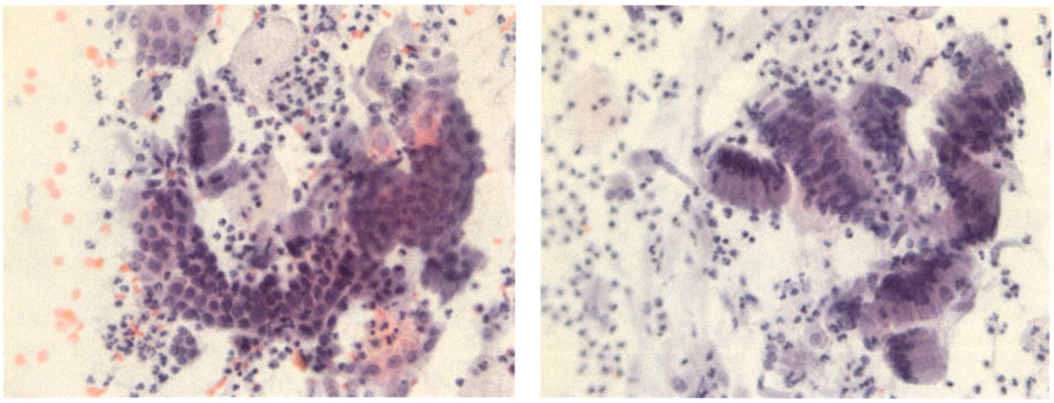

Fig. 6.2.1.2. In sheets and palisades pseudostratification of endocervical cells is present. Nuclei are slightly enlarged. (Papanicolaou x 100, x 400)

6.2.2 Atypical Glandular Cells (AGC), favouring intraepithelial lesions (glandular dysplasia)

Apearance of cytological atypias of the endocervical epithelium falls between those seen in normal glands and in AIS.

Mild (GIL1) and moderate (GIL2) glandular intraepithelial lesions have not been clearly defined, while reproducibility of the cytological and histological criteria for their identification has not been fully explored. Cellular alterations in GIL1 and GIL2 are similar to but less pronounced than those in AIS. The type of desquamation is also similar, except that the cylindrical cells are slightly packed showing a palisading pattern with mild pseudostratification, with less pronounced nuclear overlapping and observable feathering, rosettes, and glandular opening. (Fig.6.2.2.1.; Fig.6.2.2.2.; Fig.6.2.2.3.)

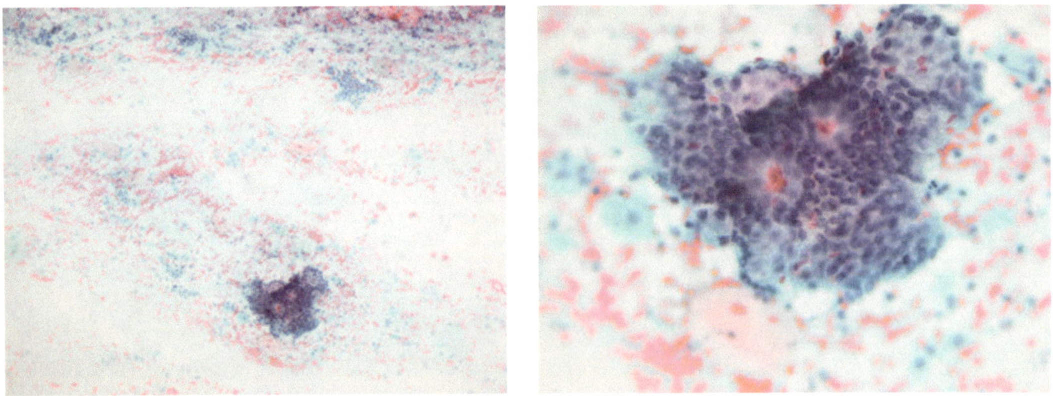

Fig. 6.2.2.1. A cluster of atypical endocervical cells (GIL 1) with glandular opening, with slight nuclear enlargement and overlapping. (Papanicolaou x100, x400)

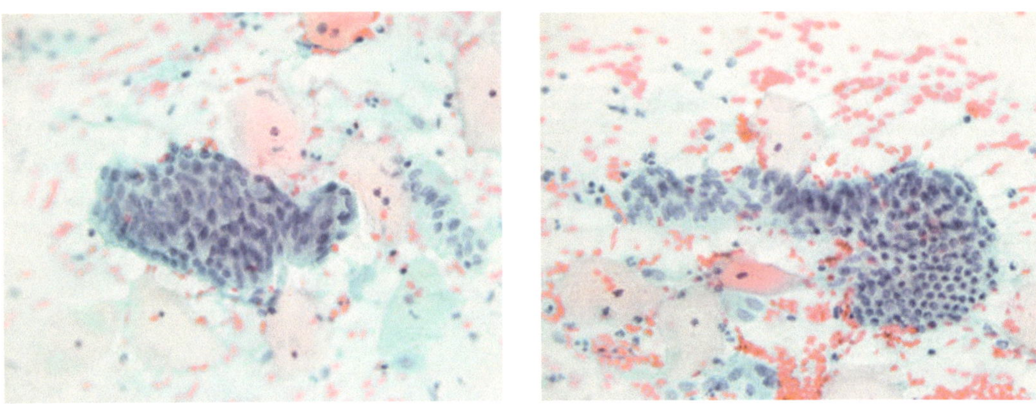

Fig. 6.2.2.2. Sheet of cells (left field) with slight nuclear enlargement and overlapping (GIL1) Note sheet of normal endocervical cells (right field) and palisade with slight nuclear enlargement and pseudostratification (GIL 1). (Papanicolaou x400)

According to the results some studies (Rabelo-Santos et al., 2008), feathering was the best criterion for predicting glandular neoplasia. Feathering was the criterion for distinguishing glandular from squamous neoplasia and also for distinguishing between glandular and . non-neoplastic diagnosis.

Rosettes and pseudostratified strips did not perfom as well. Some rosette formations can be seen in non-neoplastic cases. Squamous neoplasia, especially CIN 3 (cervical intraepithelial neoplasia), is frequently found to have rudimentary gland formation or micro-acinar structures, which can mimic AIS. These facts might help to explain the lower perfomance of the rosette when compared with feathering in the prediction of glandular neoplasia.

The cell size is like that in normal findings or slightly enlarged. **Nuclear size within a cluster varies to a greater extent than in the AIS** (Bousfield et al., 1980). The nucleus is round or oval, hyperchromasia is less pronounced, chromatin is finely granular and evenly distributed, and nucleoli are small and round. Mitoses are rare.

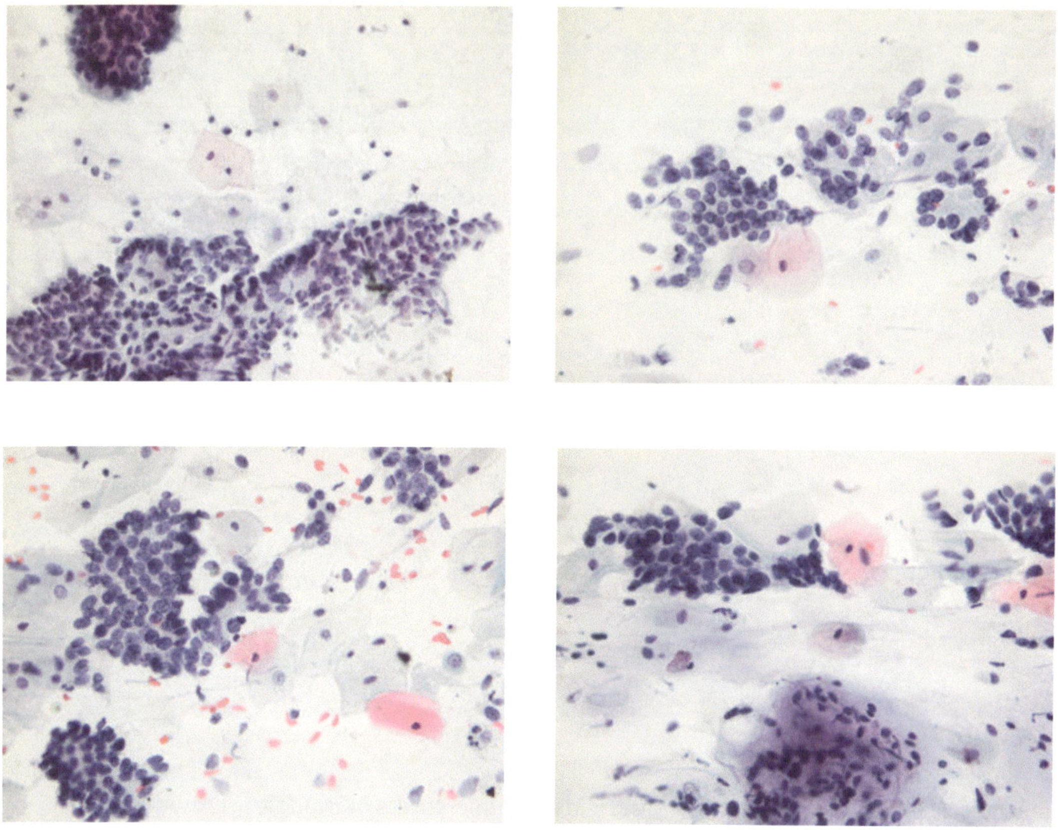

Fig. 6.2.2.3. The cervical smears contains sheets of crowded mild and moderate hyperchromatic endocervical cells with partial rosette and feathering.(GIL1, GIL2) A cluster of atypical cells (down right field) compared with normal cells in the same fields. (Papanicolaou x400).

Recognition of the characteristic architectural features in cell groups is very important in diagnosis. Without obvious and unequivocal nuclear change in endocervical cells, cytological diagnosis of GIL should not be made in the absence of these architectural features. Three-dimensional cell groups with disorderly cell arrangements, coarse grainy chromatin, and hyperchromasia with intercellular variation in nuclear staining intensity may be seen. None of the architectural abnormalities characteristic of GIL is present. . (Bousfield et al., 1980; Gloor & Hurlimann, 1986; vanAspert-van Erp et al., 1995; diTomassso et al., 1996; Golstein et al., 1998; Zaino, 2000).

Examples of abnormalities can usually be seen repeatedly in abnormal cellular material. This means that if the cellular material in question is scanty in a smear, a confident diagnosis of GIL may not be possible

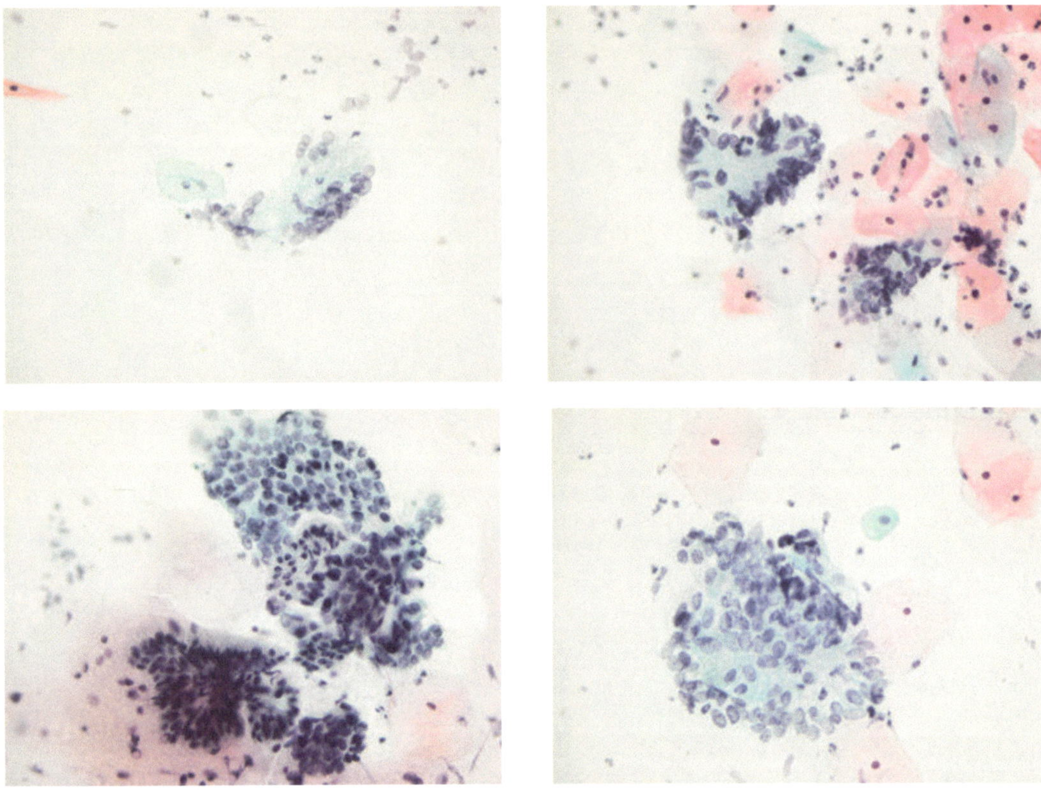

Fig. 6.2.6. The cervical smears (all four fields) contain sheets of moderate crowded endocervical cells with rosettes, partial rosettes and feathering with enlarged hyperchromatic nuclei. (GIL 2) A cluster of atypical cells compared with normal cells (pseudorosette and sheet) in the same fields (down left). Note the different nuclear size within a cluster (Papanicolaou x400).

6.2.3 Atypical Glandular Cells (AGC), favouring invasive lesions

The number of exfoliated diagnostic cells in smears varies according to the site, type, and size of the tumor and the technique used. Although generally larger than normal, the tumor cells, with few exceptions, imitate the appearance of the benign columnar cells from which they originate. In loose clusters or tight three-dimensional formations, abnormal degenerating columnar cells are identified in the "dirty" background of fresh and old degenerating blood cells, and cellular debris, consistent with the tumour diathesis.

The nuclei are enlarged, oval or round with eosinophilic granular cytoplasm. There is considerable nuclear overlapping and pleomorphism, and the chromatin pattern is coarsely granular, irregularly distributed and nucleoli are identifiable.

Unlike adenocarcinoma of the endometrium, the cells retain, especially at the periphery of clusters, their columnar configuration. A definitive cytological diagnosis cannot be made, mostly due to **poor specimen preparation.** (Fig.6.2.3.1.). Mitotic figures are occasionally seen.

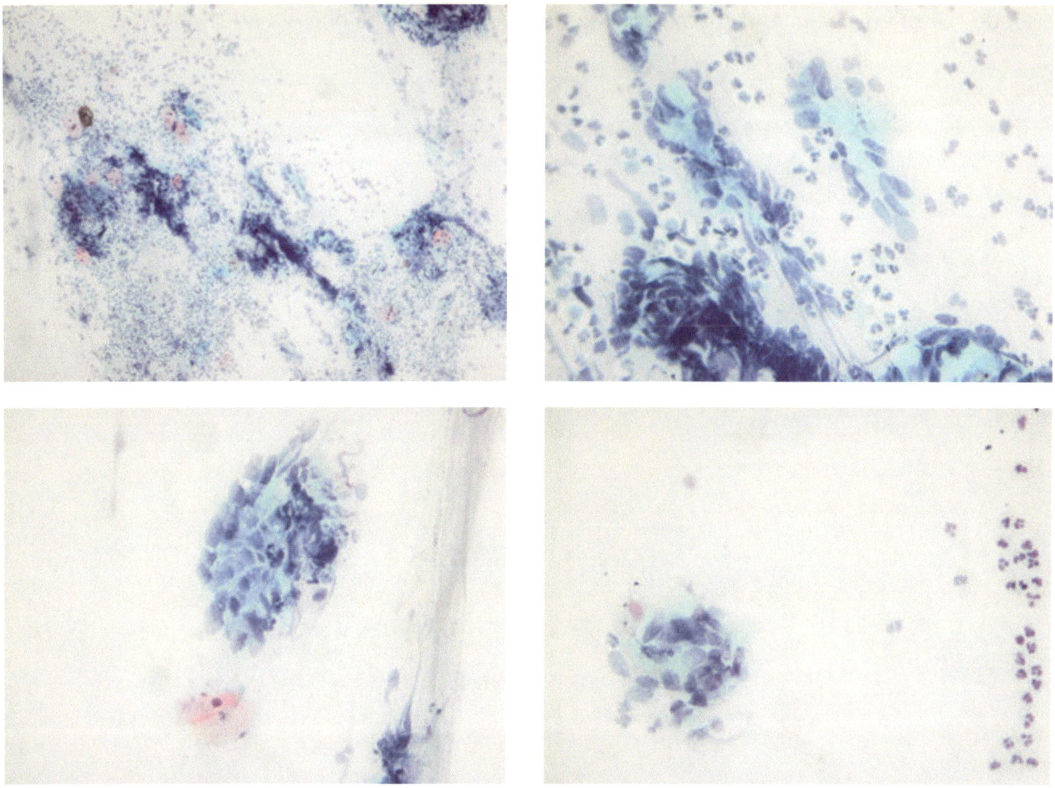

Fig. 6.2.3.1. Crowded and loose clusters, end rosettes of markedly atypical and degenerating endocervical cells. The nuclei are large, show irregular contours and coarse chromatin. Note the poor specimen preparation (Papanicolaou x100, x400 x400 x400).

6.3 Adenocarcinoma in situ

The cytomorphological criteria for diagnosis of AIS refers to changes in architectural features (sheet of cells, "strips", "rosettes", gland opening, "feathering"), and in the cells themselves. The cell size is uniform and enlarged. The cytoplasm is cyanophilic and occasionally vacuolated.

Examination of the sheets of cells does not reveal the typical honeycomb formation of normal endocervical epithelium due to crowding and overlapping of the nuclei. (Krumins et al., 1977; Bousfield et al., 1980; Gloor & Hurlimann, 1986; Betstil & Clark, 1987; Ayer et al., 1987; Pacey & Ng, 1997;Biscotti et al., 1997; Waddell,2003).

The columnar origin of cells can be recognized when lacunae, corresponding to glandular orifices, are present. At the edge of the sheets of cells, pseudo stratification of the nuclei may be observed. The glandular cells at the edge of a sheet are oriented with their long axis perpendicular to the edge. Some nuclei may have lost their surrounding cytoplasm and form irregular margins, resembling feathers at the edge of a bird's wing.

The smallest fragment is the case for 'strips' containing cells arranged in parallel with pseudo stratified nuclei and for 'rosettes', small round groups of cells with peripheral nuclei.

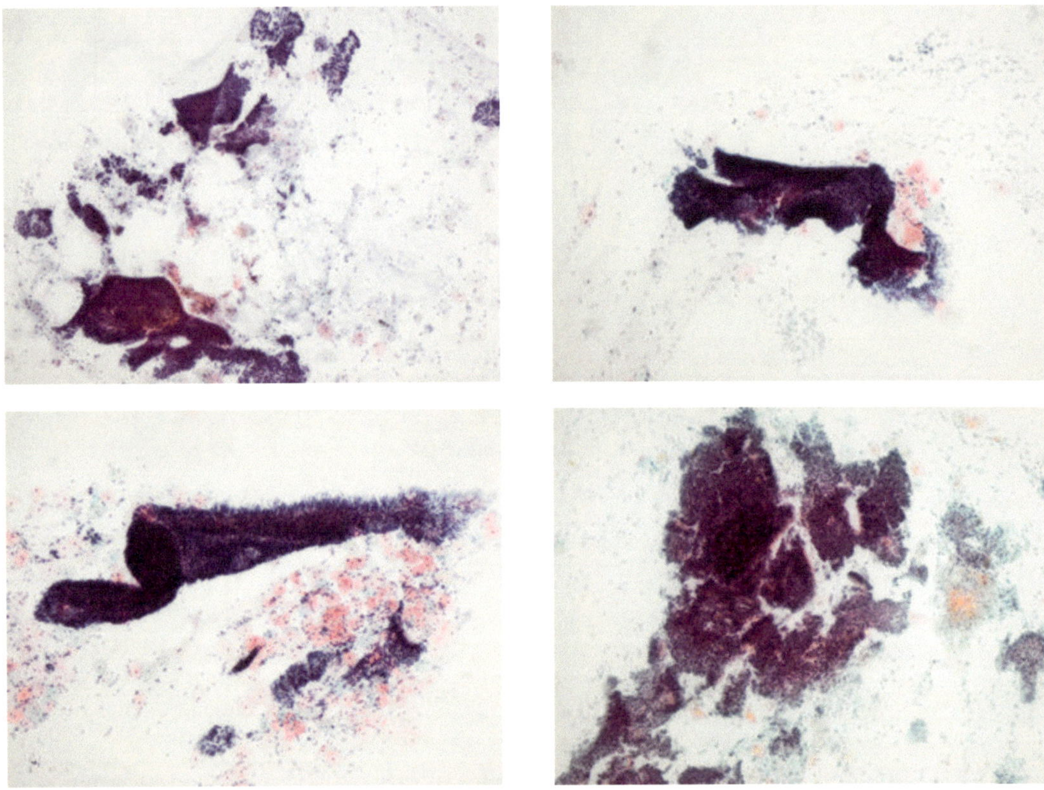

Fig. 6.3.1. AIS. Tightly crowded sheets, strips, rosettes, palisade, gland opening, feathering, of the malignant endocervical cells. The cell size is uniform and enlarged. Note crowding and overlapping of the nuclei. [Papanicolaou x 100 (all four fields)]

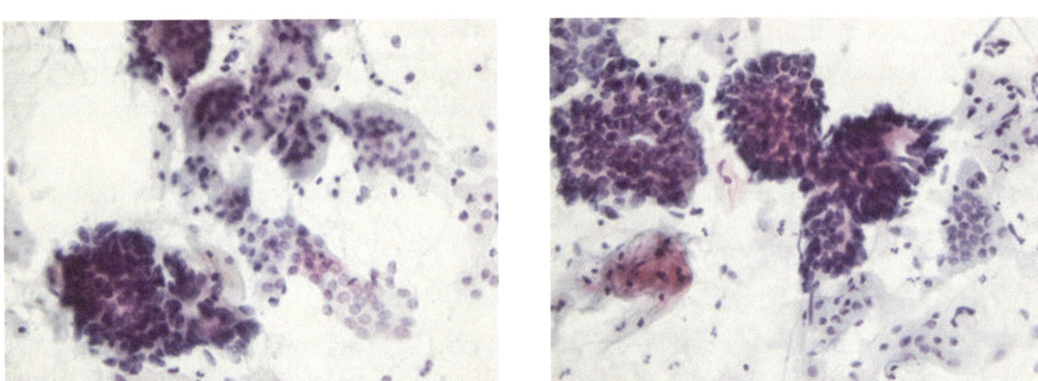

Fig. 6.3.2. AIS. Clusters of uniform small dark neoplastic cells and sheets of normal endocervical cells on the same field. (Papanicolaou x400)

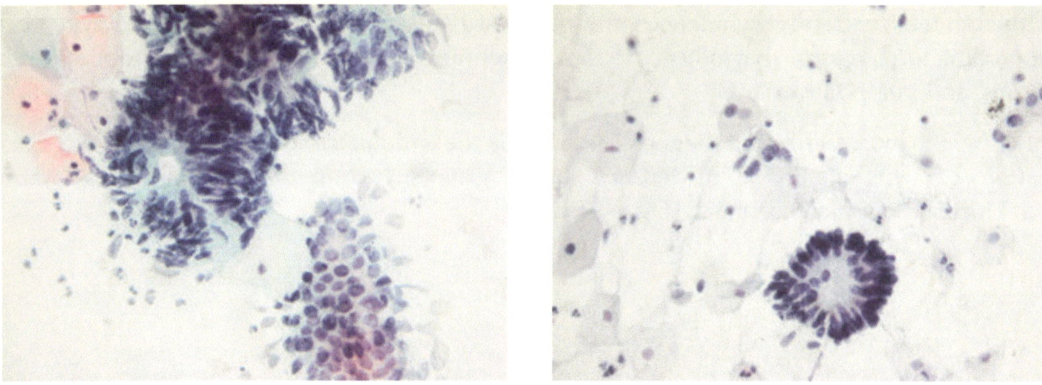

Fig. 6.3.3. AIS. Crowded sheet with "gland opening" and "rosette" of neoplastic cells. The nuclei are elongated, cigar-shaped, and hyperchromatic. Note a sheet of endocervical cells (left field) with slight nuclear enlargement and overlapping (GIL 1). (Papanicolaou x400)

The distinction between well differentiated and poorly differentiated AIS is based on nuclear features. In cell groups, the nuclei of cells of well-differentiated AIS are enlarged, oval or round, uniform, and have a regular nuclear membrane. When the cells are crowded the nuclei may be elongated, cigar-shaped, and hyper chromatic.

The chromatin is granular and evenly distributed. The nuclei in a portion of cells contain small nucleoli. Mitotic figures and apoptotic bodies are occasionally present.

Poorly differentiated AIS occurs less frequently then the well-differentiated type. (Fig.6.3.4.)

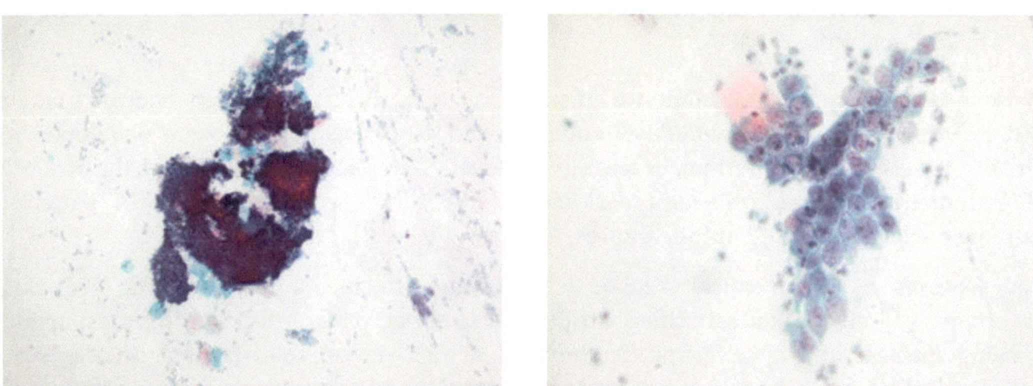

Fig. 6.3.4 Poorly differentiated AIS. The nuclei of the cells are round or irregular in shape and greatly enlarged, but less hyperchromatic and with finely granular chromatin. Nucleoli are multiple, irregular and enlarged. (Papanicolaou x100, x400).

In comparison to the cytological features of well-differentiated AIS, the nuclei of these cells are larger, but less hyperchromatic and with finely granular chromatin. The nuclei may be round and always contain nucleoli which may be multiple, irregular and/or enlarged. Mitotic figures can be seen. (Ayer et al., 1987; Pacey & Ng, 1997).

Although most endocervical adenocarcinoma in situ are of the usual 'endocervical' type, it is important to recognize that other variants sometimes occur. These include endometrioid, serous, and intestinal variants.

Of these, the most significant diagnostic variant is the endometrioid pattern (Lee, 1999). This pattern contains small cells in densely packed groups, having coarse nuclear chromatin exhibiting lack of pleomorphism (Fig.6.3.5.).

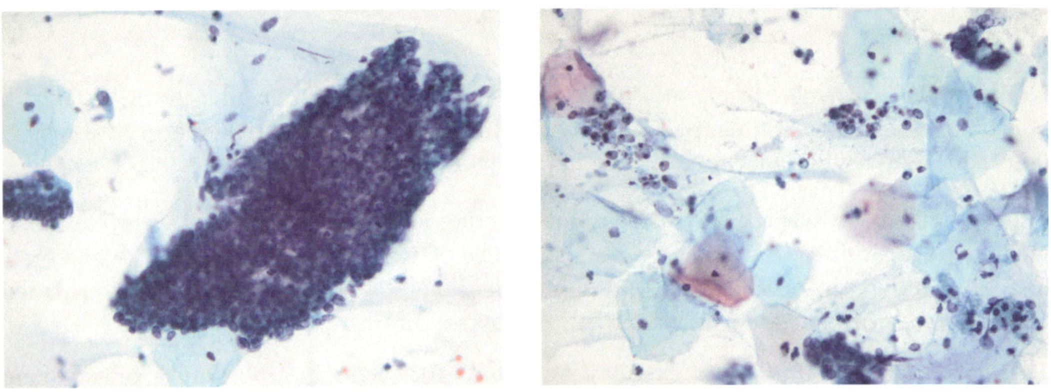

Fig. 6.3.5. AIS, endometrioid pattern, contains small cells in densely packet groups, having corse nuclear chromatin, exhibiting lack of pleomorphisam. Note apoptotic bodies on the right field (Papanicolaou x400).

These groups were more commonly misinterpreted as being of benign endometrial or endocervical origin (tubal metaplasia endometrioid variants). Criteria were developed to identify these cases as abnormal, at least to the level of atypical glandular cells: the absence of endometrial stromal cells and endometrial-like tubules, coarse chromatin patterns, extreme nuclear crowding, mitotic figures, and marginal feathering.

Key features of endocervical adenocarcinoma in situ are: hyperchromatic crowded groupings of cells, pseudostratified strips of columnar cells, epithelial rosettes, gland opening, nuclear and cytoplasmic 'feathering', twofold larger than normal nuclear size, endocervical nuclei, beyond normal increase of nucleus to cytoplasmic ratio, endocervical cells, coarsely granular and evenly distributed hyperchromatic chromatin, possible presence of small nucleoli, presence of mitotic figures and apoptotic bodies not associated with a background tumor diathesis

In a significant number of cases, abnormal squamous cells are present in association. (Fig.6.3.6) Focusing on these more commonly seen lesions can lead to a lack of identification of extant abnormal glandular processes. Careful observation and analysis of cervical cell samples should be exercised to identify these cells. Single malignant columnar cells may be mistaken as undifferentiated basal cells.

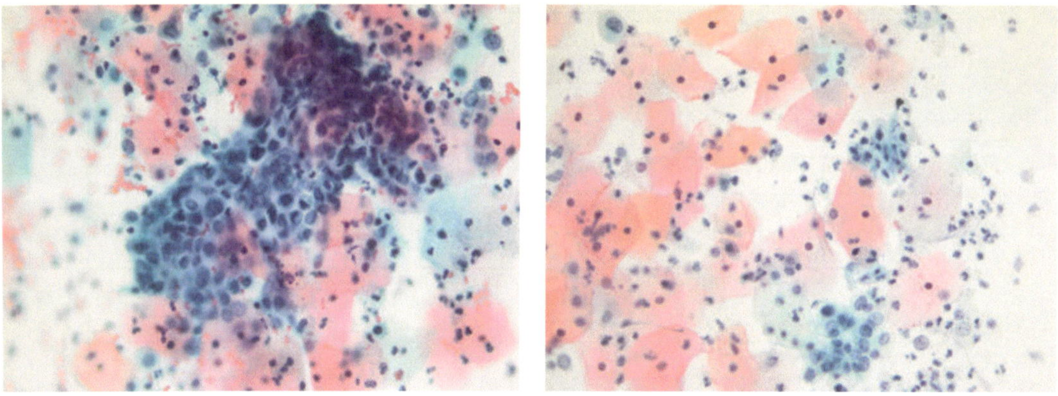

Fig. 6.3.6 CIS. A cluster of malignant squamous cells is present in association with small strip and single abnormal glandular cells (leading to lack of identification) (Papanicolaou x400).

7. Accuracy of cervical cytology

Intraepithelial lesions of the endocervical epithelium are more difficult to detect by cytology. However, cellular changes may frequently be less pronounced than those in squamous lesions and are difficult to observe unless architectural alterations call for attention. In mixed lesions, the glandular component may be eclipsed in abnormal cell count and intensity by the squamous component. (Boon et al., 1981; Di Tomasso et al., 1996).

In order to reach as accurate and precise a cytological diagnosis of intraepithelial lesions of endocervical cylindrical epithelium as possible, the cytological findings of patients with histologically verified adenocarcinoma in situ and mild to moderate glandular intraepithelial lesions were analyzed.(Ovanin-Rakic et al., 2010)

During the period 1993-2007, the value of cytology in the detection and differential diagnosis considering lesion severity and/or type of altered epithelium was assessed in 123 patients with a definite histological diagnosis of glandular lesions (AIS - n=13; GIL1 - n=11; GIL 2 - n7), glandular lesion associated with a squamous component (AIS+CIN/CI - n=58; GIL 1/GIL 2+CIN - n=28; GIL + MIC - n=6) (Table 2.).

Intraepithelial endocervical cylindrical lesions, with or without intraepithelial or invasive squamous component, were diagnosed in histological samples (78 biopsy specimens, 82 excochleation specimens, 70 conization specimens and 24 hysterectomy materials) from 123 patients aged 22-73 (mean 40).

The patients were divided into two categories : the first including 71 patients who were histologically diagnosed as AIS or AIS + CIN/CI, while the second included 52 patients who were histologically diagnosed as mild or moderate glandular intraepithelial lesions with squamous component (GIL1/ GIL2 + CIN, GIL + MIC) or without it (GIL1, GIL 2) .

In the first group, (table 2) cytological findings indicated epithelial abnormalities in 98.6% (70/71) patients. Considering lesion severity, the cytological and histological diagnoses were identical in 93% (66/71) patients.

Cytology	n	Histology					
		AIS		AIS + CIN	AIS + CI	AIS+CIN/CI	
		n	%	n	n	n	%
AIS	9	**8**	**61,5**	1		1	1,7
AIS + CIN	15	1	7,7	**12**	2	14	24,2
AC/Abnormal	6	3	23,1	3		3	5,2
AI + CIN	2			2		2	3,4
AI + CI	4			3	1	4	6,9
GIL + CIN	9			8	1	9	15,6
CIN	21			20	1	21	36,2
MIC	2			1	1	2	3,4
Abnormal	2			2		2	3,4
Inflammation	1	1	7,7				
Total	71	13 (100,0)		52	6	58	100,0
%	100,0	18,3		81,7			

Table 2. Cytohistologic correlation of either pure adenocarcinoma in situ (AIS) or a mixed AIS/squamous abnormality

The accuracy of cytological diagnosis according to lesion severity and type of epithelium was 92.3% (12/13) for glandular lesions and 56.9% (33/58) for mixed lesions.

In predicting the type of epithelium involved, the agreement between cytological and histological diagnosis was recorded in 61.5% (8/13) of histologically pure (AIS) and 20.7% (12/58) of mixed lesions (AIS + CIN / CI).

The accuracy of cytological identification of abnormalities of a particular type of epithelium, histologically diagnosed as either pure or mixed lesions, was 92.3% (12/13) and 96.6% (56/58) for cylindrical and squamous epithelium.

In the second group, (table 3), cytological findings indicated epithelial abnormality in 90.4% (47/52) patients. Considering lesion severity, the cytological and histological diagnoses were identical in 80.8% (42/52) patients.

The accuracy of cytologic diagnosis according to lesion severity and type of epithelium was 61.1% (11/18) for glandular lesions and 35.3% (12/34) for mixed lesions.

In predicting the type of epithelium involved, the agreement between the cytological and histological diagnosis was recorded in 22.2% (4/18) of histologically pure (GIL I) and 20.6% (7/34) of mixed lesions (GIL1,2 + CIN / MIC).

The accuracy of cytologic diagnosis according to lesion severity and type of epithelium was 61.1% (11/18) for glandular lesions and 35.3% (12/34) for mixed lesions.

In predicting the type of epithelium involved, the agreement between the cytological and histological diagnosis was recorded in 22.2% (4/18) of histologically pure (GIL I) and 20.6% (7/34) of mixed lesions (GIL1,2 + CIN / MIC).

Cytology	n	Histology								
		GIL I	GIL II	Total		GIL I + CIN	GIL II + CIN	GIL + MIC	Total	
		n	n	n	%	n	n	n	n	%
GIL I	4	**4**		4	22,2					
GIL I + CIN	8	2	2	4	22,2	3		1	4	11,8
GIL II+ CIN	5	1		1	5,6	1	**3**		4	1,8
AIS + CIN	4		2	2	11,1	1	1		2	5,9
GIL + MIC	2					1		**1**	2	5,9
CIN	24	1	1	2	11,1	8	10	4	22	64,6
Inflammation	5	3	2	5	27,8					
Total	52	11	7	18	100,0	14	14	6	34	100,0
%	100,0			34,6				65,4		

Table 3. Cytohistologic correlation of either pure gladular ysplasia (GIL) or a mixed GIL/squamous sbnormality

The rate of cytological identification of abnormalities of a particular type of epithelium, histologically diagnosed as either pure or mixed lesions, was 61.1% (11/18) and 100% (34/34) for cylindrical and squamous epithelium, respectively.

However, the fact that AIS patients are older than women with squamous CIS (Brown & Wells, 1986) and that the reverse is true for AI and CI could imply that the progression of GIL to AIS must be slower than the progression of CIN lesions to CIS.

In contrast, AIS should progress to AI significantly more rapidly than does CIS into CI That , indeed, seems to be the case. This would leave ample time for detection of glandular dysplasia, but not necessarily AIS (Plaxe & Saltzstein, 1999).

A coexisting SIL may obscure the presence of glandular lesion because abnormalities involving exclusively squamous components were quite frequently observed in the latter, either because of more distinct criteria and easier recognition, or due to more pronounced cellular lesions, or because of the predominant population of abnormal squamous cells, especially when extensive or high grade.

Historically, only sporadic cases of AIS were reported after it was first defined in 1953 by Friedell & McKay, 1953, who described only its histological appearance.

In the 1970s and 1980s, descriptive studies detailing the cytological criteria necessary for the prospective cytological diagnosis of AIS of the cervix uteri were published, increasing awareness and the diagnostic skill of cytologists.

For the cytologist intraepithelial glandular lesions pose possibly the greatest challenge in cervical sreening.

In a number of cases published over the period of 15 years, Papanicolaou smear screening detected a glandular abnormality before confirmation of AIS on cone biopsy or hysterectomy in 32- 79% cases. (Ayer et al., 1987; Azodi et al., 1999; Östör et al., 2000; Shin et al., 2002; Ovanin-Rakic et al., 2010).

Our observation has been that the number of AIS cases we identified has increased with time after our first identification in 1986.

The Papanicolaou smear in our patients had a sensitivity of 74.2% in detecting a glandular abnormality preoperatively. The cytological differential diagnosis of AIS showed a 61.5% and of GIL 1 22.2% accuracy. These results are similar to other reports (Ayer et al., 1987; Ioffe et al., 2003). Ioffe et al., 2003 have shown that the application of a semiquantitative system for the diagnosis of noninvasive endocervical glandular lesions results in better diagnostic reproducibility even in diagnostically problematic cases. Papanicolaou smear that includes adequate material from the transformation zone and endocervix can be a useful method for detecting precursor lesions of adenocarcinoma of the cervix. It bears remembering that cytology should not be recommended as the definitive diagnostic investigation for adenocarcinoma of the cervix uteri. If a clinician is suspicious of cancer during clinical examination, then he or she should proceed to colposcopy and biopsy regardless of the cytologic findings (Pacey & Ng, 1997).

8. Differential diagnosis

Cytological analysis of glandular lesion abnormalities in vaginal-cervical-endocervical (VCE) smears is associated with a number of diagnostic difficulties. Interpretation of the results must be based on scientific knowledge, meticulous training and experience, and demands dedication. To reach a definitive diagnosis utilizing cells that have desquamated freely from epithelial surfaces or cells that have been forcibly removed from various tissues, requires detailed examination of all available evidence. In this case, consideration must be given to both procedural aspects of the cytology laboratory and to changes that modify individual cells or cell groups.

There is overlap between the cytological criteria for various glandular lesions of the cervix, thus requiring more rigorous criteria for defining both benign and malignant cervical glandular lesions.

The emphasis is on criteria that discriminate among non-neoplastic conditions, benign neoplasms that may mimic malignancy, and malignant neoplasms that may pose as benign entities. Appropriate clinical data are certainly of great help in solving some of these diagnostic issues. Awarwness of cellular changes, together with pertinent clinical information , will prevent diagnostic errors.

8.1 Non-neoplastic lesions

8.1.1 Inflammatory changes in endocervical cells

Endocervical cells are usually present in small clusters, sheets, strips and pseudorosettes (small round groups of cells with peripheral cytoplasm), with minimal nuclear overlapping.

Hyperchromasia and mild anisonucleosis may be present in round or oval nuclei. Chromatin is finely stippled and may be smudged in the texture. Reactive/reparative atypical glandular cells are uniform in size and shape with small to medium-sized regular nucleoli and abundant cytoplasm. They are typically arranged in groups, rather than singly.

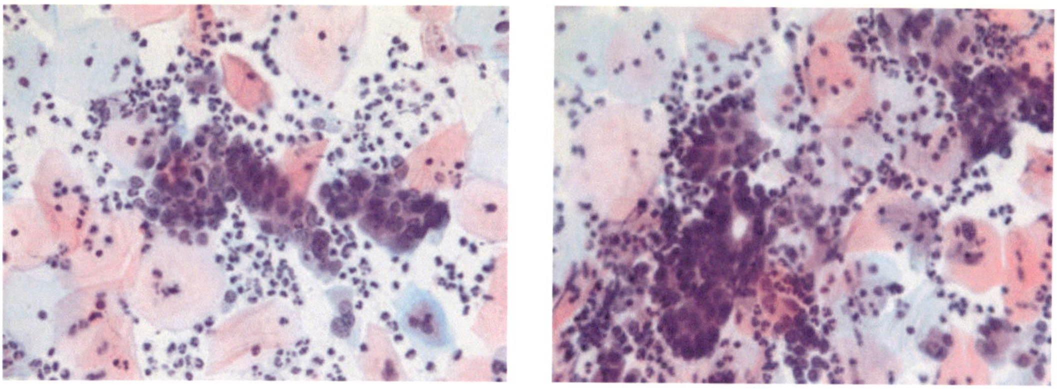

Fig. 8.1.1.1. A sheet of rective endocervical cells infiltrated by neutrophils with enlarged nuclei. Note a mitotic figure (left field) and gland opening (right field). These cells simulate glandular displasia.

The nucleoli are prominent, massive, spheroidal, and usually single, but they may vary in number. The cells can be multinucleated, variable in their size and shape, moulding, or overlapping each other, with very occasional mitoses seen in regenerating epithelial cells. There is a danger of mistaking these cells for endocervical adenocarcinoma cells. They differ by the regular distribution of their clumped chromatin and their smooth nuclear membrane. The most important feature which distinguishes sheets and clusters of endocervical cells with inflammatory changes from those of GIL is the exfoliation pattern. Nuclear stratification and feathering at the edge of sheets are features of GIL, which are rarely present in inflammatory smears. However, the cells seen in reactive conditions are usually monolayered with abundant cytoplasm. There is no stratification or 'feathering' of nuclei. Cells with marked nuclear enlargement, hyperchromasia and prominent nucleoli may be seen in polyps.

During pregnancy or the postpartum period, as a result of acute or chronic irritation, groups of endocervical cells can become considerably larger, with monstrous nuclei. They can be confused with anaplastic malignant cells, except for the persisting regularity of their smooth nuclear membrane and the abundance of their benign-appearing cytoplasm.

It is important to obtain clinical information in these situations and appraise cytological criteria for AIS with care (Naib, 1996; Pacey & Ng, 1997; Waddell, 2003).

8.1.2 Atypical repair

Reactive changes in epithelial cells are well described and generally well recognized as such by cytologists. Under some circumstances cells react to some injury of the epithelium. This condition of extreme reactivity, also known as atypical epithelial repair, can be problematic.

The cells seen in this condition may mimic a glandular abnormality, specifically invasive adenocarcinoma of the endocervix. (Fig. 8.1.2.1.) Cytoplasmic boundaries are well-defined and can clearly be seen in the overlapping or syncytial appearance of the groups noted in many neoplastic processes. Nuclei may be large with coarse chromatin and regular macro nucleoli are noted in virtually all nuclei. When repair becomes atypical, the nuclei begin to show variable degrees of pleomorphism of size and shape within the groups, often taking on nuclear contour irregularities. Chromatin patterns can turn from uniformly distributed to irregular and show coarse granularity. (Naib, 1996; Pacey & Ng, 1997; Waddell, 2003).

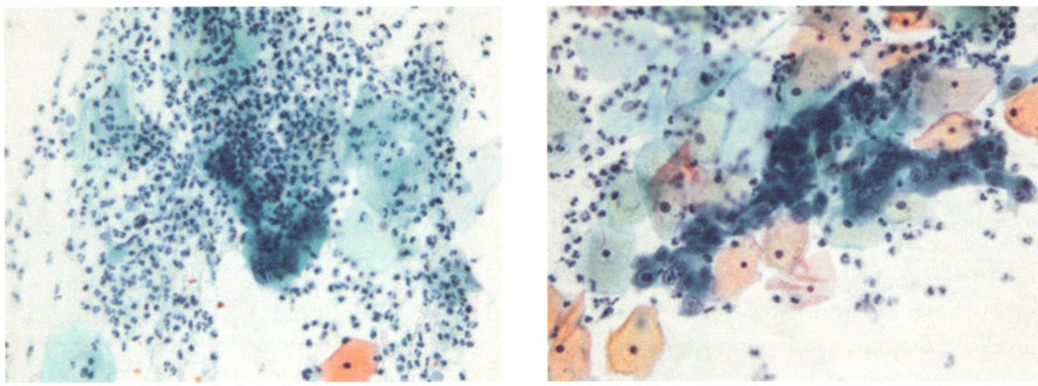

Fig. 8.1.2.1. This strips of atypical epithelial repair with enlarged nuclei. Some appear hyperchromatic and other have prominent nucleoli simulating adenocarcinoma. (Papanicolaou x400).

In determining diagnosis between atypical repair and invasive carcinoma, a designation of atypical glandular cells is warranted and an endocervical sampling procedure is required, as will be discussed below under management options.

8.1.3 Micro glandular endocervical hyperplasia

Micro glandular endocervical hyperplasia (MEH) is a localized proliferation of endocervical cells that can be mistaken for adenocarcinoma. MEH represents a non-neoplastic endocervical change usually related to progesterone effect or oral contraceptives. It is rarely seen in postmenopausal women.

The cytological manifestations of MEH falls in the spectrum of 'glandular atypia'. (Fig.8.1.3.1.)

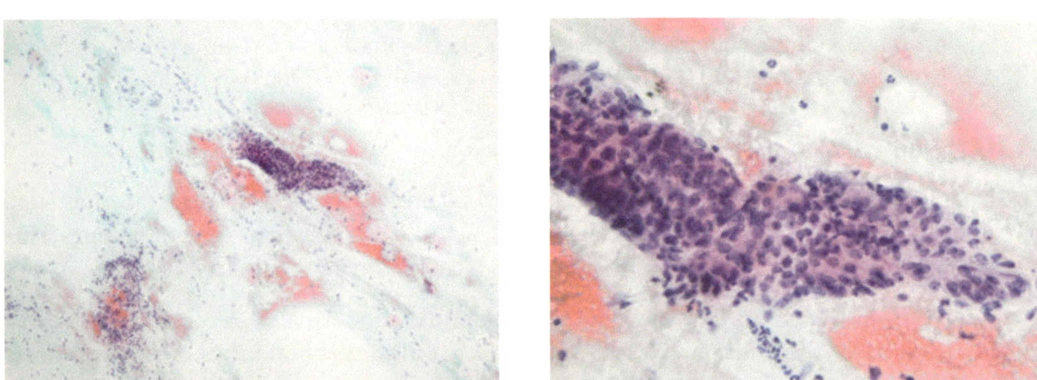

Fig. 8.1.3.1. A pseudostratified strip of endocervical cells is present. Nucleolar feathering at the periphery of the cluster, and nuclei are slightly enlarged. (Papanicolaou x 100, x 400).

The most common cytological findings are nuclear enlargement, nuclear hyperchromasia with fine nuclear chromatin, and nuclear overlap (Selvaggi and Haefner, 1997)

These are the presence of two- and three-dimensional fenestrated large sheets of cuboidal and columnar glandular cells, with finely vacuolated cytoplasm and with micro-rosette in sheets. Immature metaplastic cells, with dense basaloid cytoplasm, and reserve cells with little or no cytoplasm may also be seen. Reactive changes resulting in anisonucleosis, nuclear enlargement and prominent nuclei may lead to suspicion of either glandular or squamous neoplasia. The absence of chromatin heterogeneity, macro nucleolus formation, and tumour diathesis are the best discriminators in avoiding erroneous interpretation.

8.1.4 Sampling of the lower uterine segment, or post cone biopsy smears.

A cone biopsy shortens the endocervical canal allowing easier access to endometrial cells. Post cone biopsy smears may contain cells from this region which are referred to as lower uterine segment or LUS cells. Charateristic here is the presence of long tubular, branching glands embedded in loose monomorphic stroma. This is best observed on low power magnification.

Sampling of the lower uterine segment (LUS) following conisation is a result of endocervical brush or broom sampling of the endometrial cavity secondary to a shortened endocervical canal. This may occur following a conisation procedure or vigorous use of endocervical brushes in patients who have not undergone conisation. (Fig.8.1.4.1.)

Post cone biopsy smears are screened with a high index of suspicion, so the unwary can overreact to the presence of high endocervical cells or debrided endometrial cells in the smears.

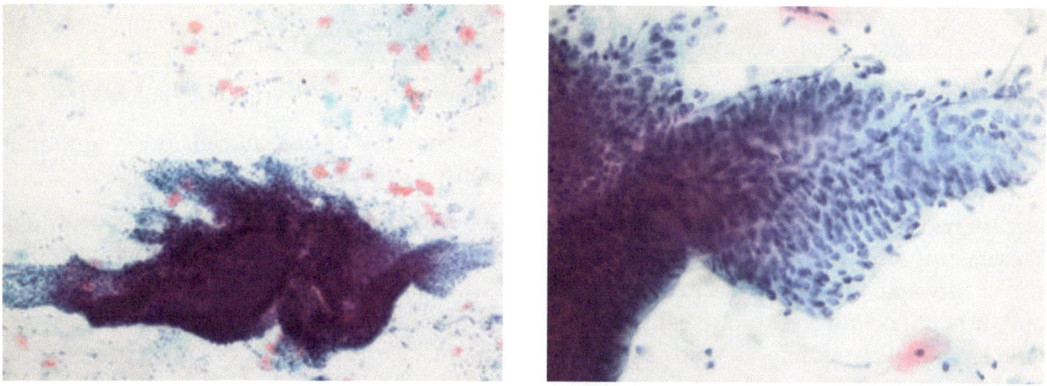

Fig. 8.1.4.1. Tightly crowded large group with pseudostratification and peripheral streaming of nuclei mimicking feathering (low uterine segment sampling) (Papanicolaou x100, x400).

Smears from the LUS show cellular two- or three-dimensional fragments with branching tubular glands that are embedded in stroma that is composed of round to spindle-shaped cells. In such circumstances, it is advisable to review the smear with the histology of the cone biopsy and with the previous abnormal Papanicolaou smear samples that led to the cone biopsy.

When compared with AIS smears, LUS sampling smears show smaller nuclei with less distinct nuclear membranes; densely dispersed, but finely granular chromatin, less frequent mitotic figures, and abundant endometrial-type stromal cells in the background (Hong et al., 2001). Presence of the endometrial-type stromal cells is significant; it is absent from the background of all cases of AIS.

Most false-positive interpretations are secondary to the presence of groups of nonciliated small glandular cells from either the upper endocervical canal or lower uterine segment of the endometrium (Lee, 1993, 1999).

These tightly crowded groups differ from AIS by having smaller, less hyperchromatic nuclei with finer chromatin, and by being intermixed with benign epithelial cells, and, occasionally, endometrial stromal cells. (Fig.8.1.4.2).

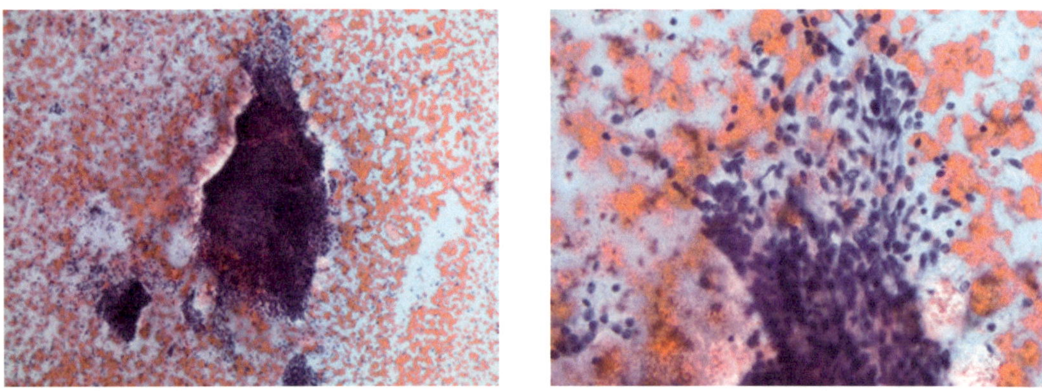

Fig. 8.1.4.2. Tightly crowded groups with benign epithelial cells, and, occasionally, endometrial stromal cells (post cone biopsy smears). (Papanicolaou x100, x400)..

More striking are the large and branching fragments of crowded glandular tissue.

Appreciation of the cytological features of LUS cells is essential to avoid misdiagnosis.

Presence of glandular cells of endometrial origin showing round nuclei, finely granular chromatin and nuclear crowding. Nucleoli are inconspicuous.

Occasional peripheral palisading of cells is noted and glandular openings are often visible. Presence of stromal cells showing uniform round to spindle-shaped nuclei, fine granular chromatin and scant cytoplasm. Peripheral cells are loosely attached and appear 'strung out'. It is important to exercise caution in examining post cone smears especially in women who have had a previous diagnosis of adenocarcinoma. Residual tumor may be present and careful scrutiny is required to differentiate abnormal from LUS cells.

8.1.5 Tubal metaplasia

Tubal metaplasia may pose a cytological problem. This refers to the replacement of normal endocervical glandular epithelium by foci of benign epithelium resembling that of normal fallopian tube epithelium. Apart from the smooth chromatin pattern of the nuclei, the most valuable feature for identification of tubal metaplasia is the density of cell cytoplasm, with blunted luminal edges bearing terminal bars and cilia. (Fig.8.1.5.1)

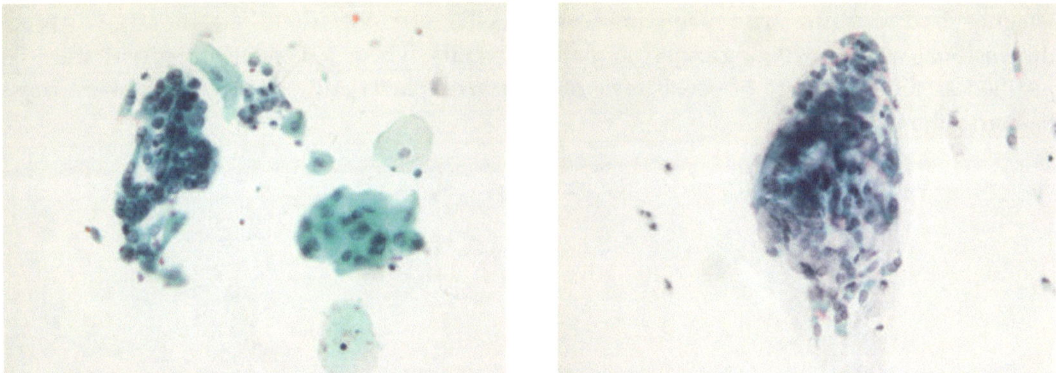

Fig. 8.1.5.1. Groups of cells with nuclear crowding, but the nuclear chromatin is finely granular. Note the terminal cilia. (Papanicolaou x400).

However, this may be a significant cause of false-positive smears for glandular neoplasia. When seen, it appears as flat sheets or cohesive clusters, and in palisade or mosaic patterns. It can mimic AIS because of nuclear crowding, nuclear overlap, nuclear feathering and nuclear palisading. Rosettes are uncommon, and, most importantly, the nuclear chromatin is finely granular and evenly distributed. Mitotic figures and apoptosis are rare. The identification of terminal bars and cilia is the most helpful cytological finding, but these features may not be present in some cases (Lee, 1993, 1999; Salvaggi & Haefner, 1997), since they may be lost during processing. Conversely, terminal bars and cilia are rarely seen in AIS.

The key to distinguishing difficult presentations of tubal metaplasia where cilia are absent is a careful review of nuclear chromatin. Most often the cells of tubal metaplasia will have normal 'endocervical' chromatin.(Fig.8.1.5.2.; Fig.8.1.5.3.; Fig 8.1.5.4.)

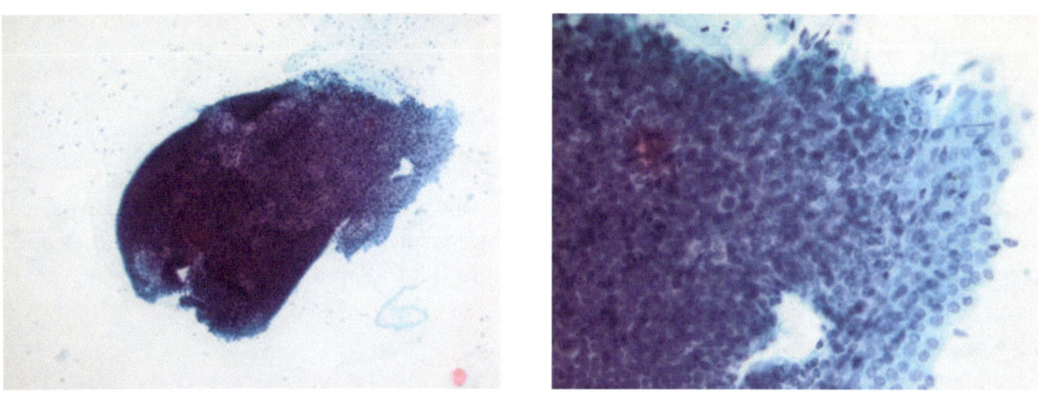

Fig. 8.1.5.2. Large three-dimensional and crowded groups of glandular cells. The cells at the edge of the fragments retain their cytoplasm and have a relatively smooth border and there is slight nuclear overlapping. (Papanicolaou x100, x400).

The typical chromatin pattern of AIS is coarse and evenly distributed. In addition, apoptotic nuclear fragments are not generally found in cases of benign tubal metaplasia, but may be commonly noted in neoplasias.

Diagnostic difficulties arise sometimes when cilia are not identified in large three-dimensional and crowded groups of glandular cells. Then, a borderline report may be justified as the possibility of coexistence of tubal metaplasia and glandular neoplasia must be borne in mind.

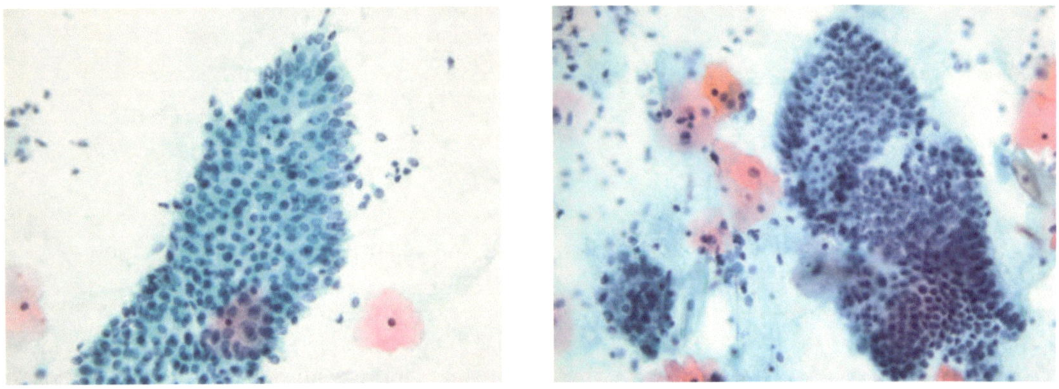

Fig. 8.1.5.3. Large groups of glandular cells with pseudo-stratification et the edge od the clusters. that mimicking feathering. The nuclear chromatin is finely granular and evenly distributed. (Papanicolaou x400).

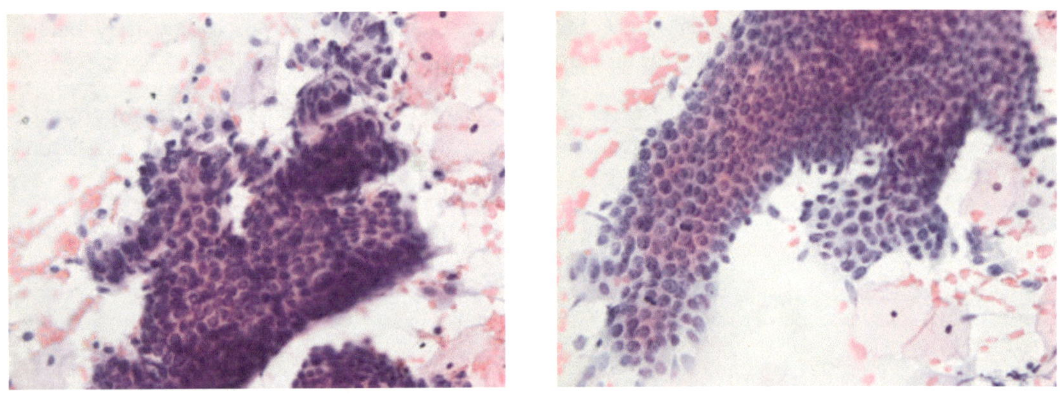

Fig. 8.1.5.4. . Large group and strips of glandular cells with palisading (left field). Large cluster that mimicking feathering (right field) . The nuclear chromatin is finely granular and evenly distributed. Note a mitotic figure on the right field. (Papanicolaou x400).

8.2 Neoplastic lesions

8.2.1 Carcinoma in situ

One of the major differential cytological diagnoses of AIS is endocervical gland involvement by CIS. In these cases, highly atypical nuclei are identified in the center of the cell aggregate, and some of the cells at the periphery of the aggregate appear to be endocervical cells. Involvement of endocervical glands by squamous CIS shows a syncytial arrangement, loss of cell polarity, and nuclear overlapping within the center of cell clusters whereas AIS cells generally maintain cell polarity. (Fig.8.2.1.1.)

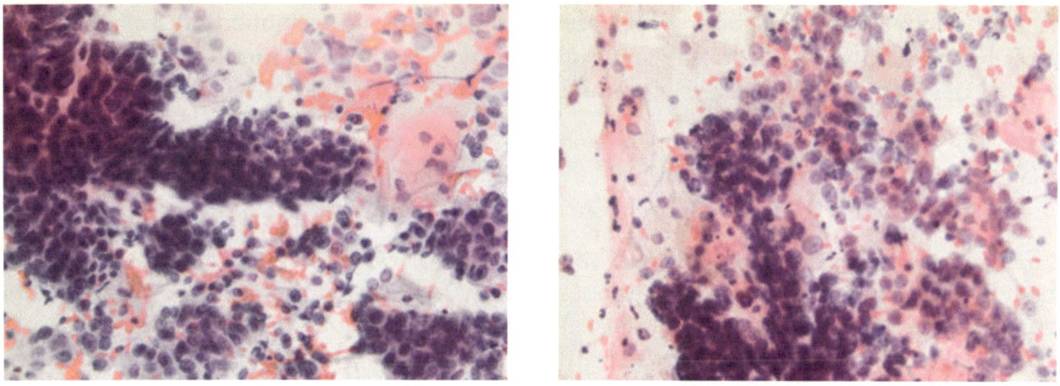

Fig. 8.2.1.1. CIS. A syncytial arrangement, loss of cell polarity, and nuclear overlapping within the center of cell clusters. Some of the cells at the periphery appear to be endocervical. (Papanicolaou x400).

The identification of occasional cells with dense eosinophilic cytoplasm and hyper chromatic cigar-shaped nuclei favors squamous CIS over AIS.

The identification of occasional cells with dense eosinophilic cytoplasm and hyper chromatic cigar-shaped nuclei favors squamous CIS over AIS.

Strips, rosettes, and gland formations, which are characteristic of AIS, are not observed in squamous CIS. In the infrequent cases that defy the above distinction, a diagnosis of atypical endocervical cells favouring AIS with a notation that squamous CIS cannot be excluded may be considered.

8.2.2 Adenocarcinoma in situ and invasive carcinoma

The most serious error is mistaking AIS for a benign process: small cell 'endometrioid' AIS, mistaken for direct sampling of the lower uterine segment endometrial cells; AIS mimicking tubal/tubo-endometrial metaplasia cells. This differential diagnosis may be extremely difficult or, in some cases, impossible in Papanicolaou smears. (Lee, 1993, 1999)

Endometrial adenocarcinoma may be mistaken for AIS if there is extension into the cervix and if the lesion is directly sampled.

Squamous carcinoma may be mistaken for adenocarcinoma if poorly differentiated.

9. New methods

A number of new technologies have been developed to improve the detection of cervical lesions, and a wide array of immuno-histochemical markers have been evaluated with respect to their specificity in staining abnormal cells in cervical cytological smears. However, there is still a significant demand for better biomarkers to identify neoplastic cervical glandular epithelial cells precisely. The most important advancement in cervical cytology has been the introduction of **liquid-based cytology (LBC)**. The advantages of LBC - compared to conventional cytology - are its increased sensitivity for detecting epithelial cell abnormality, reduced number of specimens with obscuring blood and inflammation, and the possibility of performing **molecular assay** directly from liquid-based specimens when a diagnosis of atypical cells is made (Bishop, 2002).

Human Papillomavirus (HPV DNA) detection is a potential biomarker of a neoplastic diagnosis in women with glandular abnormalities in their cervical smears. A positive HPV test is more strongly associated with squamous neoplasia than with glandular lesions.

Studies have shown that the prevalence of HPV in adenocarcinoma may be underestimated because the glandular epithelium does not support productive viral infections. HPV DNA in endocervical neoplasia is usually present in integrated form and not in the episomal particles. This integration may result in deletion of the viral genome. Detection of HPV DNA in the assay could depend on the presence of intact episomal HPV copies (Pirog et al., 2000).

Tumor suppressor protein (p16INK4a). Some studies have shown increased high-risk viral oncogene expression in dysplastic cervical epithelia, and have demonstrated that p16INK4a protein as a specific biomarker for the identification of dysplastic cervical epithelia in sections of cervical biopsy samples or cervical smears and in thin-layer LBC specimens (Murphy et al., 2002, Juric et al., 2006, 2010). The use of p16INK4a protein as a definitive marker for cervical neoplasia would be a valuable supplementary test in gynecologic cytology. A test result is considered positive if brownish granules are found in the nuclei and/or cytoplasm of dysplastic or malignant cells. (Fig.9.1.)

Murphy et al. 2004, compared the expression patterns of p16INK4a in benign and neoplastic glandular lesions and tubo-endometrioid metaplasia. All cases in each category displayed some p16INK4a expression.

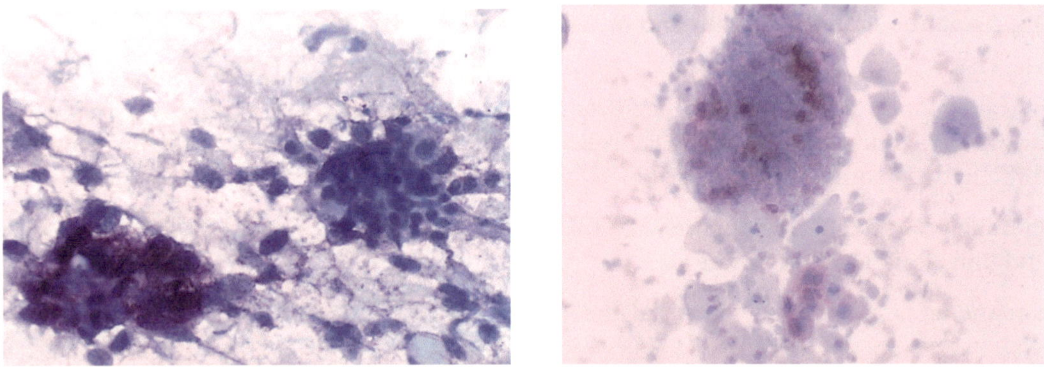

Fig. 9.1. p16INK4a postive staining of cluster malignant edocervical cells (AIS) left field, and of atypical endocervical cells (GIL2) and of high-grade squamous intraepthelial lesions (HSIL) on right field. Note a cluster of normal glandular cells p16INK4a negative staining on the left field. (x400, 100)

While p16INK4a has been demonstrated to be an excellent marker of cervical dysplasia in squamous neoplastic lesions of the cervix, it has potential pitfalls in cervical glandular lesions that may limit the utility of this biomarker in resolving the nature of suspicious glandular lesions, particularly in cytopathology.

Based on our results in detecting SIL lesions and carcinoma of the uterine cervix (Juric et al.,2010), immunocytochemical expressions of p16INK4a in ThinPrep cervical specimens correlate closely with the HPV-high-risk typed specimens through the polymerase chain reaction method (PCR) in the same samples.

We can assume that the combination of these tests can identify two groups within low-grade lesions, i.e. one with low risk for the development of premalignant cervical lesions, for which both of these tests are negative, and another group with both tests positive and with an increased risk of squamous intraepithelial lesions.

The value of immunocytochemical expressions of p16INK4a as adjunct methods for detection and differential diagnosis of glandular lesions has been investigated.

Imaging of silver-stained nucleolar organizer regions (AgNORs) is one of the more recent methods (Ploton et al. 1986). Nucleolar Organizer Regions (NORs) are structured from loops of ribosomal deoxyribonucleic acid (rDNA). Under the influence of RNA polymerase I, they are transcribed to ribosomes and proteins sited on the short arms of acrocentric chromosomes 13, 14, 15, 21, and 22. Since they have the central role in the transcription of nucleic acid into proteins, their number and size can be a reflection of cell proliferation, transformation or overt malignancy (Crocker, 1990). This method reveals AgNORs in the form of brown-black dots of different sizes within the nucleus. In numerous papers, the differential diagnostic and prognostic value of AgNOR analysis has been emphasized, on histological (Crocker, 1990; Darne et al., 1990) as well as cytological

(Fiorella et al., 1994; Audy i sur. 1995; Ovanin-Rakic & Audy-Jurkovic, 1998; Mahovlic et al., 1999) samples of benign, borderline and malignant lesions at various locations, and its significance has rarely been disputed.

Automated image analysis is applied to avoid the subjective error of an observer and to decrease the time necessary for data processing. This automated process was applied **in 1996** as a fast, reproducible method on archival cytological specimens from cervix uteri stained by the Papanicolaou method (Ovanin-Rakic & Audy-Jurkovic, 1998) from 16 patients with a histological diagnosis (4 endocervical glandular dysplasia, 5 adenocarcinoma in situ, 7 adenocarcinoma invasivum) and 10 patients with benign endocervcal cells at the Institute of Gynecological Cytology, Department of Obstetrics and Gynecology, Medical School, University of Zagreb.

AgNORs are shown in the nucleus as dark brown to black dots. The count, area and size of AgNOR per square micrometer (minute <0.24; small 0.25 - 0.74; medium 0.75 - 1.4; large 1.5 - 2.4; extra large > 2.25) were analyzed in 50 cells per smears magnified 1,000x, on the focal plane. The SFORM system was used for digital image analysis (VAMS, Zagreb, Croatia) at the Institute of Pathology and Pathological Anatomy, Medical School, University of Zagreb. The system includes a high-resolution CCD color TV camera transferring images from the microscope (Olympus BHS, Tokyo, Japan) to a PC-compatible computer via a picture digitizer, with a resolution of 512 x 512 pixels, whereby each of them can assume a value described by 24 bits.

While measuring, the results of parameters measured are automatically transferred and logged in previously defined tables. The data obtained were processed on a PC by the

SPSS/PC+ 3.0 program (Chicago, Illinois, U.S.A.). Mann-Whitney and x2 tests were applied to test the differences between the groups, while statistical significance was tested at the level P= .05.

Our results showed that the mean values of AgNOR count and area per nucleus increased from benign endocervical cells (1.9; 2.17 μ2), and dysplasia (2.11; 2.53 μ2), and AIS (3.1; 3.27 μ2) to AI (3.,7; 5.49 μ2). The differences between all groups are statistically significant (P<.05)

Regarding AgNOR size and histological diagnosis, most frequently found were minute AgNORs in AIS (7.8%) and AI (6.7%), then benign (2,1%), and dysplasia (1.9%), while extra large AgNORs most frequently found in AI (15.9%). The differences between groups are statistically significant (P<.05) except for the pairs benign endocervical glandular cells and dysplasia.

One AgNOR per nucleus was usually present in benign endocervical cells (43.6%), and four or more in adenocarcinoma, especially adenocarcinoma invasivum (37.6%; 51.7%) with the differences between all groups being statistically significant (P<.05). (Fig.9.2.)

The AgNOR technique is a simple, inexpensive and reliable method applicable to both histological and cytological samples. AgNOR number is considered to be a reflection of cell proliferation. According to the literature, digital AgNOR image analysis of endocervical benign and abnormal glandular cells has not been performed before.

Our results indicate an increase in the mean value of AgNOR count from normal to intraepithelial and invasive glandular lesions, corresponding to the results on histological samples (Allen & Galimore, 1992; Darne et al., 1990; Miller et al., 1994), and cytological smears (Fiorella et al., 1994; Audy-Jurkovic et al., 1995). A significant finding of four or more AgNORs in 51,7% indicating adenocarcinoma invasivum that correlates to the results on histological samples (Miller et al., 1994).

Digital AgNOR image analysis (count, size and area) in cytological specimens of the cervix uteri indicated that the method is helpful in differentiating benign, intraepithelial and invasive lesions of the endocervical cylindrical epithelium, because statistically significant differences were obtained among all groups except for the benign state - dysplasia pair according to AgNOR size (p=0.8946).

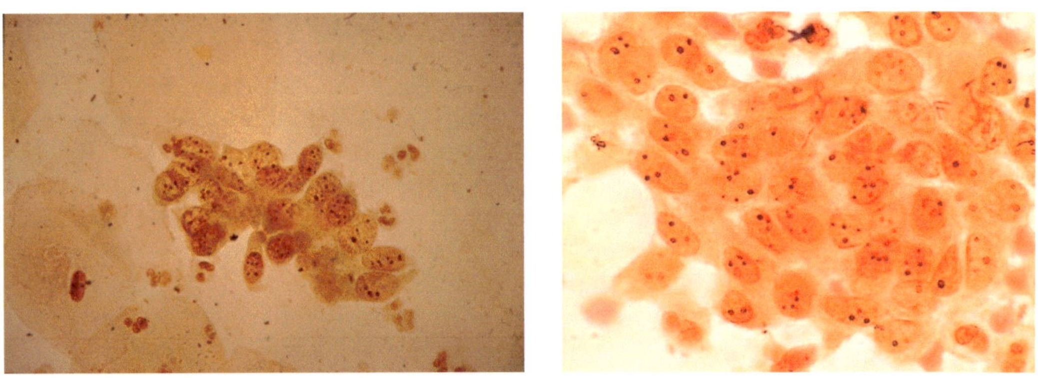

Fig. 9.2. AgNOR-stained. Cluster of adenocarcinoma in situ (left field), and adenocarcinoma invasivum (right fields). Note different types of brown-black dots within the nucleus.

10. Conclusion

Intraepithelial lesions of the endocervical epithelium are difficult to detect by cytology. However, recent studies show some favourable trends. In our study, the cytological differential diagnosis of AIS showed a 61.5% accuracy. The diagnostic accuracy of cytology is by far higher for pure (cylindrical only) than for mixed (cylindrical + squamous) lesions, because the abnormalities involving exclusively squamous component were quite frequently observed in the latter, either because of more distinct criteria and easier recognition, or due to more pronounced cellular lesions, or because of the predominant population of abnormal squamous cells.

The cytodiagnosis of cervical cylindrical epithelial lesions lags behind the cytodiagnosis of squamous epithelial lesions both in terms of screening and differential diagnosis. As data continue to accumulate, the clinical characteristics of pre-invasive glandular cervical lesions are becoming progressively better defined. Cytological screening for these lesions is imprecise. A major problem is the relative infrequency of glandular lesions and inexperience with sometimes difficult differentiation between benign glandular cells and the endocervix or lower segment of the endometrium. However, modifications to current classification systems may improve overall diagnostic accuracy. Nevertheless, all glandular abnormalities on the Papanicolaou smear require judicious evaluation and careful follow-up.

At present, the solution lies in better education. When in the hands of experienced cytologists, difficult cases of intraepithelial glandular lesions can be reliably distinguished from benign processes most of the time. The problem is in translating this experience to the entire community of cytologists, including cytotechnologists. Experience demands increased sensitivity, and cytologists and cytotechnologists both play a critical role in attempts to increase sensitivity in the face of demands for diagnostic specificity.

As our understanding of glandular lesions continues to expand and cervical sampling techniques continue to improve, we may expect continued enhancement in our ability to detect and treat intraepithelial glandular lesions, and thus help to decrease morbidity and mortality from cervical adenocarcinoma

11. References

Allen JP. & Gallimore AP. (1992). Nucleolar organizer regions in benign and malignant glandular lesions of the cervix. *The Journal of Pathology,* Vol.166, No.4 (February 1992), pp. 153-6, ISSN: 1096-9896

Audy-Jurković S. (1986). Citološka klasifikacija cerviksa uterusa. *Medicinska enciklopedija, II. Dopunski svezak,* Zagreb: Jugoslavenski leksikografski zavod, 93.

Audy-Jurković S, Singer Z, Pajtler M, Dražančić A & Grizelj V. (1992). Jedinstvena klasifikacija citoloških nalaza vrata maternice u Hrvatskoj. *Gynecol Perinatol,* Vol.1, No.4 (April 1992), pp. 185-8. ISSN: 1330-0091

Audy-Jurković S, Ovanin-Rakić A, Mahovlić V, Molnar Stantic B, Ilic-Forko J, Milicic D, Strelec M & Dimitrovski V. (1995). Citomorfologija argirofilnih nukleolarnih organizacijskih regija (AgNOR) u razlikovanju lezija endocervikalnih cilindričnih stanica. *Proceedings of the first Croatian congress of clinical cytology "Prvi hrvatski kongres kliničke citologije".* Zagreb, March 1995

Ayer B, Pacey F, Greenberg M & Bousfield L. (1987). The cytologic diagnosis of adenocarcinoma in situ of the cervix uteri and related lesions. I. Adenocarcinoma in situ. *Acta Cytologica*, Vol.31, No.3, (May-June 1987), pp.397-411. ISSN: 0001-5547

Azodi M, Chambers SK, Rutherford TJ, Kohorn EI, Schwartz PE & Chambers JT. (1999). Adenocarcinoma in situ of the cervix: management and outcome. *Gynecologic Oncology*, Vol.73, No.3, (Jun 1999), pp. 348-53. ISSN: 0090-8258

Betsill WL,jr. & Clark AH. (1987). Early endocervical glandular neoplasia. Hystomorphology and cytomorphology. *Acta Cytologica*, Vol.30, No. 2, (March-April 1987), pp.115-26 ISSN: 0001-5547

Bertrand M, Lickrish GM & Colgan TJ. (1987). The anatomic distribution of cervical adenocarcinoma in situ implications for treatment. *American Journal of Obstetrics & Gynecolog*, Vol.157, No.1, (Juy 1987), pp. 21-25. ISSN: 0002-9378

Bharucha H, McCluggage G, Lee J & al. (1993). Grading cervical dysplasia with AgNORs using a semiautomated image analysis system. *Analytical & Quantitative Cytology & Hystology*,Vol15, No.5, (Octobar 1993), pp. 323-8. ISSN: 0884-6812

Biscotti CV, Gero MA, Toddy SM, Fischler DF & Easley KA. (1997). Endocervical adenocarcinoma in situ: an analysis of cellular features. *Diagnostic Cytopathology*, Vol.17, No.5, (November 1997), pp.326-32. ISSN: 8755-1039

Bishop JW. (2002). Cellularity of liquid-based, thin-layer cervical cytology slides. *Acta Cytologica*, Vol.46, No.4 (July-August 2002), pp.633-6. ISSN: 0001-5547

Boon ME, Baak JP, Kurver PJ & al. (1981). Adenocarcinoma in situ of the cervix: an underdiagnosed lesion. *Cancer*, Vol.48, No.3, (August 1981), pp. 768-773. ISSN: 0008-543x

Boon ME & Gray W(2003) Glandular Neoplasms of the Uterine Cervix, In: *Diagnostic Cytopathology*, Gray W & McKee GT, pp 651-7o5, Churchill Livingstone, ISBN 0 443 06473 3, China

Bousfield L, Pacey F, Young Q, Krumins I & Osborn R. (1980). Expanded cytologic criteria for the diagnosis of adenocarcinoma in situ of the cervix and related lesions. *Acta Cytologica*, Vol.24, No.2. (March-April 1980), pp. 283-96. ISSN: 0001-5547

Brown LJR & Wells M. (1986). Cervical glandular atypia associated with squamous intraepithelial neoplasia: a premalignant lesion? *Journal of Clinical Pathology*, Vol.39, No.1 (January 1986), pp. 22-8. ISSN: 0021-9746

Casper GR, Ostor AG & Quinn MA. (1997). A clinicopathologic study of glandular dysplasia of the cervix. *Gynecologic Oncology*, Vol.64, No.1, (January 1997), pp. 166-170. ISSN: 0090-8258

Chieng DC & Cangiarella JF. (2003). Atypical glandular cells. *Clinics in Laboratory Medicine* , Vol.23, No.5, (May 2003), pp. 633-7. ISSN: 0272-2712

Crocker J. (1990). Nucleolar organizer regions. *Current topics in pathology,* Vol.82, No.1, (January 1990), pp. 91 - 149. ISSN: 0070-2188

Darne JF, Polacarz SV, Sheridan E, Anderson D, Ginsberg R & Sharp F. (1990). Nucleolar organizer regions in adenocarcinoma in situ and invasive adenocarcinoma of the cervix. *Journal of Clinical Pathology,* Vol.43, No.8, (August 1990), pp. 657 - 660. ISSN. 0021-9746

DiTomasso JP, Ramazy I & Mody DR. (1996). Glandular lesions of the cervix. *Acta Cytologica,* Vol.40, No.6, (November-December 1996), pp. 1127-1135. ISSN: 0001-5547

Fiorela RS, Saran B & Kragel PJ. (1994). AgNOR counts as a discriminator of lesions of the endocervix. *Acta Cytologica,* Vol.38, No.3: (May-June 1994), pp. 527-30. ISSN: 0001-5547

Friedell GH & McKay DG. (1953). Adenocarcinoma in situ of the endocervix. *Cancer,* Vol.6, No.5, (September 1953), pp.887-97. ISSN: 0008-543x

Gloor E & Hurlimann J. (1986). Cervical intraepithelial glandular neoplasia (adenocarcinoma in situ and glandular dysplasia). A correlative study of 23 cases with histologic grading, histochemical analysis of mucins and immunohistochemical determination of the affinity for four lectins. *Cancer* (Phila), Vol.58, No.6, (September), pp. 1272-80. ISSN: 0008-543x

Goldstein NS, Ahmad E, Hussain M, Hankin RC & Perez-Reyes N. (1998). Endocervical Glandular atypia: Does a preneoplastic lesion of adenocarcinoma in situ exist? *American Journal of Clinical Pathology* , Vol.110, No.2, (August 1998), pp. 200-209. ISSN: 0002-9173

Hirschowitz Eckford SD, Phillpotts B & Midwinter A. (1994). Cytologic changes Associated with Tubo-Endometroid Metaplasia of the Uterine Cervix. *Cytopathology,* Vol.5, No.1, (February 1994), pp. 1 - 8. ISSN: 0956-5507

Higgins GD, Uzelin DM, Phillips GE, McEvoy P, Marin R & Burrell CJ. (1992). Transcription patterns of human papillomavirus type 16 in genital intraepithelial neoplasia: evidence for promoter usage within the E7 open reading frame during epithelial differentiation. Journal of General Virology , Vol.73, No.8, (August 1992), pp. 2047-57. ISSN: 0022-1317

Im DD, Duska LR & Rosenshein NB. (1995). Adequacy of conisation margins in adenocarcinoma in situ of cervix as a predictor of residual disease. *Gynecologic Oncology* Vol.59, No.2, (November 1995), pp. 179-82. ISSN: 0090-8258

Ioffe OB, Sagae S, Moritani S, Dahmoush L, Chen TT & Silverberg SG. (2003) Should Pathologists Diagnose Endocervical preneoplastic Lesions "Less Then" Adenocarcinoma In Situ?: Point. *International Journal of Gynecological Pathology,* Vol.22, No.1, (January 2003), pp. 18-21. ISSN: 0277-169

Juric D, Audy-Jurkovic S, Ovanin-Rakic A, Mahovlic V & Babic D. Introduction of p16 ink4a biomarker on fresh and archival cervical smears. (abstract). *Pathologica,* Vol.98, No.5, (October 2006) pp. 425.

Juric D, Mahovlic V, Rajhvajn S, Ovanin-Rakic A, Skopljanac-Macina L, Barisic A, Samija Prolic I, Babic D, Susa M, Corusic A & Oreskovic S. (2010). Liquid-based cytology - new possibilities in the diagnosis of cervical lesions. *Collegium Antropologicum,* Vol.34, N.1, (January 2010), pp 19 - 24. ISSN: 0350-6134

Krane JF, Lee KR, Sun D & Yuan L Crum CP. (2004). Atypical glandular cells of undetermined significance. Outcome predictions based on human papillomavirus testng. *American Journal of Clinical Pathology* , Vol.121, No.1 (January 2004), pp. 87-92. ISSN: 0002-9173

Krumins I, Young Q, Pacey F, Bousfield L & Mulhearn L. (1977). The cytologic diagnosis of adenocarcinoma in situ of the cervix uteri. *Acta Cytologica,* Vol.21, No.2 (March-April 1977), pp. 320-9. ISSN: 0001-5547

Kurian K & al-Nafussi A. (1999). Relation of cervical glandular intraepithelial neoplasia to microinvasive and invasive adenocarcinoma of the uterine cervix: a study of 121 cases. *Journal of Clinical Pathology,* Vol.52, No.2 (February 1999), pp.112-7. ISSN. 0021-9746

Kurman R & Solomon D. (1994) The Bethesda System for reporting cervical/vaginal cytologic diagnoses. Definitions, criteria, and explanatory notes for terminology and specimen adequacy. *Springer-Verlag,* New York ISBN: 0-387-94077-4

Lee KR. *(1993).* Atypical glandular cells in cervical smears from women who have undergone cone biopsy. A potential diagnostic pitfall. *Acta Cytologica, Vol.*37, No.5 (September-October 1993), pp. 705–9. ISSN: 0001-5547

Lee KR, (1999). Adenocarcinoma in situ with a small (endometrioid) pattern in cervical smers: a test of the distinction from benign mimics using specific criteria. C*ancer Cytopathology,* Vol25. No.87 (October 1999), pp 254-8. ISSN 1934-662X

Ljubojevic N, Babic S, Audy-Jurkovic S, Ovanin-Rakic A, Jukic S, Babic D, Grubisic G, Radakovic B & Ljubojevic-Grgec D. (2001). Improved national Croatian diagnostic and therapeutic guidelines for premalignant lesions of the uterine cervix with some cost-benefit aspects. *Collegium Antropologicum,* Vol.25, N.2 (December 2001)*,pp* 467-74. ISSN: 0350-6134

Mahovlic V, Audy-Jurkovic S, Ovanin-Rakic A, Bilusic M, Veldic M, Babic D, Bozikov J & Danilovic Z. (1999). Digital image analysis of silver-stained nucleolar organizer region associated proteins in endometrial cytologic samples. *Analytical & Quantitative Cytology & Histology* Vol.21. No.1 (January 1999),pp 47- 53. ISSN: 0884-6812

Miller B, Flax S, Dockter M & Photopulos G. (1994). Nucleolar organizer regions in adenocarcinoma of the uterine cervix. *Cancer,* Vol.15. No.73.(12) (december 1994), pp 3142 - *3145.* ISSN: 0008-543x.

Murphy N, Ring M, Killalea AG, Uhlmann V, O'Donovan M, Mulcahy F, Turner M, McGuinnes E, Griffin M, Martin C, Sheils O & O'Leary JJ. (2003). p16INK4A as a markea cervical dyskaryosis: CIN and GIN in cervical biopsies and ThinPrep smears of Clinical Pathology; Vol.56, No.1 (January 2003), pp.56-63. ISSN: 0021-9746.

Naib ZM. (1996). Cytology of the normal female genital tract. In: *Cytopathology, fourth edition* by Little, brown and Company. ISBN: 0-316-59674-4

National Cancer Institute Workshop. (1993). The revised Bethesda System for reporting cervical/vaginal cytologic diagnoses. *Acta Cytologica,* Vol.37, No.1, (January-February 1993), pp.115-24. ISSN: 0001-5547

National Cancer Institute Workshop. (1989). The 1988 Bethesda System for reporting cervical/vaginal cytologic diagnoses. Developed and approved at the National Cancer Institute Workshop. Bethesda, Maryland, USA, December 12-13. *Acta Cytologica,* Vol.33, No.4 (July-August 1989), pp. 567-74. ISSN: 0001-5547

National Cancer Institute Workshop. (1993). The revised Bethesda System for reporting cervical/vaginal cytologic diagnoses. *Acta Cytologica,* Vol.37, No.1, (January-February 1993), pp.115-24. ISSN: 0001-5547

NCI Bethesda System 2001. website http://bethesda 2001.cancer.gov

Nieminen P, Kallio M & Hakama M. (1995). The effect of mass screening on incidence and mortality of squamos and adenocarcinomaof the cervix uteri. *Obstet Gynecol,* VOL.85. No.6. (Jun 1995), pp. 1017-21. ISSN: 0029-7844

Östör AG, Duncan A, Quinn M & Rome R. (2000). Adenocarcinoma in situ of the uterine cervix: An experience with 100 cases. *Gynecologic Oncology,* Vol.79, pp. 207-210. ISSN: 0090-8258

Ovanin-Rakić A & Audy-Jurković S. (1988). Novije metode u citodijagnostici vrata maternice. In: Eljuga D, Dražančić A i sur. Prevencija i dijagnstika tumora ženskih spolnih organa. *Naknadni zavod Globus, Hrvatsko društvo ginekologa i opstetričara, Klinika za tumore i Hrvatska liga protiv raka, Zagreb,* 114-22. ISBN: 953-167-111-7

Ovanin-Rakić A, Pajtler M, Stanković T, Audy-Jurković S, Ljubojević N, Grubišić G & Kuvačić I. (2003). Klasifikacija citoloških nalaza vrata maternice "Zagreb 2002" Modifikacija klasifikacija "Zagreb 1990" i "NCI Bethesda System 2001 ". *Gynaecologia et Perinatologia,*Vol.12.No.4 (October-December 2003), pp 148-53. ISSN: 1330-0091

Ovanin-Rakic A, Mahovlic V, Audy-jurkovic S, Barisic A, Skopljanac-Macina L, Juric D, Rajhvajn S, Ilic-Forko J, Babic D, Folnovic D & Kani D. (2010). Cytology of cervical intraepithelial glandular lesions. *Collegium Antropologicum,* Vol.34, N.2 (Jun 2010), pp 401-406. ISSN: 0350-6134

Pacey NF, Ayer B & Greenberg M. (1988). The cytologic diagnosis of adenocarcinoma in situ of the cervix uteri and related lesions III. Pitfalls in diagnosis. *Acta Cytologica,* Vol.32, No.2 (March-April 1988), pp. 325-9. ISSN: 0001-5547

Pacey NF & Ng. ABP (1997). Glandular Neoplasms of the Uterine Cervix. Chapter 10. In: Bibbo M ed. *Comprehensive Cytopathology.* Philadelphia: Saunders.

Pajtler M & Audy-Jurković S. (2002). Pap smear adequacy: is the assessing criterion including endocervical cells really valid? *Collegium Antropologicum,* Vol.26, N.2 (December 2002), pp. 565-570. ISSN: 0350-6134

Park JS, Hwang ES, Park SN, Ahn HK, Um SJ, Kim CJ, Kim SJ & Namkoong SE. (1997). Physical status and expression of HPV genes in cervical cancers. Gynecologic Oncology, Vol.65. No.4 (April 1997), pp. 121-129. ISSN: 0090-8258

Pirog EC, Kleter B, Olgac S, Bobkiewicz P, Lindeman J, Quint WG, Richart RM & Isacson C. (2000). Prevalence of human papillomavirus DNA in different istological subtypes of cervical adenocarcinoma. American Journal of Pathology ,Vol.157. No.4 (October 2000), pp. 1055-1062. ISSN: 0002-9173

Plaxe SC & Saltzstein SL. (1999). Estimation of the duration of the preclinical phase of cervical adenocarcinoma suggests that there is ample opportunity for screening. *Gynecologic Oncology* Vol.75. No.1 (October 1999); pp. 55-61. ISSN: 0090-8258

Ploton D, Manager M, Jeannesson P, Himberg G, Pigeon F & Adnet JJ. (1986). Improvement in the staining and in the visualization of the AgNOR proteins (argyrophilic proteins of the

nucleolar organizer region) et the optical level. Histochemical Jurnal, Vol. 18 (, 1986),pp. *5-14. ISSN: 1681-715x*

Rabelo-Santos SH, Derchain SFM, Amaral Westin MC, Angelo-Andrade LAL, Sarian LOZ, Oliveira ERZM, Morais SS & Zeferino LC. (2008). Endocervical glandular cell abnormalities in conventional cervical smears: evaluation of the performance of cytomorphological criteria and HPV testing in predicting neoplasia. *Cytopathology,* Vol.19. No.1 (February 2008) pp 34-43. ISSN: 0956-5507

Roberts JM, Thurloe JK, Bowditch RC & Laverty CR. (2000). Subdividing atypical glandular cells of undetermined significance according to the Australian modified Bethesda system. *Cancer,*Vol.90. No.2 (April 2000), pp. 87-95. ISSN: 0008-543x

Ruba S, Schooland M, Allpress S & Sterrett G. (1994). Adenocarcinoma in situ of the uterine cervix. Screening and diagnostic errors in Papanicolaou smears. *Cancer (Cancer Cytopathol),* Vol.102. No.5 (October 1994) pp. 280-7. ISSN: 0008-543x

Selvaggi SM. (1994). Cytologic features of squamous cell carcinoma in situ involving endocervical glands in endocervical brush specimens. *Acta Cytologica,* Vol.38, No.4, (July-August 1994), pp. 687 - 692. ISSN: 0001-5547

Selvaggi SM & Haefner HK. *(1997).* Microglandular hyperplasia and tubal metaplasia: pitfalls in the diagnosis of adenocarcinoma on cervical smears. *Diagnostic Cytopathology,* Vol.16. No.2 (February 1997) pp 168–73. ISSN: 8755-1039

Shin CH, Shorge JO, Lee KR & Sheets EE. (2002). Cytologic and biopsy findings leading to conization in adenocarcinoma in situ of the cervix. *Obstetrics & Gynecology,* Vol.100. No.2 (August 2002) pp 271-6. ISSN: 0029-7844

Singer A & Monaghan JM. (2000). Lower Genital Tract Precancer. Colposcopy, Pathology and Treatment. *Blackwel Science,* pp. 153-60 ISBN: 0-0632-04769-0

Solomon D, Davey D, Kurman R et al. (2002). The 2001 Bethesda System: terminology for reporting results of cervical cytology. *JAMA,* Vol. 287. No.16 (April 2002) pp 2114-9. ISSN: 0098-7484

Stoler MH, Rhodes CR, Whitbeck A, Wolinsky SM, Chow LT & Broker TR. (1992). Human papillomavirus type 16 and 18 gene expression in cervical neoplasias. Human Pathology, Vol. 23. No.2 (February 1992), pp. 117-28. ISSN: 0046-8177

Tase T, Okagaki T, Clark BA et al. (1989). Human papillomavirus DNA in glandular dysplasia and microglandular hyperplasia: Presumed precursors of adenocarcinoma of the uterine cervix. *Obstetrics & Gynecology,* Vol. 73. No.6 (June 1989) pp1005-1008. ISSN: 0029-7844

van Aspert - van Erp AJ, van t Hof-Grootenboer AB, Brugal G & Vooijs GP. (1995). Endocervical columnar cell intraepithelial neoplasia. *Acta Cytologica,* Vol.39, No.6, (November-December 1995), pp. 1199-1215. ISSN: 0001-5547

Waddell C. (2003) Glandular Neoplasms of the Uterine Cervix, In: *Diagnostic Cytopathology,* Gray W & McKee GT, pp 769-789, Churchill Livingstone, ISBN 0 443 06473 3, China

Willson C & Jones H. (2004). An audit of cervical smears reported to contain atypical glandular cells. *Cytopathology,* Vol.15. pp. 181-187. ISSN: 0956-5507

Zaino RJ. (2000). Glandular lesions of the uterine cervix. *Mod Pathology,* Vol.13. pp. 261-274. ISSN: 0893-3952

Part 7

Intraepithelial Neoplasia of Vulva

17

Expression of Vascular Endothelial Growth Factors VEGF- C and D, VEGFR-3, and Comparison of Lymphatic Vessels Density Labeled with D2-40 Antibodies as a Prognostic Factors in Vulvar Intraepithelial Neoplasia (VIN) and Invasive Vulvar Cancer

Robert Jach et al*,
Department of Obstetrics and Gynecology,
Jagiellonian University Medical College, Kraków,
Poland

1. Introduction

Vulvar cancer consists of 2.5-5% of all cancers of the female genital tract. Poland is a country with an average occurrence of this tumor. Most women suffer from this disease between the ages of 60 and 70 years. Recently conducted epidemiological studies indicate that the incidence of intraepithelial neoplasia and vulvar cancer is increasing particularly in women under 50 years of age. The epidemiological model of vulvar cancer in young women involves the role of sexually transmitted infections (sexually transmitted diseases), especially HPV infection with high oncogenic potential, such as HPV 16, 18, 45, 56, 66 and 69; also considered is the importance of habitual smoking in the process of disease genesis.

In older women, vulvar cancer coexists in a high percentage of cases with hyperplasia, lichen sclerosus and squamous cell carcinoma. In 60% of women, vulvar cancer develops in the labia majora, to a lesser percentage of the labia minora, the clitoris and posterior labial commissure. The method of choice in the treatment of vulvar cancer is surgery. Radiation and chemotherapy treatment are usually combined with surgical treatment. Radical excision of the vulva, together with regional lymph nodes, is an operation that involves early and late complications (Judson et al., 2006). Removal of lymph nodes in which metastatic cells are present leads to a reduction in tumor mass, which can have a positive therapeutic effect.

---

* Grzegorz Dyduch[2], Małgorzata Radoń-Pokracka[1], Paulina Przybylska[1], Marcin Mika[1], Klaudia Stangel-Wojcikiewicz[5], Joanna Dulińska-Litewka[3], Krzysztof Zając[1], Hubert Huras[1], Joanna Streb[4] and Olivia Dziadek[1]

[1] *Department of Obstetrics and Gynecology, Jagiellonian University Medical College, Kraków, Poland*
[2] *Department of Pathology, Jagiellonian University Medical College, Kraków, Poland*
[3] *Department of Medical Biochemistry Jagiellonian University Medical College, Kraków, Poland*
[4] *Department of Oncology, Jagiellonian University Medical College, Kraków, Poland*
[5] *Department of Gynecology and Oncology, Jagiellonian University Medical College, Krakow, Poland*

Cancer metastases present in the lymph nodes removed (lymphadenectomy) is also important for the final classification of the clinical stage of cancer and to decide on how to continue therapy.

Histopathologic assessment of lymph nodes removed in the vulvar cancer operation shows that metastatic cancer cells are found in the I ° stage of cancer in about 16%, grade II clinical stage in about 36%, an average of approximately 28 to 33% of cases. Thus, in approximately 70% of the women operated on with vulvar cancer, whereby there is no evidence of metastasis to the lymph nodes, removal does not improve treatment results (Markowska, 2006). Furthermore, the removal of normal lymph nodes may also have an adverse impact on the local immune status, which is important to the treatment of cancer.

Vulvar intraepithelial neoplasia (VIN) and its classification remains controversial. There are currently three systems of classification VIN:

1. The 3-staged, WHO classification system: VIN1-3
2. The Bethesda system type classification, two-staged, dividing the low-VIN and high degree VIN, and
3. The 2004 established ISSVD classification (International Society for the Study of Vulvovaginal Disease) does not stage VIN. The incidence of VIN has increased in recent decades, while the incidence of invasive vulvar cancer has remained at the same level or even declined in some countries. For example, the U.S. prevalence of VIN3 (vulvar carcinoma in situ) increased by 411% between 1973 and 2000, while the incidence of invasive vulvar cancer increased by only 20% during the same period of time (Judson et al., 2006).

Women with the immunodeficiency virus are approximately four times more vulnerable to HPV infection. However, the incidence of VIN in HIV-positive women ranges from 0.5 to 37% (Kuhn et al., 1999). Thus, a high percentage of HIV infection in women with VIN suggests recommended HIV testing for women with VIN. The lifetime risk of developing invasive cancer in women previously treated for VIN3 is between 2.5-7% (Iversen & Treli, 1998; Jones & Rowan, 1994; Thuis et al., 2000). (Figure 1).

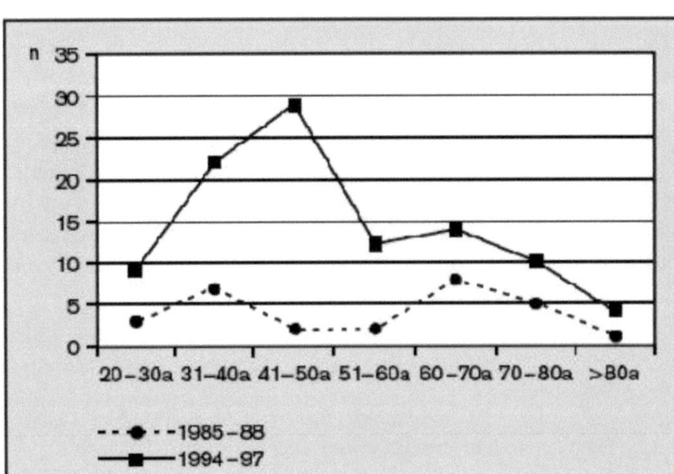

Fig. 1. VIN 2/3 incidence.

VIN is also an independent predictor of relapse (relative risk 3.06) as demonstrated in a study of 101 patients and 33 recurrences Preti (Preti et al., 2000).

In recent years, it has been observed that there is an increased incidence of vulvar cancer in women of younger ages leading to the search for less radical, but also effective surgical methods. These methods have allowed, on one hand, the reduction of injury, reduction of surgery time and reduction in the rate of postoperative complications and importantly, improvement in the quality of life for these women. To achieve this goal, it is equally important to recognize new prognostic factors, among which molecular factors are an attractive model, both in terms of diagnostics and therapeutic potential.

Lymphatic vessels play a key role in the spread of cancer. In recent years, several markers have been identified specific for lymphatic endothelium, which allowed for improved knowledge of the interaction between lymph vessels and lung cancer, but many issues in relation to their prognostic significance remains unclear (Judson et al., 2006; Markowska, 2006).

Proteins belonging to the family of glycoprotein endothelial growth factor (VEGF), referred to as VEGF-C and VEGF-D, are considered the most important regulatory factors in lymphangiogenesis. These factors are potent mitogens to the lymphatic and vascular endothelium. Furthermore, VEGF-C causes an increase in vascular permeability. These regulatory factors are ligands for the receptor VEGFR-3, whose expression is restricted to the endothelium of lymphatic vessels, and in the formation of blood vessels during embryogenesis. Factors VEGF-C and VEGF-D have been identified as stimulators of lymphatic endothelial proliferation, acting through the activation of the receptor 3 VEGF (VEGFR-3), which functions as a specific receptor in mature tissues and shows strong expression within the endothelial cells (Wissmann & Detmar, 2006; Najda & Detmar, 2006). Many clinical studies have shown a positive correlation between expression of VEGF-C and VEGF-D in the primary tumor and lymph node metastases (Donoghue et al., 2007; Nisato et al., 2003).

2. Aim

The aim of the study is to compare the immunohistochemical expression of vascular endothelial growth factors VEGF-C and D, and the expression of VEGFR-3, in VIN and vulvar invasive cancer, and to also compare the density of lymphatic marker D2-40 antibody in both groups, as prognostic factors, and to compare them with other clinicopathologic features.

3. Material and methods

The study was based on tissue material obtained during surgical procedures performed in the Department of Gynecology and Oncology at Jagiellonian University from 2006-2008. This tissue was in the form of cubes stored in paraffin, kept in the archives of the Department of Pathology. The clinical data of patients treated was obtained from the Department of Gynecology and Obstetrics. (Figure 2-6). The material was fixed in formalin on a routine basis. The analysis included 100 cases of vulvar dysplasia (30 - VIN I, 10 - VIN2, 60-VIN3) of which the average age of the patient was 65 years, and 10 cases of vulvar cancer of which the average age was 71 years. Patients were observed in the Gynecology Oncology Clinic of Jagiellonian University, Krakow from 12 to 48 months. At intervals of 4 - 6 months, patients were evaluated by history and physical examination, undergoing cytologic-colposcopic screening, and assessment of HPV DNA. In case of recurrence, a second operation was performed. The average age of women with vulvar cancer was 71.1 (59-79) years of age and was significantly higher than the average age of women with VIN, which was 56.6 (43-78) years at $p = 0.003$. (Table 1, Figure 7)

Type	n	Average mean	SD	min	max
VIN3	60	56,0	14,4	43	78
VIN2	10	67,0		67	67
ViN1	30	54,3	3,8	50	57
All groups VIN	100	56,6	11,5	43	78
Ca	100	71,1	7,2	59	79

Table 1. Charakteristics of women studied with VIN and vulvar cancer.

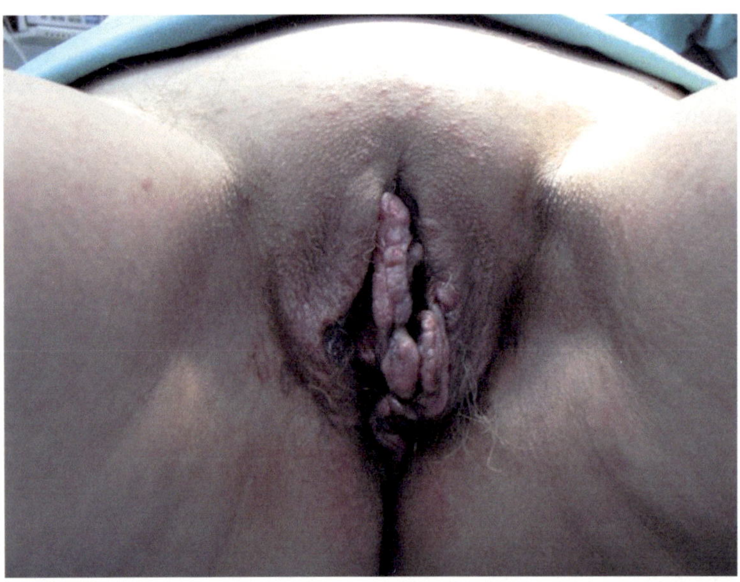

Fig. 2. VIN3 clinical manifestation.

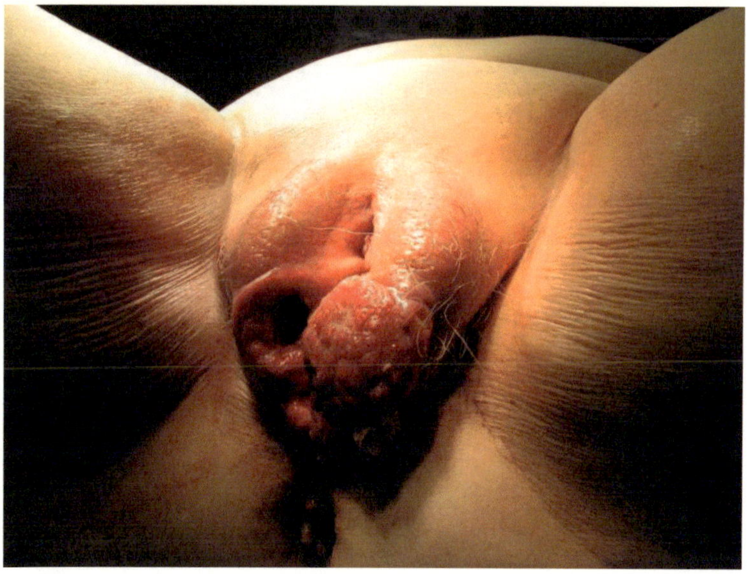

Fig. 3. Vulvar cancer. Clinical presentation.

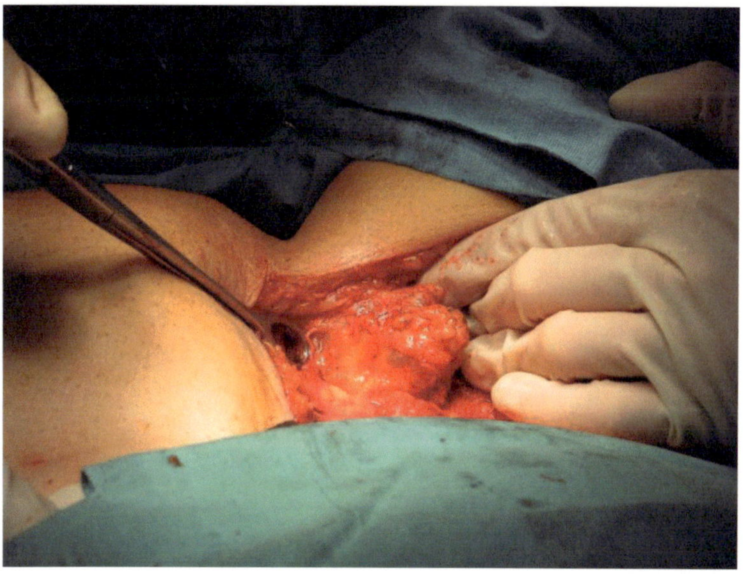

Fig. 4. Metastatic inguinal lymphnodes in vulvar cancer.

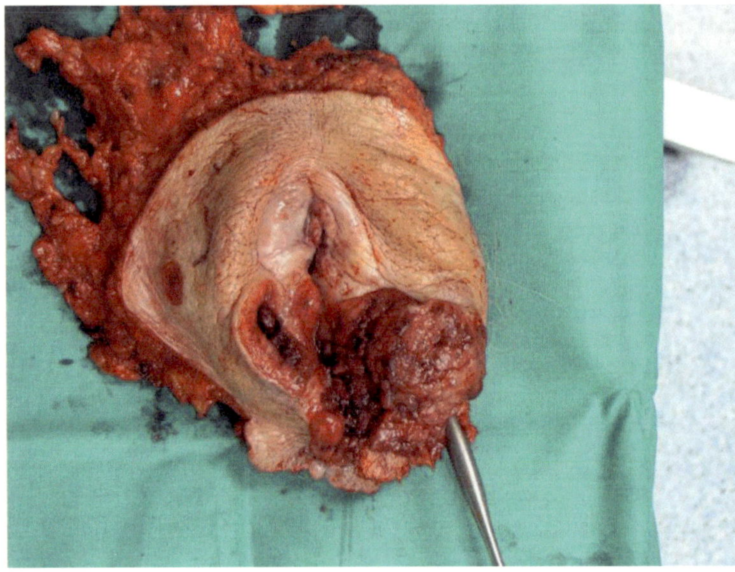

Fig. 5. Postoperative speciemen

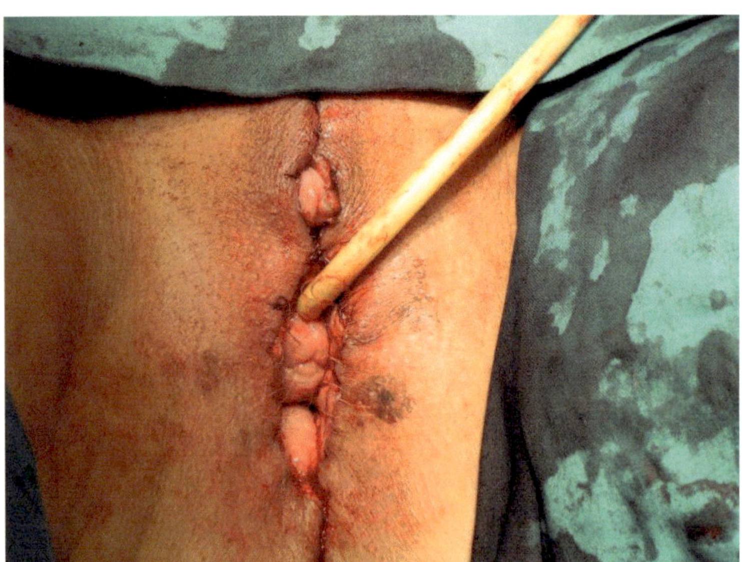

Fig. 6. Clinical presentation after surgery in vulvar cancer.

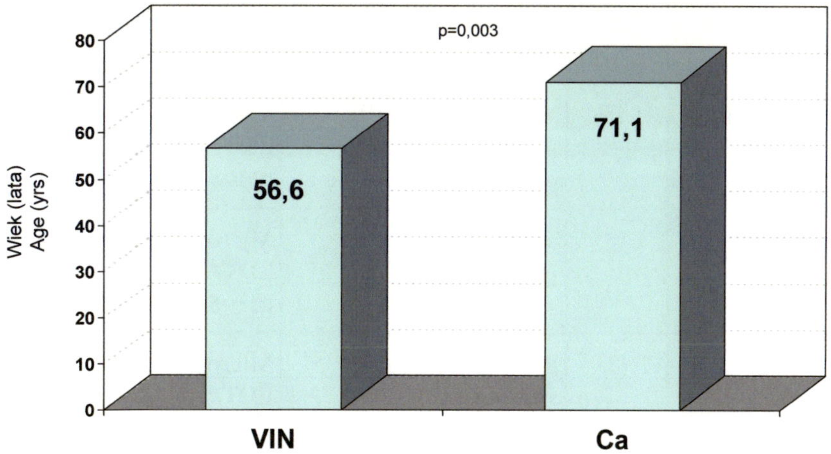

Fig. 7. Age distribution in VIN and vulvar cancer.

The diagnosis of VIN and vulvar cancer was based on histological evaluation of specimens taken from the vulva with guidance of the colposcope. In every case, specimens were also assessed in the presence of the HPV DNA test using Hybrid Capture II (DIGENE Corp.) with the material taken directly from the vulvar brush made of Dacron. The sample was also assessed histologically for metastasis in lymph nodes (superficial inguinal and deep) collected bilaterally in all 100 cases of vulvar cancer and 100 cases of VIN (clinically examined enlarged lymph nodes) during surgical treatment.

For immunohistochemical studies, samples were selected individually and made into paraffin blocks, each representative of a specific case.

From the selected paraffin cubes, 4 microns thick, samples were placed on glass slides coated with silanized basic Super Frost + (SuperFrost Inc.). Deparafinization involved placing the sample for 10 minutes in xylene and then dehydrated lead through three changes of ethyl alcohol of increasing concentration (70%, 86% and 96%), each lasting 5 minutes. In order to inhibit endogenous peroxidase activity, preparations were placed for 10 min in 3% H202 solution. Antigen unmasking was achieved by heating in a microwave oven Whirlpool, 3 times for 5 minutes in a 750W preparation placed in citrate buffer (pH 6.0, 0.01m), or EDTA buffer (pH 8.0, 0.01M).

After incubation, preparations were washed with TBS buffer (50 mM Tris-Hcl, 150 mM NaCl, pH 7.6, DAKO Corporation). To visualize the antigen-antibody complex, we used the En Vision system (DAKO Corporation) and Lab Vision (LabVision) (see the table) with 3-amino-9-ethylcarbazole (AEC) (DAKO Corporation) as a chromogen. Nuclei were contrasted with *Mayer* Hematoxylin for 1 minute and then covered with slide coverslips in glycerol. Basic data on the antibody used in the work is presented in Table 2.

Positive control preparations were: tonsil - for D2-40, placenta- for VEGFR-3 and VEGF-C and VEGF-D, ductal carcinoma of the breast - for VEGF-C and VEGF-D, the small intestine - for D2-40. Negative controls were the same antibody preparations as the original.

Antibody	Type	Clone	Manufact urer	Dilution	Unmasking	Time	Detection system
VEGFR-3	monoclonal	KLT9	Novocastra	1:50	Microwave EDTA, pH=8,0	60 min	Lab Vision
VEGF-C	polyclonal		Santa Cruz	1:100	Microwave EDTA, pH=8,0	12 hrs	En Vision
VEGF-D	monoclonal	78923	R&D systems	1:200	Microwave EDTA, pH=8,0	12 hrs	En Vision
D2-40	monoclonal	D2-40	Covance	Ready-to-use	Microvave citrate buffer ph=6,0	30 min	En Vision

Table 2. Antibodies, their dilution and incubadion time

4. Evaluation of immunohistochemistry

Lymphatic vessel density was evaluated using high power (40x). (Figure 8-10) All D2-40 positive vessels within the area of 0,5mm width beneath the dysplastic epithelium (VIN) or invasive edge of the tumor were counted and the result has been provided. All vessels were counted and the result is given as the number of vessels per 2mm. (Figure 11, 12).

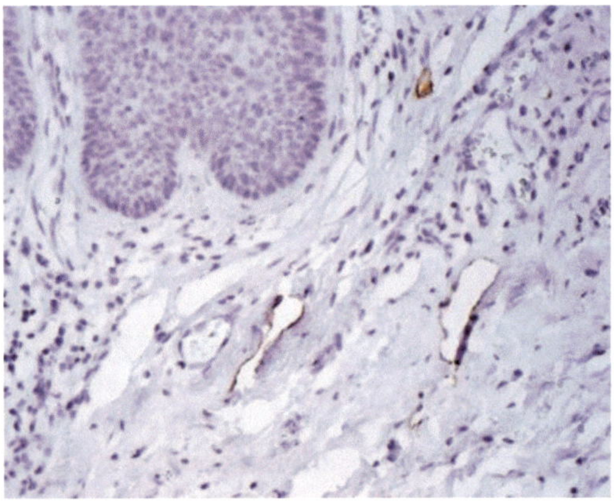

Fig. 8. Histologic picture of VIN I. Immunohistochemical staining with D2-40 antibody. Magnification 40x.

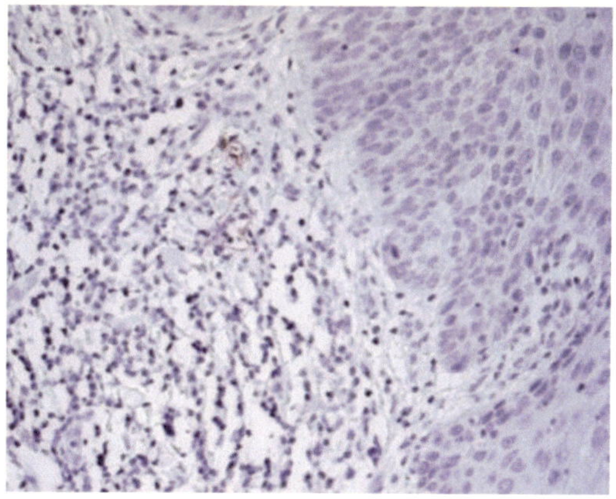

Fig. 9. VIN II . Small lymphatic vessels. Immunohistochemical staining with D2-40 antibody. Magnification 40x.

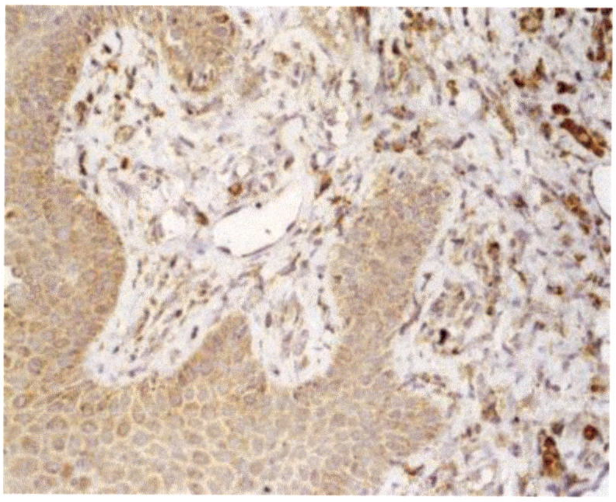

Fig. 10. Histologic picture of VIN. Strong VEGF-D expression in dysplastic epithelium. VEGF-D positive, magnification 40x.

The staining for VEGF-C, VEGF-D, and VEGFR-3 expression was assessed by semiquantitative method, at high (400x) magnification. The severity of expression was evaluated on a scale from 0 to 3; 0-lack of staining, 1-weak, 2-moderate, 3-strong). The number of cells expressing VEGF-C and D and VEGFR-3 were classified to four groups: 0 - no staining or staining in individual cells at the edge of the preparation, 1 - less than 20% positive cells, 2 - 20-50%, 3 - above 50%. Points earned for staining intensity and number of positive cells finally summed 4 groups:

0: 0-1 points
I: 2-3 points
II - 4 points
III - 5-6 points

5. Results

The results are presented in Table 3-10.

DGN	n	VEGF-C	
		0	1
VIN3	60	30	30
		50,00%	50,00%
VIN2	10	10	0
		100,00%	0,00%
VIN1	30	30	0
		100,00%	0,00%
All Grps VIN	100	70	30
		70,00%	30,00%
CA	100	90	10
		90,00%	10,00%

Table 3. Expression of VEGF-C in studied groups of women.

DGN	n	VEGF-D			
		0	1	2	3
VIN3	60	10	20	30	0
		16,67%	33,33%	50,00%	0,00%
VIN2	10	0	10	0	0
		0,00%	100,00%	0,00%	0,00%
VIN1	30	20	1	0	0
		66,67%	33,33%	0,00%	0,00%
All Grps VIN	100	30	40	30	0
		30,00%	40,00%	30,00%	0,00%
CA	100	0	30	60	10
		0,00%	30,00%	60,00%	10,00%

Table 4. Expression of VEGF-D in groups of women studied.

DGN	n	VEGFR-3 0	VEGFR-3 1	VEGFR-3 2	VEGFR-3 3
VIN3	60	0	0	60	0
		0,00%	0,00%	100,00%	0,00%
VIN2	10	0	0	0	10
		0,00%	0,00%	0,00%	100,00%
VIN1	30	0	20	10	0
		0,00%	66,67%	33,33%	0,00%
All Grps VIN	100	0	20	70	10
		0,00%	20,00%	70,00%	10,00%
CA	100	10	0	30	60
		10,00%	0,00%	30,00%	60,00%

Table 5. Expression of VEGFR-3 in the studied groups of women.

Identification	n	D2-40 Average mean	SD	min	max	
VIN3	6	4,88	0,81	4,0	6,0	
VIN2	1	3,90		3,9	3,9	
VIN1	3	2,00	0,00	2,0	2,0	
All Grps VIN	10	3,92	1,49	2,0	6,0	NS
Ca	10	3,80	1,76	1,7	7,0	

Table 6. The density of D2-40 vessel in the examined groups of women.

Identification	n	Recurrence NO	Recurrence YES	
VIN3	6	2	4	
		33,33%	66,67%	
VIN2	1	1	0	
		100,00%	0,00%	
VIN1	3	3	0	
		100,00%	0,00%	
All Grps VIN	10	6	4	
		60,00%	40,00%	
CA	10	7	3	
		70,00%	30,00%	p=0,639

Table 7. Presence of recurrences in examined groups of women.

Indentification	n	Metastasises to lymph nodes		
		NO	YES	
VIN3	6	6	0	
		100,00%	0,00%	
VIN2	1	1	0	
		100,00%	0,00%	
VIN1	3	3	0	
		100,00%	0,00%	
All Grps VIN	10	10	0	
		100,00%	0,00%	
CA	10	8	2	
		80,00%	20,00%	p=0,136

Table 8. Presence of metastasises in examined groups of women.

Identification	n	HPVDNA		
		NO	Yes	
VIN3	6	2	4	
		33,33%	66,67%	
VIN2	1	1	0	
		100,00%	0,00%	
VIN1	3	2	1	
		66,67%	33,33%	
All Grps VIN	10	5	5	
		50,00%	50,00%	
CA	10	6	4	p=0,653

Table 9. Presence of HPV DNA in examined groups of women.

The statistical analysis (statistical package Statistica 8.0, Statsoft. Inc. USA) showed no significant differences in the expression of VEGF-C and D and VEGFR-3 between the VIN group and invasive vulvar cancer group. Weak expression of VEGF-C was found only in two cases of the analyzed series, and in all cases, the expression of VEGF-D and VEGFR-3 was observed. The strongest expression of VEGF-D and VEGFR-3 was observed in the group of invasive cancers. Similarly, the differences in the amount of lymphatic vessels between the group of invasive cancers and VIN group did not reach statistical significance.

The highest density of lymphatic vessels per 2 mm was observed in VIN. In this group, and in most cases, sections of lymphatic vessels were irregular and slightly expanded. In the cancer group, we observed small lymphatic vessels with a narrow, oval lumen. Moreover, in two cases, the presence of lymphovascular space invasion (LVSI) was observed.

The evaluation of recurrence in women treated showed a statistical difference between the group VIN3 and VIN1 at $p = 0.058$ (ie. 5.8%, with the conclusion that VIN3 and VIN1 differ by the presence of recurrence), which is an interesting trend and needs further investigation in more cases, with specific attention to the literature citing similar occurrence of relapses and VIN1 and VIN2 / 3 (Table 7).

The median survival time without recurrence was the longest in the group of patients with vulvar cancer, in which it was followed by 45.2 months; in women with VIN, it was followed by 37.2 months The shortest survival time without recurrence was among women with VIN3-28.7 months, 95% CI (Table 10). In our opinion, this trend may result from the heterogeneity of women diagnos ed with VIN3, location and multiplicity of the disease.

Group	Median survival time without recurrence	95% CI (95% Confidence Interval)
VIN3	28,7 mos.	14,4 mos. - 43,0 mos.
VIN	37,2 mos.	25,8 mos. - 48,6 mos.
Ca	45,2 mos.	37,6 mos. - 52,8 mos

Table 10. Comparison of average survival time without recurrence in the treated groups of patients.

Disease-free survival curves were compared using log-rank tests. There were no statistically significant differences between survival without recurrence in groups of Ca. and VIN. Two-year survival among patients with VIN was 60%, and for patients with vulvar cancer, 70% (Figure 13). No statistically significant differences in the prevalence of HPV DNA in the test groups and the presence of lymph node metastases in the groin were observed. (Table 8, 9).

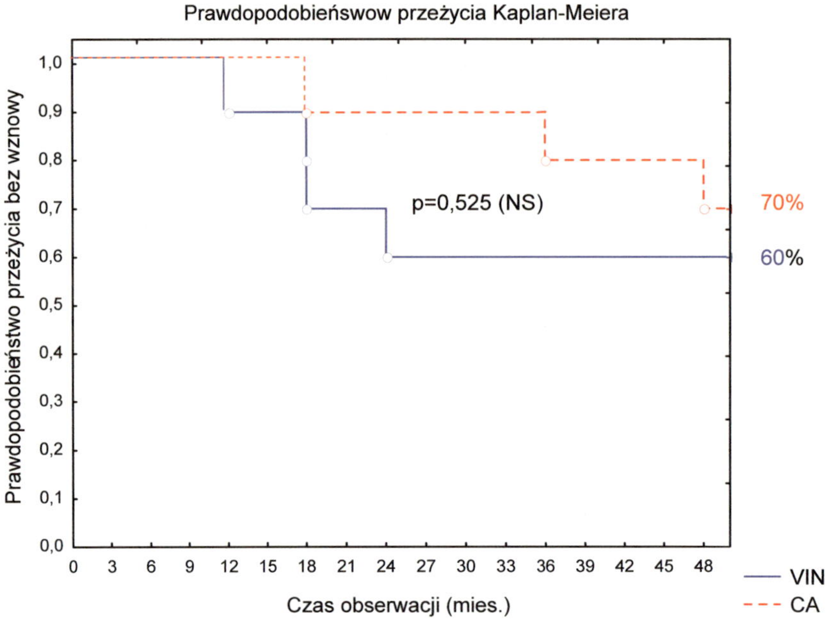

Fig. 13. Recurrence- free survival rate in cancerous and VIN patients.

6. Discussion

Lymphatic vessels play a key role in the spread of cancer. In recent years, several markers specific to lymphatic endothelium have been identified, which allowed for a deeper insight into the relationship between lymph vessels and cancer, although there are still a lot of questions for which there is no clear answer (Hillen & Griffioen, 2007; Sundar & Ganesan, 2007).

The idea that cancer cells spread to already existing lymphatic vessels is still present in the literature, although it seems that there is a belief about the presence of active lymphangiogenesis in tumors (Beasley et al., 2002; Maula et al., 2003; Nathanson, 2003). Currently, though one does not deny the presence of lymphatic vessels in tumors, the problem of the existence of active lymphangiogenesis, and the prognostic value of lymphatic vessel density inside or at the periphery of the tumor has not been completely resolved (Nathanson, 2003; Stacker et al., 2001; Ji, 2006). The functionality of the lymphatic vessels, and their role in metastasis is the subject of discussion (Maula et al., 2003; Ji, 2006; Padera et al., 2002).

In the presence of primary tumors, the extent of lymphangiogenesis can serve as a prognostic indicator of survival. A positive correlation is observed in the density of lymphatic vessels with lymph node metastasis; this has been reported in cases of squamous cell carcinoma of the head and neck (Beasley et al., 2002), gastric carcinomas (Kitadai et al., 2005) and pancreatic tumors (Rubbia-Brandt et al., 2004). In breast cancer, no correlation has been found between the number of lymphatic vessels and lymph node status, to the survival of patients (Bono et al., 2004). The multivariate analysis showed that high-density peritumoral lymphatic vessels were associated with higher risk of metastasis to lymph nodes in squamous cell carcinomas of the head and neck (Kyzas et al., 2005). In other studies, no correlation was found between the density of lymphatic vessels and lymphatic vessel invasion, lymph node status, and survival of patients as in cases of hepatocellular carcinoma and pancreatic cancer (Mouta Carreira et al., 2001; Sipos et al., 2005). In prostate cancer, or in some case series of breast cancer, there was no opportunity to determine the presence of lymphatic vessels inside the tumor. A lot of work highlights significant changes in the lymph vessels - the proliferation, budding of new blood vessels and expansion in the vicinity of the tumor.

As in physiological conditions, vascular growth factors VEGF-C and-D, activating receptor VEGFR-3, play an essential role in this process. VEGF-C and-D exhibit lymphangiogenic functions through the stimulation of VEGFR-3. They are produced as pre-propeptides that undergo proteolytic processing in the extracellular matrix. Their mature forms exhibit a greater affinity for VEGFR-3, but can also bind VEGFR-2 and induce angiogenesis. Overexpression of VEGF-C and-D in experimental tumor models was accompanied by intensive growth of new lymphatic vessels (Skobe et al. 2001), but in human tumors, these molecules involved in angiogenesis and lymphangiogenesis, are a controversial subject. Some authors state a significant correlation between expression of VEGF-C and-D and lymphangiogenesis and lymph node status, as well as an increase in the density of blood vessels in tumors (Mohammed et al., 2007; Nakamura et al., 2003; Nakamura et al., 2003) although there are also works in which this relationship is not stated (Currie et al., 2004).

In the mouse model of VEGF-C and VEGF-D secreted by tumor cells, there is induced formation of lymphatic vessels in, and around the tumor, which promotes the development of metastasis to regional lymph nodes. These processes have undergone deceleration under the influence of antibodies against VEGFR-3, blocking the activity of the ligands VEGF-D and C (Kitadai et al., 2005). Expression of VEGF-C was observed in many human cancers: breast cancer, cervical and bronchial and prostate and stomach cancers (Roskoski, 2007).

In a study of a small number of patients, including 17 cases of VIN and 26 cases of vulvar cancer, MacLean and colleagues demonstrated the presence of VEGF in 96% of vulvar cancer and only 6% of cases of VIN, not expressing this factor in healthy tissue (MacLean et al., 2000). In experimental models, tumor cells exhibiting overexpression of VEGF-C induced the formation of lymphatic vessels around the tumor (Saharinen et al., 2004; He et al., 2004). An additional issue is the relationship of lymphangiogenesis parameters such as density of lymph vessels, VEGF-C and D, and invasion of lymphatic vessels in tumor progression and prognosis.

In numerous trials, there has been a positive correlation between expression of VEGF-C and the invasion of lymphatic vessels, the presence of lymph node metastases and survival (He et al., 2004). Increased expression of VEGF-D was observed in breast, colorectal, gastric and thyroid multiforme and gliomas, and it has a positive correlation with the presence of lymph node metastases as reported in colorectal cancer, ovarian and bronchus (Roskoski, 2007). In malignant melanoma, VEGF-D likely has an important role both in lymphocytes and angiogenesis (Achen et al., 2001). Similarly, in many tumors, there has been a significant positive correlation between expression of VEGF- C, D in the primary tumor and lymph node status. However, in highly differentiated gastric cancers, this association is not found, and in cases of breast cancer and small cell lung cancer the results were inconclusive.

Increased expression of VEGF-C is a negative prognostic factor in many types of cancer, with the exception of Neuroblastoma, pancreatic cancer and colon cancer. A statistically significant correlation between VEGF-D expression in tumors and shorter overall survival was observed in endometrial cancer, ovarian and pancreatic cancers, in contrast to breast cancer or colorectal cancer (Thiele & Sleeman, 2006). Expression of VEGF-C in tumor cells in many types of cancer generally increases the risk of spread to the lymph nodes, and has some negative effect on survival (Hirakawa et al., 2007).

In gynecological tumors, one also considers the characteristics of lymphangiogenesis. In cervical cancer, a higher density of lymphatic vessels is observed in the periphery of the tumor and in the interior of the tumor in comparison with the normal cervix. The density of blood vessels in the periphery of the tumor correlates positively with higher tumor stage, lymphatic vessel invasion and metastases to lymph nodes, also an independent prognostic factor in multi-and one-dimensional analysis (Gombos et al., 2005). New development of lymphatic vessels has already been concluded in the early stages of carcinogenesis in cervical cancer. Longatto-Filho and colleagues observed that higher density of lymphatic vessels was characterized by changes in invasive cancers (squamous cell carcinoma and adenocarcinoma) compared with changes in preinvasive cancers (CIN I, CIN II, CIN III). However, not found in this study, was a statistically significant correlation between lymphatic vessel density and lymph node status (longatto-Filho et al., 2007). A widely used marker of lymphatic vessels is the D2-40. The expression of this marker was also found in cancer cells and cervical epithelium with features of CIN. Although D2-40 expression in the epithelium did not correlate with clinical features and histological changes, a significant relationship between low expression of D2-40 with invasion of lymphatic vessels and metastases in lymph nodes was observed. This may suggest participation of M2A antigen recognized by D2-40 in the interaction of tumor cells and endothelial cells of lymphatic vessels (Dumoff et al., 2005).

Similarly, expression of vascular growth factors essential for lymphangiogenesis in tumor cells is a phenomenon often described in cases of cervical cancer (Ueda et al., 2001). Increased expression of VEGF-C is attributed to the formation of lymph node metastases (Hashimoto et al., 2001).

A clear and statistically significant difference in the expression of VEGF-C and-D and their receptor VEGFR-3 was observed between (changes in) CIN I and CIN II, CIN III and invasive cancer. A higher degree of dysplasia was associated with increased expression of growth factors and their receptors. This may suggest, in addition to pro-lymphangiogenic activity, autocrine effects of VEGF-C and-D directly on tumor cells via receptor VEGFR-3 (Van Trappen et al., 2003). In cases of vulvar cancer and VIN-type changes described, we see the adverse effect that lymphangiogenic factors have on prognosis and their relationship with the progression of dysplastic lesions (Näyhä & Stenbäck, 2007; Lewy-Trenda et al., 2005). For many years, it was believed that the true VIN3 precursor of invasive vulvar cancer, created a higher risk for women over 40 years of age. Time from VIN3 diagnosis to invasive cancer is estimated to be about 4 years (1.1 to 7.3).

Recently, dominated by many views and defended by clinical data, is the belief that the potential for malignant changes in low grade VIN does not fully reflect the true behavior of these changes, but rather the survival of patients with this disease. (Rotmensch & Yamada, 2003; Van Seters et al., 2005; Jones et al., 2005). However, there are few reports analyzing the parameters of lymphangiogenesis in these diseases. In the present study, the presence of lymphatic vessels was observed along with changes in the type and degree of dysplasia. It was also found that expression of VEGF-C, VEGF-D and VEGFR-3 in both groups was correlated with the progression of the disease. No statistically significant difference between groups is most likely related to the small size of the analyzed series.

Taking into account the fact that lymph node involvement is an important prognostic factor in vulvar cancer (Raspagliesi et al., 2006), also having been described in other tumor lymphangiogenesis parameters, there is a strong gynecological association with progression and prognosis (Bednarek et al., 2008; Bednarek et al., 2009). One would expect that with vulvar cancer precursors and changes toward progressive disease, it is possible to determine similar relationships. Therefore, also bearing in mind the small number of publications on this matter, it seems that further analysis of lymphangiogenesis in the present group of cases of vulvar cancer is justified and purposeful. Due to the relatively small number of studies that have examined biomarkers (VEGF-C, VEGF-D and VEGFR-3) in carcinogenesis of the vulvar area and the lack of multivariate analysis in these studies, and taking into account the presence of small vulvar cancer and its precursors, one can not establish clear conclusions regarding their prognostic value.

7. References

Achen, MG., Williams, RA., Minekus, MP., Thornton, GE., Stenvers, K. &Rogers, PA. (2001). Localization of vascular endothelial growth factor-D in malignant melanoma suggests a role in tumour angiogenesis. *Journal of Pathology,* Vol.193, No.2, (February 2001), pp. 147-154.

Beasley, NJ., Prevo, R., Banerji, S., Leek, RD., Moore, J. &Van Trappen, P. (2002). Intratumoral lymphangiogenesis and lymph node metastasis in head and neck cancer. *Cancer Research,* Vol.62, (March 2002), pp. 1315-1320.

Bednarek, W., Mazurek, M. & Ćwiklińska, A. (2009). Ekspresja wybranych markerów i modulatorów angiogenezy u chorych na raka jajnika w okresie przed-, około- i pomenopauzalnym. *Ginekologia Polska,* Vol.80, No.2, (February 2009), pp. 93-98.

Bednarek, W., Wertel, I. & Kotarski, J. (2008). Limfangiogeneza w guzach nowotworowych. *Ginekologia Polska,* Vol.79, pp. 625-629.

Bono. P., Wasenius, VM., Heikkilä, P., Lundin, J., Jackson, DG. & Joensuu, H. (2004). High LYVE-1-positive lymphatic vessel numbers are associated with poor outcome in breast cancer. *Clinal Cancer Research,* Vol.10, No.21, (2004), pp. 7144-7149.

Currie, MJ., Hanrahan, V., Gunningham, SP., Morrin, HR., Frampton, C. & Han, C. (2004). Expression of vascular endothelial growth factor D is associated with hypoxia inducible factor (HIF-1alpha) and the HIF-1alpha target gene DEC1, but not lymph node metastasis in primary human breast carcinomas. *Journal of Clinal Pathology,* Vol.57, No.8, (August 2004), pp. 829-834.

Donoghue, JF., Lederman, FL., Susil, BJ. & Rogers, PA. (2007). Lymphangiogenesisof normal endometrium and endometrial adenocarcinoma. *Human Reproduction.,* Vol.22, No.6, (June 2007), pp. 1705-13.

Dumoff, KL., Chu, C., Xu, X., Pasha, T., Zhang, PJ. & Acs, G. (2005). Low D2-40 immunoreactivity correlates with lymphatic invasion and nodal metastasis in early-stage squamous cell carcinoma of the uterine cervix. *Modern Pathology*, Vol.18, No.1, (Jabuary 2005), pp. 97-104.

Gombos, Z., Xu, X., Chu, CS. & Acs, G. (2005). Peritumoral lymphatic vessel density and vascular endothelial growth factor C expression in early-stage squamous cell carcinoma of the uterine cervix. *Clinal Cancer Research*, Vol.11, (December 2005), pp. 8364-71.

Hashimoto, I., Kodama, J., Seki, N., Hongo, A., Yoshinouchi, M., & Okuda, H. (2001). Vascular endothelial growth factor-C expression and its relationship to pelvic lymph node status in invasive cervical cancer. *British Journal of Cancer*, Vol.85, No.1, (July 2001), pp. 93-7.

He, Y., Karpanen, T. & Alitalo, K. (2004). Role of lymphangiogenic factors in tumor metastasis. *Biochimica and Biophysia Acta*, Vol.1654, No.1, (March 2004), pp. 3-12.

Hillen, F. & Griffioen, AW. (2007). Tumour vascularization: sprouting angiogenesis and beyond. *Cancer Metastasis Review*, Vol.26, No.3-4, (December 2007), pp. 489-502.

Hirakawa, S., Brown, LF., Kodama, S., Paavonen, K., Alitalo, K. & Detmar, M. (2007). VEGF-C-induced lymphangiogenesis in sentinel lymph nodes promotes tumor metastasis to distant sites. *Blood*, Vol.109, No.3, (February 2007), pp. 1010-1017.

Iversen, T. & Tretli, S. (1998). Intraepithelial and invasive squamous cell neoplasia of thevulva: trends in incidence, recurrence, and survival rate in Norway. *Obstetrics & Gynecology*, Vol.91, No.6, (June 1998), pp. 969-972.

Ji, RC. (2006). Lymphatic endothelial cells, tumor lymphangiogenesis and metastasis: New insights into intratumoral and peritumoral lymphatics. *Cancer Metastasis Review*, Vol.25, No.4, (December 2006), pp. 677-694.

Jones, RW. & Rowan, DM. (1994). Vulvar intraepithelial neoplasia III: a clinical study of the outcome in 113 cases with relation to the later development of invasive vulvar carcinoma. *Obstetrics & Gynecology*, Vol.84, No.5, (November 1994), pp. 741-745.

Jones, RW., Rowan, DM. & Stewart, AW. (2005). Vulvar intraepithelial neoplasia: aspects of the natural history and outcome in 405 women. *Obstetrics & Gynecology*, Vol.106, No.6, (December 2005), pp. 1319-26.

Joura, EA. (2002). Epidemiology, diagnosis and treatment of vulvar intraepithelial neoplasia. *Current Opinion in Obstetrics and Gynecology*, Vol.14, No.1, (February 2002), pp. 39-43.

Judson, PL., Habermann, EB., Baxter, NN., Durham, SB. & Virnig, BA. (2006). Trends in the incidence of invasive and in situ vulvar carcinoma. *Obstetrics & Gynecology*, Vol.107, No.5, (May 2006), pp. 1834-22.

Kitadai, Y., Kodama, M., Cho, S., Kuroda, T., Ochiumi, T. & Kimura, S. (2005). Quantitative analysis of lymphangiogenic markers for predicting metastasis of human gastric carcinoma to lymph nodes. *International Journal of Cancer*, Vol.115, No.3, (June 2005), pp. 388-392.

Kuhn, L., Sun, XW. &Wright, Jr. TC (1999). Human immunodefficiency virus infection and female Lower genital tract malignancy. *Current Opinion in Obstetrics and Gynecology*, Vol.11, No.1, (Febryary 1999), pp. 35-39.

Kyzas, PA., Geleff, S., Batistatou, A., Agnantis, NJ. & Stefanou, D. (2005). Evidence for lymphangiogenesis and its prognostic implications in head and neck squamous cell carcinoma. *Journal of Pathology*, Vol.206, No.2, (June 2005), pp. 170-177.

Lewy-Trenda, I., Wierzchniewska-ławska, A. & Papierz, W. (2005). Expression of vascular endothelial growth factor (VEGF) in vulvar squamous cancer and VIN. *Polish Journal of Pathology*, Vol.56, No.1, pp. 5-8.

Longatto-Filho, A., Pinheiro, C., Pereira, SM., Etlinger, D., Moreira, MA. & Jubé, LF. (2007). Lymphatic vessel density and epithelial D2-40 immunoreactivity in pre-invasive and invasive lesions of the uterine cervix. *Gynecologic Oncology*, Vol.107, No.1, (October 2007), pp. 45-51.

MacLean, AB., Reid, WM., Rolfe, KJ., Gammell, SJ., Pugh, HE. & Gatter, KC. (2000). Role of angiogenesis in benign,premalignant and malignant vulvar lesions. *Journal of Reproductive Medicine*, Vol.45, No.8, pp. 609-612.

Markowska, J. (2006). Oncologia ginekologiczna. Wydawnictwo Medyczne Urban&Partner. Wrocław, Poland.

Maula, SM., Luukkaa, M., Grénman, R., Jackson, D., Jalkanen, S. & Ristamäki, R. (2003). Intratumoral lymphatics are essentialfor the metastatic spread and prognosis in squamous cell carcinomas of the head and neck region. *Cancer Research*, Vol.63, No.8, (April 2003), pp. 1920-1926.

Mohammed, RA., Green, A., El-Shikh, S., Paish, EC., Ellis, IO. & Martin, SG. (2007). Prognostic significance of vascular endothelial cell growth factors -A, -C and -D in breast cancer and their relationship with angio- and lymphangiogenesis. *British Journal of Cancer*, Vol.96, (March 2007), pp. 1092-1100.

Mouta Carreira, C., Nasser, SM., di Tomaso, E., Padera, TP., Boucher, Y. & Tomarev, SI. (2001). LYVE-1 is not restricted to the lymph vessels: expression in normal liver blood sinusoids and down-regulation in human liver cancer and cirrhosis. *Cancer Research*, Vol.61, No.22, (November 2001), pp. 8079-8084.

Nadja, ET. & Detmar, M. (2006). Tumor and lymph node lymphangiogenesis – impact on cancer metastasis. *Journal of Leucocyte Biology*, Vol.80, No.4, (October 2006), pp. 691-6.

Nakamura, Y., Yasuoka, H., Tsujimoto, M., Yang, Q., Imabun, S. & Nakahara, M. (2003). Flt-4-positive vessel density correlates with vascular endothelial growth factor-d expression, nodal status, and prognosis in breast cancer. *Clinal Cancer Research*, Vol.9, No.14, (November 2003), pp. 5313-5317.

Nakamura, Y., Yasuoka, H., Tsujimoto, M., Yang, Q., Imabun, S. & Nakahara, M. (2003). Prognostic significance of vascular endothelial growth factor D in breast carcinoma with longterm follow-up. *Clinical Cancer Research*, Vol.9, No.2, (February 2003), pp. 716-721.

Nathanson, SD. (2003). Insights into the mechanisms of lymph node metastasis. *Cancer*. Vol.98, No.2, (July 2003), pp. 413-23.

Näyhä, VV. & Stenbäck, FG. (2007). Increased angiogenesis is associated with poor prognosis of squamous cell carcinoma of the vulva. *Acta Obstetrica et Gynecologica Skandinavica*. Vol.86, No.11, (October 2007), pp. 1392-7.

Nisato, RE., Tille, JC. & Pepper, MS. (2003). Lymphangiogenesis and tumor metastasis. *Thrombosis and Haemostasis*, Vol.90, No.4, (2003), pp. 591-7.

Padera, TP., Kadambi, A., di Tomaso, E., Carreira, CM., Brown, EB. & Boucher, Y. (2002). Lymphatic metastasis in the absence of functional intratumor lymphatics. *Science*, Vol.296, No.5574, (June 2002), pp. 1883-1886.

Preti, M., Ronco, G., Ghiringhello, B. & Micheletti, L. (2000). Recurrent squamous cell carcinoma of the vulva: clinicopathologic determinants identifying low risk patients. *Cancer*, Vol.88, No.8, (April 2000), pp. 1869-1876.

Raspagliesi, F., Hanozet, F., Ditto, A., Solima, E., Zanaboni, F. & Vecchione, F. (2006). Clinical and pathological prognostic factors in squamous cell carcinoma of the vulva. *Gynecological Oncology*, Vol.102, No.2, (August 2008), pp. 333-7.

Roskoski, R. (2007). Vascular endothelial growth factor (VEGF) signaling in tumor progression. *Critical Reviews in Oncology/Hematology*. Vol.62, No.3, (June 2007), pp. 179-213.

Rotmensch, J. &Yamad, SD. (2003). Neoplasms oft he Vulva and Vagina. In: Kufe DW, Pollock RE, Weichselbaum RR, Bast JrR, Gansler TSHJFea, editors. Holland- Frei Cancer Medicine. 6th ed. Hamilton, Ontario: B.C. Decker, Inc.

Rubbia-Brandt, L., Terris, B., Giostra, E., Dousset, B., Morel, P. & Pepper, MS. (2004). Lymphatic vessel density and vascular endothelial growth factor-C expression correlate with malignant behavior in human pancreatic endocrine tumors. *Clinical Cancer Research*, Vol.10, No.20. (October 2004), pp. 919-6928.

Saharinen, P., Tammela, T., Karkkainen, MJ., Alitalo, K. (2004).Lymphatic vasculature: development, molecular regulation and role in tumor metastasis and inflammation. *Trends in Immunology*, Vol.25, No.7, (July 2004), pp. 387-95.

Sipos, B., Kojima, M., Tiemann, K., Klapper, W., Kruse, ML. & Kalthoff, H. (2005). Lymphatic spread of ductal pancreatic adenocarcinoma is independent of lymphangiogenesis. *Journal of Pathology*, Vol.207, No.3, (November 2005), pp.: 301-312.

Skobe, M., Hawighorst, T., Jackson, DG., Prevo, R., Janes, L. & Velasco, P. (2001). Induction of tumor lymphangiogenesis by VEGF-C promotes breast cancer metastasis. *Nature Medicine*, Vol.7, No.2, (February 2001), pp. 192-198.

Stacker SA, Caesar C, Baldwin ME, Thornton GE, Williams RA, Prevo R et al (2001). VEGF-D promotes the metastatic spread of tumor cells via the lymphatics. *Nature Medicine*, Vol.7, No.2, (February 2001), pp. 186-191.

Sundar, SS. & Ganesan, TS. (2007). Role of lymphangiogenesis in cancer. *Journal of Clinical Oncology*, Vol.25, No.27, (September 2007), pp. 4298-4307.

Thiele, W. & Sleeman, JP. (2006). Tumor-induced lymphangiogenesis: a target for cancer therapy? *Journal of Biotechnology*, Vol.124, No.1, (June 2006), pp. 224-241.

Thuis, YN., Campion, M., Fox. H, & Hacker, NF. (2000).Contemporary experience with the management of vulvar intraepithelial neoplasia. *International Journal of Gynecological Cancer*, Vol.10, No.3, (May 2000), pp. 223-227.

Ueda, M., Terai, Y., Kumagai, K., Ueki, K., Yamaguchi, H. & Akise, D. (2001). Vascular endothelial growth factor C gene expression is closely related to invasion phenotype in gynecological tumor cells. *Gynecological Oncology*, Vol.82, No.1, (July 2001), pp. 162-6.

Wissmann, C. & Detmar, M. (2006). Pathways targeting tumor lymphangiogenesis. *Clinical Cancer Research*, Vol.12, No.23, (2006), pp. 6865-8.

Van Seters, M., Van Beurden, M. & de Craen, AJ. (2005). Is the asssumed natural history of vulvar intraepithelial neoplasia III based on enough evidence? A systemic review of 3322 published patients. *Gynecological Oncology*, Vol.97, No.2, (May 2007), pp. 645-51.

Van Trappen, PO., Steele, D., Lowe, DG., Baithun, S., Beasley, N. & Thiele, W. (2003). Expression of vascular endothelial growth factor (VEGF)-C and VEGF-D, and their receptor VEGFR-3, during different stages of cervical carcinogenesis. *Journal of Pathology*, Vol.201, No.4, (December 2003), pp. 544-54.

18

Current Insight into Specific Cellular Immunity of Women Presenting with HPV16-Related Vulvar Intra-Epithelial Neoplasia and Their Partners

Isabelle Bourgault-Villada
AP-HP, Hôpital Ambroise Paré, Boulogne Billancourt,
UVSQ, Versailles,
France

1. Introduction

The premalignant lesions of vulvar intraepithelial neoplasia (VIN) involve the mucosal and/or cutaneous epithelium of the vulva. VIN may be HPV-related VIN (usual VIN) or -unrelated and represents the most frequent vulvar cancer precursors. Usual VIN occurs in adult women and commonly resembles persistent anogenital warts which are often multifocal pigmented papular lesions. It is caused by high-risk HPV (HR-HPV) types, essentially 16 in up to 91% of the cases (Srodon et al, 2006), and histologically, it is made of poorly to undifferentiated basal cells and/or highly atypical squamous epithelial cells (McClugagge et al, 2009). The involvement of the entire thickness of the epithelium defines the grade 3 of the disease (VIN3). The disease progresses towards invasion in about 3% of treated patients and 9% of the untreated ones according to a review of over 3,000 cases (van Seters et al, 2005) whereas evolution towards invasive carcinoma is observed in about 30% of untreated grade 3 cervical intraepithelial neoplasia (CIN3) patients (Ostor et al, 1993).

2. Virology

HPVs are DNA viruses with a circular double strain genome including 8 000 base pairs. The genome is divided into three regions: a Long Control Region which controls viral replication, a region coding for Early proteins (E1 to E7, including the E6 and E7 proteins that share oncogenic and transforming properties), and a region coding for Late proteins such as L1 and L2 proteins that constitute 80% and 20% of the viral capside, respectively. More than 150 HPV have been sequenced, one HPV being considered different from another when there is a difference in 10% of nucleotides coding for L1 genes.

Following a breach in the malpighian pluristratified epithelium, HPVs infect basal stem cells of keratinocytes. The virus initially remains in episomal form with synthesis of E2 protein. This protein is a major regulator of viral vegetative cycle and is required for transcriptional regulation as well as viral DNA replication together with the E1 helicase (Desaintes et al, 1996). In contrast, E2 is generally undetectable in cancers due to a preferential integration of the viral genome in the cell genome and disruption of the E2 open reading frame (Berumen et al, 1994; Collins et al, 2009). Therefore E2 is a marker of viral infection and is specific for the early stages of the viral gene expression in infected cells. This was formally demonstrated in a recent work that showed a strong staining of the E2 protein in the intermediate differentiated layers of HPV16-infected tissues and low grade CIN (Xue et al, 2010). The high expression of HPV16 E2 in low grade lesions therefore represents a marker for HPV infection even before any clinical manifestation.

After integration of the genome of oncogenic HPVs such as HPV16 into the host genome, viral oncogenic E6 and E7 proteins are synthesized in large quantities in the inner third of the epithelium. E6 links to p53 and induces its degradation by the ubiquitin pathway and E7 links to pRB and allows the release of growth factors such as E2F.

During maturation of keratinocytes from the basal layer to the epithelial surface, viral capside proteins L1 and L2 are synthesized and expressed at the surface of mature keratinocytes in order to form a new viral particle which is able to infect adjacent healthy epithelium and to contaminate sexual partners.

3. Epidemiology of HPV16 related VIN

HPV infections occur preferentially in young women under 25 years of age (Boulanger et al, 2004). Several stages of lesions can be observed following oncogenic HPV infection. The first stage is a simple infection of keratinocytes that become koilocytes. The following stages are related to the transformation of infected keratinocytes into malignant cells. The depth at which malignant cells are found defines the disease stage. High grade squamous intraepithelial lesions as VIN3 are diagnosed on the basis of biopsy, with malignant cells in entire thickness of the epithelium

The premalignant lesions of HPV-related grade 3 intraepithelial neoplasia involve the mucosal and/or cutaneous epithelium of the vulva (usual VIN or VIN3), perineal and perianal region. Usual VIN occurs in adult women and commonly resembles persistent anogenital warts that are more often multifocal pigmented papular lesions disseminated on the vulva and/or the perianal skin than monofocal unique lesion (Figure 1).

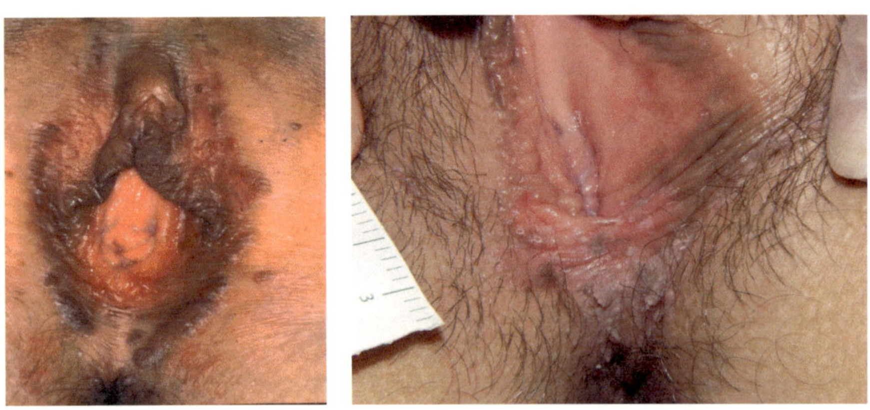

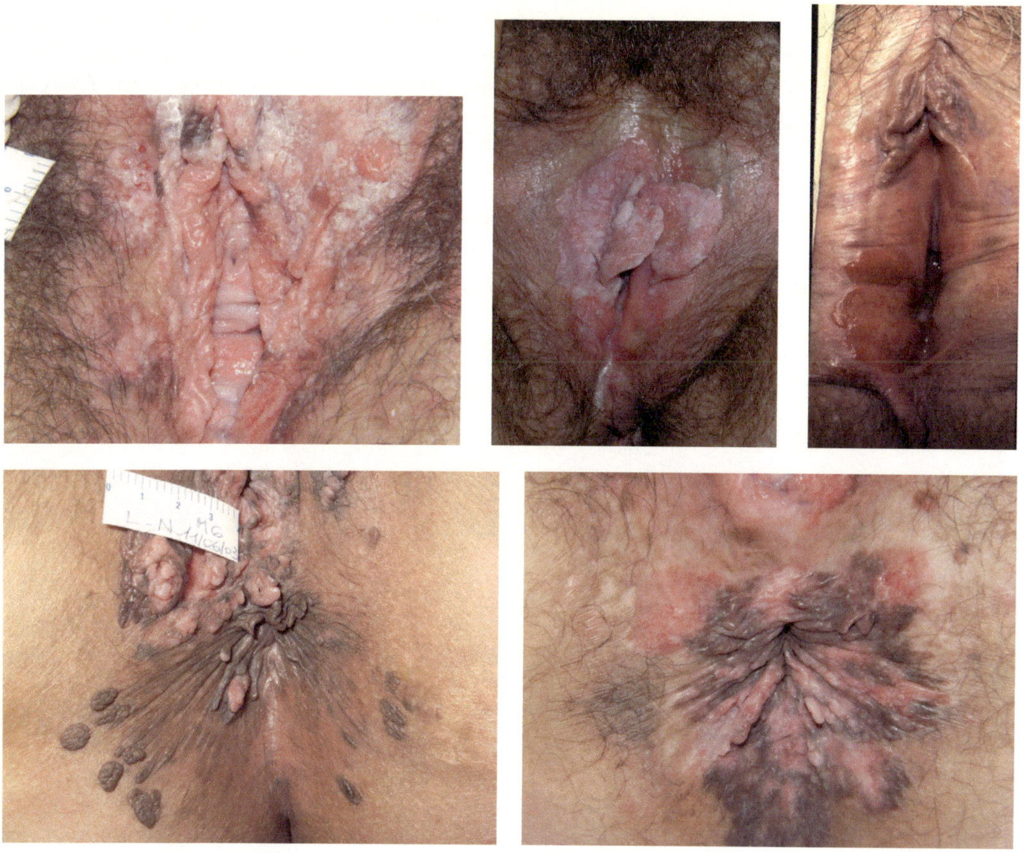

Fig. 1. Clinical presentations of usual multifocal or monofocal vulvar and preineal intraepithelial neoplasia

4. Why does usual VIN can spontaneously regress?

Although usual VIN lesions are often chronic and recurrent, they can regress spontaneously in up to 35% of young (less than 30 years) women presenting with multiple pigmented lesions within a median duration of 9.5 months (Jones et al, 2005} (Bourgault Villada, 2010). We previously studied a patient who presented with multifocal usual VIN and showed a complete clearance of viral lesions eight months after disease onset and two months after electrocoagulation of less than 50% of the usual VIN lesions (Bourgault Villada et al, 2004). Immunohistochemical study of her initial vulvar biopsy revealed a marked dermal infiltrate containing a majority of CD4+ T lymphocytes and an epidermal infiltrate made up of both $CD4^+$ and $CD8^+$ T cells (Figure 2). She showed also a proliferating response against one peptide from E6 protein and a high frequency anti-E6 and anti-E7 effector blood T cells by *ex vivo* IFNγ– ELISpot assay just before clinical regression (Figure 3). Such a study of blood cellular immune responses together with the analysis of vulvar biopsies obtained simultaneously and correlated to clinical outcome was not previously reported. In an anti-HPV vaccine trial conducted by Davidson and al (Davidson et al, 2003), usual VIN lesions completely regressed in a patient following vaccination. Interestingly, immunostaining of vulvar biopsy prior to the vaccine showed a marked CD4+ and CD8+ T lymphocyte infiltrate of both epithelial and sub-epithelial sheets. One may wonder whether the regression of these patient lesions could be related to a spontaneous regression. Therefore, the observation of a CD4+ and CD8+ infiltrate within sub-epithelial and epithelial sheets in the biopsy and the visualization of very strong blood anti-HPV T cell responses in patient with usual VIN could be predictive of spontaneous clinical outcome. It may also be thought that high numbers of blood $CD4^+$ and $CD8^+$ lymphocytes after therapeutic vaccination could allow clearance of HPV-16 lesions in usual VIN, assuming that anti-HPV vaccine-induced T effector cells could home in the HPV cutaneous and mucosal lesions.

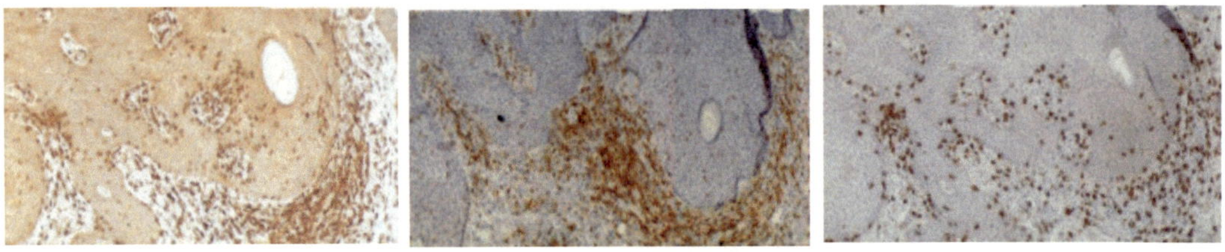

Fig. 2. Immunohistochemical study of the vulvar biopsy just before spontaneous regression

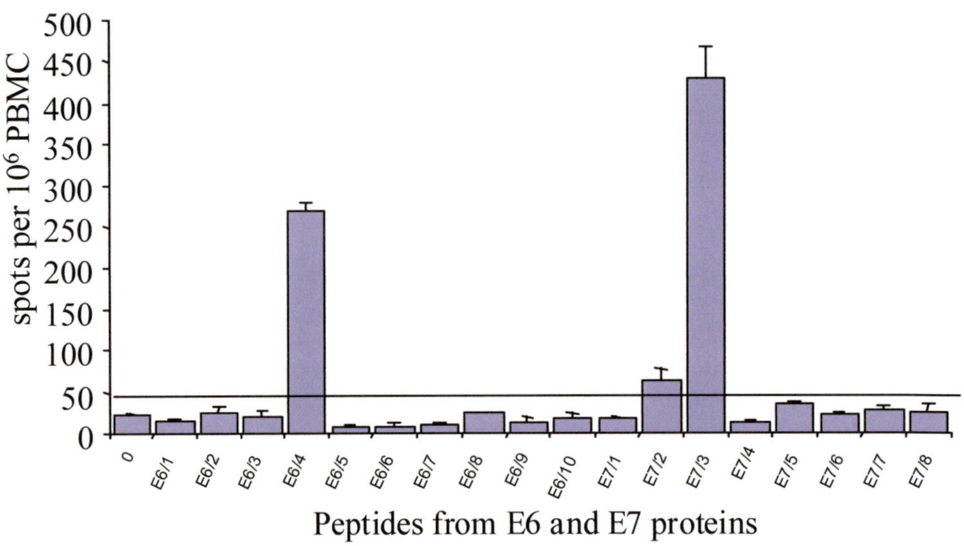

Fig. 3. IFNγ–ELISpot assay performed just before clinical regression

5. What is the exact role of cellular HPV16-specific T-cell responses?

Cellular immunity (CD4+ and CD8+ T-cells) plays a key role in the defense against all HPV-induced infections or lesions by destroying HPV-infected or -transformed keratinocytes. Indeed, the incidence of HPV infections and diseases significantly increases with $CD4^+$ T cell impairment in immunosuppressed such as transplanted (Arends et al, 1997) or HIV-infected patients (Sun et al, 1997). In asymptomatic HPV16 infections, most women resolve spontaneously their infection without clinical disease concomitantly with blood anti-HPV16 Th1 CD4+ T cell responses (Welters et al, 2003). Similarly, regression of condyloma is associated with a dense epithelial cellular infiltrate made up of both CD4+ and CD8+ T lymphocytes with a Th1 cytokine profile as measured by cytokine mRNAs in interferon (IFN)-treated condylomas (Coleman et al, 1994). Proliferative CD4+ T cell responses are also associated with spontaneously regressive CIN3 (Kadish et al, 1997). The evolution of CIN3 towards invasive cancers is featured by a decrease of CD4+ cellular infiltrate, an increase of CD8+ T lymphocytes (Ghosh et al, 1992) with impairment of HPV16-specific CTL responses which could be related to a down- regulation of MHC class I molecules on HPV-16-infected cells and to the appearance of suppressive T lymphocytes (Treg) and a loss of blood anti-HPV-16 CD4+ activity. In high grade cervical intraepithelial neoplasia (CIN), positive intra-dermal reaction after intra-dermal injection of 5 HPV-16 E7 large peptides correlated with the spontaneous clearance of the lesions, which further indicates the presence and the very important role of HPV specific CD4+ T lymphocytes (Hopfl et al, 2000).

6. Anti-E2 T-cell responses are a marker of clinical viral control

We recently tested in a longitudinal study of 18 months, by proliferative assays, intracellular cytokines synthesis and IFNγ–ELISpot, the cellular immune responses against the HPV16 E2 protein that is early synthesized after HPV infection when the virus is episomal in eight women presenting with HPV16-related usual VIN and their healthy male partners (Jacobelli et al, 2011, unpublished data). In six women, we showed that anti-E2 polyfunctional CD4 T-cell responses (proliferative responses and synthesis of IFNγ and/or IL2) appear when the clinical lesions heal after treatment or when the HPV infection remains silent. In the women presenting with persistent lesions, no proliferation was observed.

Blood proliferative T-cell responses against HPV16 E2 peptides have been also observed in 50% of healthy women, who presumably previously cleared HPV16 infection (de Jong et al, 2004) and in 9 out of 22 regressive CIN3 cases (Dillon et al, 2007). In another studies, the lack of anti-E2 proliferative responses was reported in 16 of 18 patients (89%) affected with usual VIN lesions (Davidson et al, 2003) and in 7 of 8 and 9 of 12 women affected with CIN3 (Dillon et al, 2007; de Jong et al, 2004).These observations reinforce the strong role of T-cells in the control of HPV replication.

7. Why the male partners do not have any HPV16-related lesions?

Men are vectors of oncogenic HPV infection (Buckley et al, 1981; Giuliano et al, 2011). However, while HPV infection was found in 71 to 90% of the partners of HPV-infected women (Hippelainen et al, 1994; Nicolau et al, 2005), only 52% harbored the same HPV subtypes (Reiter et al, 2010). Moreover, penile intra-epithelial neoplasia is rare and detected in less than 2% of the men in contact with oncogenic HPV (Giraldo et al, 2008). We thus analyzed HPV infection and anti-HPV16 E2 blood T-cell responses in asymptomatic male partners chronically exposed to HPV16 during sexual intercourses with their wives affected with usual VIN (Jacobelli et al, 2011, unpublished data). We had hypothesized that male partners exposed to replicative HPV16 could develop immunologic responses against the early E2 viral protein and thus clear infection. In the absence of condom usage for at least 6 months, the male partners of women presenting with usual VIN could be contaminated by HPV16. HPV16 and HPV27 (a cutaneous HPV) were identified in genital sampling gathered by cytobrush in only two of the eight healthy partners. Such a prevalence of contamination by HPV16 is similar to the one usually observed in male partner of oncogenic HPV-infected women (Reiter et al, 2010). In this male population, we have chosen to study anti-HPV16 E2 T-cell responses because E2 protein is an early highly expressed protein. E2 is bigger than E6 and E7 proteins and induces more T-cell responses than E6 and E7. Therefore looking for an E2-specific response is then more sensitive. In addition, E2 is required for replication and the detection of E2-specific T cell responses is the signature of viral replication. The study of anti-E2 T-cell responses is then more appropriate for the early phases of HPV16 infection as supposed in male partners of women having usual VIN. We have observed HPV16-E2-specific proliferative responses in seven and intracellular cytokine synthesis of single IFNγ, dual IFNγ/IL2 and single IL2 in six out of the seven partners. Since there is no E2 protein in the viral particle, the high frequency of E2-specific T cells responses in partners of women with usual VIN demonstrates that the virus replicate in males.

These E2 specific T-cell responses indicate a striking correlation in all male partners but two between the absence of the HPV-related lesion. The presence of spontaneous E2-specific proliferative T-cell responses and single IFNγ, dual IFNγ/IL2, single IL2 T-cell producers was previously described in other viral systems (Harari et al, 2006; Pantaleo et al, 2006). These polyfunctional anti-E2 T-cell responses could be due to an efficient presentation of viral antigens by dendritic cells present in mucosal tissue and it is tempting to speculate that E2-specific responses are responsible for the clearing of the lesion. Therefore, spontaneously HPV control is related to the presence of memory polyfunctional CD4+ T-cells in male partners.

8. Why the prophylactic vaccine could be useful in men?

The analysis of E2 specific T cell responses is a sensitive and reliable tool to analyze disease progression and the natural history of HPV infection. In six out of eight male partners, the presence of T-cell proliferative responses and single IL2, dual IFNγ/IL2, single IFNγ memory T-cells against HPV16 E2 peptides was concomitant to the control of genital HPV lesions despite HPV16 exposure. These results are reminiscent of those described in Gambian prostitutes exposed to HIV with presence of anti-HIV cytotoxic T lymphocytes without any detectable HIV (Rowland-Jones et al, 1995). Such anti-viral immune T cells responses thus reflect an undetectable viral infection. Our experimental results demonstrate for the first time that, although not clinically detectable, HPV16 can replicate in men and can induce a strong memory T cell response against one of an early viral protein. The presence of polyfunctional (IL2, IFNγ/IL2 and IFNγ secretions and proliferation) anti E2 CD4+ T-cell responses in asymptomatic men unambiguously establishes that E2 is a marker of HPV infection even when undetectable lesions. Responses represent correlates of protective antiviral immunity in HPV infection. Monofunctional (production of IFNγ by IFNγ-ELISpot) "anti-E2 T-cell" responses does not allow HPV16 control. These results suggest that male are an important reservoir of HPV and provide a strong argument in favor of prophylactic HPV vaccination of young men with VLPs to decrease HPV16 infection in men, viral transmission from men to women and thus fight against the spread of mucosal HPV diseases in the population.

9. How to cure usual VIN? Therapeutic vaccines

Preventive vaccines do not address the current need for better treatment for women previously infected by HPV 16 or 18. Other types of vaccines must be used to increase or induce new specific anti-HPV cellular immunity (CD4+ and CD8+ T lymphocytes) in order to kill transformed epithelial cells. Several approaches can be used in this aim. To stimulate cytotoxic or antiviral CD8+ T lymphocytes, the vaccines must target the cytoplasm of dendritic cells. The degradation of vaccine antigens by proteasomes results in short peptides that can bind to HLA class I molecules and migrate at the surface of dendritic cells. To stimulate CD4+ T lymphocytes, endocytosis of vaccinal antigens is essential, followed by degradation of antigens by lysosome/endosome in large peptides that associate with HLA class II molecules before migrating at the surface of dendritic cells. All these therapeutic vaccines must target E6 and E7 viral proteins and contain recombinant viruses (vaccinia viruses for example), DNA or peptides.

Recently, an open clinical trial was performed by the Melief's group (Kenter et al, 2009) in twenty women presenting with usual VIN using 13 large peptides spanning the whole E6 and E7 proteins. Forty five percent of complete (9/20 women) and 25 % (5/20) of partial remission were observed 12 months after immunization. These important results would be even more interesting if the investigators had included a placebo group (Bourgault Villada, 2010a). A new trial with a placebo group is currently under way.

Vaccinia virus was also used in a recombinant vaccine containing E6 and E7 genes from HPV16 and HPV18 (TA-HPV) to vaccinate usual VIN patients. A clinical complete or partial response was observed in 8/18 treated women (Davidson et al, 2003). More recently, vaccination against usual VIN was also performed with another recombinant vaccinia virus, TA-L2E6E7 from HPV16 (Daayana et al, 2010). Two months before vaccination, 19 women were treated by topical imiquimod and then vaccinated by intramuscular route with 3 doses of recombinant vaccinia virus. Imiquimod is an immunomodulator that increases the synthesis of type I IFN by dendritic cells after its fixation to the TLR7 in human dendritic cells. Complete remission was obtained in 58% of vaccinated women.

10. How to determine the epitopic regions for a therapeutic vaccine?

In a study including 16 women presenting with usual VIN, we have determined the strongly immunogenic regions from HPV16 E6 and E7 proteins for CD4+ and/or CD8+ T lymphocytes (Bourgault Villada et al, 2010b). Among 18 large peptides of the proteins E6 and E7, two were recognized in proliferative assays as immunodominant by T cells from 10 out of 16 women (62%) at the entry in the study, namely E6/2 (aa 14-34) and E6/4 (aa 45-68) peptides. Four other peptides, E6/7 (aa 91-110), E7/2 (aa 7-27), E7/3 (aa 21-40) and E7/7 (aa 65-87) were recognized by only 12% of the women in proliferative or IFNγ–ELISpot tests. The regions of E6 and E7 proteins implicated in T cell recognition during HPV infection were not yet well defined because of the usually low frequency of anti-HPV blood T cell responses and of the difficulties of their study.

In protein E6, some peptides included in, including or overlapping our peptides E6/2 (aa 14-34) and E6/4 (aa 45-68) have already been described as preferentially recognized by CD4+ T cells. Among them, peptide E6 42-57 that is restricted by HLA-DR7 has already been identified (Strang et al, 1990). Regions E6 1-31, 22-51 and 24-45 can be also immunogenic for CD4+ T cells as shown in CIN or sexually active healthy women (Kadish et al, 1997). The region E6 42-71, which includes peptide E6/4 (aa 45-68), has also been described as a target of proliferative responses in CIN patients (Kadish et al, 1997). Another E6 111-158 region was previously described as inducing proliferative responses in infected asymptomatic subjects or in patients with CIN3 (Kadish et al, 1997; Strang et al, 1990) as well as E6 127-141 peptide in healthy young women (Gallagher et al, 2007). Similarly, peptides E7 43-77, E7 50-62 and E7 58-68 which are restricted by DR3, DR15 and DR17, respectively, were defined as epitopic peptides for CD4 + T cells (Strang et al, 1990; van der Burg et al, 2001; Wang et al, 2009). E7 region 51-98, including our E7/7 (aa 65-87) peptide, is also very immunogenic for proliferating T lymphocytes (de Gruijl et al, 1998; Luxton et al, 1996; Nakagawa et al, 1996).

The characterization of E6 and E7 HPV-16 epitopes and the HLA restriction of their recognition by CD8+ T lymphocytes are more precise: E6 29-38, E7 11-20, E7 82-90 and E7 86-93 epitopes are presented by HLA-A2 (Evans et al, 2001; Ressing et al, 1995, 1996), E6 80-88 and E7 44-52 by HLA-B18 (Bourgault Villada et al, 2000) and E6 49-57 by HLA-A24 (Morishima et al, 2007). In women who cleared HPV 16 infection, cytotoxic T lymphocytes (CTL) responses are directed against epitopes preferentially located in the N-terminal half of the E6 protein (region 16-40) (Nakagawa et al, 2005). In this fragment, the dominant epitope E6 29-37 is restricted by HLA-B48, E6 31-38 by HLA-B4002 and the subdominant epitope E6 52-61 by HLA-B35 (Nakagawa et al, 2007). The same group had also shown that the peptide E6 33-42 61 is recognized by CD8+ T lymphocytes in association with HLA-A68, peptide E6 52-61 in association with HLA-B57 and –B35, peptide E6 75-83 in association with HLA-B62, peptide E7 7-15 in association with HLA-B48 and peptide E7 79-87 in association with HLA-B60 (Nakagawa et al, 2004, 2007; Wang et al, 2008). In addition, E7 7-15 is also able to bind HLA-A2 and -B8 to be recognized by CTL (Oerke et al, 2005; Ressing et al, 1995). From the latter results, two hot spots of CD8+ T-cell epitopes in protein E6 may be located in the regions E6 29-38 and 52-61 and another one in protein E7 (E7 7-15) (Nakagawa et al, 2007). Nevertheless, a poor immunogenicity of E7 protein was observed in many studies during both HPV 16 infection and after peptidic vaccination using long peptides spanning both E6 and E7 (Kenter et al, 2008; Welters et al, 2008) such as those used in our study.

The epitopes E6/2 (aa 14-34) and E6/4(aa 45-68) hence could be strongly recognized by CD4+ and / or CD8+ T lymphocytes and could be particularly relevant in the design of a peptide vaccination. We may hypothesize that the T cell responses that we observed were able to contain the tumor cells into the epithelium. Therefore, E6/2 (aa 14-34) and E6/4 (aa 45-68) peptides could play a major role in the protection against invasive cancer by stimulating T lymphocytes. Specific CD4+ T-cells play an essential role in the defense against HPV in particular in women presenting with usual VIN and their male partners.

11. References

Arends, M. J., Benton, E. C., Mclaren, K. M., Stark, L. A., Hunter, J. A., & Bird, C. C. (1997). Renal allograft recipients with high susceptibility to cutaneous malignancy have an increased prevalence of human papillomavirus DNA in skin tumours and a greater risk of anogenital malignancy. *Br J Cancer* 75:722-8.

Berumen, J., Casas, L., Segura, E., Amezcua, J. L., & Garcia-Carranca, A. (1994). Genome amplification of human papillomavirus types 16 and 18 in cervical carcinomas is related to the retention of E1/E2 genes. *Int J Cancer* 56:640-5.

Boulanger, J. C., Sevestre, H., Bauville, E., Ghighi, C., Harlicot, J. P., & Gondry, J. (2004). [Epidemiology of HPV infection]. *Gynecol Obstet Fertil* 32:218-23.

Bourgault Villada, I., Beneton, N., Bony, C., Connan, F., Monsonego, J., Bianchi, A., Saiag, P., Levy, J. P., Guillet, J. G., & Choppin, J. (2000). Identification in humans of HPV-16 E6 and E7 protein epitopes recognized by cytolytic T lymphocytes in association with HLA-B18 and determination of the HLA-B18-specific binding motif. *Eur J Immunol* 30:2281-9.

Bourgault Villada, I., Moyal Barracco, M., Ziol, M., Chaboissier, A., Barget, N., Berville, S., Paniel, B., Jullian, E., Clerici, T., Maillere, B., & Guillet, J. G. (2004). Spontaneous regression of grade 3 vulvar intraepithelial neoplasia associated with human papillomavirus-16-specific CD4(+) and CD8(+) T-cell responses. *Cancer Res* 64:8761-6.

Bourgault Villada, I. (2010a). Vaccination against HPV-16 for vulvar intraepithelial neoplasia. *N Engl J Med* 362:655-6.

Bourgault Villada, I., Moyal Barracco, M., Berville, S., Bafounta, M. L., Longvert, C., Premel, V., Villefroy, P., Jullian, E., Clerici, T., Paniel, B., Maillere, B., Choppin, J., & Guillet, J. G. (2010b). Human papillomavirus 16-specific T cell responses in classic HPV-related vulvar intra-epithelial neoplasia. Determination of strongly immunogenic regions from E6 and E7 proteins. *Clin Exp Immunol* 159:45-56.

Buckley, J. D., Harris, R. W., Doll, R., Vessey, M. P., & Williams, P. T. (1981). Case-control study of the husbands of women with dysplasia or carcinoma of the cervix uteri. *Lancet* 2:1010-5.

Coleman, N. H., Birley D, Renton, A. M., Hanna, N. F., Ryait, B. K., Byrne, M., Taylor-Robinson, D., & Stanley, M. A. (1994). Immunological events in regressing genital warts. *Am J Clin Pathol* 102: 768-74.

Collins, S. I., Constandinou-Williams, C., Wen, K., Young, L. S., Roberts, S., Murray, P. G., & Woodman, C. B. (2009). Disruption of the E2 gene is a common and early event in the natural history of cervical human papillomavirus infection: a longitudinal cohort study. *Cancer Res* 69:3828-32.

Daayana, S., Elkord, E., Winters, U., Pawlita, M., Roden, R., Stern, P. L., & Kitchener, H. C. (2010). Phase II trial of imiquimod and HPV therapeutic vaccination in patients with vulval intraepithelial neoplasia. *Br J Cancer* 102:1129-36.

Davidson, E. J., Boswell, C. M., Sehr, P., Pawlita, M., Tomlinson, A. E., Mcvey, R. J., Dobson, J., Roberts, J. S., Hickling, J., Kitchener, H. C., & Stern, P. L. (2003). Immunological and clinical responses in women with vulval intraepithelial neoplasia vaccinated with a vaccinia virus encoding human papillomavirus 16/18 oncoproteins. *Cancer Res* 63:6032-41.

De Gruijl, T. D., Bontkes, H. J., Walboomers, J. M., Stukart, M. J., Doekhie, F. S., Remmink, A. J., Helmerhorst, T. J., Verheijen, R. H., Duggan-Keen, M. F., Stern, P. L., Meijer, C. J., & Scheper, R. J. (1998). Differential T helper cell responses to human papillomavirus type 16 E7 related to viral clearance or persistence in patients with cervical neoplasia: a longitudinal study. *Cancer Res* 58:1700-6.

De Jong, A., Van Poelgeest, M. I., Van Der Hulst, J. M., Drijfhout, J. W., Fleuren, G. J., Melief, C. J., Kenter, G., Offringa, R., & Van Der Burg, S. H. (2004). Human papillomavirus type 16-positive cervical cancer is associated with impaired CD4+ T-cell immunity against early antigens E2 and E6. *Cancer Res* 64:5449-55.

Desaintes, C., & Demeret, C. (1996). Control of papillomavirus DNA replication and transcription. *Semin Cancer Biol* 7:339-47.

Dillon, S., Sasagawa, T., Crawford, A., Prestidge, J., Inder, M. K., Jerram, J., Mercer, A. A., & Hibma, M. (2007). Resolution of cervical dysplasia is associated with T-cell proliferative responses to human papillomavirus type 16 E2. *J Gen Virol* 88:803-13.

Evans, M., Borysiewicz, L. K., Evans, A. S., Rowe, M., Jones, M., Gileadi, U., Cerundolo, V., & Man, S. (2001). Antigen processing defects in cervical carcinomas limit the presentation of a CTL epitope from human papillomavirus 16 E6. *J Immunol* 167:5420-8.

Fausch, S. C., Da Silva, D. M., & Kast, W. M. (2005). Heterologous papillomavirus virus-like particles and human papillomavirus virus-like particle immune complexes activate human Langerhans cells. *Vaccine* 23:1720-9.

Gallagher, K. M., & Man, S. (2007). Identification of HLA-DR1- and HLA-DR15-restricted human papillomavirus type 16 (HPV16) and HPV18 E6 epitopes recognized by CD4+ T cells from healthy young women. *J Gen Virol* 88:1470-8.

Ghosh, A. K., & Moore M. (1992). Tumour-infiltrating lymphocytes in cervical carcinoma. *Eur J Cancer* 28A: 1910-6.

Giraldo, P. C., Eleuterio, J., Jr., Cavalcante, D. I., Goncalves, A. K., Romao, J. A., & Eleuterio, R. M. (2008). The role of high-risk HPV-DNA testing in the male sexual partners of women with HPV-induced lesions. *Eur J Obstet Gynecol Reprod Biol* 137:88-91.

Giuliano, A. R., Lee J. H., Fulp, W., Villa, L. L., Lazcano, E., Papenfuss, M. R., Abrahamsen, M., Salmeron, J., Anic, G. M., Rollison, D. E., & Smith, D. (2011). Incidence and clearance of genital human papillomavirus infection in men (HIM): a cohort study. *Lancet* 377: 932-40.

Harari, A., Dutoit V., Cellerai, C., Bart, P. A., Du Pasquier, R. A., & Pantaleo, G et al. (2006). Functional signatures of protective antiviral T-cell immunity in human virus infections. *Immunol Rev* 211: 236-54.

Hippelainen, M. I., Yliskoski, M., Syrjanen, S., Saastamoinen, J., Hippelainen, M., Saarikoski, S., & Syrjanen, K. (1994). Low concordance of genital human papillomavirus (HPV) lesions and viral types in HPV-infected women and their male sexual partners. *Sex Transm Dis* 21:76-82.

Hopfl, R., Heim K., Christensen, N., Zumbach, K., Wieland, U., Volgger, B., Widschwendter, A., Haimbuchner, S., Muller-Holzner, E., Pawlita, M., Pfister, H., &Fritsch, P. (2000). Spontaneous regression of CIN and delayed-type hypersensitivity to HPV-16 oncoprotein E7. *Lancet* 356: 1985-6.

Jacobelli S., Sanaa. F.., Moyal Barracco M., Pelisse M., Berville S., Villefroy P., North M.O., Figueiredo S., Charmeteau B., Clerici T., Plantier F., Dupin N., Avril M.F., Guillet J.G., & Bourgault Villada I. (2011). Anti-HPV16 E2 protein T-cell responses and viral control in women with usual vulvar intraepithelial neoplasia and their healthy partners. *Submitted.*

Kadish, A. S., Ho, G. Y., Burk, R. D., Wang, Y., Romney, S. L., Ledwidge, R., & Angeletti, R. H. (1997). Lymphoproliferative responses to human papillomavirus (HPV) type 16 proteins E6 and E7: outcome of HPV infection and associated neoplasia. *J Natl Cancer Inst* 89:1285-93.

Kenter, G. G., Welters, M. J., Valentijn, A. R., Lowik, M. J., Berends-Van Der Meer, D. M., Vloon, A. P., Drijfhout, J. W., Wafelman, A. R., Oostendorp, J., Fleuren, G. J., Offringa, R., Van Der Burg, S. H., & Melief, C. J. (2008). Phase I immunotherapeutic trial with long peptides spanning the E6 and E7 sequences of high-risk human papillomavirus 16 in end-stage cervical cancer patients shows low toxicity and robust immunogenicity. *Clin Cancer Res* 14:169-77.

Kenter, G. G., Welters, M. J., Valentijn, A. R., Lowik, M. J., Berends-Van Der Meer, D. M., Vloon, A. P., Essahsah, F., Fathers, L. M., Offringa, R., Drijfhout, J. W., Wafelman, A. R., Oostendorp, J., Fleuren, G. J., Van Der Burg, S. H., & Melief, C. J. (2009). Vaccination against HPV-16 oncoproteins for vulvar intraepithelial neoplasia. *N Engl J Med* 361:1838-47.

Luxton, J. C., Rowe, A. J., Cridland, J. C., Coletart, T., Wilson, P., & Shepherd, P. S. (1996). Proliferative T cell responses to the human papillomavirus type 16 E7 protein in women with cervical dysplasia and cervical carcinoma and in healthy individuals. *J Gen Virol* 77 (Pt 7):1585-93.

Morishima, S., Akatsuka, Y., Nawa, A., Kondo, E., Kiyono, T., Torikai, H., Nakanishi, T., Ito, Y., Tsujimura, K., Iwata, K., Ito, K., Kodera, Y., Morishima, Y., Kuzushima, K., & Takahashi, T. (2007). Identification of an HLA-A24-restricted cytotoxic T lymphocyte epitope from human papillomavirus type-16 E6: the combined effects of bortezomib and interferon-gamma on the presentation of a cryptic epitope. *Int J Cancer* 120:594-604.

Nakagawa, M., Stites, D. P., Farhat, S., Judd, A., Moscicki, A. B., Canchola, A. J., Hilton, J. F., & Palefsky, J. M. (1996). T-cell proliferative response to human papillomavirus type 16 peptides: relationship to cervical intraepithelial neoplasia. *Clin Diagn Lab Immunol* 3:205-10.

Nakagawa, M., Kim, K. H., & Moscicki, A. B. (2004). Different methods of identifying new antigenic epitopes of human papillomavirus type 16 E6 and E7 proteins. *Clin Diagn Lab Immunol* 11:889-96.

Nakagawa, M., Kim, K. H., & Moscicki, A. B. (2005). Patterns of CD8 T-cell epitopes within the human papillomavirus type 16 (HPV 16) E6 protein among young women whose HPV 16 infection has become undetectable. *Clin Diagn Lab Immunol* 12:1003-5.

Nakagawa, M., Kim, K. H., Gillam, T. M., & Moscicki, A. B. (2007). HLA class I binding promiscuity of the CD8 T-cell epitopes of human papillomavirus type 16 E6 protein. *J Virol* 81:1412-23.

Nicolau, S. M., Camargo, C. G., Stavale, J. N., Castelo, A., Dores, G. B., Lorincz, A., & De Lima, G. R. (2005). Human papillomavirus DNA detection in male sexual partners of women with genital human papillomavirus infection. *Urology* 65:251-5.

Oerke, S., Hohn, H., Zehbe, I., Pilch, H., Schicketanz, K. H., Hitzler, W. E., Neukirch, C., Freitag, K., & Maeurer, M. J. (2005). Naturally processed and HLA-B8-presented HPV16 E7 epitope recognized by T cells from patients with cervical cancer. *Int J Cancer* 114:766-78.

Ostor, A. G. (1993). Natural history of cervical intraepithelial neoplasia: a critical review. *Int J Gynecol Pathol* 12:186-92.

Pantaleo, G., & Harari A. (2006). Functional signatures in antiviral T-cell immunity for monitoring virus-associated diseases. *Nat Rev Immunol* 6: 417-23.

Reiter, P. L., Pendergraft, W. F., 3rd, & Brewer, N. T. (2010). Meta-analysis of human papillomavirus infection concordance. *Cancer Epidemiol Biomarkers Prev* 19:2916-31.

Reiter, P. L., Pendergraft, W. F., 3rd, & Brewer, N. T. (2010). Meta-analysis of human papillomavirus infection concordance. *Cancer Epidemiol Biomarkers Prev* 19:2916-31.

Rowland-Jones, S., Sutton J., Ariyoshi, K., Dong, T., Gotch, F., McAdam, S., Whitby, D., Sabally, S., Gallimore, A., & Corrah, T. (1995). HIV-specific cytotoxic T-cells in HIV-exposed but uninfected Gambian women. *Nat Med* 1: 59-64.

Srodon, M., Stoler, M. H., Baber, G. B., & Kurman, R. J. (2006). The distribution of low and high-risk HPV types in vulvar and vaginal intraepithelial neoplasia (VIN and VaIN). *Am J Surg Pathol* 30:1513-8.

Strang, G., Hickling, J. K., Mcindoe, G. A., Howland, K., Wilkinson, D., Ikeda, H., & Rothbard, J. B. (1990). Human T cell responses to human papillomavirus type 16 L1 and E6 synthetic peptides: identification of T cell determinants, HLA-DR restriction and virus type specificity. *J Gen Virol* 71 (Pt 2):423-31.

Sun, X. W., Kuhn, L., Ellerbrock, T. V., Chiasson, M. A., Bush, T. J., & Wright, T. C., Jr. (1997). Human papillomavirus infection in women infected with the human immunodeficiency virus. *N Engl J Med* 337:1343-9.

Van Der Burg, S. H., Ressing, M. E., Kwappenberg, K. M., De Jong, A., Straathof, K., De Jong, J., Geluk, A., Van Meijgaarden, K. E., Franken, K. L., Ottenhoff, T. H., Fleuren, G. J., Kenter, G., Melief, C. J., & Offringa, R. (2001). Natural T-helper immunity against human papillomavirus type 16 (HPV16) E7-derived peptide epitopes in patients with HPV16-positive cervical lesions: identification of 3 human leukocyte antigen class II-restricted epitopes. *Int J Cancer* 91:612-8.

van Seters, M., van Beurden M., & de Craen, A. J (2005). Is the assumed natural history of vulvar intraepithelial neoplasia III based on enough evidence? A systematic review of 3322 published patients.*Gynecol Oncol* 97(2): 645-51.

Wang, X., Moscicki, A. B., Tsang, L., Brockman, A., & Nakagawa, M. (2008). Memory T cells specific for novel human papillomavirus type 16 (HPV16) E6 epitopes in women whose HPV16 infection has become undetectable. *Clin Vaccine Immunol* 15:937-45.

Wang, X., Santin, A. D., Bellone, S., Gupta, S., & Nakagawa, M. (2009). A novel CD4 T-cell epitope described from one of the cervical cancer patients vaccinated with HPV 16 or 18 E7-pulsed dendritic cells. *Cancer Immunol Immunother* 58:301-8.

Welters, M. J., de Jong A., van den Eeden, S. J., van der Hulst, J. M., Kwappenberg, K. M., Hassane, S., Franken, K. L., Drijfhout, J. W., Fleuren, G. J., Kenter, G., Melief, C. J., Offringa, R., & van der Burg, S. H. (2003). Frequent display of human papillomavirus type 16 E6-specific memory t-Helper cells in the healthy population as witness of previous viral encounter. *Cancer Res* 63(3): 636-41.

Welters, M. J., Kenter, G. G., Piersma, S. J., Vloon, A. P., Lowik, M. J., Berends-Van Der Meer, D. M., Drijfhout, J. W., Valentijn, A. R., Wafelman, A. R., Oostendorp, J., Fleuren, G. J., Offringa, R., Melief, C. J., & Van Der Burg, S. H. (2008). Induction of tumor-specific CD4+ and CD8+ T-cell immunity in cervical cancer patients by a human papillomavirus type 16 E6 and E7 long peptides vaccine. *Clin Cancer Res* 14:178-87.

Xue, Y., Bellanger, S., Zhang, W., Lim, D., Low, J., Lunny, D., & Thierry, F. (2010). HPV16 E2 is an immediate early marker of viral infection, preceding E7 expression in precursor structures of cervical carcinoma. *Cancer Res* 70:5316-25.